Workbook

Workbook in Practical Neonatology

Fourth Edition

Richard A. Polin, MD

Professor of Pediatrics
College of Physicians and Surgeons
Columbia University
Director, Division of Neonatology
Morgan Stanley Children's Hospital of New York–Presbyterian
New York, New York

Mervin C. Yoder, MD

Richard and Pauline Klingler Professor of Pediatrics
Professor of Bichemistry and Molecular Biology
Professor of Cellular and Integrative Physiology
Indiana University School of Medicine
Attending Physician
James Whitcomb Riley Hospital for Children
Indianapolis, Indiana

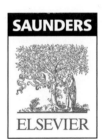

SAUNDERS

ELSEVIER

SAUNDERS
ELSEVIER

1600 John F. Kennedy Blvd.
Ste 1800
Philadelphia, PA 19103–2899

WORKBOOK IN PRACTICAL NEONATOLOGY   ISBN: 978-1-4160-2637-2

Library of Congress Cataloging-in-Publication Data

Workbook in practical neonatology / [edited by] Richard A. Polin, Mervin C. Yoder.—4th ed.
    p. ; cm.
  Rev. ed. of: Workbook in practical neonatology / Richard A. Polin. 3rd ed. c2001.
  Includes bibliographical references and index.
  ISBN 978-1-4160-2637-2
  1. Newborn infants–Diseases. 2. Neonatology. I. Polin, Richard A. (Richard Alan).
Workbook in practical neonatology. II. Polin, Richard A. (Richard Alan), III. Yoder, Mervin C.
  [DNLM: 1. Infant, Newborn, Diseases—Programmed Instruction. WS 18.2 W926 2007]
RJ254.W66 2007
618.9201—dc22   2007019288

Publishing Director: Judith Fletcher
Editorial Assistant: Colleen McGonigal
Senior Project Manager: David Saltzberg
Design Direction: Lou Forgione

Printed in the United States of America.

Last digit is the print number: 9   8   7   6   5   4   3   2   1

Contributors

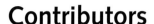

Matthew E. Abrams, MD
Neonatologist, Pediatrix Medical Group
Phoenix Children's Hospital, Phoenix, Arizona
Principles of Mechanical Ventilation

Sharon P. Andreoli, MD
Byron P. and Frances D. Hollett Professor of
Pediatrics, Indiana University, Indianapolis,
Indiana; James Whitcomb Riley
Hospital for Children, Indianapolis,
Indiana
Renal Failure in the Newborn Infant

William E. Benitz, MD
Philip Sunshine Professor of Neonatology,
Division of Neonatal and Developmental Medicine,
Pediatrics, Stanford University School of Medicine,
Stanford, California; Director of Nurseries,
Johnson Center for Pregnancy and Newborn
Services, Lucile Packard Children's Hospital,
Palo Alto, California
Neonatal Sepsis

Ricardo A. Caicedo, MD
Clinical Instructor, Pediatric Gastroenterology
and Nutrition, Wake Forest University Baptist
Medical Center, Winston-Salem, North Carolina;
Clinical Instructor, Pediatric Gastroenterology
and Nutrition, Brenner Children's Hospital,
Winston-Salem, North Carolina
Necrotizing Enterocolitis

Robert A. Cowles, MD
Assistant Professor of Surgery
(Pediatric Surgery), Department of Surgery,
Columbia University College of Physicians
and Surgeons, New York, New York;
Assistant Attending Surgeon, Department of
Surgery, Morgan Stanley Children's Hospital of
New York–Presbyterian, New York, New York
Surgical Emergencies in the Newborn

Robert A. Darnall, MD
Professor, Pediatrics and Physiology,
Dartmouth Medical School, Lebanon,
New Hampshire; Attending Neonatologist,
Pediatrics, Dartmouth-Hitchcock Medical Center,
Lebanon, New Hampshire
Breathing Disorders

Steven M. Donn, MD
Professor of Pediatrics, Chief, Division
of Neonatal-Perinatal Medicine, University of
Michigan Health System, Ann Arbor, Michigan;
Staff Neonatologist, Holden Neonatal Intensive
Care Unit, C.S. Mott Children's Hospital,
Ann Arbor, Michigan
Principles of Mechanical Ventilation

Eric C. Eichenwald, MD
Associate Professor, Pediatrics, Baylor
College of Medicine, Houston, Texas; Medical
Director, Newborn Intensive Care Unit,
Pediatrics/Neonatology, Texas Children's Hospital,
Houston, Texas
Early Discharge of the Premature Infant

William A. Engle, MD

Erik T. Ragan Professor of Pediatrics,
James Whitcomb Riley Hospital for Children,
Indianapolis, Indiana

Persistent Pulmonary Hypertension of
the Newborn

Nick Evans, DM, MRCPCH

Clinical Associate Professor, Neonatology,
University of Sydney, Sydney, New South Wales,
Australia; Senior Staff Specialist and Director of
NICU, Neonatology, Royal Prince Alfred Hospital,
Sydney, New South Wales, Australia

Patent Ductus Arteriosus

Neil N. Finer, MD

Professor of Pediatrics, Director, Division of
Neonatology, Pediatrics, University of California
San Diego, San Diego, California

Principles of Neonatal Resuscitation

Jeffrey S. Gerdes, MD

Associate Professor, Pediatrics, University of
Pennsylvania School of Medicine, Philadelphia,
Pennsylvania; Chief, Section of Newborn
Pediatrics, Pennsylvania Hospital of the University
of Pennsylvania Health System, Philadelphia,
Pennsylvania; Director, Neonatology Network,
Pediatrics, Children's Hospital of Philadelphia,
Philadelphia, Pennsylvania

Bronchopulmonary Dysplasia

Frank R. Greer, MD

Professor, Pediatrics/Nutritional Science,
University of Wisconsin, School of Medicine
and Public Health, Madison, Wisconsin

Disorders of Calcium, Phosphorus, and
Magnesium in the Newborn Period

Martin Kluckow, FRACP, PhD

Senior Lecturer, Obstetrics and Gynaecology,
University of Sydney, Sydney, New South Wales,
Australia; Senior Staff Neonatologist, Neonatology,
Royal North Shore Hospital, Sydney, New South
Wales, Australia

Hypotension in the Newborn Infant

Tina A. Leone, MD

Assistant Professor, Pediatrics, Division of
Neonatology, University of California San Diego,
San Diego, California

Principles of Neonatal Resuscitation

John M. Lorenz, MD

Professor of Clinical Pediatrics, Pediatrics,
College of Physicians and Surgeons,
Columbia University, New York,
New York; Attending Neonatologist,
Pediatrics, Morgan Stanley Children's
Hospital of New York–Presbyterian,
New York, New York

Fluid and Electrolyte Management in
the Newborn Intensive Care Unit

M. Jeffrey Maisels, MB, BCh

Clinical Professor, Pediatrics, Wayne State
University School of Medicine, Detroit,
Michigan; Adjunct Clinical Professor,
Pediatrics and Communicable Diseases,
University of Michigan Medical School,
Ann Arbor, Michigan; Chairman, Pediatrics,
William Beaumont Hospital, Royal Oak, Michigan

Neonatal Hyperbilirubinemia

**Colin J. Morley, MA, MD, DCH, FRCP, FRCPCH,
FRACP**

Professor of Neonatal Medicine, Obstetrics,
University of Melbourne, Melbourne, Victoria,
Australia; Director of Neonatal Medicine,
Neonatal Services, Royal Women's Hospital,
Melbourne, Victoria, Australia; Professorial
Fellow, Neonatal Research, Murdock Children's
Research Institute, Melborne, Victoria, Australia

Respiratory Distress Syndrome

Josef Neu, MD

Professor, Pediatrics, Division of Neonatology,
University of Florida, Gainesville, Florida

Necrotizing Enterocolitis

Robin K. Ohls, MD

Professor, Pediatrics, University of New Mexico,
Albuquerque, New Mexico

Anemia in the Newborn Infant

Gilberto R. Pereira, MD

Professor, Pediatrics, University of Pennsylvania
School of Medicine, Philadelphia, Pennsylvania;
Neonatologist, Pediatrics/Neonatology, Children's
Hospital of Philadelphia, Philadelphia,
Pennsylvania

Parenteral Nutrition

Jeffrey M. Perlman, MB, ChB

Professor, Pediatrics, Weill Cornell Medical College, New York, New York; Chief, Newborn Medicine, Pediatrics, New York–Presbyterian Hospital, New York, New York

Intraventricular Hemorrhage

Brenda B. Poindexter, MD, MS

Associate Professor of Clinical Pediatrics, Section of Neonatal-Perinatal Medicine, Indiana University School of Medicine, Riley Hospital for Children, Indianapolis, Indiana

Enteral Nutrition in the High-Risk Neonate

S. David Rubenstein, MD

Professor of Clinical Pediatrics, Pediatrics, College of Physicians and Surgeons, Columbia University, New York, New York; Director, Neonatal Intensive Care Unit and Fellowship Training Program in Neonatal Medicine, Pediatrics, Morgan Stanley Children's Hospital of New York–Presbyterian, New York, New York

The Recognition and Management of Congenital Heart Disease in the Neonate

Mark S. Scher, MD

Professor of Pediatrics and Neurology, Pediatrics, Case Western Reserve University School of Medicine, Cleveland, Ohio; Division Chief, Pediatric Neurology, Director, Pediatric Sleep/Epilepsy and Fetal/Neonatal Neurology Programs, Pediatrics, Rainbow Babies and Children's Hospital, University Hospitals of Cleveland, Cleveland, Ohio

Neonatal Seizures

Rebecca A. Simmons, MD

Associate Professor, Pediatrics, Children's Hospital of Philadelphia, Philadelphia, Pennsylvania; Attending Neonatologist, Pediatrics, Children's Hospital of Philadelphia, Hospital of the University of Pennsylvania, Philadelphia, Pennsylvania

Glucose Metabolism in the Newborn Infant

Steven Stylianos, MD

Professor of Surgery, University of Miami Miller School of Medicine, Miami, Florida; Chief, Pediatric Surgery, Miami Children's Hospital, Miami, Florida

Surgical Emergencies in the Newborn

David D. Weaver, MS, MD

Professor Emeritus, Medical and Molecular Genetics, Indiana University School of Medicine, Indianapolis, Indiana

Birth Defects and Genetic Disorders

Michael D. Weiss, MD

Assistant Professor of Pediatrics, Division of Neonatology, University of Florida, Gainesville, Florida

Necrotizing Enterocolitis

Gil Wernovsky, MD, FACC, FAAP

Professor of Pediatrics, Children's Hospital of Philadelphia, University of Pennsylvania School of Medicine, Philadelphia, Pennsylvania; Staff Cardiologist, Cardiac Intensive Care Unit, Director, Program Development, Cardiac Center, Children's Hospital of Philadelphia, Philadelphia, Pennsylvania

The Recognition and Management of Congenital Heart Disease in the Neonate

Preface

This is the fourth edition of the *Workbook in Practical Neonatology*. Our enthusiasm for writing this edition remains as great as it was when writing the first nearly 24 years ago. In 1983, our goal was to create a textbook format that was as engaging as it was informative. Each chapter was centered around case histories in which the reader was asked to make management decisions. True-to-life clinical scenarios were chosen to involve the reader in the care of the babies described in each chapter. We still believe that providing active learning is a better way to promote reader comprehension than presenting concepts in a strictly didactic fashion.

For this edition, we have added five entirely new chapters—"Enteral Nutrition in the High-Risk Neonate," "Patent Ductus Arteriosus," "Hypotension in the Newborn Infant," "Congenital Heart Disease in the Neonate" and "Early Discharge of the Premature Infant"—and six chapters have new authorship. Each of the new authors (like those that remain from the previous edition) was chosen for his or her expertise and recognition as an expert. They were challenged to provide a comprehensive and state-of-the-art review that used actual cases from their own nurseries. We hope that the readers of this book will take away as much about the style of teaching as about the book's content. The interactive, case-oriented format is as readily adaptable to bedside teaching as it is to lecturing to large audiences. We hope that this book will serve as an example that education (even about serious topics) can be delivered in an interesting way.

There are several individuals to whom we owe thanks. These include the phenomenal group of contributors who have provided us with well-written, absorbing, and informative chapters; Judy Fletcher and the staff at Elsevier; and Heidi Kleinbart for her technical, editorial, and organizational help. Most importantly, we would like to thank the great teachers of our past who taught us the importance of being effective teachers.

Special Dedication

During the preparation of this edition of the *Workbook in Practical Neonatology*, Dr. Frederic Burg suddenly passed away at the age of 66. Fred had a distinguished academic career at the University of Pennsylvania and the University of Alabama. He was instrumental in the development of the first edition of the Workbook and served as co-editor for three subsequent editions. Fred was a remarkable human being who genuinely cared about the health and welfare of children. He brought that caring and enthusiasm to every part of his professional life. The world has lost a wonderful pediatrician, an advocate for children, an educational innovator, and a leader in pediatrics—and we have lost a good friend.

He will be remembered by
all of us who worked with him.

RICHARD A. POLIN
MERVIN C. YODER

Contents

Principles of Neonatal Resuscitation

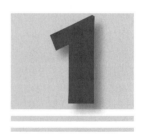

Tina A. Leone, MD, and Neil N. Finer, MD

The birth of an infant is a dynamic process that entails extensive physiologic changes in the newborn for successful transition from intrauterine to extrauterine life. If problems occur prior to, during, or immediately after birth, the infant may suffer devastating consequences. Approximately 10% of newborns will require some form of resuscitation upon birth. Of those, 10% to 20% will require more advanced resuscitation measures in order to achieve stability. A neonatal resuscitation team must be immediately at hand for the delivery of all newborns in order to perform emergent resuscitation.

The procedures involved in neonatal resuscitation are taught by the Neonatal Resuscitation Program (NRP)[1] that was jointly developed by the American Academy of Pediatrics and the American Heart Association as a method of teaching large numbers of individuals an organized approach to newborn resuscitative measures. The program recommendations are regularly reviewed and revised based on current evidence and a consensus of expert opinion. The most recent version was released in 2006 and included updates in preterm infant care, methods of improving thermoregulation, and types of equipment available for resuscitation. All medical personnel who attend deliveries should be thoroughly familiar with NRP and capable of performing the appropriate steps. Neonatologists and neonatal trainees should also become NRP instructors. This chapter will concentrate on areas of resuscitation that are frequently problematic. It is not intended in any way to substitute for NRP training. Some of the issues discussed in this chapter are not specifically outlined by the NRP but may be useful when performing resuscitation.

An understanding of the physiology of normal transition from intrauterine to extrauterine life is essential to understanding the rationale for the approach to resuscitation. In utero, the fetus receives oxygen through the placenta and has a normal Pao_2 of 20 to 30 torr. Throughout gestation the fetal lung is fluid-filled and receives only 10% of fetal cardiac output because in fetal life the lungs are not used as the organ of gas exchange. Lung fluid is absorbed through a process that begins with the onset of labor and is not complete until after birth. The majority of lung fluid is cleared as an infant takes its first breaths of life and the lungs inflate with air. In the first few minutes of life the newborn's pulmonary vascular resistance falls, allowing blood to flow through the lungs, increasing the pulmonary perfusion to the now air-filled lungs. When this entire process occurs normally, the infant breathes spontaneously, the lungs become inflated and perfused, the arterial oxygenation increases, and the infant becomes pink.

These normal, occurrences may not take place properly for several reasons and the infant will then need assistance transitioning to extrauterine life. Providers must recognize the need for help and be capable of providing that assistance to the infant who is having a difficult transition.

Preparedness

All institutions where infants are delivered should have staff able to initiate neonatal resuscitation quickly, even when unexpected. Anticipating the need for resuscitation should come from communication with the obstetric team.

However, any situation in which an infant may be depressed at birth can be a predictor of the need for resuscitation. Knowing which infants will require resuscitation enables providers to prepare adequately and initiate resuscitation promptly.

Neonatal depression and the lack of spontaneous respiration may be related to acidosis (which can lead to apnea), maternal medications depressing neonatal respiration, congenital neuromuscular diseases, or anomalies preventing adequate respiration. Conditions that lead to acidosis include those resulting in blood or volume loss (such as placental abruption, cord accidents or compression), sepsis, chronic placental insufficiency (as seen in maternal hypertension), or chronic anemia (as seen in fetal maternal transfusion, or Rh isoimmunization). A list of conditions often associated with resuscitation is included in Table 1-1.

All the necessary equipment for resuscitation should be available in every delivery area. The environment should provide adequate warmth for the newborn, enough space for a radiant warmer and the individuals performing the resuscitation, and adequate light for evaluation of the infant. The minimum necessary equipment includes a radiant warmer and warming blankets, apparatus for suctioning, devices for providing positive pressure and performing intubation, and equipment for placement of an umbilical line and a chest tube. The use of room air or oxygen for initial resuscitation is still under debate, but evidence favors the use of room air as initial resuscitation for the term infant. There should be oxygen, compressed air, and blender (to allow titration of F_{IO_2} and medications used in resuscitation) readily available.

The resuscitation team should include a minimum of three individuals to assess the infant and perform the procedures required for resuscitation. A team leader should be clearly identified, and capable of overseeing the entire process, directly assigning tasks to individuals, and intervening if tasks are not being performed appropriately. The team should have open communication and participate in a debriefing after the resuscitation is complete.

TABLE 1-1

RISK FACTORS FOR NEED FOR RESUSCITATION AT BIRTH

Maternal Factors
Diabetes mellitus
Preeclampsia
Chronic illness
Poor prenatal care
Substance abuse
Uterine rupture
General anesthesia
Chorioamnionitis

Fetal Factors
Intrauterine growth restriction
Known fetal anomalies
Multiple gestation
Hydrops fetalis
Oligohydramnios
Polyhydramnios
Preterm birth
Premature rupture of membranes
Fetal distress as indicated by fetal heart rate
    monitoring or tests of fetal well-being
Breech presentation
Decreased fetal movement

Placental Factors
Placenta previa
Placenta accreta
Vasa previa
Placental abruption

Case Study 1

An 18-year-old gravida 1 para 0 woman presents to the emergency room in labor with delivery imminent for a fetus of unknown gestational age. You are called to attend the delivery and arrive just as the baby is born. The baby is initially blue, with weak spontaneous respiratory effort.

Exercise 1

QUESTIONS

1. The intensive care unit and labor and delivery area are four floors from the emergency room. Where will you resuscitate this infant?

2. What pieces of equipment are essential to have available immediately?

3. What are your initial steps in resuscitating this infant?

4. After you have completed the initial steps of resuscitation, the infant is crying vigorously and is now pink centrally. What will be your main focus in the next several minutes?

ANSWERS

1. You need to resuscitate the newborn immediately in the emergency room. If a radiant warmer is not available, find a flat surface on which to place the baby so that you may provide care. This surface can be an empty stretcher or an infant transporter.

2. You will need a form of suction and a device for providing positive pressure ventilation with a face mask. The most accessible suction device will probably be a bulb syringe. Remember that if you are attempting resuscitation in an area where there is no gas flow available it is still possible to provide positive pressure with a self-inflating bag. This is not necessarily the device of choice, but when in an area where gas flow is not available it may be the only option. Although equipment for intubation may be necessary, you should be able to provide positive pressure ventilation with a face mask until intubation equipment can be retrieved and prepared. It is critical to provide warmth for the infant, who should be dried immediately to reduce heat loss. Warming blankets are useful, and a portable warmer should be obtained. Heat packs are available in most emergency rooms and can be used with caution, until a warmer can be supplied. If no warmer is available and the baby is stable, warmth may be provided by placing the infant in skin-to-skin contact.

3. The oropharynx should be suctioned and the baby dried. Brief stimulation should be done because the baby has weak respiratory effort. The heart rate must be evaluated quickly. If the heart rate is less than 100 bpm or the baby has inadequate respiratory effort, positive pressure ventilation should be initiated.

4. The next most important task is to provide adequate warmth for this infant. This may be accomplished as discussed in answer 2, but the infant should also be transported to an area where more stable care can be provided. An overall evaluation of the infant should be performed, including a clinical assessment of gestational age so that appropriate care is provided.

Assessment

Immediately after birth the infant's condition is evaluated by general observation as well as specific parameters. The newborn adapting well to extrauterine life will cry vigorously and maintain adequate respirations. The color will transition from blue to pink, the heart rate will remain in the 140s to the 160s, and the infant will demonstrate adequate muscle tone with some flexion of the extremities. The overall assessment of an infant who does not adapt well to extrauterine life will often reveal apnea, cyanotic color, and poor tone. Resuscitation interventions are based mainly on the respiratory effort and heart rate evaluation. These gauges need to be continually evaluated throughout the resuscitation. Heart rate can be monitored by auscultation or by palpation of the cord pulsations and should be done every 30 seconds. For an infant who does not show an immediate response, one caregiver should have the responsibility of obtaining a continuous heart rate and should communicate this to the other team members (using finger signals or audible exchange). The early placement of a pulse oximeter can provide a continuous heart rate signal within 30 seconds of application.

The overall assessment of a newborn was quantified by Virginia Apgar in the 1950s with the Apgar score. The score consists of a 10-point scale with a maximum of 2 points assigned for each of the following five categories: respirations, heart rate, color, tone, and reflex irritability. The score was initially intended to assess the infant's response to intrapartum anesthesia.[2] It is currently used as an assessment of the infant's overall condition at 1 and 5 minutes of age, and every 5 minutes thereafter if the infant continues to require resuscitation. The score has not been predictive of neurodevelopmental outcome.[3]

Initial Steps

After birth the infant should be placed on a radiant warmer and dried, the mouth suctioned, respiratory effort evaluated, and the heart rate assessed by palpation or auscultation. The provision of warmth is particularly important for the extremely preterm infant. Infants of less than 26 weeks' gestation with an initial intensive care admission temperature of less than 35°C have an increased risk of death.[4] Vohra and associates have shown that admission temperatures may be improved in infants less than 28 weeks' gestation by immediately wrapping the body with polyethylene wrap prior to drying the infant.[5,6] In their studies, only the infant's head was dried prior to application of the wrap. Other measures for maintaining infant temperature include performing resuscitations in a room that is kept at an ambient temperature of approximately greater than 26°C, using modern radiant warmers, which produce adequate heat when utilized with their servo controlled temperature probes applied to the infant immediately after birth, and the use of a prewarmed mattress/heating pad. It is important to note that as a required safety feature, radiant warmers that are not used in servo control mode will decrease their power output after 15 minutes of continuous operation.

When amniotic fluid is meconium stained, the initial steps of resuscitation are modified. In this situation if the infant is vigorous with good respiratory effort, the steps of resuscitation should proceed as usual. However, if the infant is floppy and nonvigorous, it is currently recommended that endotracheal intubation for airway suctioning should be done immediately in an effort to remove meconium that may have been aspirated.[7] We recommend avoiding frequent intubation attempts and proceeding with airway suctioning followed by bag and mask ventilation.

Case Study 2

A 28-year-old gravida 2 para 1 woman at 30 weeks' gestation with twins presents in labor. She is administered betamethasone, antibiotics, and tocolytics. Labor continues to progress with one twin in breech presentation. The decision is made to deliver the twins by cesarean section.

Exercise 2

QUESTIONS

1. How many people from your neonatal team would attend this delivery and what would be the general composition of the team?

2. What would your initial steps entail?

3. After performing the initial steps of resuscitation Twin A has good respiratory effort and a heart rate of 140 bpm. He begins to have mild grunting and retractions but a saturation probe placed on his right hand shows an oxygen saturation of 95% at 5 minutes of life on room air. How would you treat this infant at this point?

4. Twin B is handed to you floppy with minimal respiratory effort. You dry, suction, and stimulate the baby and the initial heart rate is found to be 80 bpm. How do you proceed?

ANSWERS

1. A minimum of three individuals per infant would be appropriate in this situation. These twins are at risk for being depressed at birth because they were preterm and the mother received magnesium prenatally. At least one member of the team should focus on clearing and establishing the airway, another individual should be assigned to monitor the heart rate, and a third should lead the resuscitation. It is important that both twins be assigned their own team so that resuscitation may proceed without delay for each baby.

2. Each twin should be placed on a separate radiant warmer, dried, and suctioned. An overall assessment of adequacy of respirations should be made and the heart rate should be measured. Subsequent steps will be determined by these findings.

3. Twin A has adequate respiration and heart rate but is beginning to display increased work of breathing. It is not necessary to provide oxygen to this infant, but the application of continuous positive airway pressure would likely be beneficial. Although not specifically recommended by NRP, the use of continuous positive airway pressure (CPAP) in this situation may be beneficial by assisting in the establishment and maintenance of functional residual capacity and may prevent the need for intubation. The use of CPAP for the treatment of respiratory distress syndrome compared with intubation and administration of surfactant is still under investigation. However, in this baby of 30 weeks' gestation who is having normal oxygen saturation on room air it would be reasonable to use CPAP as initial therapy. The infant must be monitored closely thereafter to detect any deterioration in respiratory status and the possible need for intubation and surfactant administration.

4. Twin B is depressed with a heart rate less than 100 bpm; therefore, positive pressure ventilation via face mask must be administered. During positive pressure ventilation it is important to continually monitor the heart rate so that the direction of change may be detected with each intervention. The heart rate should increase and the infant should begin making spontaneous respirations. If this does not occur, ensure that ventilation is adequate by suctioning the oropharynx,

checking the seal, and attempting to reposition the head and mask. If these adjustments do not improve the heart rate, it may be necessary to provide a prolonged breath or increase the inspiratory pressure (see further discussion later). In this case the heart rate improved after suctioning the oropharynx again and repositioning the head.

Positive Pressure Ventilation

As the newborn infant begins breathing and replaces the lung fluid with air, the lung becomes inflated and a functional residual capacity (FRC) (air remaining in the lung at the end of expiration) is developed and maintained. Many of the problems encountered during resuscitation occur because of lack of inflation and inadequate development of FRC. The steps involved in performing resuscitation include providing assisted positive pressure ventilation when the infant shows signs of inadequate lung inflation. Indications for positive pressure ventilation include apnea, inadequate respiratory effort, and heart rate less than 100 bpm. Bradycardia is often a result of poor lung inflation leading to hypoxia.

Positive pressure ventilation is usually begun using a pressure delivery device with a face mask. Pressure delivery devices include self-inflating bags, flow-inflating or anesthesia bags, and t-piece resuscitators; each has its own advantages and disadvantages. A self-inflating bag requires a reservoir to provide nearly 100% oxygen and may deliver very high pressure if not used carefully. However, self-inflating bags are easy to use for less experienced personnel and will work in the absence of a gas source. These devices have pressure blow-off valves, but these valves do not always open at the target blow-off pressures.[8] An anesthesia bag or flow-inflating bag requires a gas source for use, allows the operator to "instinctively" vary delivery pressures, but requires significant practice to develop expertise. A t-piece resuscitator is easy to use, requires a gas source for use, delivers the most consistent levels of pressure, but requires intentional effort to vary pressure levels.[9] The flow-inflating bag and t-piece resuscitator allow the operator to deliver continuous positive airway pressure (CPAP) or positive end expiratory pressure (PEEP) relatively easily.[10,11]

A certain amount of experience is required to perform assisted ventilation using a face mask and resuscitation device. It is important to maintain a patent airway in order for the air to reach the lungs. Obtaining and maintaining patency of the airway includes at minimum clearing the mouth and pharynx of fluid with a suction device, holding the head in a neutral position, and sometimes lifting the jaw anteriorly. The face mask must make an adequate seal with the face in order for air to pass to the lungs effectively. No device will adequately inflate the lungs if there is a large leak present between the mask and the face. Signs that the airway is patent and air is being delivered to the lungs include visual inspection of chest rise with each breath and improvement in clinical condition, including heart rate and color. The use of a colorimetric carbon dioxide detector during bagging will confirm that gas exchange is occurring and will alert the operator of an obstructed airway.[12] It is important to remember that these devices will not change color in the absence of a circulating rhythm. It can at times be very difficult to achieve airway patency and this may require multiple maneuvers such as readjusting the head and mask positions, choosing a mask of more appropriate size, and further suctioning of the pharynx. Alternate methods of providing a patent airway include the use of a nasopharyngeal tube[13] or of a laryngeal mask airway device.[14]

Although it is important to provide adequate pressure for ventilation, excessive pressure can contribute to lung damage. The exact pressure to be given with assisted breaths has not been unequivocally determined and it is likely that the right pressure for one baby may not be appropriate for another. It has been shown that using enough pressure to produce visible chest rise may be associated with hypocarbia on the admission blood gas evaluation[15] and excessive pressure may decrease the effectiveness of surfactant therapy.[16] It may be possible to establish FRC without increasing peak inspiratory pressures by providing a few prolonged inflations (3 to 5 seconds inspiration), and this may be a useful maneuver before increasing ventilating pressures.[17] Such prolonged inflations have not been associated with better outcomes than conventional breaths during resuscitation.[18] It is also clear that assisted ventilation with PEEP or the use of CPAP is beneficial for the establishment and maintenance of FRC and improvement in surfactant function, and there are current randomized trials evaluating the use of early CPAP initiated following delivery.[19–22]

If assisted ventilation is necessary for a prolonged period of time or other resuscitative measures have been unsuccessful, endotracheal intubation should be performed. If it has been difficult to maintain a patent airway ventilating via a face mask, the endotracheal tube will provide a stable airway. This will allow more consistent delivery of gas to the lungs and establishment and maintenance of FRC. Intubation is also necessary to deliver surfactant and other medications that may be needed for resuscitation. Finally, for depressed infants born through meconium-stained amniotic fluid, intubation is performed for suctioning of the airway.

The intubation procedure requires a significant amount of skill and experience to perform reliably and can be associated with serious complications. The procedure entails using a laryngoscope to visualize the vocal cords and passing the endotracheal tube through the vocal cords. The placement of the laryngoscope in the pharynx often produces vagal stimulation which leads to bradycardia. During intubation, assisted ventilation must be paused. If intubation is prolonged, it can lead to hypoxia and bradycardia. The procedure has been shown to increase blood pressure and intracranial pressure.[23] Trauma to the mouth, pharynx, vocal cords, and trachea are all possible complications of intubation. If misplacement of the endotracheal tube in the esophagus goes unrecognized, the infant may experience further clinical deterioration. Clinical signs that the endotracheal tube has been correctly placed in the trachea include auscultation of breath sounds over the anterolateral aspects of the lungs (near the axilla), mist visible on the endotracheal tube, chest rise, and clinical improvement in heart rate and color or saturation. The use of a colorimetric carbon dioxide detector to confirm intubation decreases the amount of time necessary to determine correct placement of the endotracheal tube, and we recommend the routine use of such detectors.[24,25]

Oxygen Use

Although it has been routinely recommended that 100% oxygen be delivered to infants who are centrally cyanotic or are being given positive pressure ventilation, extensive research comparing pure oxygen with room air suggests that resuscitation with room air is associated with improved outcome.[26–28] The World Health Organization does not recommend the use of supplemental oxygen for the resuscitation of newborns unless color does not improve with adequate ventilation.[29] The most recent NRP textbook recommends initiating resuscitation with 100% oxygen but recognizes that individual physicians may choose to provide varying oxygen concentrations.[1] The use of varied oxygen levels requires a compressed air source and a blender (that may not always be available) and has yet to be evaluated systematically. Nevertheless, our recommendation is that all delivery areas be equipped with compressed air, oxygen, and blenders so that infants can receive the appropriate amount of oxygen. In keeping with previous observations during resuscitation.[26,30] a reasonable target for oxygen delivery would be to achieve an oxygen saturation of no more than 90% at 5 minutes of life. Such precision in oxygen delivery will require the early use of pulse oximeters. Because preterm infants are at increased risk of oxygen toxicity, hospitals where such infants are regularly delivered should have the necessary equipment in the delivery room for providing lower concentrations of oxygen and for monitoring.

Case Study 3

You are called because a 26-year-old gravida 1 para 0 woman at 24 weeks' estimated gestational age presents to labor and delivery with contractions and bulging membranes. There have been no prenatal complications and antenatal laboratory testing is unremarkable. An ultrasound was done at 8 weeks' gestation, at which time size was consistent with dates. Another ultrasound at 18 weeks showed normal anatomy. Despite attempts to stop labor, it progresses and delivery is imminent. Betamethasone is administered to the mother. You walk to labor and delivery to meet the mother and prepare for the delivery. The labor continues to progress and the baby is delivered vaginally. The mouth is suctioned by the obstetrician, and the baby, making minimal respiratory effort, is handed to you blue.

Exercise 3

QUESTIONS

1. What preparations will you make prior to the delivery?

2. What are your initial steps in resuscitating this baby?

3. After completing your initial resuscitation steps you find that the baby is still not making good respiratory effort and the heart rate is 80. What is your next step?

ANSWERS

1. Preparations that should be occurring prior to the delivery include ensuring that the equipment is accessible and functioning and that a warm environment is created. The bed should be set up with all the necessary equipment within easy access to the resuscitators. Although equipment varies at different hospitals, the resuscitation team should be familiar with the equipment and should test it and prepare it appropriately. A critical step in pre-resuscitation preparation is for team members to be identified and for the leader to provide a general plan and distribute tasks to individuals. For an infant of this degree of prematurity, there should be at least one experienced team member who has successfully resuscitated such infants, and there should be a selection of small face masks for the delivery of bag mask ventilation, which is needed in over 80% of such deliveries. If time allows, it is best to meet the mother and other family members prior to delivery. This meeting may serve both to prepare the mother for the immediate postnatal events and to discuss issues of resuscitation decisions at this level of prematurity. Hospitals may have different practices regarding resuscitation at different gestational ages, but discussing these issues with the family prior to birth can facilitate decision making.

2. The infant should be placed on the radiant warmer and wrapped in plastic to retain warmth. One team member should suction the mouth with a bulb syringe while another team member obtains a heart rate and visibly displays it. Because the baby is not making good respiratory effort, positive pressure ventilation should be initiated. In a baby of this gestational age, time should not be spent attempting to stimulate breath by indirect measures. When giving positive pressure ventilation it is important to ensure that a seal is established between the mask and the face, and that air is moving into the baby's lungs. A third team member should be placing a pulse oximeter on the baby (if available) or assisting with airway maintenance and ventilation.

3. Once positive pressure has been initiated, if the heart rate remains low and is not improving it is essential to recheck that a seal was created between the mask and the face, and ensure that the airway is not obstructed with fluid or by positioning. A 3- to 5-second prolonged breath may be given once or twice to improve FRC followed by an increase in the targeted peak inspiratory pressure. If these procedures are not effective in improving the heart rate, it may be necessary to intubate the baby or use an alternate method to establish an airway (such as a nasopharyngeal tube). Although intubation may be performed in this setting, whenever possible it is preferable to stabilize the baby prior to intubation. It is also important to remember that if the face mask is pressing too hard on the face, the baby may experience a reflex bradycardia from stimulation of the trigeminal nerve.

Bradycardia

Bradycardia is usually the result of poor oxygenation and improves with adequate positive pressure ventilation. However, if the heart rate is less than 60 bpm despite adequate positive pressure ventilation for 30 seconds, chest compressions should be initiated. The recommended method of performing chest compressions includes using two thumbs on the sternum with the hands wrapped around the chest and thumbs compressing the sternum about one third the anterior-posterior depth of the chest. Chest compressions are provided in a 3:1 ratio with ventilation breaths. If the infant does not respond to chest compressions and ventilation, further action may include intubation and administration of epinephrine. Epinephrine acts on alpha- and beta-adrenergic receptors and increases blood pressure and cardiac contractility. Epinephrine may be administered by endotracheal tube or intravenously in a dose of 0.01 to 0.03 mg/kg (0.1 to 0.3 mL/kg of 1:10,000 solution). The intratracheal route will, most likely, not be well absorbed because it is being delivered to a fluid-filled lung with possible intra- and extrapulmonary shunts.

However, if no intravenous access is immediately available, it is beneficial to initiate epinephrine therapy through the endotracheal tube while intravenous access is being established. Doses can be repeated every 3 to 5 minutes if no response has occurred.

Emergency intravenous access can be achieved by placing an umbilical venous catheter in the infant. The catheter should only be placed a short distance (just beyond the abdominal wall at a point where good blood return is achieved) to avoid problems with infusion into the liver through a misplaced line. The catheter may be used for emergency purposes safely in this way without confirming placement with an x-ray.

Volume Replacement

When it is suspected that an infant has suffered significant volume loss, or when an infant is not responding to standard resuscitation measures, placing an umbilical venous catheter for fluid therapy may be necessary. This possibility should be considered when the infant is not responding to ventilation and bradycardia persists despite chest compressions. Infants who are born after placental abruption or a cord accident are particularly at risk for having blood loss leading to significant hypovolemia. In that situation, placing an umbilical venous catheter for fluid replacement may be a lifesaving measure. It is important to remember that blood loss at the time of delivery may not be obvious in the newborn because it may occur into the placenta or the blood present at delivery may be confused with maternal blood. The fluid used for volume replacement should be an isotonic solution such as normal saline. However, significant blood loss may need to be replaced with either emergent type O negative blood from the blood bank or blood drawn up from the placenta.

Case Study 4

A 32-year-old gravida 3 para 2 woman presents at 38 weeks' gestation in labor. After her membranes ruptured, she began having contractions regularly, and is dilated 3 cm. Routine labor and delivery care is initiated, including external fetal monitoring. After several hours of labor, the fetal heart rate has started to increase with intermittent variable decelerations. Within the next 30 minutes the fetal heart tones are lost altogether and the mother is having vaginal bleeding. An emergent cesarean section is performed and the baby is delivered 15 minutes from the time fetal heart tones were lost. The baby is handed to you floppy with no respiratory effort and no heart rate.

Exercise 4

QUESTIONS

1. What do you think is the cause of this infant's distress?

2. What steps would your initial resuscitative efforts include?

3. If the infant does not respond to your initial resuscitative efforts, what further measures would you take?

4. If your resuscitation is successful, how would you evaluate this infant after resuscitation?

ANSWERS

1. From the description of the prenatal course including fetal heart rate findings and maternal vaginal bleeding it is likely that this mother had a sudden placental abruption or the infant suffered a cord accident. Therefore, blood loss and hypovolemia are likely to have contributed to the infant's distress.

2. The infant should be placed on the radiant warmer and dried; the oropharynx should be "bulb suctioned" and positive pressure ventilation initiated immediately. If the heart rate remains undetectable, chest compressions should be initiated.

3. If the infant has not improved with these initial measures, intubation should be performed; and if the heart rate remains less than 60 bpm, the baby should be given epinephrine. The epinephrine may be given in the endotracheal tube initially, but this infant should have an umbilical venous catheter placed quickly for both epinephrine and volume replacement because it is likely that this infant had a

significant volume loss. Normal saline may be given initially, but if maternal blood loss has been excessive, it is appropriate to give blood to the baby as well. Unmatched type O negative blood from the blood bank could be given urgently, but in this situation an attempt should be made to aspirate blood from the placenta for infusion into the baby. A second choice in extreme situations is to use the mother's blood (if possible).

4. Because this infant had a significant resuscitation it would be best to monitor the baby in the neonatal intensive care unit. The baby may be acidotic from the hypovolemia and a blood gas should be obtained. If the infant appears encephalopathic, with evidence of altered tone, primitive reflexes, or early seizures after resuscitation, it would be important to consider the possibility of providing hypothermia therapy for hypoxic ischemic encephalopathy. Evaluation of the infant for other organ dysfunction secondary to hypoxia-ischemia—including the heart, liver, and kidneys—may be necessary. Disseminated intravascular coagulation should be considered as well because of the history of blood loss.

Resuscitative Medications

Few medications are used in neonatal resuscitation. The most critical medication for resuscitation is epinephrine (see prior discussion of bradycardia). However, occasionally if an infant is apneic and a recent history of maternal narcotic administration during labor is known, naloxone may be used to reverse respiratory depression of the prenatally dosed narcotic. However, if the mother has been using chronic narcotics for any reason (recreational or therapeutic), naloxone should not be given to the infant because it may potentiate a sudden opiate withdrawal syndrome that can induce seizures. Prior to dosing naloxone, and if an effect is not apparent, it is important to continue to provide assisted ventilation to the infant. The use of naloxone should not supplant the provision of adequate ventilation.

Finally, sodium bicarbonate has been used in resuscitation in an attempt to reverse the acidosis that is caused by poor cardiac output and poor perfusion. However, there are many concerns about the use of bicarbonate because of its high osmolarity and conversion to carbon dioxide. The current guidelines recommend using sodium bicarbonate only for prolonged resuscitation if other measures are not leading to improvement, and even this use lacks convincing evidence of benefit.

Case Study 5

A 35-year-old gravida 1 para 0 woman with good prenatal care presents at 32 weeks' estimated gestational age with a sudden increase in swelling and is evaluated for preeclampsia. She is found to have an elevated blood pressure and is started on magnesium sulfate. It is determined that she has severe preeclampsia and the infant is delivered by cesarean section. The infant is handed to you floppy and blue without any respiratory effort. You place the infant on the warmer and suction the mouth, then dry and stimulate the infant. The nurse auscultates the heart rate and displays a rate of approximately 100 bpm.

Exercise 5

QUESTIONS

1. What is your next step in resuscitation?
2. After you have initiated positive pressure ventilation, the heart rate improves but the infant does not begin to make independent respiratory effort. Would you give naloxone for this infant's apnea?
3. How would you treat this infant's continued apnea?
4. What other physical findings would you expect?

ANSWERS

1. The next step in resuscitation would be to initiate positive pressure ventilation. The infant is apneic and the heart rate is approximately 100 bpm; therefore, positive pressure ventilation is necessary.
2. It would not be appropriate to give naloxone to this infant because the apnea is most likely related to increased magnesium sulfate levels. If the mother had received narcotics prior to delivery it would be reasonable to

try naloxone, but this mother did not receive narcotics.

3. If the infant does not initiate independent breathing, it is necessary to continue providing ventilation and to intubate. It is not common for infants exposed to magnesium sulfate to require intubation for prolonged apnea, but if apnea is persistent it will be necessary because there is no agent to reverse the effects of magnesium. Because this infant is preterm, surfactant deficiency is possible, and respiratory distress syndrome should be considered.

4. This infant will most likely have very poor tone, possibly a poor suck and decreased bowel sounds. Even if apnea is not persistent, the other findings will make it unlikely that this baby will tolerate feeding. The hypotonia and feeding intolerance may persist for several days.

After Resuscitation

Resuscitation can be a trying experience for both the newborn and the resuscitation team. A calm and organized approach can make the process run smoothly even in difficult clinical circumstances. The team leader should generate confidence and direction for the entire team. After resuscitation, a team debriefing will help identify areas that can be performed more effectively as well as reinforce good individual performances. If each team member is encouraged to speak openly and a nonpunitive approach is taken, this discussion will encourage the process of performance improvement for the entire resuscitation team. The resuscitation should be carefully documented.

If resuscitation has not been successful at regaining spontaneous circulation by 15 minutes of effective resuscitative measures, efforts should be discontinued. It is also considered appropriate not to initiate resuscitation in infants with trisomy 13, trisomy 18, or anencephaly and infants of less than 400 g birth weight. Local practices for routine resuscitation may vary from institution to institution, and according to gestational age. The newborn who has survived a prolonged resuscitation should be monitored for further organ system compromise.

A 20-year-old gravida 2 para 1 woman without any prenatal care presents in labor and precipitously delivers an infant who appears to be 36 weeks' gestation. Although the infant is vigorous, he is blue and begins having signs of respiratory distress, including nasal flaring and subcostal and intercostal retractions shortly after birth. You begin providing CPAP with 100% oxygen and place a pulse oximeter on the right hand. The oxygen saturation is initially 40% but begins increasing slowly. You note that the infant continues to have significant deep retractions.

Exercise 6

QUESTIONS

1. What are you considering as possible causes of this infant's cyanosis and respiratory distress?

2. How would you differentiate these etiologies?

3. On further evaluation you realize that the abdomen appears scaphoid and you cannot hear breath sounds over the left hemithorax. How would you adjust the resuscitation?

ANSWERS

1. Cyanosis may be related to pulmonary or cardiac causes. In general, infants with cyanotic congenital heart disease will initially appear well. They usually do not have severe respiratory distress, as is seen in this case. A wide variety of pulmonary diseases may cause cyanosis and respiratory distress including surfactant deficiency, pneumonia, meconium aspiration syndrome, pulmonary hypoplasia, pneumothorax, pleural effusion, congenital diaphragmatic hernia, airway obstruction, and retained fetal lung fluid.

2. With this history, cyanotic congenital heart disease is less likely because of the severe respiratory distress as mentioned above, although some lesions such as transposition of the great arteries (TGA) or total anomalous pulmonary venous return can cause pulmonary congestion leading to respiratory distress. The infant's response to oxygen can help with the differential diagnosis. Many of the pulmonary causes of cyanosis will have

dramatic improvement in oxygen saturation when oxygen and continuous positive airway pressure are provided. Infants with cyanotic congenital heart disease may have a small improvement in oxygen saturation with such measures, but in infants with fixed right-to-left shunts, such as pulmonary atresia, or TGA, the oxygen saturation will not increase beyond 85% to 90%. Most of the pulmonary causes of cyanosis with respiratory distress can be differentiated based on physical examination, chest radiographs, and clinical response to treatment. Surfactant deficiency, pneumonia, meconium aspiration, and retained fetal lung fluid all should begin to show signs of improvement with the basic resuscitative support that has already been initiated. When these measures do not lead to clinical improvement, other more complicated problems must be considered. A history of prolonged oligohydramnios would suggest the possibility of pulmonary hypoplasia. However, in this case with its lack of prenatal care, there is no documented history. Airway obstruction would result in severe muscle retractions with no audible air movement and could be caused by choanal atresia, a mucus plug, extreme micrognathia, or other obstructive lesions.

A physical examination with absent breath sounds over one side can be indicative of a pneumothorax, a pleural effusion, or congenital diaphragmatic hernia. Prenatal care with advanced ultrasound technology has made delivery room diagnosis of congenital anomalies such as congenital heart disease and congenital diaphragmatic hernia uncommon. The clinician must, therefore, have a high index of suspicion when evaluating infants not responding to routine treatment.

3. The absent breath sounds with a scaphoid abdomen can indicate congenital diaphragmatic hernia. You decide that the baby should be intubated to prevent further air distention of the bowel within the chest. An orogastric tube should be placed to decompress the bowel. It may be necessary to give a muscle relaxant to prevent the baby from continually swallowing air. This will require early placement of an umbilical venous catheter. An oxygen saturation monitor should be placed and lower saturations (70s) and higher Pa_{CO_2} (up to approximately 70 mm Hg) should be initially accepted to prevent barotrauma from excessive ventilating pressures.[29] This infant will need complex and sophisticated management and should be stabilized and transferred to an appropriate facility as soon as possible.

The Practice of Resuscitation

Although neonatologists and many pediatricians perform neonatal resuscitation routinely, it is an area of neonatal care that is often given minimal attention but can have lasting impact on a child's life. Centers that care for complex neonatal problems requiring highly skilled personnel and advanced equipment differ from facilities that primarily deliver term newborns and are not equipped to care for neonatal complications. It is imperative that all institutions adequately provide the expertise and equipment to resuscitate and stabilize newborn infants. Each center should prospectively evaluate its facilities, equipment, and training of personnel. Where resuscitation is infrequent it may be necessary to run mock codes for continued staff training, and to work with larger regional centers to assure the provision of skilled resuscitative care. The process should be reviewed on a regular basis and all complicated resuscitations should be evaluated to identify areas requiring improvement, as well as recognizing individual competencies. Well-planned resuscitations in adequately equipped facilities with skilled personnel provide the best chance for optimal resuscitation outcomes and healthy children.

References

1. Kattwinkel J (ed): The Textbook of Neonatal Resuscitation, 5th ed. Elk Grove Village, IL, American Academy of Pediatrics and American Heart Association, 2006.
2. Apgar V: A proposal for a new method of evaluation of the newborn infant. Curr Res Anesth Analg 1953;32:260–267.
3. Nelson KB, Ellenberg JH: Apgar scores as predictors of chronic neurologic disability. Pediatrics 1981;68:36–44.
4. Costeloe K, Hennessy E, Gibson AT, et al: The EPICure study: Outcomes to discharge from the hospital for infants born at the threshold of viability. Pediatrics 2000;106:659–671.
5. Vohra S, Frent G, Campbell V, et al: Effect of polyethylene occlusive skin wrapping on heat loss in very low birth weight infants at delivery: A randomized trial. J Pediatr 1999;134:547–551.

6. Vohra S, Roberts RS, Zhang B, et al: Heat Loss Prevention (HeLP) in the delivery room: A randomized controlled trial of polyethylene occlusive skin wrapping in very preterm infants. J Pediatr 2004;145:750–753.

7. Halliday HL, Sweet D: Endotracheal intubation at birth for preventing morbidity and mortality in vigorous, meconium-stained infants born at term (Cochrane Review). In: The Cochrane Library Issue 4. Chichester, UK, John Wiley & Sons, 2003.

8. Finer NN, Barrington KJ, Al-Fadley F, Peters KL: Limitations of self-inflating resuscitators. Pediatrics 1986;77:417–420.

9. Hoskyns EW, Milner AD, Hopkin IE: A simple method of face mask resuscitation at birth. Arch Dis Child 1987;62:376–378.

10. Bennett SC, Rich W, Vaucher Y, Finer NN: An in vitro comparison of three neonatal resuscitation devices. Pediatr Res 2004;55–537A.

11. Finer NN, Rich W, Craft A, Henderson C: Comparison of methods of bag and mask ventilation for neonatal resuscitation. Resuscitation 2001;49:299–305.

12. Leone TA, Lange A, Rich W, Finer NN: Disposable colorimetric carbon dioxide detector use as an indicator of a patent airway during non-invasive mask ventilation. Pediatrics 2006;118:e202–e204.

13. Lindner W, Vossbeck S, Hummler H, Pohlandt F: Delivery room management of extremely low birthweight infants: Spontaneous breathing or intubation? Pediatrics 1999;103:961–967.

14. Grein AJ, Weiner GM: Laryngeal mask airway versus bag-mask ventilation or endotracheal intubation for neonatal resuscitation. Cochrane Database Syst Rev 2005.

15. Tracy M, Downe L, Holberton J: How safe is intermittent positive pressure ventilation in preterm babies ventilated from delivery to newborn intensive care unit? Arch Dis Child Fetal Neonatal Ed 2004;89:F84–F87.

16. Bjorklund LJ, Ingimarsson J, Curstedt T, et al: Manual ventilation with a few large breaths at birth compromises the therapeutic effect of subsequent surfactant replacement in immature lambs. Pediatr Res 1997; 42:348–355.

17. Milner AD: Resuscitation at birth. Eur J Pediatr 1998;157:524–527.

18. Lindner W, Hogel J, Pohlandt F: Sustained pressure-controlled inflation or intermittent mandatory ventilation in preterm infants in the delivery room? A randomized, controlled trial on initial respiratory support via nasopharyngeal tube. Acta Paediatr 2005;94:303–309.

19. Hevesi ZG, Thrush DN, Downs JB, Smith RA: Cardiopulmonary resuscitation—Effect of CPAP on gas exchange during chest compressions. Anesthesiology 1999;90:1078–1083.

20. Ho JJ, Subramaniam P, Hendersen-Smart DJ, Davis PG: Continuous distending airway pressure for respiratory distress syndrome in preterm infants (Cochrane Review). The Cochrane Library, Issue 3. Oxford, Update Software, 2002.

21. Hartog A, Gommers D, Haitsma JJ, Lachmann B: Improvement of lung mechanics by exogenous surfactant: Effect of prior application of high positive end-expiratory pressure. Br J Anaesth 2000;85: 752–756.

22. Michna J, Jobe AH, Ikegami M: Positive end-expiratory pressure preserves surfactant function in preterm lambs. Am J Respir Crit Care Med 1999; 160:634–639.

23. Kelly MA, Finer NN: Nasotracheal intubation in the neonate: Physiologic responses and effects of atropine and pancuronium. J Pediatr 1984;105: 303–309.

24. Repetto JE, Donohue PK, Baker SF, et al: Use of capnography in the delivery room for assessment of endotracheal tube placement. J Perinatol 2001; 21:284–287.

25. Aziz HF, Martin JB, Moore JJ: The pediatric disposable end-tidal carbon dioxide detector role in endotracheal intubation in newborns. J Perinatol 1999; 19:110–113.

26. Saugstad OD, Rootwelt T, Aalen O: Resuscitation of asphyxiated newborn infants with room air or oxygen: An international controlled trial: The Resair 2 study. Pediatrics 1998;102:e1.

27. Saugstad OD, Ramji S, Vento M: Resuscitation of depressed newborn infants with ambient air or pure oxygen: A meta-analysis. Biol Neonate 2005;87: 27–34.

28. Tan A, Schulze A, O'Donnell CP, Davis PG: Air versus oxygen for resuscitation of infants at birth. Cochrane Database Syst Rev 2004.

29. Basic newborn resuscitation: A practical guide. World Health Organization. Accessed at www. who.int/reproductive-health/publications/ MSM_98_1/MSM_98_1_chapter2.en.html 1997.

30. Kamlin COF, O'Donnell CPF, Davis PG, Morley CJ: Oxygen saturations in healthy newborn infants during the first minutes of life: Defining the normal range. Pediatr Acad Soc 2005;58:205.

31. Finer NN, Tierney A, Etches PC, et al: Congenital diaphragmatic hernia: Developing a protocolized approach. J Pediatr Surg 1998;33:1331–1337.

Fluid and Electrolyte Management in the Newborn Intensive Care Unit

John M. Lorenz, MD

Fluid and electrolyte management is an important and challenging part of the initial management of any very premature or critically ill newborn. The transition from fetal to neonatal life is associated with major changes in fluid and electrolyte homeostasis and total body balance. Before birth the fetus has a constant and ready supply of water and electrolytes, and homeostasis is largely a function of maternal and placental mechanisms. After birth, newborns must rapidly assume responsibility for their own fluid and electrolyte homeostasis in an environment in which water and electrolyte availability and losses are much more variable and less subject to feedback control than in utero. Moreover, significant contraction of the extracellular fluid (ECF) space occurs with the transition from fetal to neonatal life. In very premature newborns, this transition is also associated with a significant change in internal potassium (K) balance: K shifts from the intracellular fluid (ICF) space to the ECF space. The goal of fluid and electrolyte therapy in the immediate postnatal period is not to maintain fluid and electrolyte balance but to allow the appropriate changes in balance to occur without detrimental perturbations in fluid and electrolyte status.

Body Water and Sodium

A weight loss of about 5% to 15% is almost invariable during the first week of life in preterm infants.[1-3] Although inadequate caloric intake may contribute to this weight loss, it results in large part from contraction of the ECF space after birth[3-7] (Fig. 2-1). The reason for this contraction is not completely understood. However, relatively large increases in water and sodium intake are necessary to attenuate the contraction of the ECF space.[1,8,9] Moreover, higher intakes of sodium and water have been associated with increased incidences of patent ductus arteriosus, necrotizing enterocolitis, more prolonged oxygen dependence, and bronchopulmonary dysplasia.[10-14] Finally, aggressive parenteral nutrition in the first week of life lessens weight loss, but contraction of the ECF space still occurs.[6] The negative total body water (TBW) and total body sodium (TBNa) balances are associated with the contraction of ECF space and are believed to be physiologically appropriate in the first week of life.

Potassium

The serum potassium concentration ($[K^+]$) rises in the first 24 to 72 hours after birth in very premature infants, even in the absence of exogenous K intake or renal failure.[15-17] This increase results from the shift of K from the ICF space to the ECF space. The magnitude of this shift correlates roughly with the degree of prematurity, but it does not seem to occur (or at least is not clinically significant) after 30 to 32 weeks of gestation[16] (Fig. 2-2). The reason for and appropriateness of this shift are not understood. However, it is known to result in hyperkalemia in 25% to 50% of infants weighing less than 1000 g at birth or born before 28 weeks' gestation.[17-23]

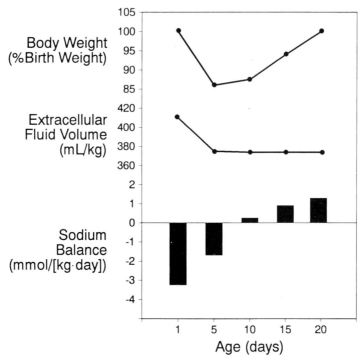

Figure 2-1 Postnatal changes in body weight, extracellular fluid volume, and sodium balance in very premature infants. (From Shaffer SG, Weismann DN: Fluid requirements in the preterm infant. Clin Perinatol 1992;19:233–250. Used with permission.)

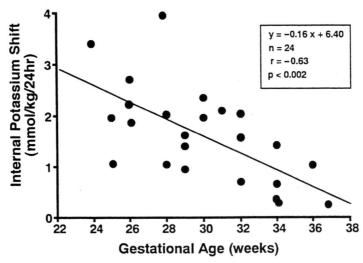

Figure 2-2 Magnitude of the shift in potassium from the intracellular fluid to the extracellular fluid space during the first 24 hours of life as a function of gestational age. (From Sato K, Kondo T, Iwao H, et al: Internal potassium shift in premature infants: Cause of nonoliguric hyperkalemia. J Pediatr 1995;126:109–113. Used with permission.)

Glucose

With the clamping of the umbilical cord at birth, the supply of glucose and other nutrients from the mother ceases. As a result, serum glucose concentrations fall sharply over the first 60 to 90 minutes of life.[24,25] In response, there are abrupt increases in the levels of epinephrine, norepinephrine, and glucagon with a concomitant fall in insulin. Together, these responses mobilize glucose from glycogen stores and promote gluconeogenesis.[26] Glucose utilization averages 4 to 8 mg/kg/minute in term and preterm newborns.[27,28] Endogenous glucose production may be inadequate or may not be sustained at a sufficient rate in infants with perinatal stress, prematurity, or intrauterine growth restriction.[29] Exogenous administration of glucose at a rate that matches the rate of glucose utilization is necessary to prevent hypoglycemia and to conserve glycogen stores. However, premature infants are also at increased risk for hyperglycemia with exogenous glucose infusions because of a sluggish insulin response to rising plasma glucose concentrations.[30,31]

Diuresis and Natriuresis

In most infants, the excretion of water and sodium (Na) that occurs as a result of contraction of the ECF space in the first few days of life is not gradual. In fact, a characteristic pattern of fluid and electrolyte adaptation, which is largely independent of fluid and electrolyte intake, is observed in the first week of life in the majority of very low birth weight newborns.[1,32-34] Usually, three phases can be distinguished. Table 2-1 summarizes the changes in fluid and electrolyte balance, ECF volume, and renal function associated with each phase.

TABLE 2-1

POSTNATAL RENAL, FLUID, AND ELECTROLYTE ADAPTATION IN VERY PREMATURE NEWBORNS

Parameter	Prediuretic Phase	Diuretic/Natriuretic Phase	Homeostatic Phase
Age	From birth to 2 days	1–5 days	After 2–5 days
Urine output	Low	Abrupt ↑↑	↓ then α intake
Sodium excretion	Minimal	Abrupt ↑↑	↓ then α intake
Potassium excretion	Minimal	Abrupt ↑↑	↓ then α intake
Water balance	< Intake–IWL	Markedly negative	~ α sodium balance
Sodium balance	~ Negative	Markedly negative	Stable, then positive w/ growth
Potassium balance	~ Negative	Markedly negative	Stable, then positive w/ growth
ECF volume (mL)	Stable or ~ ↓	Abrupt ↓↓	1. α sodium balance 2. ↑ w/ growth
Creatinine clearance	Low	Abrupt ↑↑	± ↓, then gradual ↑ with maturation
FENa	Variable	↑	Gradual ↓
FEK	Variable	No change	No change
Urine osmolality	Moderately hyposmotic	Moderately hyposmotic	Moderately hyposmotic
Water intake	~ IWL	↑ to allow 2–5% weight loss per day up to total of 5–15%	Volume to optimize caloric intake without fluid retention
Sodium intake	None	Begin when serum [Na$^+$] is stable with weight loss or falling; ↑ as necessary to maintain serum [Na$^+$] normal	Approximate sodium loss ± growth allowance; sodium requirement will be inversely proportional to gestational age
Potassium intake	None	1–2 mmol/kg/d if serum [K$^+$] <5–6 mmol/L *and not rising*	≥2–3 mmol/kg/d to maintain serum [K$^+$] normal
Glucose intake	4–8 mg/kg/min; adjust to maintain plasma glucose concentration normal	↑ fluid requirement may require ↓ dextrose concentration	↑ as tolerated to maximize caloric intake
Common problems			
Water balance	Water intoxication with lower IWL than anticipated		Water and sodium retention with PDA, CLD
Sodium balance	Hypernatremia with higher IWL than anticipated	Hypernatremia	Water and sodium depletion with or without hyponatremia
Potassium balance	Hyperkalemia		Hypokalemia
Glucose balance		Hyperglycemia	

α, proportional to; CLD, chronic lung disease; ECF, extracellular fluid; FE, fractional excretion; GFR, glomerular filtration rate; IWL, insensible water loss; PDA, patent ductus arteriosus.

During the first 12 to 48 hours of life, the urine flow rate is low (0.5 to 3 mL/kg/hour), regardless of intake. Therefore, during this pre-diuretic phase, excretion of Na and K is also quite low; insensible water loss (IWL) is the major route of water loss. The low glomerular filtration rate (GFR) in the immediate perinatal period limits the infant's ability to excrete water and electrolyte loads.

As the diuretic/natriuretic phase begins, an abrupt increase in urinary water and Na occurs independent of water and Na intake, and her-alds contraction of the ECF space.[3] Early in the diuretic/natriuretic phase, sodium concen-tration ([Na^+]) often rises because water bal-ance is more negative than sodium balance. The majority of body weight loss occurs during this phase. A fall in plasma [K^+] can be antici-pated as increased delivery of water and Na to the distal nephron stimulates K secretion and kaliuresis. As the ECF space stabilizes at an appropriately reduced volume, urinary water and electrolyte excretion decreases and begins to vary appropriately with intake.

Case Study 1

Baby girl A is a 610-g, 28-week-old infant delivered by cesarean section because of maternal preeclampsia. She is placed on nasal continuous positive airway pressure in an incubator with 50% relative humidity and started on 5% dextrose in water at 140 mL/kg/day. At 12 hours of age, plasma [Na^+] is 128 mmol/L. The only sodium intake has been via the umbilical artery catheter (UAC) as normal saline at 1 mL/hour. Urine output has been 1.1 mL/kg/hour.

Exercise 1

QUESTIONS

1. Why is the baby hyponatremic?
2. What are the risks of hyponatremia?
3. What fluid and sodium intake should the baby receive today?

ANSWERS

1. Plasma [Na^+] is determined by TBW volume and TBNa content. Plasma [Na^+] may be low because either TBW is increased or TBNa is low, or both. In evaluating TBW balance, the following equation is conceptually helpful.

$$\text{TBW balance} = \text{fluid intake} - [\text{insensible water loss} + \text{urine output} + \text{stool water loss}]$$

Stool water loss under the conditions above is usually negligible. Therefore, in this case, for water balance to be negative, fluid intake must be less than IWL + urine output. Thus, fluid intake – urine output must be less than IWL. Insensible water loss is a function of gestational age and postnatal age[35,36] (Table 2-2) and environmental conditions, especially ambient humidity[37] (Fig. 2-3). In the case presented here, fluid intake – urine output was 127 mL for the first 12 hours of life. Although highly variable at any given gestational age (even under the same envi-ronmental conditions), it is unlikely that IWL was greater than 127 mL over 12 hours. Therefore, it is likely that TBW bal-ance is positive. Although this infant is very small, she is not extremely premature. IWL (normalized for body weight or surface area)

TABLE 2-2								
INSENSIBLE WATER LOSS INAPPROPRIATE FOR GESTATIONAL AGE NEWBORNS*								
GA	**PA < 1**	**PA 1**	**PA 3**	**PA 5**	**PA 7**	**PA 14**	**PA 21**	**PA 28**
25–27[†]	57–214	62–171	59–96	43–72	31–68	18–59	14–55	8–53
28–30	22–75	23–68	20–57	19–48	16–45	12–37	9–34	9–34
31–36	8–29	8–28	10–27	10–27	10–27	9–22	10–19	11–16
37–41	8–18	11–14	11–14	11–14	11–14	11–14	12–13	11–16

*Nursed naked in an incubator with 50% ambient humidity, ambient air temperature in the neutral thermal range, and constant airflow of 8 L/minute.
†Ninety-five percent confidence intervals.
GA, gestational age in weeks; PA, Postnatal age in days.
Calculated from data in references 35 and 36.

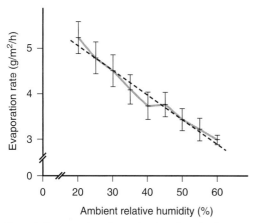

Figure 2-3 Transepidermal water loss (IWL from the skin) as a function of ambient humidity. Mean ± SE; dashed line = regression line (R = −0.986). (From Hammarlund K, Nilsson GE, Oberg PA, et al: Transepidermal water loss in newborn infants. Relation to ambient humidity and site of measurement and estimation of total transepidermal water loss. Acta Paediatr Scand 1977;66:553–562. Used with permission.)

is a function of maturity, not size. Therefore, this infant very likely received more fluid on the first day of life than she should have. This conclusion would be supported by an increase in body weight, although this information was not available in this case.

Could TBNa be low as well? There are two possible reasons that TBNa could be low at this age. First, if maternal plasma [Na⁺] were low at birth, neonatal TBNa (and therefore plasma [Na⁺]) would be low at birth. This is because fetal extracellular [Na⁺] is determined by maternal plasma [Na⁺]. If there had been a maternal value (plasma [Na⁺]) recorded in the perinatal period, this possibility could have been confirmed.

The second cause of a low TBNa is that TBNa balance could have been more negative than TBW balance for the first 12 hours of life.

TBNa balance = Na intake − (urinary Na
loss + stool Na loss)

Urinary sodium losses would be expected to be less than 2 to 3 mmol/day prior to diuresis/natriuresis at this gestational age,[21,31] and stool sodium losses should be negligible. Therefore, with a sodium intake of 3 mmol/day (= 1 mL/hour normal saline × 154 mmol/1000 mL normal saline × 12 hours/0.61 kg) via the UAC, it is unlikely that TBNa balance is significantly negative.

Thus, although decreased fetal TBNa cannot be excluded, the likely magnitude of

the increase in TBW due to excessive water intake is sufficient to explain the hyponatremia.

2. The distribution of water between the ECF space and ICF space is determined by ECF osmolality. An acute decrease in ECF osmolality (due in this case to hyponatremia) causes water to move from the ECF space to the ICF space. In the brain, this results in cerebral edema. The likelihood of signs and sequelae of hyponatremia depend on the magnitude and rapidity of the decrease in plasma [Na⁺]. Acute hyponatremia (defined in adults as a decrease in plasma [Na⁺] of more than 12 mmol/L/day with a low plasma [Na⁺] for <48 hours) may cause vomiting, seizures, impaired consciousness, brain stem herniation, long-term neurodevelopmental disability, or death. In newborns, cerebral palsy[38] and sensorineural hearing loss[39] have been associated with hyponatremia.

3. Fluid restriction to 60 to 90 mL/kg/day (at least until the onset of diuresis, natriuresis) should be sufficient to correct this moderate degree of hyponatremia in this infant without signs of central nervous system disturbance. No sodium intake is required because the baby is asymptomatic and TBNa has been judged as not low. Plasma [Na⁺] should be followed every 8 hours to be sure it is increasing, but it should not increase too rapidly. The maximum rate of increase recommended in asymptomatic adults is 12 mmol/L during the first 24 hours and 6 mmol/L in the next 24 hours. More rapid correction may cause *osmotic demyelination syndrome*,[40] which can result in death or long-term neurodevelopmental disability. Chronic, asymptomatic hyponatremia should be corrected even more slowly.

If acute hyponatremia is more severe (<115 to 120 mmol/L in adults; there are no data in newborns) or there are associated neurologic signs, more rapid correction is recommended, but no more than 2 mmol/L/hour until plasma [Na⁺] has increased 6 to 8 mmol/L and symptoms have abated. This may be accomplished by inducing a diuresis with furosemide and replacing urine output volume for volume with hypertonic saline. Thereafter, the total correction should be no more than 12 mmol/L in the first 24 hours, and 18 mmol/L in the first 48 hours. In the immediate neonatal period, especially in premature infants, furosemide diuresis with hypertonic saline replacement may be less effective because the response to furosemide may be blunted by the low GFR.

Fluid intake was decreased to 60 mL/kg/day. Later in the afternoon, urine flow rate has increased to 1.8 mL/kg/hour and plasma [Na$^+$] is 131 mmol/L. Urine output will be followed closely and plasma [Na$^+$] and body weight will be rechecked in 8 hours. Should the diuretic phase appear to begin in the interim, fluid intake will be increased to 100 to 120 mL/kg/day to ensure that the rise in plasma [Na$^+$] is not too rapid.

Case Study 2

Baby boy M is a 3-day-old infant of 29 weeks' gestation who delivered precipitously in the emergency room. Apgar score was estimated, in retrospect, to be 3 at 1 minute and 5 at 5 minutes. He has required continued, low ventilatory support. He has no murmur and a quiet precordium. His plasma sodium this morning is 155 mmol/L. Neurologic status has been normal since admission. You review his nursing flow sheets (DOL, day of life):

	DOL 1	DOL 2	DOL 3	DOL 4
Body weight (g)	850	880	800	800
Fluid intake (mL/kg/day)	101	86	127	
Urine output (mL/kg/day)	26	25	66	
Sodium intake (mmol/kg/day)	2.1 (via UAC)	2.1 (via UAC)	2.1 + 5 mmol/kg NaHCO$_3$	
Plasma [Na$^+$] (mmol/L)	137	138	150	155

Exercise 2

QUESTIONS

1. Why did this baby become hypernatremic?
2. What are the risks of hypernatremia?

3. What fluid and sodium intake should the baby receive today?
4. Would it have been better to give tris (hydroxymethyl)aminomethane (THAM) instead of NaHCO$_3$ on DOL 3?
5. When should the plasma [Na$^+$] be checked again?

ANSWERS

1. Plasma [Na$^+$] may be high either because TBW is decreased or because TBNa is increased, or both. Therefore, the question to be addressed in this case is whether TBW should be increased or TBNa decreased, or both. The loss of 6% of the birth weight reflects in part a decrease in ECF volume. Some of the increase in plasma [Na$^+$], especially from the morning of day 2 to the morning of DOL 3, is due to a decrease in TBW. However, the decrease in ECF volume (and TBW) is not excessive. It is noteworthy that the infant also received over 17 mmol/kg of Na over 3 days, which was apparently too much to keep plasma [Na$^+$] in a normal range for the expected and appropriate decrease in TBW. Therefore, the increase in plasma [Na$^+$] from DOL 2 to DOL 3 was due to appropriate net water loss plus inappropriately positive TBNa balance. This was then compounded by the administration of a large amount of NaHCO$_3$ on DOL 3 for metabolic acidosis. Therefore, the primary cause of the hypernatremia is abnormally high TBNa content as the result of excessive Na intake.

2. The distribution of water between the ECF space and ICF space is determined by ECF osmolality. Increase in ECF osmolality (due in this case to hypernatremia) causes water to move from the ICF space to the ECF space. This is particularly problematic in the brain, where decrease in ICF volume may result in neurologic abnormalities such as high-pitched cry, irritability, seizures, impaired consciousness, intracranial hemorrhage, cerebral infarction, long-term neurodevelopmental disability, or death.

3. First, sodium intake should be withheld, which will necessitate changing the UAC infusate to 5% dextrose in water. The increased urinary Na excretion that is likely with the increasing urine output will then

lead to a more negative Na balance and decrease in plasma [Na$^+$]. In addition, further decrease in TBW should be prevented. Consideration could be given to increasing TBW, particularly in the presence of neurologic signs, although a very substantial increase in fluid intake would probably be required and could increase the risk of cardiopulmonary problems. Because there has been no change in the baby's neurologic status, body weight had been stable on the prior day's fluid intake, and urine (and very likely urinary Na) output was increasing, fluid intake was continued at 125 mL/kg/day with no Na intake.

4. No. THAM is hyperosmolar (1 mmol/3.3 mL). The increase in the concentration of cation, THAM, and the bicarbonate ion formed would still increase plasma osmolality. This increase in osmolality is associated with the same risk of increased osmolality due to hypernatremia, but the increase in plasma osmolality is not apparent from the plasma [Na$^+$].

5. The baby's neurologic status should be followed closely and fluid and electrolyte balance should be reassessed in 6 to 8 hours. It is important to document that plasma [Na$^+$] is falling, but it should not fall too rapidly. Too rapid a fall in brain interstitial fluid osmolality will cause water to move intracellularly, causing cerebral edema. In adults, the recommended rate of decrease in plasma [Na$^+$] in acute hypernatremia is 2 mmol/L/hour. If there are neurologic signs, they should improve as plasma [Na$^+$] decreases toward normal. If neurologic signs appear or worsen as plasma [Na$^+$] falls, suspect cerebral edema secondary to too rapid correction.

Later in the evening, there has been no change in the baby's neurologic status, urine flow rate has remained about the same as the previous day, and plasma [Na$^+$] has fallen to 146 mmol/L. The glucose concentration in the sample indicates there has not been significant dilution of the blood sample by the UAC infusate (now Na free, 5% dextrose in water), which would spuriously lower the plasma [Na$^+$].[41] No change in fluid and electrolyte administration is made. Fluid and electrolyte balance will be reassessed in 8 to 12 hours.

Case Study 3

Baby boy F was born by cesarean section at 23 weeks' gestation for a placental abruption. His mother had not received antenatal steroids. Apgar scores were 1 at 1 minute, 3 at 5 minutes, and 5 at 10 minutes, after intubation, positive pressure ventilation, external cardiac massage, and 30 mL/kg of normal saline. The birth weight was 680 g. The first hematocrit was 30%. After two packed red blood cell transfusions (15 mL/kg) the hematocrit was 45%. He required mechanical ventilation. During the first 2 days of life the baby received 172 mL/kg/day of fluid intake (exclusive of the normal saline in the delivery room and the transfusions) without sodium or potassium. There has been no urine output since birth. The weight is now 623 g. Heart rate, blood pressure, and perfusion are normal. Plasma sodium has increased from 135 to 146 mmol/L. Plasma [K$^+$] values at 14, 21, and 28 hours of age were 6.2, 7.2, and 7.0 mmol/L (samples from the UAC). The plasma creatinine concentration, [Creat], has risen from 1.1 mg/dL at 14 hours of age to 1.3 mg/dL at 28 hours of age. Arterial pH is 7.36, P$_{CO_2}$ 39 mm Hg, P$_{O_2}$ 70 mm Hg, and base excess −2.7. Plasma ionized calcium is normal.

Exercise 3

QUESTIONS

1. Is this baby in acute renal failure?
2. Is this nonoliguric hyperkalemia?
3. What adjustments should be made in fluid and electrolyte administration?
4. What other interventions are indicated?

ANSWERS

1. Perhaps. The plasma [Creat] at this age is still a function of maternal plasma [Creat].[42] A single plasma [Creat], therefore, indicates nothing about the baby's GFR at this age. The best criterion for acute renal failure in the first week of life is the change in plasma [Creat] over time.[43] However, the rate of change that is normal depends upon what GFR is normal. Because GFR increases with gestational age, the rate of change in plasma [Creat] after birth is proportional to

gestational age[44] (Fig. 2-4). In very preterm infants, plasma creatinine may rise 0.1 to 0.3 mg/dL/day in the first few days of life, then return to the original base line and decrease slowly[43] (Fig. 2-5). Thus, the small observed increase in plasma [Creat] is not abnormal for this extremely premature infant. However, 29 hours of anuria is certainly suggestive of acute renal failure. Urinary catheterization should be considered to rule out urinary retention. Sequential measurements of plasma [Creat] and urine output will clarify this baby's renal status.

If there is a possibility of acute renal failure that can be remediated, causes must be considered now. Oligoanuria may be prerenal, intrinsic (due to renal parenchymal maldevelopment or injury), or postrenal in origin. Prerenal failure (e.g., secondary to hypovolemia, decreased effective blood volume, decreased cardiac output) is very often difficult to exclude and may result in intrinsic renal failure if the cause is not promptly treated. If prerenal failure is suspected, a 10- to 20-mL/kg intravenous bolus of normal saline or 5% albumin should be administered over 10 to 20 minutes, unless ECF volume expansion is strongly contraindicated by a concomitant condition. If there is no response, this can be followed by a dose

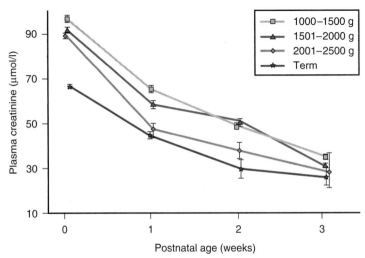

Figure 2-4 Change in plasma [Creat] in the first 3 weeks of life in healthy full-term infants and premature infants with uncomplicated postnatal courses (88 μmol/L creatinine = 1 mg/dL). (From Bueva A, Guignard JP: Renal function in pre-term neonates. Pediatr Res 1994;36:572–577. Used with permission.)

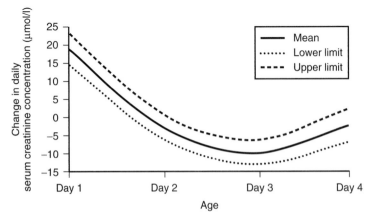

Figure 2-5 Daily change in plasma [Creat] in newborns at 32 weeks' gestation or less without risk factors for acute renal failure. Mean and 99th percentile confidence intervals (88 μmol/L creatinine = 1 mg/dL). (From Choker G, Gouyon JB: Diagnosis of acute renal failure in very preterm infants. Biol Neonate 2004;86:212–216. Used with permission.)

of a loop diuretic, such as furosemide (2 mg/kg intravenously). If there is still no response with a urethral catheter in place or intrinsic renal failure is likely, low-dose dopamine (0.5 to 4 μg/kg/minute) is widely recommended. Although there is some evidence that this improves urine output in prerenal failure,[45] there are no data regarding its effectiveness in intrinsic renal failure. Urethral catheterization will exclude the possibility of urinary retention and posterior urethral valves. Postrenal failure due to congenital obstruction of the urinary tract proximal to the bladder can usually be diagnosed by ultrasonography.

The baby appears to be normovolemic at this time and the history is consistent with acute intrinsic renal failure secondary to hypovolemia due to acute blood loss in the perinatal period. It is possible that 8.4% weight loss indicates excessive contraction of the ECF volume, but this degree of weight loss is not unusual and the weight loss is due to free (insensible) water loss, because there has been no urinary sodium loss. Moreover, with the resulting increase in plasma $[Na^+]$ (and ECF osmolality) water has shifted from the ICF space to the ECF space, attenuating the decrease in ECF volume. Thus, excessive contraction of the ECF space was judged unlikely.

2. If the baby is anuric, this is, by definition, not nonoliguric hyperkalemia. However, the baby has no urinary K loss as the result of acute renal failure, and therefore, the increase in plasma $[K^+]$ must be the result of the ICF to ECF shift of K, because the baby has received no exogenous potassium. The packed red blood cell transfusions would not increase plasma $[K^+]$ significantly.[46] The source of the K in the plasma in the packed red blood cells is leakage of K from the erythrocytes during storage. After transfusion, the red blood cells take up K.

3. The change in body weight of 8.4% in 1 day suggests that intake is less than IWL, because there has been no urinary water loss. The fluid administration rate should be increased (to ~200 mL/kg/day) and the baby reweighed in 8 to 12 hours. Sodium should not be started until it is confirmed that there has been compensation for free (insensible) water loss.

4. Although Table 2-3 summarizes the management options for nonoliguric hyperkalemia, these are for the most part applicable to acute management of hyperkalemia of any cause. Plasma ionized calcium is normal, there is no metabolic acidosis, and no arrhythmia, so neither intravenous calcium nor $NaHCO_3$ are indicated at this time. An insulin drip should be started as soon as

TABLE 2-3

MANAGEMENT OF NONOLIGURIC HYPERKALEMIA IN VERY PREMATURE NEWBORNS

1. Antagonize cardiac toxicity
   - Administer 0.5–1.0 mEq/kg elemental calcium (1–2 mL/kg of 10% calcium gluconate) by slow IV push for acute arrhythmia; if no arrhythmia, treat hypocalcemia of prematurity aggressively.
2. Stimulate cellular uptake of potassium from the ECF space
   - Administer $NaHCO_3$ 1–2 mmol/kg by slow IV push, for acute arrhythmia; otherwise administer $NaHCO_3$ only as indicated for metabolic acidosis.
   - Administer glucose and insulin.[47,48]
   - Administer nebulized albuterol (400 μg in 2 mL normal saline).[49]
     Note: Transient, paradoxical increase in plasma $[K^+]$ has been associated with the administration of β_2-sympathomimetic amines to animals and adults with acute renal failure.
3. Remove potassium from the body
   - $NaHCO_3$ administration will also stimulate renal potassium secretion.
   - Give sodium polystyrene sulfonate (1g in 10% sucrose in a 1 g: 4 mL ratio) by orogastric tube or retention enema. May be repeated every 4 to 6 hours as indicated.
     Notes:
     — This is an ion exchange resin (Na for K) and, thus, may cause or exacerbate expansion of the extracellular fluid space or hypernatremia.
     — This solution is very hyperosmolar. Exchange resins have been associated with the development of intragastric masses and intestinal perforation.[50–52]
   - Perform peritoneal dialysis.

From Mildenberger E, Versmold HT: Pathogenesis and therapy of non-oliguric hyperkalaemia of the premature infant. Eur J Pediatr 2002;161;415–422.

possible. Sodium polystyrene sulfonate (Kayexalate) could be considered, but if so, it should be in addition to the insulin drip because alone it will not be effective in lowering plasma $[K^+]$ as quickly as an insulin drip.[47,48]

No normal saline was given, but fluid intake was increased to 200 mL/kg/day. By 40 hours of age, the baby has begun to pass urine. Urine output has been 1.1 mL/kg/hour. Body weight is now 599 g. Plasma $[Na^+]$ is 141 mmol/L, plasma $[K^+]$ is 7.7 mmol/L, and plasma [Creat] is 1.6 mg/dL. The arterial blood gas is essentially unchanged. Heart rate remains normal, but T waves are now peaked on the cardiorespiratory monitor.

QUESTIONS

5. Is this baby in acute renal failure?
6. What adjustments should be made in fluid and electrolyte administration?
7. What other interventions are indicated?

ANSWERS

5. Probably. Even though the baby is no longer oliguric, the increase in plasma [Creat] is at least at the upper limit of normal, even for an extremely premature infant. If the fractional excretion (FE) of Na (FENa) were significantly elevated *with this relative low urine flow rate*, that would support this diagnosis. In fact, urine $[Na^+]$ was 132 mmol/L and urine [Creat] was 18 mg/dL.

$$FENa = (urine[Na^+]/plasma[Na^+]) \times (plasma[Creat]/urine[Creat]) = 132/141 \times 1.5/18 = 0.078 \text{ or } 7.8\%$$

This confirms the diagnosis of acute intrinsic renal failure with tubular dysfunction.

6. None now. However, if the baby has a polyuric phase of acute renal failure, Na intake should be increased to replace urinary losses. An increase in fluid intake may also be needed. This diuresis/natriuresis would not be the normal physiologic diuresis/natriuresis of prematurity. It would be due to renal tubular injury. These urinary losses would not be under homeostatic

control and, therefore, cannot be considered normal. The baby has already lost 12% of body weight, indicating that contraction of the ECF space has occurred; further contraction due to urinary water and Na losses that are not under homeostatic control may be deleterious. If the baby does enter a polyuric phase of acute renal failure, fluid and electrolyte intake should be directed at maintaining body weight at 85% to 90% of birth weight (until caloric intake is sufficient to expect growth) and plasma $[Na^+]$ and $[K^+]$ within the normal ranges. This may well require fluid, Na, and K intakes well above usual until tubular function recovers.

7. It may be necessary to increase the amount of glucose and insulin infused because the plasma $[K^+]$ is still rising and now there are T-wave changes. Certainly, intravenous calcium and $NaHCO_3$ should be at the bedside and nebulized albuterol readily available should bradycardia develop. Nebulized albuterol should be used with caution, however, because only efficacy, and not safety, has been demonstrated.[49] Of course, K should continue to be withheld.

The rates of glucose and insulin infusion are increased. Plasma $[K^+]$ is 7.7, 7.2, and 6.3 mmol/dL at 48, 53, and 65 hours of age. The weight has decreased to 575 g. Plasma $[Na^+]$ is 132 mmol/dL. Plasma [Creat] is 1.4 mg/dL. Urine output is now 2.6 mL/kg/hour.

Case Study 4

Baby boy M is a 42-day-old term infant (born following a 37-week gestation) with chronic lung disease after persistent primary pulmonary hypertension requiring high-frequency oscillatory ventilation. This is day 9 of gentamicin for Escherichia coli urosepsis. He has been fed 160 mL/kg/day of 20 kcal/oz infant formula. He has been on daily furosemide for 2 weeks, since shortly before being extubated. He currently requires 0.30 F_{IO_2} by nasal continuous positive airway pressure. In the last week he has gained 220 g. Weekly plasma electrolytes have shown that sodium has fallen from 135 mmol/L 2 weeks ago, to 134 mmol/L 1 week ago, to 128 mmol/L today. On warmed, nonhemolyzed heel sample this morning, *pH is 7.46, P_{CO_2} is 54 mm Hg, $[HCO_3^-]$ is 39 mmol/L, and base excess $+12$ mmol/L. Other laboratory values from the same sample show plasma $[K^+]$ to be 3.5 mmol/L, plasma chloride concentration ($[Cl^-]$) 82 mmol/L, plasma bicarbonate concentration ($[HCO_3^-]$) 32 mmol/L, plasma urea nitrogen 15 mg/dL, and plasma $[Creat]$ 0.4 mg/dL.*

Exercise 4

QUESTIONS

1. What is the cause of the hyponatremia?

2. Should the hyponatremia be treated? If so, how?

3. Is the metabolic alkalosis compensatory for the respiratory acidosis?

4. Should the metabolic alkalosis be treated? If so, how?

ANSWERS

1. The hyponatremia is due to the diuretic therapy. The mechanisms by which diuretics cause hyponatremia are complex and incompletely understood[53] (Fig. 2-6). It is more likely to occur with thiazide diuretics than loop diuretics because the latter do not decrease sodium reabsorption in the distal tubule. However, it can be caused by loop diuretics as well, especially when used for treatment of water and sodium retention, as was the case here.

   As with hyponatremia of any cause, the plasma $[Na^+]$ may be low either because TBW is too high or TBNa is too low, or both. If diuretic therapy has resulted in excessive reduction in the ECF volume, the low TBNa is too low. In this case, the dosing frequency of the diuretic should be reduced to reduce renal sodium excretion and correct the TBNa depletion. If the degree of ECF volume reduction is judged to be consistent with the

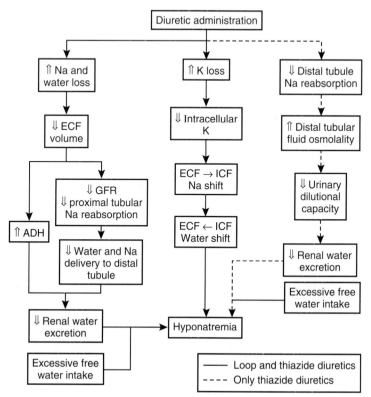

Figure 2-6 Pathophysiology of diuretic-induced hyponatremia. ADH, antidiuretic hormone; ECF, extracellular fluid; GFR, glomerular filtration rate; ICF, intracellular fluid.

TABLE 2-4

THE DIFFERENTIAL DIAGNOSIS, PATHOGENESIS, AND TREATMENT OF METABOLIC ALKALOSIS IN THE NEONATAL PERIOD

Generation of Alkalosis	Pathophysiology	Maintenance of Alkalosis	Treatment
K depletion	ECF $\Rightarrow$ ICF shift of H^+ in exchange for K	$\Uparrow$ Proximal tubular HCO_3^- reabsorption and $\Downarrow$ GFR; inhibition of aldosterone secretion	KCl
ECF volume contraction	$\Downarrow$ Extracellular water with no change in ECF HCO_3^- content	$\Downarrow$ EABV	Water and NaCl
Gastric fluid losses	Loss of acid	$\Downarrow$ EABV, K depletion	Water, NaCl, and KCl to replace deficits and ongoing losses
Administration of alkalizing salts (bicarbonate, lactate, citrate, acetate)	Addition of base	Continued alkali administration; K depletion	Discontinue or decrease alkali; KCl
Hypercapnia	$\Uparrow$ Urinary H^+ and Cl^- excretion	Continued hypercapnia; diuretics	Normalize P_{CO_2}; KCl, improve EABV, reduce diuretic
Loop and thiazide diuretic administration	$\Uparrow$ K and H^+ secretion in the distal nephron	$\Downarrow$ EABV or excessive ECF volume contraction, K depletion	KCl, improve EABV, reduce diuretic
Adrenogenital syndrome 11β-Hydroxylase deficiency	$\Uparrow$ Deoxycorticosterone	K depletion	Cortisol; KCl
17α-Hydroxylase deficiency	$\Uparrow$ Deoxycorticosterone	K depletion	Cortisol; KCl

EABV, effective arterial blood volume; ECF, extracellular fluid; ICF, intracellular fluid.

therapeutic goal of the diuretic therapy, then free water intake should be restricted. Judging the appropriateness of the ECF volume reduction during diuretic therapy is difficult. In this case, the recent weight gain was considered to be excessive for the caloric intake. The normal blood urea nitrogen (BUN) also argues against excessive ECF volume depletion. The possibility of K depletion should be investigated as well (see answer 3).

2. Free water intake should be restricted if possible. If there is concomitant K deficiency, K supplementation will also increase plasma $[Na^+]$.

3. In part! However, compensation for respiratory acidosis alone would mitigate the acidemia,* but would not result in alkalemia.* Therefore, in addition to metabolic compensation for the respiratory acidosis,* there must be a primary metabolic alkalosis* as well. Table 2-4 summarizes the pathogenesis and treatment of metabolic alkalosis. The root cause in all of these conditions is gain of

base or loss of acid from the ECF space, resulting in the generation of bicarbonate (HCO_3^-). However, in order to maintain a metabolic alkalosis, there must be an increased capacity for HCO_3^- reabsorption in the distal nephron so that the associated increase in filtered HCO_3^- load can be reabsorbed. Neither generation of HCO_3^- nor increase in HCO_3^- reabsorptive capacity alone can generate a metabolic alkalosis. Note that either K depletion or decrease in effective arterial blood volume is nearly always essential for perpetuation of metabolic alkalosis.

In this case, it has been judged that the baby's ECF volume is appropriate. Therefore, the other possibility is that the baby is K depleted. Hypokalemia cannot be excluded on the basis of a heel stick sample, because only a small degree of hemolysis is necessary to significantly raise the plasma $[K^+]$.

The relationship of metabolic alkalosis to hypokalemia and K depletion are complex. Potassium deficiency can cause metabolic alkalosis by increasing renal HCO_3^- reabsorption in the distal tubule. Metabolic alkalosis can cause hypokalemia by increasing renal K secretion in the distal tubule.

*Note that the suffix –*emia* refers to the pH of the blood; the suffix -*osis* refers to the pathologic processes that cause acid-base disturbances.

Therefore, both the compensatory metabolic alkalosis and use of furosemide increase renal K excretion. The reduction in total body potassium then causes a primary metabolic alkalosis that exacerbates the compensatory metabolic alkalosis. Although metabolic alkalosis causes K to shift from the ECF to the ICF space, the magnitude of this effect in adults and experimental animals is small—on the order of a decrease in plasma [K$^+$] of 0.1 to 0.3 mmol/L per 0.1 increase in pH. Aminoglycoside therapy can cause magnesium deficiency by increasing urinary magnesium excretion. Magnesium deficiency may also cause K depletion by increasing renal K excretion.

4. The metabolic alkalosis should be treated because it is indicative of K depletion, which will impair growth. Moreover, if K depletion becomes severe, it can cause life-threatening ventricular ectopy. Therapy should always be directed at the underlying cause, rather than at correcting the metabolic alkalosis (e.g., administering acetazolamide). In this case, KCl supplementation will correct both the K depletion and alkalemia. The plasma magnesium concentration should also be checked because hypokalemia can be refractory to K supplementation when magnesium is deficient.

In the rare situation that metabolic alkalemia itself is life-threatening, exogenous acid (arginine or L-lysine monochloride) may be administered.

The baby was started on 3 mmol/kg/day of oral KCl supplementation and feedings were changed to 145 mL/kg/day of 24 kcal/oz formula. Two days later plasma electrolytes were measured at [Na$^+$] 133 mmol/L, [K$^+$] 4.0 mmol/L, [Cl$^-$] 89 mmol/L, and [HCO$_3{}^-$] 26 mmol/L. KCl supplementation was decreased to 2 mmol/kg/day.

Clinical Summary

Careful attention to fluid and electrolyte balance in newborns requiring an intensive care period is a critical part of their management. It is important to monitor the ability of the critically ill newborn to assume fluid and electrolyte homeostasis as the transition from fetal to neonatal life occurs. Pathologic conditions for which low urine output is a hallmark can be particularly difficult to diagnose in the immediate newborn period when urine output is normally low. In every newborn, but especially those born prematurely, the ability to assume control of fluid and electrolyte homeostasis is seriously limited by increased insensible losses of water through the skin and respiratory tract. Water loss by this route is not under homeostatic control. Moreover, in the first day or two of life the ability of the newborn to excrete excessive water and Na intake is limited by a low GFR. Thus, a reasonably accurate estimation of IWL (taking into account gestational age and the environment in which the infant is cared for) is particularly important in the immediate newborn period. In extremely premature infants, a shift of potassium from the ICF to the ECF space should be anticipated during this period with the possibility of life-threatening hyperkalemia. It is also important to provide dextrose at a rate that meets requirements, so that limited glucose stores can be preserved and hypoglycemia and hyperglycemia can be avoided. Although glucose requirements are similar across gestational ages, fluid requirements are quite variable. Therefore, the glucose concentration ordered will depend upon the amount of fluid administered, so that the targeted dextrose administration rate can be achieved.

After the first one or two days of life, self-limited diuresis and natriuresis occur that are largely independent of water and Na intake and that result in physiologically appropriate postnatal contraction of the ECF space. This contraction of the ECF space should be allowed to occur at a rate that avoids hypernatremia. Failure to allow this physiologic contraction of the ECF space can predispose the premature newborn to patent ductus arteriosus, necrotizing enterocolitis, and bronchopulmonary dysplasia. During this period urinary K secretion is high, usually requiring the initiation of potassium supplementation if hypokalemia is to be avoided. It is important to distinguish physiologic diuresis/natriuresis from the polyuric phase of acute renal failure, because the latter is not self-limited and will result in dehydration and hypokalemia if the attendant water, Na, and K losses are not appropriately replaced.

Finally, with the cessation of diuresis/natriuresis, water and electrolyte excretion begin to vary appropriately with intake, although the premature infant is at risk for hyponatremia secondary to excessive urinary sodium loss as the result of renal immaturity. Fluid intake is now maximized to optimize caloric intake while avoiding fluid retention. Principles of fluid and electrolyte maintenance and management of perturbations in fluid and electrolyte homeostasis during this phase are the same as in older children.

It must be emphasized that appropriate fluid and electrolyte management during the first week of life requires *anticipation* of fluid and electrolyte losses that are likely to occur and the changes in water and electrolyte balance that are appropriate. Consideration of these factors then allows the water, Na, and K requirements to be *estimated*. These requirements are quite variable among infants. Therefore, intakes must be individualized and evaluation of fluid and electrolyte balance that results from these estimated intakes must be periodically reevaluated so that fluid and electrolyte intake can be appropriately adjusted. Parameters useful in evaluating fluid and electrolyte balance include change in body weight, intakes and outputs, and plasma and urine electrolyte and creatinine concentrations.

References

1. Lorenz JM, Kleinman LI, Kotagal UR, et al: Water balance in very low-birth-weight infants: Relationship to water and sodium intake and effect on outcome. J Pediatr 1982;101:423–432.
2. Shaffer SG, Quimiro CL, Anderson JV, et al: Postnatal weight changes in low birth weight infants. Pediatr 1987;79:702–705.
3. Bauer K, Versmold H: Postnatal weight loss in preterm neonates <1500 g is due to isotonic dehydration of the extracellular volume. Acta Paediatr Scand Suppl 1989;360:37–42.
4. Shaffer SG, Meade VM: Sodium balance and extracellular volume regulation in very low birth weight infants. J Pediatr 1989;115:285–290.
5. Shaffer SG, Weismann DN: Fluid requirements in the preterm infant. Clin Perinatol 1992;19:233–250.
6. Heimler R, Doumas BT, Jendrzejczak BM, et al: Relationship between nutrition, weight change, and fluid compartments in preterm infants during the first week of life. J Pediatr 1993;122:110–114.
7. Singhi S, Sood V, Bhakoo ON, et al: Composition of postnatal weight loss and subsequent weight gain in preterm infants. Indian J Med Res 1995;101:157–162.
8. Costarino AT, Gruskay JA, Corcoran L, et al: Sodium restriction versus daily maintenance replacement in very low birth weight premature neonates: A randomized, blind therapeutic trial. J Pediatr 1992;120:99–106.
9. Hartnoll G, Bétrémieux P, Modi N: Randomized controlled trial of postnatal sodium supplementation on body composition in 25–30 week gestational age infants. Arch Dis Child Fetal Neonatal Ed 2000;82:F24–F28.
10. Stevenson JG: Fluid administration in the association of patent ductus arteriosus complicating respiratory distress syndrome. J Pediatr 1977;90:257.
11. Brown ER, Start A, Sosenko I, et al: Bronchopulmonary dysplasia: Possible relationship to pulmonary edema. J Pediatr 1978;92:982.
12. Bell ED, Warburton D, Stonestreet B, et al: Effect of fluid administration on the development of symptomatic patent ductus arteriosus and congestive heart failure in premature infants. N Engl J Med 1980;302:598–604.
13. Spahr RC, Klein AM, Brown DR, et al: Fluid administration and bronchopulmonary dysplasia. Am J Dis Child 1980;134:958.
14. Hartnoll G, Bétrémieux P, Modi N: Randomized controlled trial of postnatal sodium supplementation on oxygen dependency and body weight in 25–30 week gestational age infants. Arch Dis Child Fetal Neonatal Ed 2000;82:F19–F23.
15. Usher R: The respiratory distress syndrome of prematurity. I. Changes in potassium in the serum and the electrocardiogram and effects of therapy. Pediatrics 1959;24:562–576.
16. Sato K, Kondo T, Iwao H, et al: Internal potassium shift in premature infants: Cause of nonoliguric hyperkalemia. J Pediatr 1995;126:109–113.
17. Lorenz JM, Kleinman LI, Markarian K: Potassium metabolism in extremely low birth weight infants in the first week of life. J Pediatr 1997;131:81–86.
18. Gruskay J, Costarino AT, Polin RA, et al: Nonoliguric hyperkalemia in the premature infant weighing less than 1000 grams. J Pediatr 1988;113:381–386.
19. Fukada Y, Kojima T, Ono A, et al: Factors causing hyperkalemia in premature infants. Am J Perinatol 1989;6:76–79.
20. Sato K, Kondo T, Iwao H, et al: Sodium and potassium in red blood cells of premature infants during the first few days: risk of hyperkalemia. Acta Paediatr Scand 1991;80:899–904.
21. Shaffer SG, Kilbride HW, Hayes LK, et al: Hyperkalemia in very low birth weight infants. J Pediatr 1992;121:275–279.
22. Stefano JL, Norman ME, Morales MC, et al: Decreased erythrocyte Na^+-K^+-ATPase activity associated with cellular potassium loss in extremely low birth weight infants with nonoliguric hyperkalemia. J Pediatr 1993;122:276–284.
23. Stefano JL, Norman ME: Nitrogen balance in extremely low birth weight infants with nonoliguric hyperkalemia. J Pediatr 1993;123:632–635.
24. Srinivasan G, Pildes RS, Cattamanchi G, et al: Plasma glucose values in normal neonates: A new look. J Pediatr 1984;105:114–119.
25. Heck LJ, Erenberg A: Serum glucose values during the first 48 hours of life. J Pediatr 1987;110:119–122.
26. Ogata ES: Carbohydrate metabolism in the fetus and neonate and altered neonatal glucoregulation. Pediatr Clin North Am 1986;33:25–45.
27. Bier DM, Leake RD, Haymond MW, et al: Measurement of true glucose production rates in infancy and childhood with 6,6-dideuteroglucose. Diabetes 1977;26:1016–1023.
28. Sunehag A, Ewald U, Larsson A, et al: Glucose production rate in extremely immature neonates (<28 weeks) studied with use of deuterated glucose. Pediatr Res 1993;33:97–100.
29. Tyrala EE, Chen X, Boden G: Glucose metabolism in the infant weighing less than 1100 grams. J Pediatr 1994;125:283–287.

30. Louik C, Mitchell AA, Epstein MF: Risk factors for neonatal hyperglycemia associated with 10% dextrose infusion. Am J Dis Child 1985;139:783–786.

31. Grasso S, Messina A, Distefano G: Insulin secretion in the premature infant: response to glucose and amino acids. Diabetes 1973;22:349–353.

32. Costarino AT, Baumgart S, Norman ME, et al: Renal adaptation to extrauterine life in patients with respiratory distress syndrome. Am J Dis Child 1985;139:1060–1063.

33. Bidiwala KS, Lorenz JM, Kleinman LI: Renal function correlates of postnatal diuresis in preterm infants. Pediatrics 1988;82:50–58.

34. Lorenz JM, Kleinman LI, Ahmed G, et al: Phases of fluid and electrolyte homeostasis in the extremely low birth weight infant. Pediatrics 1995;96:484–489.

35. Hammarlund K, Sedin G, Stromberg B: Transepidermal water loss in newborn infants VIII. Relation to gestational age and post-natal age in appropriate and small for gestational age infants. Acta Paediatr Scand 1983;72:721–728.

36. Riesenfeld T, Hammarlund K, Sedin G: Respiratory water loss in relation to gestational age in infants on their first day after birth. Acta Paediatr Scand 1995;84:1056–1059.

37. Hammarlund K, Nilsson GE, Oberg PA, et al: Transepidermal water loss in newborn infants. Relation to ambient humidity and site of measurement and estimation of total transepidermal water loss. Acta Paediatr Scand 1977;66:553–562.

38. Murphy DJ, Hope PL, Johnson A: Neonatal risk factors for cerebral palsy in very preterm babies: A case-control study. Br Med J 1997;314:404–408.

39. Ertl T, Hadzeiv K, Vincze O, et al: Hyponatremia and sensorineural hearing loss in preterm infants. Biol Neonate 2001;79:109.

40. Sterns RH, Riggs JE, Schochet SS Jr: Osmotic demyelination syndrome following correction of hyponatremia. N Engl J Med 1986;314:1535–1542.

41. Brown DR, Fenton LJ, Tsang RC: Blood sampling through umbilical catheters. Pediatrics 1975;55:257–260.

42. Pitkin RM, Reynolds WA: Creatinine exchange between mother, fetus and amniotic fluid. Am J Physiol 1975;228:231–235.

43. Choker G, Gouyon JB: Diagnosis of acute renal failure in very preterm infants. Biol Neonate 2004;86:212–216.

44. Bueva A, Guignard JP: Renal function in pre-term neonates. Pediatr Res 1994;36:572–577.

45. Tulassay T, Seri I, Machay T, et al: Effects of dopamine on renal function in premature infants with respiratory distress syndrome. Int J Pediatr Nephrol 1983;4:19–23.

46. Lee DA, Slagle TA, Jackson TM, et al: Reducing blood donor exposure in low birth weight infants by the use of older, unwashed packed red blood cells. J Pediatr 1995;126:280–286.

47. Malone TA: Glucose and insulin versus cation-exchange resin for the treatment of hyperkalemia in very low birth weight infants. J Pediatr 1991;118:121–123.

48. Hu PS, Su BH, Peng CT, et al: Glucose and insulin infusion versus kayexalate for early treatment of non-oliguric hyperkalemia in very-low-birth-weight infants. Acta Paediatr Taiwan 1999;40:314–318.

49. Singh DS, Sadiq HF, Noguchi A, et al: Efficacy of albuterol inhalation in treatment of hyperkalemia in premature infants. J Pediatr 2002;141:16–20.

50. Ohlsson A, Hosking M: Complications following oral administration of exchange resins in extremely low-birth-weight infants. Eur J Pediatr 1987;146:571–574.

51. Bennet LN, Myers TF, Lambert GH: Cecal perforation associated with sodium polystyrene sulfonate-sorbitol enemas in a 650 gram infant with hyperkalemia. Am J Perinatol 1996;13:167–170.

52. Grammatikopoulos T, Greenough A, Pallidis C, et al: Benefits and risks of calcium resonium therapy in hyperkalaemic preterm infants. Acta Paediatr 2003;92:118–127.

53. Spital A: Diuretic-induced hyponatremia. Am J Nephrol 1999;19:447.

Disorders of Calcium, Phosphorus, and Magnesium in the Newborn Period

Frank R. Greer, MD

The skeleton is the major reservoir for calcium, phosphorus, and magnesium in newborn infants as well as in adults. It is estimated that the skeleton contains 99% of total body calcium, 80% to 85% of total body phosphorus, and 60% to 65% of total body magnesium. Circulating calcium, phosphorus, and magnesium account for less than 1% of total body stores of each mineral. Relatively large amounts of phosphorus and magnesium are contained in soft tissue. During human fetal life, most of these mineral stores (up to 80%) are accumulated during the last trimester of pregnancy.

Calcium (Ca) circulates in blood in three different fractions: bound to albumin (45%); complexed with bicarbonate, phosphate, or citrate (5%); and ionized (50%). The ionized fraction is the only one that is physiologically active. As a general rule, the serum concentration of calcium in newborns, as in older children and adults, is under tight control with an elaborate mechanism of homeostasis. Phosphorus (P) is very important in calcium homeostasis, as it is required for calcium deposition in bone; however, few direct homeostatic regulatory mechanisms are recognized for phosphorus. As for magnesium (Mg), one third is protein bound, and two thirds is free and ionized in the circulation. Serum magnesium concentrations are kept within a narrow range, but unlike calcium, there is no known homeostatic system.[1,2]

Calcium homeostasis is regulated by serum 1,25-dihydroxyvitamin D [1,25(OH)$_2$D] produced in the renal tubular cells (Fig. 3-1). This hormone controls the transcellular absorption of Ca and P from the intestine. The concentration of circulating Ca controls the secretion of parathyroid hormone (PTH), which in turn can promote the synthesis of 1,25(OH)$_2$D by the renal tubular cells when more Ca is needed. There is also a negative feedback of 1,25(OH)$_2$D on the parathyroid cells to decrease the synthesis of PTH. It is now well known that the effects of 1,25(OH)$_2$D on the cell nucleus are mediated by specific vitamin D receptors, similar in structure to steroid receptors. 1,25(OH)$_2$D circulates in the plasma attached to a vitamin D binding protein. Once inside the cell, 1,25(OH)$_2$D binds to the vitamin D receptor (VDR), activating the receptor to translocate from the cytosol to the nucleus, where it heterodimerizes with its partner the retinoid X receptor (RXR). The VDR/RXR complex then binds specific sequences in the promoter region of the vitamin D responsive genes in the nucleus, and either increases or suppresses the rate of gene transcription by RNA polymerase. In the case of intestinal cells, 1,25(OH)$_2$D increases the rate of gene transcription to promote the synthesis of Ca binding protein. In the case of parathyroid cells, 1,25(OH)$_2$D results in transcriptional repression of the PTH gene.[3] In passing, it is now known that vitamin D acts through the VDRs in many cell types, and has many more actions than Ca regulation. These actions include widespread effects on cellular differentiation and proliferation, and modulation of immune responsiveness and central nervous system function.[4]

A variety of perinatal factors can cause disturbances of homeostasis of these three minerals in the newborn period. Because serum mineral concentrations represent only a minute portion of the total mineral pool, significant variations in total body mineral content may

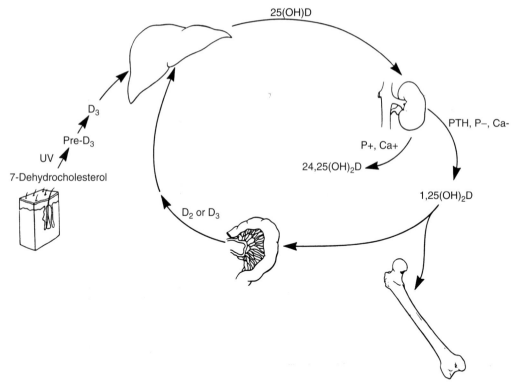

Figure 3-1 Vitamin D_3, which is normally produced in the skin, is converted to 25(OH)D (25-hydroxyvitamin D) in the liver; 25-hydroxyvitamin D is further converted to 1,25(OH)$_2$D (1,25-dihydroxyvitamin D) in the kidney. This conversion is stimulated by hypocalcemia (Ca−), hypophosphatemia (P−), and parathyroid hormone (PTH); 1,25-dihydroxyvitamin D then stimulates intestinal calcium and phosphate absorption and mobilization of calcium from bone.

occur with little or no alteration in serum concentration; not uncommonly, even abnormal serum concentrations may not produce any obvious clinical symptoms. The purpose of this chapter is to review mineral homeostasis and the disturbances that may arise during fetal and neonatal life, using clinical cases to illustrate major points.

Hypocalcemia in Newborns

Case Study 1

A 1000-g male infant was born at 28 weeks' gestation to a 21-year-old primigravida by spontaneous vaginal delivery after a week of magnesium sulfate therapy and 7 days after a 48-hour course of maternal betamethasone therapy. The infant had minimal respiratory distress but was placed on nasal continuous positive airway pressure (CPAP) at 2 hours of age when the F_{IO_2} exceeded 30%. An umbilical venous
catheter was placed at this time after unsuccessful attempts to place an umbilical arterial catheter. An x-ray of the chest and abdomen was consistent with mild respiratory distress syndrome and revealed that the umbilical catheter was in the liver (subsequently pulled back to the 4-cm mark). The infant was started on 110 mL/kg/day of 5% dextrose and 25% normal saline. Urine output was 60 mL during the first 24 hours of life. Serum electrolytes at 24 hours of age revealed sodium at 135 mg/dL, potassium at 4.5 mg/dL, and calcium at 7.2 mg/dL. By 36 hours of age, the serum calcium was 6.5 mg/dL. No seizures, jitteriness, or cardiac arrhythmias were noted.

Exercise 1

QUESTIONS

Which of the following statements are true or false?

1. The cause of hypocalcemia in this infant is "early hypocalcemia of prematurity."

2. There is a direct correlation between gestational age and fall in serum calcium after birth.

3. Any decline in serum calcium after birth in term or preterm neonates is not physiologic.

ANSWERS

1. True

2. True

3. False

This infant has early hypocalcemia of prematurity (EHP). Even in term infants, there is a physiologic decline in serum calcium during the first 48 hours of life (Fig. 3-2). Approximately 3% of healthy term neonates have calcium levels less than 8 mg/dL at 24 hours of age. However, in preterm infants, this decline is exaggerated, and there is a direct correlation between serum calcium and gestational age: the lower the gestational age, the greater the decline in serum calcium. From 30% to 57% of premature infants exhibit EHP,[5,6] which by definition is a serum calcium level below 7 mg/dL (1.75 mmol/dL). Gestational age is more important than actual birth weight with respect to the development of EHP. Suggested causes of EHP include decreased calcium intake,[7] hypomagnesemia,[8] increased urinary losses,[6] hyperphosphatemia,[6] vitamin D deficiency,[9] abnormalities in vitamin D metabolism,[9–12] elevated serum calcitonin,[13] alkali therapy, functional hypoparathyroidism,[6,8,14] and end-organ unresponsiveness to PTH.[6,8–12,14–16]

There are several ways to treat this infant, as typified by the responses of three pediatric residents.

Resident A. No changes were made in the intravenous (IV) fluids; however, the rate was increased to 120 mL/kg at 48 hours of age, and potassium chloride was added. Serum sodium was 136 mg/dL, potassium 3.5 mg/dL, and calcium 6 mg/dL at this time. At 72 hours, the infant was begun on total parenteral nutrition (TPN) through a peripheral line containing 2 mEq/kg/day of calcium gluconate. On day 7, the infant was begun on small enteral feedings of human milk. Serum calcium slowly increased to 7.7 mg/dL by the eighth day of life.

Resident B. This resident took a different approach to the treatment of hypocalcemia of prematurity. When the serum calcium decreased to 6.5 mg/dL at 36 hours, 200 mg/kg/day of calcium gluconate was added to the umbilical venous fluids. By 48 hours, serum calcium was 6.8 mg/dL. At 72 hours, the infant was started on peripheral TPN (containing the same amount of calcium as described by resident A), and calcium was removed from the umbilical venous catheter by 96 hours. Enteral feedings of breast milk were begun on day 7, and the infant's serum calcium on day 8 had increased to 7.9 mg/dL.

Resident C. When the serum calcium at 48 hours was 6 mg/dL, a 0.5-mg dose of calcitriol (1,25-dihydroxyvitamin D_3) was given IV for 5 days. TPN and breast milk feedings were begun

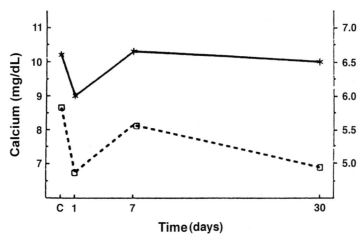

Figure 3-2 Serum total (*solid line*) and ionized (*dotted line*) calcium concentrations in term infants measured in cord blood (C) or venous blood during the first month of life. (From Loughead JL, Tsang RC: Neonatal mineral metabolism. In Cowett RM [ed]: Principles of Perinatal-Neonatal Metabolism, 2nd ed. New York, Springer-Verlag, 1998, p. 882. With kind permission of Springer Science and Business Media.)

as in the treatment plans of residents A and B. Serum calcium on day 8 was 7.8 mg/dL.

QUESTION

4. Which of the residents' treatment plans is correct?

ANSWER

4. Resident B's treatment plan is correct. However, if you answered resident A you are not too far off the mark (see following discussion).

Note that the infant had almost the same serum calcium concentration on the eighth day of life regardless of the treatment plan used. Resident A had done lots of reading and was aware of the following regarding EHP: (1) It is asymptomatic most of the time; (2) in nearly all cases, it resolves spontaneously over time; (3) long-term follow-up studies have never shown any benefit of treating EHP; (4) total serum calcium is a poor predictor of ionized serum calcium in this population; and (5) IV calcium therapy involves complications that must be considered.

Resident B knows that despite the frequency of the problem, there are relatively few studies regarding EHP management. Furthermore, this resident hypothesized that low serum calcium would have an adverse effect on the premature infant, because calcium is essential for the functioning of all living cells, including providing potential benefits for both the cardiac and the central nervous systems. However, the efficacy of calcium therapy in asymptomatic premature infants remains to be demonstrated. Recommended doses of calcium replacement have ranged from 24 to 75 mg/kg/day. It is also very difficult to determine the exact morbidity and mortality rates from hypocalcemia because of other complicating clinical variables that usually occur in infants with the lowest serum calcium levels (e.g., severe respiratory disease, birth asphyxia, hypotension, metabolic acidosis). Calcium therapy for EHP does not take into consideration the premature infant's own physiologic response to hypocalcemia. Thus, replacement therapy may block the normal physiologic adaptation. It has been shown that an increase in PTH concentration on the first day of life can be blunted in premature infants who receive an IV infusion of 18 to 70 mg/kg/day of elemental calcium.[17,18] There are also a number of reports on the hazards of calcium therapy in newborns. Oral calcium supplements have been associated with an increased incidence of necrotizing enterocolitis[19] and increased stool frequency.[7] Parenteral infusions of calcium have produced intestinal necrosis in animals,[20] as well as inflammation and necrosis following infiltration of calcium into the skin. Calcifications have been reported in the liver following bolus therapy when the umbilical catheter is in or below the liver, as in the case described. Thus, the umbilical venous catheter in this infant is not an option for TPN therapy.

There is no good evidence to support the vitamin D therapy chosen by resident C. Numerous investigators have attempted to treat or prevent early hypocalcemia with supplements of vitamin D or its metabolites. Very few studies, however, used parenteral vitamin D therapy in premature infants receiving oral calcium. In one study of 19 low-birth-weight infants (<1500 g) born at or before 32 weeks' gestation, hypocalcemia did not respond to large pharmacologic doses of 1,25-dihydroxyvitamin D (0.05 to 3 mg/kg) given intramuscularly on three occasions between 6 and 60 hours after birth.[21] In these infants, no changes in PTH serum concentrations were observed during the therapy. Oral doses of vitamin D (parent compound), 25-hydroxyvitamin D, 1α-hydroxyvitamin D, and 1,25-dihydroxyvitamin D have also been used with mixed results in EHP, both with and without oral feedings containing calcium.[10,22–26] One can reasonably conclude from these studies that in infants receiving no oral intake of calcium, vitamin D therapy is not indicated. This is logical, given that the primary method of action of vitamin D is to increase intestinal absorption of calcium.

In summary, treatment of all symptomatic hypocalcemia (seizures, jitteriness, cardiac arrhythmias) in premature infants is indicated. In light of the present incomplete knowledge base regarding EHP, treatment of preterm infants with serum calcium levels less than 6 mg/dL may be indicated, regardless of symptomatology. In this population, at this level of total serum calcium, most serum ionized calcium values are less than 4.4 mg/dL (<1.10 mmol/L). However, the efficacy of treatment of asymptomatic preterm infants has not been demonstrated.

Case Study 2

A 2460-g, small-for-gestational-age male infant was born at 41 weeks' gestation to a 20-year-old primigravida by cesarean section performed for fetal distress following a Pitocin induction of labor for a post-dates pregnancy. The pregnancy was complicated by intrauterine growth restriction. The delivery was otherwise uncomplicated, though a significant cardiac murmur was noted in the delivery room. Apgar scores were 8 and 10. The infant was taken to the NICU for observation and subsequently developed mild respiratory distress with borderline hypoglycemia (blood sugar levels 30 to 40 mg/dL). A pulse oximeter reading was 85% oxygen saturation.

On physical examination, the axillary temperature was 98.1°F, the pulse was 127/minute, and the respiratory rate was 70/minute. Systolic blood pressure was measured between 60 and 70 mm Hg. On examining the chest, a prominent cardiac point of maximal impulse and a palpable thrill were noted. There was a grade IV/VI continuous, harsh murmur over most of the chest, with a loud second heart sound. Femoral pulses were noted to be decreased but present. There was no abdominal organomegaly. The remainder of the physical examination was unremarkable.

Laboratory studies included a chest x-ray demonstrating diminished pulmonary vasculature and a slightly enlarged heart. The possibility of a right-sided aortic arch was noted. No thymic shadow was noted (Fig. 3-3). A capillary blood gas revealed a pH of 7.36, P_{CO_2} of 47 mm Hg, P_{O_2} of 29 mm Hg, a bicarbonate of 25.0 mmol/L, and a base deficit of −0.1. Serum Na was 132 mmol/L, K 4.5 mmol/L, Cl 103 mmol/L, and total CO_2 26 mmol/L. A total serum Ca was 6.6 mg/dL with an ionized Ca of 1.05 mmol/L (normal 1.15 to 1.40 mmol/L). The hemoglobin concentration was 18.8 g/dL, the hematocrit was 54%, the white blood cell count was 13.1/mm³, and the platelet count was 164,000/mL.

An echocardiogram revealed a truncus arteriosus type I with a moderate truncal valve stenosis. There was a severe, truncal valve regurgitation. A right-sided aortic arch was confirmed.

During the first 2 days of life, the infant's cardiorespiratory status continued to deteriorate. Oral feedings were not well tolerated and the infant was fed by a nasogastric tube. In addition, the infant was started on calcium glubionate, 400 mg every 6 hours, which stabilized the serum calcium in the normal range. At 48 hours of age he was

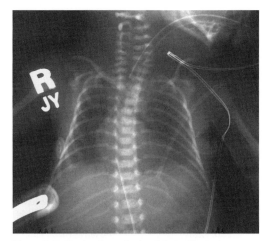

Figure 3-3 Chest radiograph of an infant with classic DiGeorge syndrome with truncus arteriosus and a right sided aortic arch. The pulmonary vasculature is decreased. No thymic shadow is present.

begun on digoxin and furosemide. At the end of the third hospital day, the infant's respiratory status underwent an acute deterioration. A capillary blood gas revealed a pH 6.77, P_{CO_2} 117 mm Hg, P_{O_2} 38 mm Hg, and BE −23.0. The infant was intubated, stabilized on a ventilator, and taken to the operating room for open heart surgery.

Exercise 2

QUESTIONS

1. What was this infant's underlying diagnosis and the etiology of both the hypocalcemia and the congenital heart defect, and what additional laboratory test would confirm the diagnosis?

2. What is the typical course and etiology of the hypocalcemia of DiGeorge syndrome?

3. What is the long-term prognosis for this infant?

4. Which of the following conditions are associated with early hypocalcemia in a term neonate?

   a. Maternal diabetes mellitus

   b. Birth asphyxia

   c. Systemic alkali therapy

   d. Hypomagnesemia

ANSWERS

1. This infant has DiGeorge syndrome, now more correctly known as 22q11 microdeletion syndrome.[27] Historically, DiGeorge syndrome is a congenital disorder in which the defective development of the third and fourth pharyngeal pouches results in hypoplasia or aplasia of the thymus and parathyroid glands, usually associated with congenital heart defects (conotruncal anomalies of the great vessels) and typically, facial anomalies. It is also associated with neonatal hypocalcemia and disorders of cell-mediated immunity.[28] The syndrome of microdeletion of 22q11 now also includes velocardiofacial syndrome (cleft palate, cardiac anomalies, typical facies), which is less commonly associated with hypocalcemia compared to the classic DiGeorge syndrome.[27] The 22q11 microdeletion syndrome has a prevalence between 13 and 26 per 100,000 live births, making it the most frequent contiguous gene deletion syndrome in humans, and second only to trisomy 21 as a chromosomal cause of significant congenital heart disease.[27] This disorder can now be rapidly diagnosed with chromosomal analysis for 22q11 microdeletions using fluorescent in situ hybridization (90% of patients are FISH positive), which confirmed the diagnosis in this infant.[29]

2. DiGeorge syndrome is a cause of transient hypocalcemia of the neonatal period, but can also present as neonatal seizures (and occasionally seizures can occur in older children with the syndrome). About 60% of children with a 22q11 microdeletion have hypocalcemia, usually in the subgroup of infants with classic cases of DiGeorge syndrome. It is thought to be a result of hypoparathyroidism, though the natural history of the hypocalcemia and hypoparathyroidism in these patients is not well described. Hypoparathyroidism has been diagnosed in older children and adults with a 22q11 deletion with minimal or no symptoms of a mild hypocalcemia.

3. There is growing concern about long-term developmental delays and learning disabilities in this population, which should be discussed with the family. Such developmental delays may be related to the complications of the severe cardiac malformations with subsequent operative repair, or related to an effect of the 22q11 deletion itself. Chronic hypoparathyroidism has also been described. Thus, a careful long-term follow-up of these patients is needed.[30]

4. All of the above. Other conditions causing neonatal hypocalcemia include maternal diabetes mellitus[1,2] and birth asphyxia.[31] Miscellaneous disorders also associated with neonatal hypocalcemia include late infantile tetany associated with cow milk formula feeding,[32] acid-base disturbances such as those associated with systemic alkali therapy and hyperventilation (treatment for pulmonary hypertension), exchange transfusions,[33] and hypomagnesemia.[34,35] Acute hypomagnesemia increases PTH secretion, whereas chronic hypomagnesemia suppresses PTH secretion, induces bone resistance to the action of PTH, and is associated with either a decrease in synthesis of or bone resistance to 1,25-dihydroxyvitamin D. Magnesium deficiency leading to early neonatal hypocalcemia has been observed in infants born to diabetic mothers (maternal urinary magnesium wastage causes a fetal deficiency state), intrauterine growth restricted infants, and infants born to preeclamptic mothers. The magnesium deficiency in these infants must be treated before the hypocalcemia corrects with calcium infusion. The normal serum magnesium concentration of a neonate (1.5 to 2.8 mg/dL) is similar to that of an older child and adult.

Hypophosphatemia with Normocalcemia in Premature Infants

Case Study 3

A 3-month-old breastfed infant is brought to the emergency room following a fall from a sofa. The parents note that the infant seems to have a tender right forearm. An x-ray of the wrist is shown in Figure 3-4.

Past medical history reveals that the infant was born at 27 weeks' gestation weighing 970 g. Otherwise, pregnancy, labor, and delivery were unremarkable. There is no family history of rickets

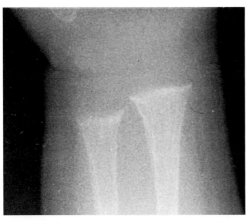

Figure 3-4 X-ray showing osteopenia with cupping and flaring of the distal metaphyses of the ulna and radius in a growing premature infant fed unsupplemented human milk.

or other metabolic bone disease. Mild respiratory distress syndrome developed in the first 24 hours of life requiring head-hood oxygen for the first 10 days. At 1 week, the infant received expressed breast milk with a daily multivitamin supplement that contained 400 IU of vitamin D. Breast milk intake averaged 165 mL/kg/day by 2 weeks of life.

During weeks 4 and 5, a patent ductus arteriosus required treatment with fluid restriction (90 mL/kg/day) and intermittent oral furosemide therapy (2 mg/kg). Milk intake averaged 160 mL/kg/day between weeks 5 and 9 of life, after which time the baby nursed directly from the breast, preventing routine assessment of daily milk intake. At 8 weeks, the serum calcium was 8.8 mg/dL, serum phosphorus was 3.5 mg/dL, and alkaline phosphatase was 475 IU/L. At 10 weeks of age, the infant was discharged on breast milk, and supplemental vitamins were continued.

At the time of presentation in the emergency room, the infant weighs 3500 g, and marked swellings of the costochondral junctions on the chest are noted. Skull bones are described as soft and "thin." A slight swelling of both wrists is noted, although movement of all extremities produces no obvious discomfort. The remainder of the physical examination is unremarkable.

Laboratory studies showed a serum calcium of 10.2 mg/dL, phosphorus 2.6 mg/dL, magnesium 2.1 mg/dL, and alkaline phosphatase 835 IU/L. Subsequently, serum 25-hydroxyvitamin D was 40 ng/mL (normal, 25 to 60 ng/mL), and serum 1,25-dihydroxyvitamin D was 120 pg/mL (normal, 17 to 44 pg/mL). Serum PTH was

30 mEq/mL (normal, 33 to 117 mEq/mL), and urinary calcium was 20 mg/kg/24 hours (normal, up to 4 mg/kg/24 hours).

Exercise 3

QUESTIONS

1. Which of the following statements are true?

   a. The x-ray findings in Figure 3-4 are consistent with the diagnosis of rickets.

   b. Furosemide use in preterm infants may disrupt calcium homeostasis.

   c. Administration of vitamin D to a premature breastfed infant is unnecessary.

   d. Very low birth weight preterm infants require mineral intakes greater than that provided by breast milk alone, even at volumes of 160 mL/kg/day.

2. Which plan should you choose for treatment of this infant, resident A or B?

Resident A

This resident started daily oral supplements of calcium glubionate and potassium phosphate, supplying 60 mg of elemental calcium and 30 mg of elemental phosphorus per kilogram of body weight. These supplements plus 400 IU vitamin D were continued for 4 months (until 7 months of age). Two weeks after initiating therapy, the serum phosphate had increased to 5.3 mg/dL. By 7 months of age, x-rays demonstrated a complete resolution of the rachitic findings. Serum 1,25-dihydroxyvitamin D had decreased to 90 pg/mL, and alkaline phosphatase to 210 IU/L.

Resident B

This resident, responding to the laboratory evidence of severe hypophosphatemia with "normocalcemia," began a supplement of 50 mg of elemental phosphorus per kilogram of body weight per day. Within 24 hours, the infant had a grand mal seizure. A workup at this time revealed a serum calcium of 4.3 mg/dL and a serum phosphorus of 7.4 mg/dL.

3. Given that the mother elected to continue breastfeeding, which of the residents'

treatment plans is correct? Why did the infant treated by resident B develop seizures?

4. Can a similar clinical picture occur in infants maintained exclusively on TPN?

ANSWERS

1. a, b, and c are true. This infant has the form of clinical rickets observed in very low birth weight infants exclusively fed breast milk without mineral supplementation. In most cases, this problem occurs after 6 to 8 weeks of life with severe hypophosphatemia and hypercalciuria that is far more dramatic on x-ray than the "relative hypercalcemia" observed biochemically.[36–40] As in this case, these infants usually have normal 25-hydroxyvitamin D and very high concentrations of 1,25-dihydroxyvitamin D. The low mineral intake and hypophosphatemia are stimuli for 1,25-dihydroxyvitamin D synthesis with increased intestinal absorption of calcium. Hypercalcemia and hypercalciuria presumably occur because the very low intake of phosphorus severely limits deposition of calcium in bone. PTH is also suppressed in these infants by the normal or elevated serum calcium concentrations. Even at 8 weeks of age, this infant's serum phosphorus level of 3.5 mg/dL was an indication that this clinical condition was developing.

2. Resident A's treatment plan is correct.

3. Resident A's treatment plan is correct. With the treatment plan of resident B, the phosphorus supplement, combined with the underlying calcium deficiency, resulted in a rapid deposition of calcium and phosphorus into the skeleton, causing the development of severe hypocalcemia and the seizure. After IV bolus therapy with 10% calcium gluconate (2 mL/kg), the infant was begun on a treatment plan similar to that of resident A.

4. Yes, this is certainly possible. In these cases, the cause of the severe hypophosphatemia is iatrogenic, as when phosphate is inadvertently deleted from or decreased in TPN solutions.[41] This may occur when potassium phosphate salts are replaced with potassium acetate to treat metabolic acidosis. These infants may develop severe hypercalcemia combined with severe hypophosphatemia and become critically ill.

Metabolic Bone Disease in Premature Infants

Case Study 4

A 600-g male infant was born at 25 weeks' gestation, the second of twins. The hospital course was complicated by severe respiratory distress syndrome, which progressed to chronic lung disease despite prenatal steroids and surfactant therapy. The infant required supplemental oxygen therapy until 91 days of age. Nutritional status was a major concern throughout his hospitalization, with pulmonary fluid retention and episodes of congestive heart failure requiring repeated restrictions of fluids and modification of dietary intake. Infant nutrition included TPN, which provided 200 IU vitamin D per day for most of the first month of life. At 1 month of age, enteral feedings via a nasogastric tube were begun with a standard infant formula (20 kcal/oz). Full enteral feedings (120 kcal/kg/day) were achieved by the sixth week of life, and TPN was discontinued. However, because of poor growth, feedings were changed to a 24 kcal/oz formula for preterm infants (Ca = 133 mg/dL, P = 70 mg/dL, vitamin D = 218 IU/dL) by the seventh week of life, and medium chain triglycerides (1 mL) were added to each feeding to maximize calories but keep fluid intake at a minimum. In addition, alternate day furosemide was instituted as treatment for chronic lung disease. A routine chest x-ray obtained during the eighth week of life can be seen in Figure 3-5.

Exercise 4

QUESTIONS

1. What factors contributed to the multiple healing rib fractures seen in this x-ray? Choose all that apply:

   a. Prematurity

   b. Diuretic therapy

   c. Inadequate calcium and phosphorus intake

   d. Inadequate vitamin D intake

   e. Chest physiotherapy

2. How could you have prevented the severe degree of osteopenia in this infant?

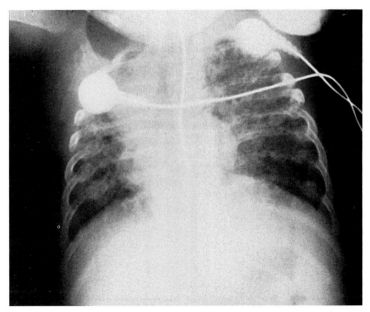

Figure 3-5 X-ray showing osteopenia and multiple healing rib fractures in a growing premature infant with severe bronchopulmonary dysplasia.

ANSWERS

1. a, b, c, and e. This infant has severe osteopenia with subsequent bone fractures related to poor nutritional status and the chest physical therapy administered by caretakers. The diagnosis is osteopenia of prematurity, commonly referred to as rickets of prematurity.[42] This condition refers to a hypomineralized skeleton that occurs almost exclusively in growing very low birth weight infants (birth weight < 1000 g). The high incidence of this disorder in preterm infants is not surprising, considering that 80% of fetal skeletal mineralization takes place during the last trimester of pregnancy. The cause of this disorder is multifactorial, however, and is summarized in Figure 3-6. The primary deficiency is of calcium and phosphorus, not vitamin D. The diuretic therapy used to ameliorate the symptoms of the chronic lung disease in this infant also contributed to diminished mineral retention by increasing urinary calcium and phosphate losses. In general, the severity of osteopenia in premature infants increases with decreasing gestational age.

2. Calcium and phosphorus intake should have been optimized throughout the infant's hospital course by maximizing calcium and phosphorus intake in hyperalimentation solutions, using infant formulas designed for premature infants (containing increased amounts of vitamins and minerals) or adding commercially available human milk fortifiers to breast milk to improve calcium, phosphorus, and vitamin D intake.

   In TPN solutions, it is unlikely that enough calcium and phosphorus can be infused parenterally to achieve the in utero rate of calcium and phosphorus accretion, which is up to 150 and 85 mg/kg/day, respectively.[1] Solutions containing 60 mg/dL (15 mmol) of calcium and 46.5 mg/dL (15 mmol) of phosphorus will maintain the desired biochemical and calcitropic hormone indices of mineral homeostasis.[43–47] Overt fractures and rickets can also be prevented by using one of the commercially available formulas especially designed for premature infants with much higher concentrations of calcium, phosphorus, and vitamin D compared to standard formulas. In breastfed preterm infants, commercial supplements containing calcium, phosphorus, and vitamin D should be used to increase mineral intake.

   At 8 weeks of age, because of persistent lung disease and inability to wean from mechanical ventilation, furosemide intake was increased to once a day, and 0.25 mg of dexamethasone was started every 12 hours. By age 12 weeks he developed

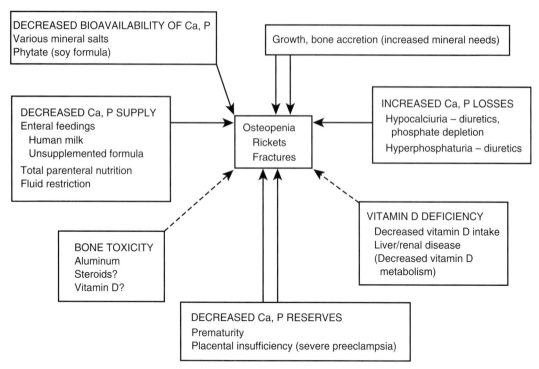

Figure 3-6 Schematic diagram of the etiology of osteopenia (rickets) of prematurity. Dotted lines show factors of less importance in most preterm infants.

hypertension, presumably due to the steroid therapy, and was treated with hydralazine. At 20 weeks of age, nursing reported 1+ hematuria, and a workup revealed moderately severe nephrocalcinosis by renal ultrasonography. The infant's weight was now 2500 g and he was still on the special formula for low-birth-weight infants at a rate of 150 mL/kg/day.

QUESTIONS

3. Which of the following are the most likely causes of this infant's nephrocalcinosis with hematuria?

    a. Diuretic therapy

    b. Steroid therapy

    c. Excessive nutritional intake of calcium

    d. Excessive vitamin D supplementation

4. Which laboratory tests of mineral homeostasis might be expected to be abnormal in this patient at this time?

    a. Calcium

    b. Magnesium

    c. Phosphorus

    d. 1,25-Dihydroxyvitamin D

    e. 25(OH) vitamin D

5. What would be the appropriate treatment for the nephrocalcinosis?

ANSWERS

3. a, c, and d. The nephrocalcinosis was most likely caused by the daily furosemide therapy (increasing urinary calcium excretion), in combination with high intakes of calcium and vitamin D in the preterm formula. The calcium and vitamin D intakes at this time were 200 mg/kg/day and 817 IU/day, respectively. Normal intakes at 46 weeks' postmenstrual age should be closer to 100 mg/kg/day of Ca and 200 to 400 IU/day of vitamin D.

4. a and e. Laboratory test results were as follows: serum calcium 11.0 mg/dL, phosphorus 3.5 mg/dL, alkaline phosphatase 350 IU/mL, 1,25-dihydroxyvitamin D 20 pg/mL (normal, 15 to 60 pg/mL), and 25(OH) vitamin D 140 ng/mL (normal, 14 to 42 ng/mL). The elevated levels of 25(OH) vitamin D reflect the increased vitamin D intake, and the elevated serum Ca reflects both the increased Ca intake and decreased renal excretion of Ca despite diuretic therapy,

secondary to the nephrocalcinosis (the serum creatinine has increased to 1.7 mg/dL).

5. The prudent treatment would be to stop the preterm infant formula immediately and place the infant on a standard formula. The furosemide should also be stopped if at all possible. Months of decreased calcium intake will be necessary for the nephrocalcinosis to resolve radiographically.

Hypercalcemia in Newborns

Case Study 5

A 2600-g male infant, born at term, presented to the physician's office with feeding difficulty (spitting) and irritability at 12 days of age. The infant was being exclusively breastfed with no vitamin supplements. A physical examination revealed normal vital signs. The infant was thought to be slightly "funny looking," with a long philtrum and mild mandibular hypoplasia. A grade II-III/VI short systolic murmur was heard along the left sternal border (LSB) and radiated widely. The remainder of the physical examination was normal except for irritability.

The physician ordered a complete blood count (CBC) and a metabolic panel. The CBC and electrolytes were normal. However, a serum Ca was 12.7 mg/dL with a serum phosphorus of 3.5 mg/dL.

Exercise 5

QUESTIONS

1. What is the differential diagnosis of the cause of hypercalcemia in this infant?

2. How would you distinguish between the various causes of hypercalcemia in this infant? What laboratory tests might you order?

ANSWERS

1. Compared to hypocalcemia, hypercalcemia in the newborn infant is uncommon. Thus, the differential diagnosis would be difficult for the average resident but would include

subcutaneous fat necrosis, Williams-Beuren syndrome, maternal hypoparathyroidism, congenital hyperparathyroidism, and vitamin D intoxication.

2. Subcutaneous fat necrosis can largely be eliminated by a careful physical examination. Though the timing is right, 1 to 2 weeks after birth, a lack of the characteristic erythematous indurated skin rash (sometimes with a bluish discoloration), typical of the subcutaneous calcifications, eliminates the diagnosis.[48–51] In addition, the hypercalcemia is usually more severe and can be life-threatening at times (serum Ca up to 22 mg/dL). The pathogenesis of this disorder is unknown. Both elevated and normal concentrations of $1,25(OH)_2D$ have been reported in infants with this disorder.[52–55]

Williams-Beuren syndrome is characterized by hypercalcemia, elfin facies, mental retardation, and supravalvular aortic stenosis. The facies have been described as a prominent upper lip and philtrum, underdeveloped mandible, depressed nasal bridge, hypertelorism, epicanthic folds, and low-set ears. Interestingly, the phenotypic facies become more evident beyond the infancy period.[56] A cardiac ultrasound will diagnose the typical cardiac lesions. Only about 15% of the patients diagnosed with this disorder (usually after the newborn period) have documented hypercalcemia in infancy, which typically is mild and resolves over time with minimal treatment. These infants demonstrated increased calcium absorption, hypercalciuria, and nephrocalcinosis; an excess of circulating vitamin D has been suggested as a cause, though this finding has not been consistently documented in these patients.[57] It is now known that this syndrome is the result of a hemizygous submicroscopic deletion of 7q11.2. More than 20 genes, most without well-defined functions, are found in this region of chromosome 7. The gene encoding the extracellular matrix protein elastin is found here and elastin deficiency likely accounts for the vascular and connective tissue abnormalities (facies) observed.[58] Subjects found to have very small deletions of the elastin gene do not have typical facial features, hypercalcemia, or mental retardation. None of the genes in this area have been identified as having a role in calcium metabolism to date. The diagnosis of this syndrome can now be confirmed in 90% of patients with fluorescent in situ hybridization (FISH) of this chromosomal region.

In this infant, a cardiac ultrasound revealed a moderate sized muscular ventricular septal defect, which made the diagnosis of Williams-Beuren syndrome less likely. This was confirmed by a negative FISH study for 7q11.2.

Another cause of hypercalcemia in the newborn is poorly controlled maternal hypoparathyroidism with subsequent maternal hypocalcemia. As maternal hypocalcemia stimulates hypercalcemia in the fetus and the newborn, a medical workup of the infant should reveal osteoporosis from subperiosteal bone resorption, possible pathologic fractures, and elevated PTH levels accompanying the hypercalcemia. A spontaneous case of primary infantile hyperparathyroidism might also produce the same findings, though these cases are very rare.[59] In this infant, a radiologic skeletal survey revealed no abnormalities and a serum PTH was very low (2.5 ng/mL, normal range 10 to 65 ng/mL), thus ruling out the diagnoses of maternal hypoparathyroidism and primary infantile hyperparathyroidism.

From the initial differential diagnosis, we are left only with the diagnosis of vitamin D intoxication, which could also explain the infant's hypercalcemia with a very low serum PTH level. At first glance this does not seem to be a very likely diagnosis. However, a more careful history revealed that the mother had a long history of multiple endocrine adenomatosis. Maternal treatment of this disorder included a total thyroid-parathyroidectomy and a bilateral adrenalectomy many years before the pregnancy. Given this history, one might still suspect that maternal hypoparathyroidism was the cause of the infant's hypercalcemia, but the infant's PTH was normal, as noted above, and the mother's serum Ca and P were 8.5 mg/dL and 4.1 mg/dL, respectively. The maternal medications taken during the pregnancy included 1 g elemental Ca plus 100,000 IU vitamin D per day, and fludrocortisone acetate, thyroxine, and prednisone. After the delivery, all the maternal medications were continued, including the very large intake of vitamin D. The mother had elected to exclusively breastfeed her infant.

The most likely cause of hypercalcemia in this infant was the exposure to large amounts of vitamin D throughout pregnancy and during feedings of human milk. Vitamin D (parent compound)

and 25(OH) vitamin D both cross the placenta and are excreted readily into human milk. Cord blood was available and a 25(OH)D level was 250 ng/mL. The mother's serum 25(OH)D at the time of the infant's presentation was 545 ng/mL. A sample of breast milk was analyzed for vitamin D, revealing a concentration of 8000 IU/L. Assuming an intake of 700 mL of breast milk a day, this would give the infant an intake of 5600 IU vitamin D a day in addition to what crossed the placenta.

Exercise 5 *Continued*

QUESTION

3. How should this infant be treated?

ANSWER

3. In this case, the mother elected to discontinue breastfeeding and the infant was placed on a standard infant formula. Serum calcium returned to a normal level within 2 weeks and the infant's irritability resolved.

If the infant's hypercalcemia had been more symptomatic, he could have been treated with twice maintenance IV fluids, furosemide (1 mg/kg every 6 hours) to promote calcium diuresis, and IV hydrocortisone (1 mg/kg every 6 hours) until the symptoms resolved.

Congenital Rickets and Hypercalcemia

Case Study 6

A 4337-g female infant, born at 40 weeks' gestation, was admitted for respiratory distress shortly after birth. The mother was a 21-year-old primigravida with a reportedly normal pregnancy, labor, and delivery. Because of the respiratory distress, a chest x-ray was obtained, which revealed lung fields consistent with transient tachypnea of the newborn. However, the chest x-ray (which fortuitously included the left arm) also revealed a metabolic bone disease consistent with congenital rickets—cupping and flaring of the metaphyses of the long bones and marked periosteal reactions.

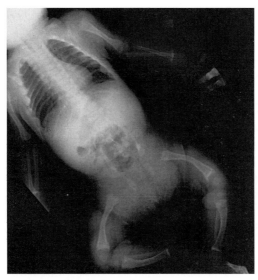

Figure 3-7 X-ray showing cupping and flaring of the distal metaphyses of the long bones in a newborn infant with asymptomatic hypercalcemia (early manifestations of Jansen's disease). Pseudofractures of the femurs are also noted.

There were also "pseudofractures" of the femurs on a subsequent skeletal survey (Fig. 3-7). The serum calcium was 10.6 mg/dL, phosphorus 5.3 mg/dL, alkaline phosphatase 209 IU/L, and PTH 0.8 pmol/L (well within normal limits). Serum calcium was normal in both parents. Diagnoses entertained included congenital I-cell disease, osteogenesis imperfecta, and hyperparathyroidism. These were ruled out with additional studies.

As the child was asymptomatic, she was discharged after 5 days of hospitalization, with instructions for her family physician to repeat the serum calcium and phosphorus in 2 weeks. When this was done, the serum calcium was up to 13.6 mg/dL, and the serum phosphorus was 4.3 mg/dL. PTH was rechecked, and it was still normal. The infant was placed on PM60/40, a low-calcium and low-phosphorus formula.

At 1 month of age, the child remained asymptomatic but was readmitted to the hospital for additional workup. The serum calcium at this time was 12.3 mg/dL, and phosphorus was 4.1 mg/dL. Alkaline phosphatase was now up to 447 IU/L. A 24-hour urine sample for calcium and phosphorus was collected. The urinary calcium was elevated at 35 mg/24 hours. Urinary phosphorus output was 30 mg/24 hours. The serum 1,25-dihydroxyvitamin D level was 47.3 pg/mL (normal range, 40 to 60 pg/mL), despite the hypercalcemia. The 25-hydroxyvitamin D was 17.5 ng/mL (normal range, 15 to 40 ng/mL). Chromosomes were within normal limits. Diagnoses considered during this admission *were congenital hypophosphatasia or pseudohypophosphatasia, as well as an abnormality in circulating parathyroid hormone–related peptide (PTH-rp).*

Over the next month, a large battery of tests (including osteocalcin, procollagen, urinary prostaglandins, urinary phosphoethanolamine, pyridoxal-5 phosphate, and PTH-rp [unmeasurable]) failed to yield a definitive diagnosis. During this period, the serum calcium remained elevated, and the infant remained asymptomatic. Serum PTH and vitamin D metabolites remained normal.

Exercise 6

QUESTION

1. What is this infant's diagnosis?

ANSWER

1. This infant has Jansen's disease, otherwise known as Jansen's metaphyseal chondro-dysplasia. Infants with this disease initially present with active rickets. Therefore, in this case, the x-ray was fortuitous.[60] Within several years radiographic appearance typifies the condition and is pathognomonic—irregular patches of partially calcified cartilage protruding into the diaphyses in all

tubular bones. By this stage, it is no longer confused with rickets, as it was in the infant described here. It has now been reported that these patients have one or more mutations of the gene encoding the receptor for PTH and PTH-rp, which belongs to a distinct family of G-protein coupled receptors.[61] In patients with Jansen's metaphyseal chondrodysplasia who are asymptomatic, ligand-independent hypercalcemia is most likely caused by a constitutive activation of PTH–PTH-rp receptors.[61]

Hypermagnesemia in Newborns

Case Study 7

A 24-year-old woman presented at 32 weeks' gestation in labor with findings consistent with preeclampsia. A 4-g bolus of magnesium sulfate (MgSO₄) was administered, and a continuous infusion was begun at 2 to 4 g/hour. A maternal magnesium level obtained 10 hours later was 9.3 mg/dL. Seventeen hours after the onset of labor and 7 hours after spontaneous rupture of membranes, a female infant was delivered vaginally. At delivery, the infant was lethargic and cyanotic, had no spontaneous respirations, and was poorly perfused. The initial heart rate was 80 beats per minute. Bag and mask ventilation was instituted, and the color and heart rate improved. The respiratory effort and tone remained depressed, however, and the infant was intubated. The admitting physical examination revealed an occipital cephalohematoma, a grade I/VI systolic ejection murmur, decreased pulse and perfusion, and poor tone. On day 2 of life, the patient's physical condition improved, and ventilatory support was discontinued.

Exercise 7

QUESTION

1. Which of the following neonatal signs and symptoms can be attributed to hypermagnesemia? Choose all that apply.

   a. Hypotonia

   b. Poor respiratory effort

   c. Low heart rate

   d. Lethargy

ANSWER

1. a, b, and d. Controversy continues regarding the effect of maternal administration of MgSO₄ on the newborn infant. The majority of symptoms observed in infants born to mothers with elevated magnesium levels (weak or absent cry, decreased reflexes, hypotonia, muscle weakness, lethargy, poor respiratory effort, poor suck, and poor swallowing) are generally mild, considering that other in utero factors may be contributing to the overall status of the infant. It does not appear that serum magnesium levels in the neonate correlate with the level of neurologic or respiratory depression. Some investigators suggest that the more prolonged the maternal administration of MgSO₄ the more likely it is that symptoms will be observed in the neonate. Interventions other than supportive care are rarely required. Renal excretion is the primary route of elimination of excess magnesium.

References

1. Greer FR Disorders of calcium homeostasis. In Spitzer AR (ed): Intensive Care of the Fetus and Neonate 2nd ed. Philadelphia, Elsevier, 2005, pp 1179–1204.
2. Loughead JL, Tsang RC: Neonatal calcium and phosphorus metabolism. In Cowett RM (ed): Principles of Perinatal-Neonatal Metabolism. New York, Springer-Verlag, 1998, pp 879–908.
3. Dusso AS, Thadhani R, Slatopolsky E: Vitamin D receptor and analogs. Semin Nephrol 2004;24: 10–16.
4. Lin R, White JH: The pleiotropic action of vitamin D. Bioessays 2004;26:21–28.
5. Rösli A, Fanconi A: Neonatal hypocalcemia: "Early type" in low birth weight newborns. Helv Paediatr Acta 1973;28:443–457.
6. Tsang RC, Light IJ, Sutherland JM, et al: Possible pathogenetic factors in neonatal hypocalcemia of prematurity. J Pediatr 1973;82:423–429.
7. Brown DR, Tsang RC, Chen IW: Oral calcium supplementation in premature and asphyxiated neonates. J Pediatr 1976;89:973–977.
8. David L, Anast CS: Calcium metabolism in newborn infants: The interrelationship of parathyroid function and calcium, magnesium, and phosphorus metabolism in normal, "sick," and hypocalcemic newborns. J Clin Invest 1974;54:287–296.
9. Rosen JF, Roginsky M, Nathenson G, et al: 25-Hydroxyvitamin D: Plasma levels in mothers and

their premature infants with neonatal hypocalcemia. Am J Dis Child 1974;127:220–223.

10. Chan GM, Tsang RC, Chen IW, et al: The effects of $1,25(OH)_2$ vitamin D supplementation in premature infants. J Pediatr 1978;93:91–96.

11. Ron M, Levitz M, Chuba J, et al: Transfer of 25-hydroxyvitamin D_3 and 1,25-dihydroxyvitamin D_3 across the perfused human placenta. Am J Obstet Gynecol 1984;148:370–374.

12. Hillman LS, Haddad GJ: Perinatal vitamin D metabolism. III. Factors influencing late gestational human serum 25-hydroxyvitamin D. Am J Obstet Gynecol 1976;125:196–200.

13. David L, Salle B, Chopard P, et al: Studies on circulating immunoreactive calcitonin in low birth weight infants during the first 48 hours of life. Helv Paediatr 1977;32:39–48.

14. Tsang RC, Chen IW, Friedman MA, et al: Neonatal parathyroid function: Role of gestational age and postnatal age. J Pediatr 1973;83:728–738.

15. Hillman LS, Rojanasathit S, Slatopolsky E, et al: Serial measurements of serum calcium, magnesium, parathyroid hormone, calcitonin, and 25-hydroxyvitamin D in premature and term infants during the first week of life. Pediatr Res 1977;11: 739–744.

16. Linerelli LG, Bobik C, Bobik J: Urinary cAMP and renal responsiveness to parathyroid hormone in premature hypocalcemic infants. Pediatr Res 1973;7:329A.

17. David L, Salle BL, Putet G, et al: Serum immunoreactive calcitonin in low birth weight infants: Description of early changes; effect of intravenous calcium infusion; relationships with early changes in serum calcium, phosphorus, magnesium, parathyroid hormone, and gastrin levels. Pediatr Res 1981;15:803–808.

18. Venkataraman PS, Wilson DA, Sheldon RE, et al: Effect of hypocalcemia on cardiac function in very-low-birth-weight preterm neonates: Studies of blood ionized calcium, echocardiography, and cardiac effect of intravenous calcium therapy. Pediatrics 1985;76:543–550.

19. Willis DM, Chabot J, Radde IC, et al: Unsuspected hyperosmolality of oral solutions contributing to necrotizing enterocolitis in very-low-birth-weight infants. Pediatrics 1977;60:535–538.

20. Book LS, Herbst JJ, Stewart D: Hazards of calcium gluconate therapy in the newborn infant: Intraarterial injection producing intestinal necrosis in rabbit ileum. J Pediatr 1978;92:793–797.

21. Venkataraman PS, Tsang RC, Steichen JJ, et al: Early neonatal hypocalcemia in extremely premature infants. Am J Dis Child 1986;140:1140–1148.

22. Fleischman AR, Rosen JF, Nathenson G: 25-Hydroxycholecalciferol for early neonatal hypocalcemia: Occurrence in premature newborns. Am J Dis Child 1978;132:973–977.

23. Lin CY, Ishida M: Calcium homeostasis in premature infants and treatment of early hypocalcemia by 1,25-dihydroxycholecalciferol. Eur J Pediatr 1987;146:383–386.

24. Salle BL, David L, Glorieux FJ, et al: Hypocalcemia in infants of diabetic mothers: Studies in circulating calcitropic hormone concentrations. Acta Paediatr Scand 1982;71:573–577.

25. Barak Y, Milbauer B, Weisman Y, et al: Response of neonatal hypocalcemia to 1-a-hydroxyvitamin D. Arch Dis Child 1979;54:642–643.

26. Petersen S, Christensen NC, Fogh-Andersen N: Effect on serum calcium of 1-a-hydroxyvitamin D supplementation in infants of low birth weight, infants with perinatal asphyxia, and infants of diabetic mothers. Acta Paediatr Scand 1981;70: 897–901.

27. Taylor SC, Morris G, Wilson D, et al: Hypoparathyroidism and 22q11 deletion syndrome. Arch Dis Child 2003;88:520–522.

28. Scriver R, Beaudet AL, Sly WS (eds): (2001). *In* The Metabolic and Molecular Gases of Inherited Disease. New York, McGraw Hill, pp 1309–1310.

29. Greenbaugh KL, Aligianis IA, Bromilow G, et al: 22q11 deletion disorder requiring multidisciplinary input. Arch Dis Child 2003;88:523–524.

30. Maharasingam M, Östman-Smith I, Pike MG: A cohort study of neurodevelopmental outcome in children with DiGeorge Syndrome following cardiac surgery. Arch Dis Child 2003;88:61–64.

31. Tsang RC, Chen I, Hayes W, et al: Neonatal hypocalcemia in infants with birth asphyxia. J Pediatr 1974;84:428–433.

32. Venkataraman PS, Tsang RC, Greer FR, et al: Late infantile tetany and secondary hyperparathyroidism in infants fed humanized cow milk formula. Am J Dis Child 1985;139:664–668.

33. Nelson N, Finnström O: Blood exchange transfusions in newborns, the effect on serum ionized calcium. Early Hum Dev 1988;18:157–164.

34. Brown JK, Cockburn F, Forfar JO: Clinical and chemical correlates in convulsions of the newborn. Lancet 1972;1:135–138.

35. Cockburn F, Brown JK, Belton NR, et al: Neonatal convulsions associated with primary disturbance of calcium, phosphorus, and magnesium metabolism. Arch Dis Child 1973;48:99–108.

36. Greer FR: Calcium, phosphorus and vitamin D requirements and TPN regimens in low-birthweight infants. Proceedings of the Abbott Conference on Parenteral Nutrition in the Pediatric Patient, Columbus, Ohio, 1983, pp 111–114.

37. Keipert JA: Rickets with multiple fractured ribs in a premature infant. Med J Aust 1970;1:672–675.

38. Koo WWK, Antony G, Stevens HS: Continuous nasogastric phosphorus infusion in hypophosphatemic rickets of prematurity. Am J Dis Child 1984;138:172–175.

39. Rowe J, Wood DH, Rowe DW, et al: Nutritional hypophosphatemic rickets in a premature infant fed breast milk. N Engl J Med 1979;300:293–296.

40. Sagy M, Birenbaum E, Balin A, et al: Phosphate-depletion syndrome in a premature infant fed human milk. J Pediatr 1980;96:683–685.

41. Miller RR, Menke JA, Mentser MI: Hypercalcemia associated with phosphate depletion in the neonate. J Pediatr 1984;105:814–816.

42. Greer FR: Osteopenia of prematurity. Ann Rev Nutr 1994;14:169–185.

43. Koo WWK, Tsang RC, Succop P, et al: Minimal vitamin D and high calcium and phosphorus needs of preterm infants receiving parenteral nutrition. J Pediatr Gastroenterol Nutr 1989;8: 225–233.

44. MacMahon P, Blair ME, Treweeke P, Kovar IA: Association of mineral composition of neonatal intravenous feeding solutions and metabolic bone disease of prematurity. Arch Dis Child 1989;64: 489–493.

45. Pelegano JF, Rowe JC, Carey DE, et al: Effect of calcium/phosphorus ratio on mineral retention in parenterally fed premature infants. J Pediatr Gastroenterol Nutr 1991;12:351–355.

46. Pelagano JF, Rowe JC, Carey DE, et al: Simultaneous infusion of calcium and phosphorus in parenteral nutrition for premature infants: Use of physiologic calcium/phosphorus ratio. J Pediatr 1989;114:115–119.

47. Chessex P, Pineault M, Brisson G, et al: Role of the source of phosphate salt in improving the mineral balance of parenterally fed low birth weight infants. J Pediatr 1990;116:765–772.

48. McAleer JK, Mercer RD: Subcutaneous fat necrosis with calcifications and hypercalcemia in an infant. Cleve Clin Q 1964;31:179–183.

49. Michael AF, Hong R, West CD: Hypercalcemia in infancy: Association with subcutaneous fat necrosis and calcification. Am J Dis Child 1962;104:235–244.

50. Norwood-Galloway A, Lebwohl M, Phelps RG, et al: Subcutaneous fat necrosis of the newborn with hypercalcemia. J Am Acad Dermatol 1987;16:435–439.

51. Sharlin DN, Koblenzer P: Necrosis of subcutaneous fat with hypercalcemia: A puzzling and multifaceted disease. Clin Pediatr 1970;9:290–294.

52. Cook JS, Stone MS, Hansen JR: Hypercalcemia in association with subcutaneous fat necrosis of the newborn: Studies of calcium-regulating hormones. Pediatrics 1992;90:93–96.

53. Finne PH, Sanderud J, Aksnes L, et al: Hypercalcemia with increased and unregulated 1,25-dihydroxyvitamin D production in a neonate with subcutaneous fat necrosis. J Pediatr 1988;112:792–794.

54. Kruse K, Irle U, Uhlig R: Elevated 1,25-dihydroxyvitamin D serum concentrations in infants with subcutaneous fat necrosis. J Pediatr 1993;122:460–463.

55. Veldhuis JD, Kulin HE, Demers LM, et al: Infantile hypercalcemia with subcutaneous fat necrosis: Endocrine studies. J Pediatr 1979;95:460–462.

56. Committee on Genetics, American Academy of Pediatrics: Health care supervision for children with Williams syndrome. Pediatrics 2001;107:1192–1204.

57. Scriver R, Beaudet AL, Sly WS (eds): The Metabolic and Molecular Gases of Inherited Disease. New York, McGraw Hill, pp 1302–1303.

58. Cagle AP, Waguespack SG, Buckingham BA, et al: Severe infantile hypercalcemia associated with Williams syndrome successfully treated with intravenously administered pamidronate. Pediatrics 2004;114:1091–1095.

59. Ross AJ III, Cooper A, Attie MF, et al: Primary hyperparathyroidism in infancy. J Pediatr Surg 1986;21:493–499.

60. Frame B, Poznanski AK: Conditions confused with rickets. In DeLuca HF, Anast CS (eds): Pediatric Diseases Related to Calcium. New York, Elsevier, 1980, pp 270–278.

61. Schipani E, Langman CB, Parfitt AM, et al: Constitutively activated receptors for parathyroid hormone and parathyroid hormone–related peptide in Jansen's metaphyseal chondrodysplasia. N Engl J Med 1996;335:708–714.

Glucose Metabolism in the Newborn Infant

Rebecca A. Simmons, MD

The fetus is completely dependent on its mother for glucose and other nutrient transfer across the placenta. In the basal nonstressed state, placental transport of glucose meets all of the fetal glucose requirements. The human fetal liver has the enzymatic capacity for gluconeogenesis and glycogenolysis as early as the third month of gestation. However, the absolute levels of gluconeogenic enzymes are far lower than those of adults, and it is unlikely that the fetus produces much glucose under normal conditions. The fetus prepares for extrauterine survival by increasing energy stores and developing enzymatic processes for rapid mobilization of stored energy. Development of carbohydrate homeostasis in the newborn infant results from a balance between hormonal, enzymatic, and neural regulation, and substrate availability. The newborn infant must supply its own substrate to meet the energy requirements for maintenance of body temperature, respiration, muscular activity, and regulation of blood glucose. The concentration of glucose in the umbilical venous blood approximates 70% to 80% of that in the mother and is higher than in the umbilical arterial blood. During the first 4 to 6 hours of postnatal life, glucose values fall, stabilizing between 50 and 60 mg/dL.[1] This decrease in glucose is even greater in preterm or small-for-gestational-age infants. By 2 or 3 days of age, plasma glucose values average 70 to 80 mg/dL.

Blood glucose concentration is normally maintained at a relatively constant level by a fine balance between hepatic glucose output and peripheral glucose uptake. Hepatic glucose output depends on adequate glycogen stores, sufficient supplies of endogenous gluconeogenic precursors, a normally functioning hepatic gluconeogenic and glycogenolytic system, and a normal endocrine system for modulating these processes.

At birth the neonate has glycogen stores that are greater than those in the adult. However, because of a twofold greater basal glucose utilization, these stores are rapidly depleted and begin to decline within 2 to 3 hours after birth, remain low for several days, and then gradually rise to adult levels. Both serum glucagon and catecholamines increase threefold to fivefold in response to umbilical cord cutting. Circulating insulin levels usually decrease in the immediate newborn period and remain low for several days. The depressed serum insulin and elevated glucagon and epinephrine levels along with elevated serum growth hormone levels at birth favor glycogenolysis, lipolysis, and gluconeogenesis. Changes in various hormone receptors also modulate these processes. Hepatic glucagon receptors increase in number and become functionally linked with cAMP responses. Neonatal glucose homeostasis also requires appropriate enzyme maturation and response in the newborn. After birth, glycogen phosphorylase activity is increased, whereas glycogen synthetase activity is decreased, thus allowing for the rapid depletion of hepatic glycogen. Phosphoenolpyruvate carboxykinase activity, the rate-limiting enzyme for gluconeogenesis, also increases during the immediate postnatal period. Thus, hormonal and enzymatic activities in the fetus provide for anabolism and substrate accretion, whereas those in the newborn period provide for the maintenance of glucose homeo-stasis in response to the abrupt interruption of maternal glucose supply.

Many pathophysiologic conditions influence neonatal glucose homeostasis, leading to hypo-glycemia. Most of these conditions are related to an increase in the utilization of glucose, a decrease in production, or hyperinsulinism. Each of these categories is associated with several different disease states (Table 4-1).

Case Study 1

Baby boy Williams is a 4500-g infant born at 38 weeks' gestation to a 21-year-old primigravida mother. Her pregnancy was complicated by lack of prenatal care. The infant was born via cesarean section for failure to progress. The infant's Apgar scores were 4 at 1 minute and 5 at 5 minutes. Owing to significant respiratory distress the infant was intubated in the delivery room. At 6 hours of age his Dextrostix reading was 40 mg/dL. A serum glucose sent to the laboratory showed a glucose level of 39 mg/dL.

Exercise 1

QUESTIONS

1. Is this infant hypoglycemic?
2. What are the signs and symptoms of hypoglycemia?
3. What is the mechanism responsible for this infant's hypoglycemia?
4. What other complications are commonly observed in infants of diabetic mothers?
5. How should this infant's hypoglycemia be managed?

ANSWERS

1. There is no consensus defining a blood glucose level diagnostic of hypoglycemia. Earlier data defining hypoglycemia as a blood glucose level less than 35 mg/dL in term infants and 25 mg/dL in preterm infants were derived from data in fasted infants and are probably invalid. Concerns about the long-term effects of asymptomatic neonatal hypoglycemia, first raised by Pildes and coworkers, have led to efforts to change the definition of hypoglycemia.[2] In newborns, brain metabolism probably accounts for at least 85% to 90% of total glucose consumption and the newborn brain is not able to adequately use other substrates for its metabolic needs. Therefore, many neonatologists and pediatricians now define hypoglycemia as a glucose level less than 50 mg/dL, regardless of gestational age. It is important to remember that a whole blood glucose concentration, such as those measured by Dextrostix, will be 10% to 15% lower than plasma glucose concentrations because of the dilutional effect of the red blood cell mass. Furthermore, it is important not to delay testing the sample, as this can result in an artificially low value due to red blood cell oxidation of glucose.

2. The signs and symptoms of neonatal hypoglycemia are often subtle and nonspe-cific (Table 4-2). In fact, some infants with low glucose values are asymptomatic. This is compounded by the occurrence of symptoms at different blood glucose concentrations in different neonates and the lack of a universal threshold below or above which symptom-atology may occur. Therefore, it is extremely important to closely monitor the high-risk infant (diabetic mother, small for gestational

TABLE 4-1

CONDITIONS ASSOCIATED WITH NEONATAL HYPOGLYCEMIA

Limited Glycogen Supply	Diminished Glucose Production
Prematurity	Small-for-gestational-age infant
Perinatal stress	Inborn errors of metabolism
Glycogen storage disease	
	Others
Hyperinsulinism	Hypothermia
Infant of a diabetic mother	Sepsis
Congenital hyperinsulinism	Polycythemia
Beckwith-Wiedemann syndrome	Hypothalamic or hypopituitary disorders
Maternal drug therapy	Adrenal insufficiency
Erythroblastosis fetalis	

TABLE 4-2

SIGNS AND SYMPTOMS OF HYPOGLYCEMIA

Apnea
Bradycardia
Cyanosis
Jitteriness
Lethargy
Poor feeding
Seizures
Tachypnea
Temperature instability

age, sepsis). The maternal and perinatal history may yield useful information in helping decide which infants may be at risk for low blood glucose. High-risk situations include the presence of diabetes mellitus, any history of glucose intolerance, use of medications (e.g., salicylates and beta-sympathomimetics), history of preterm labor, and preeclampsia. Risk factors in the perinatal history include cold stress, asphyxia, trauma, and sepsis. The symptomatic infant may be jittery, lethargic, cyanotic, apneic, bradycardic, or hypotonic. Occasionally an infant will seize or suffer a cardiac arrest.

3. Because of the lack of prenatal care, one cannot definitively make the diagnosis of gestational diabetes. However, the infant is large for gestational age (LGA) and has hypoglycemia, both common features found in infants of diabetic mothers (IDM). As yet, no single mechanism has been clearly established that can explain the diverse and numerous complications found in the IDM. Nevertheless, most of the effects can be attributed to an abnormal intrauterine milieu. Pedersen first hypothesized that maternal hyperglycemia (and aberrances in amino acid and lipid availability) causes fetal hyperglycemia, stimulating the fetal pancreas, resulting in islet cell hypertrophy and β-cell hyperplasia with increased insulin availability.[3] With the disruption of a continuous glucose supply, the infant becomes hypoglycemic after delivery. Hyperinsulinemia in utero affects many organ systems, including the placenta. Insulin is the primary anabolic hormone of fetal growth. An increase in insulin levels in the fetus will result in increased growth of insulin-sensitive tissue (e.g., heart, liver, and muscle). In the presence of excess substrate such as glucose, increased fat synthesis and deposition occur during the third trimester. Fetal macrosomia is caused by increased body fat, muscle mass, and organomegaly. Insulin-insensitive tissues, such as brain and kidney, are not affected and are normal in size.

4. The IDM is at greater risk for morbidity and death, although the rate for both has dropped substantially in the last decade. What has not fallen is the incidence of congenital malformations. These infants have a higher rate of congenital heart disease, caudal regression syndrome, small left colon syndrome, and musculoskeletal anomalies. Cardiac septal hypertrophy is also more common in IDM. It is hypothesized that alterations in maternal glucose metabolism in the first weeks of pregnancy may cause defects in organogenesis. Hyperglycemia, hyperketonemia, and hyperosmolality have all been shown to disrupt organogenesis in animal models.

In addition to disorders of carbohydrate metabolism, these infants are at risk for other types of perinatal morbidities (Table 4-3). An increased incidence of respiratory distress syndrome is likely due to the effects of insulin and glucose upon surfactant production. Polycythemia resulting from an increased red blood cell mass may further compromise these infants, who already are at risk for development of venous thrombosis. The increase in red blood cell mass is caused by many factors: elevated erythropoietin levels, perinatal stress, placental insufficiency, and hyperinsulinemia. The increased red blood cell mass in addition to hepatic dysfunction results in hyperbilirubinemia. Infants of diabetic mothers are also at risk for hypocalcemia,

TABLE 4-3

ASSOCIATED CONDITIONS IN INFANTS OF DIABETIC MOTHERS

Congenital malformations
Fetal distress
Hyperbilirubinemia
Hyperviscosity
Hypocalcemia
Hypoglycemia
Macrosomia
Respiratory distress syndrome
Sudden fetal demise

which may be related to placental dysfunction and hypoxia.

5. Typically, hypoglycemia occurs shortly after birth and can last for several days. The most effective treatment is a continuous infusion of glucose at a rate that keeps the serum glucose level above 50 mg/dL. To bring the glucose concentration into the normal range, consider a bolus of 2 mL/kg 10% dextrose in water. However, repeated boluses should be avoided as rebound hypoglycemia may occur when the hyperresponsive β-cell produces an insulin surge in response to the infused glucose.

Case Study 2

Baby boy Smith was born to a 29-year-old gravida 2 para 1 mother at 32 weeks' gestation. His birth weight was 1000 g. He was vigorous at delivery and required no resuscitation. He was placed on IV fluids of $D_{10}W$ at 80 mL/kg/day. At 6 hours of age his glucose level was 35 mg/dL.

Exercise 2

QUESTIONS

1. What is the cause of this infant's hypoglycemia?
2. How should the hypoglycemia be managed?

ANSWERS

1. Infants born prematurely and or small for gestational age (SGA) are at high risk for developing hypoglycemia. In some reports as many as 60% of premature SGA infants show evidence of hypoglycemia. SGA babies have decreased glycogen stores and impaired gluconeogenesis. It is thought that there is a functional delay in the development of phosphoenolpyruvate carboxykinase (PEPCK) activity, the rate-limiting enzyme of gluconeogenesis. In normal newborns, this enzyme is activated at birth; however, in SGA infants, there is a delay in induction of PEPCK that might be related to decreased glycogen stores or decreased sensitivity to glucagon. Although insulin and glucagon secretion are similar in appropriate in size and SGA infants, the plasma amino acid response to glucagon

may be altered in hypoglycemic SGA babies. Commonly, several days are required for these infants to attain normal glucose homeostasis; thus, they remain at risk for hypoglycemia for an extended time after birth.

2. Similar to the infant of a diabetic mother, hypoglycemic SGA infants should be treated with a constant infusion of glucose. Many of these infants will need between 8 and 10 mg/kg/minute of 10% dextrose in water solution. The rate of infusion can be titrated to achieve a normal glucose level. The use of a peripheral vein or an umbilical venous catheter is preferable to the use of an umbilical arterial catheter as infusions of glucose into an umbilical artery have been associated with hyperinsulinism via direct pancreatic stimulation by the infused glucose.

Case Study 3

Baby girl Jones was born precipitously at home to a 20-year-old gravida 1 mother who received no prenatal care. The paramedics were called and upon arrival they found the infant to have a temperature of 34°C. They brought the infant to the hospital and she was admitted to the nursery for observation. Upon arrival, the infant was lethargic and mottled. Her Dextrostix reading was 15 mg/dL. The infant was treated and her clinical status improved. Twenty-four hours later, the infant was again found to be lethargic and not feeding well. Her Dextrostix reading was 20 mg/dL. Her temperature was normal.

Exercise 3

QUESTIONS

1. What is the cause of the first episode of hypoglycemia?
2. What is the cause of the second episode of hypoglycemia?

ANSWERS

1. Hypothermia is often associated with hypoglycemia. The hypoglycemia is thought to be secondary to high levels of catecholamines which in turn result in elevated free fatty acids. It is necessary to be cognizant of the risk of hypoglycemia in cold-stressed infants

and institute therapy not only to warm the infant but also to provide an adequate glucose supply.

2. The infant is now 24 hours old and her temperature is normal. Therefore, another cause for the hypoglycemia should be considered. Neonatal sepsis is commonly linked with low blood sugar values. Several mechanisms have been identified and relate to both increased utilization and decreased production. Studies in which sepsis was induced in animal models have demonstrated a decreased rate of gluconeogenesis. Septic infants also have an increased metabolic rate and increased peripheral insulin sensitivity, both of which raise the infant's requirement for glucose.

Case Study 4

Baby boy Davis was born at 37 weeks' gestation to a 25-year-old primigravida. Both his weight and length were greater than the 95% percentile for gestational age. At delivery it was noted that the infant had an omphalocele. He was immediately taken to surgery for repair of the abdominal wall defect. After surgery, upon closer examination, it was noted that the infant had macroglossia. At 16 hours of age his blood glucose was 15 mg/dL.

Exercise 4

QUESTIONS

1. What is this infant's primary diagnosis?
2. What is the mechanism of hypoglycemia given this diagnosis?
3. What other features are associated with this condition?

ANSWERS

1. Beckwith-Wiedemann syndrome is a common overgrowth syndrome that usually presents in the neonatal period. It is estimated to occur in 1 in approximately 14,000 births. The characteristic triad of findings include macrosomia, abdominal wall defect, and macroglossia. Most of these infants are large for gestational age, and both length and weight are increased proportionately. Visceromegaly is a frequent manifestation of overgrowth in affected patients. Cytomegaly of the adrenal gland, pancreas, kidney, liver, and spleen has been demonstrated. The most distinctive facial feature of Beckwith-Wiedemann syndrome is macroglossia, which nearly all patients exhibit. Slitlike linear creases of the earlobe and indentations of the posterior helix are characteristic ear findings. Facial nevus flammeus and prominent eyes with infraorbital creases are frequently seen. Patients are at increased risk of childhood malignant tumor development, mostly intra-abdominal tumors.

2. Approximately 50% of babies with Beckwith-Wiedemann syndrome have hypoglycemia that is thought to be due to islet cell hyperplasia. Hypoglycemia is often severe and difficult to treat. However, in most cases it spontaneously resolves in infancy or early childhood.

3. Genomic imprinting appears to be important in the inheritance of Beckwith-Wiedemann syndrome. Linkage studies in familial cases have mapped the gene for Beckwith-Wiedemann syndrome to chromosome 11p15.5. Also located in this region is the gene for insulin-like growth factor type 2 (IGF-2), an important fetal growth factor. This region is subject to imprinting, i.e., the maternal allele is not expressed. Maternal suppressor genes may be present in the same region balancing the growth effect of IGF-2 expression. Overexpression of the paternal allele or underexpression of the maternal allele can result in fetal overgrowth and the propensity for tumor formation.

Case Study 5

Baby boy Davidson was born at term to a 36-year-old gravida 8 para 7 woman. The pregnancy was unremarkable, as were labor and delivery. The infant's birth weight was 4.6 kg; his Apgar scores were 9 at 1 minute and 10 at 5 minutes. There were no risk factors for infection. At approximately 6 hours of age he developed seizures. A septic workup was done (including a lumbar puncture), and antibiotics were started. His Dextrostix reading was 15 mg/dL. Over the next 24 hours he required approximately 15 mg/kg/minute of glucose. His mother reported that this was her second child with this disorder.

Exercise 5

QUESTIONS

1. What is the most likely diagnosis?
2. How should this infant be treated?

ANSWERS

1. This infant likely has congenital hyperinsulinism, the most common cause of recurrent hypoglycemia in early infancy. Affected children are usually large for gestational age and often present with seizures in the first 1 to 2 days of life due to severe hypoglycemia. The majority of cases of congenital hyperinsulinism are caused by genetic defects in the regulation of insulin secretion by pancreatic β-cells. In some children, recessively inherited mutations have been demonstrated in the gene for the plasma membrane sulfonylurea receptor (SUR 1) or its associated potassium channel of the β-cell. Other children have been described with milder, dominantly inherited forms of hyperinsulinism that are not linked to the sulfonylurea receptor locus; a mutation in the glucokinase gene has been identified in one of these families. SUR mutations have been identified in Ashkenazi Jewish patients, and two mutations account for nearly all cases. As many as a dozen private mutations have been found in patients of non-Ashkenazi Jewish origin.

2. This hypoglycemia is often very difficult to treat. Diazoxide and octreotide are the drugs of choice for treatment of this form of hyperinsulinism. Diazoxide and octreotide act by inhibiting the action potential generation of the β-cell. Remember that in these patients the ATP (adenosine triphosphate)-sensitive K^+ channels are not operational (which normally control membrane potential). Therefore, it is hypothesized that diazoxide activates a novel K^+ selective ion channel leading to inhibition of spontaneous electrical events and inhibition of insulin secretion. Unfortunately, many patients (95%) do not respond to these drugs and require a subtotal pancreatectomy. In some patients with SUR mutations who have had subtotal pancreatectomy, diabetes has been reported to develop during adolescence. Whether the diabetes is a natural consequence of the SUR defects or is caused by the surgery is unknown.

References

1. Srinivasan G, Pildes RS, Cattamanchi G, et al: Plasma glucose values in normal neonates: A new look. J Pediatr 1986;109:114–177.
2. Pildes RS, Pyati SP: Hypoglycemia and hyperglycemia in tiny infants. Clin Perinatol 1986;13:2351–2375.
3. Pedersen J, Molsted-Pedersen L, Andersen B, et al: Assessors of fetal perinatal mortality in the diabetic pregnancy. Diabetes 1974;23:302–305.

Suggested Readings

Andrews MW, Amparo EG: Wilms' tumor in patients with Beckwith Wiedemann syndrome. Am J Roentgenol 1993;160:139–140.

Beckwith JB: Extreme cytomegaly of the adrenal fetal cortex, omphalocele, hyperplasia of the kidneys and pancreas, and Leydig cell hyperplasia—Another syndrome? J Genet Hum 1964;13:232–233.

Carey BE, Zeilinger TC: Hypoglycemia due to high positioning of umbilical artery catheters. J Perinatol 1989;9:407–410.

Cowett RM: Hypoglycemia and hyperglycemia in the newborn. In Polin RA, Fox WW (eds): Fetal and Neonatal Physiology. Philadelphia, WB Saunders, 1998, p 596.

Cowett RM: The infant of the diabetic mother. In Cowett RM (ed): Principles of Perinatal-Neonatal Metabolism. New York, Springer-Verlag, 1998, p 1105.

Denne SC, Karn CA, Wang J, et al: Effect of intravenous glucose and lipid on proteolysis and glucose production in normal newborns. Am J Physiol 1995;269:E361–E367.

Frantz ID III, Medina G, Taeusch HW Jr: Correlation of Dextrostix values with true glucose in the range less than 50 mg/dL. J Pediatr 1975;87:417–420.

Fuhrmann K, Reiher H, Semmler K, et al: Prevention of congenital malformations in infants of insulin dependent diabetic mothers. Diabetes Care 1983;6:219–223.

Girard J: Gluconeogenesis in late fetal and early neonatal life. Biol Neonate 1986;50:237–258.

Hay WW: Fetal and neonatal glucose homeostasis and their relation to the small for gestational age infant. Semin Perin 1984;8:101–116.

Kalhan SC, Raghavan CV: Metabolism of glucose in the fetus and newborn. In Polin RA, Fox WW (eds): Fetal and Neonatal Physiology. Philadelphia, WB Saunders, 1998, p 543.

Kane C, Lindley KJ, Johnson PRV, et al: Therapy for persistent hyperinsulinemic hypoglycemia of infancy. J Clin Inves 1997;100:1888–1893.

Kitzmiller JL, Cloherty JP, Younger MD, et al: Diabetic pregnancy and perinatal morbidity. Am J Obstet Gynecol 1978;131:560–568.

Neave C: Congenital malformation in offspring of diabetics. Perspect Pediatr Pathol 1984;8:213–222.

Nogee L, McMahon M, Whitsett JA: Hyaline membrane disease and surfactant protein SAP 35 in diabetes in pregnancy. Am J Perinatol 1988;5:374–377.

Ogata ES: Carbohydrate metabolism in the fetus and neonate and altered neonatal glucoregulation. Pediatr Clin North Am 1986;33:25–45.

Schwartz R, Gruppuso PA, Pelzold K, et al: Hyperinsulinemia and macrosomia in the fetus of the diabetic mother. Diabetes Care 1994;17: 640–648.

Stanley CA, Lieu YK, Hsu BY, et al: Hyperinsulinism and hyperammonemia in infants with regulatory mutations of the glutamate dehydrogenase gene. N Engl J Med 1998;338:1352–1357.

Stanley CA: Hyperinsulinism in infants and children. Pediatr Clin North Am 1997;44:363–374.

Yeung CY: Hypoglycemia in neonatal sepsis. J Pediatr 1970;77:812–817.

Neonatal Hyperbilirubinemia

M. Jeffrey Maisels, MB, BCh

The bilirubin level in all newborn infants, whether term or premature, increases in the first few days after birth, and about 60% of full-term infants become visibly jaundiced. Although hyperbilirubinemia is a benign condition for most infants, the newborn infant is unique because this is the time of life when an elevation of serum bilirubin levels may be toxic to the infant's developing central nervous system (CNS).

In the last 10 to 15 years, we have seen changes that require a rethinking of our approach to the jaundiced newborn. The first is that kernicterus, thought to be nearly eradicated, is still occurring. The second is the shortened hospital stay for newborns, and the third is an increase in the incidence of neonatal jaundice, possibly related to the increase in breastfeeding.

In this chapter we discuss the physiologic mechanisms causing neonatal hyperbilirubinemia, management of the jaundiced infant, and the phenomenon of bilirubin brain injury and kernicterus. Clinical cases are presented that demonstrate the issues confronted by practitioners in dealing with jaundiced neonates.

Bilirubin Metabolism

Exercise 1

QUESTION

1. Which of the following mechanisms contribute to the rise in serum bilirubin following birth in healthy infants?

a. High circulating red blood cell mass and shortened red blood cell lifespan
b. Decreased hepatic conjugation of bilirubin
c. Inability to form photoisomers
d. Increased enterohepatic circulation
e. Presence of β-glucuronidase in the brush border of the intestine

ANSWER

1. a, b, d, and e.

Bilirubin Production

As shown in Figures 5-1 and 5-2 bilirubin is derived from the catabolism of heme proteins. About 75% of daily bilirubin production comes from the normal destruction of senescent erythrocytes in the reticuloendothelial system, and the catabolism of 1 g of hemoglobin produces 35 mg of bilirubin. The remaining 25% of bilirubin comes from sources other than circulating red blood cells. These sources include (1) ineffective erythropoiesis and the destruction of immature erythrocyte precursors either in the bone marrow or soon after release into the circulation and (2) the turnover of heme protein and free heme, primarily in the liver. These two sources form the so-called "early-labeled" bilirubin (see Fig. 5-1).

Hemoglobin is catabolized to bilirubin in the reticuloendothelial system. In the first step of the heme degradation pathway, heme is converted to biliverdin in the presence of the microsomal enzyme heme oxygenase and

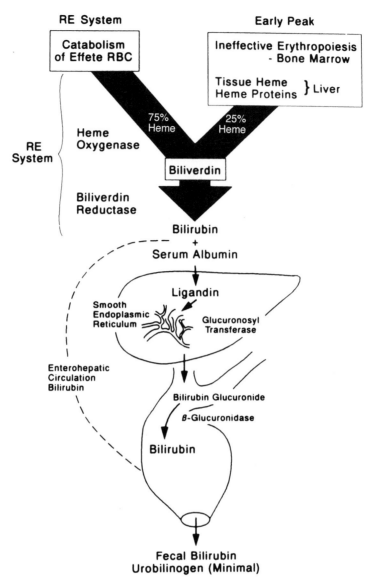

Figure 5-1 Neonatal bile pigment metabolism. RBCs, red blood cells; RE, reticuloendothelial. (From Maisels JM: Jaundice. In Avery GB, Fletcher MA, MacDonald MG [eds]: Neonatology: Pathophysiology and Management of the Newborn, 4th ed. Philadelphia, JB Lippincott, 1994, p 635.)

carbon monoxide (CO) is produced. One molecule of CO is produced for each molecule of heme catabolized and bilirubin produced (see Fig 5-2). (The concentration of CO in the blood [as carboxyhemoglobin] or in exhaled air is a useful measure of bilirubin production in jaundiced infants.) The biliverdin then undergoes reduction after its release from the microsomes to form bilirubin, a step catalyzed by biliverdin reductase (see Fig. 5-2).

Transport and Hepatic Uptake of Bilirubin

The bilirubin formed in the reticuloendothelial system is released into the circulation where it is reversibly but tightly bound to albumin. Under physiologic conditions, most bilirubin is bound to albumin in the circulation, and only very small amounts of "free" bilirubin can be detected in the circulation.

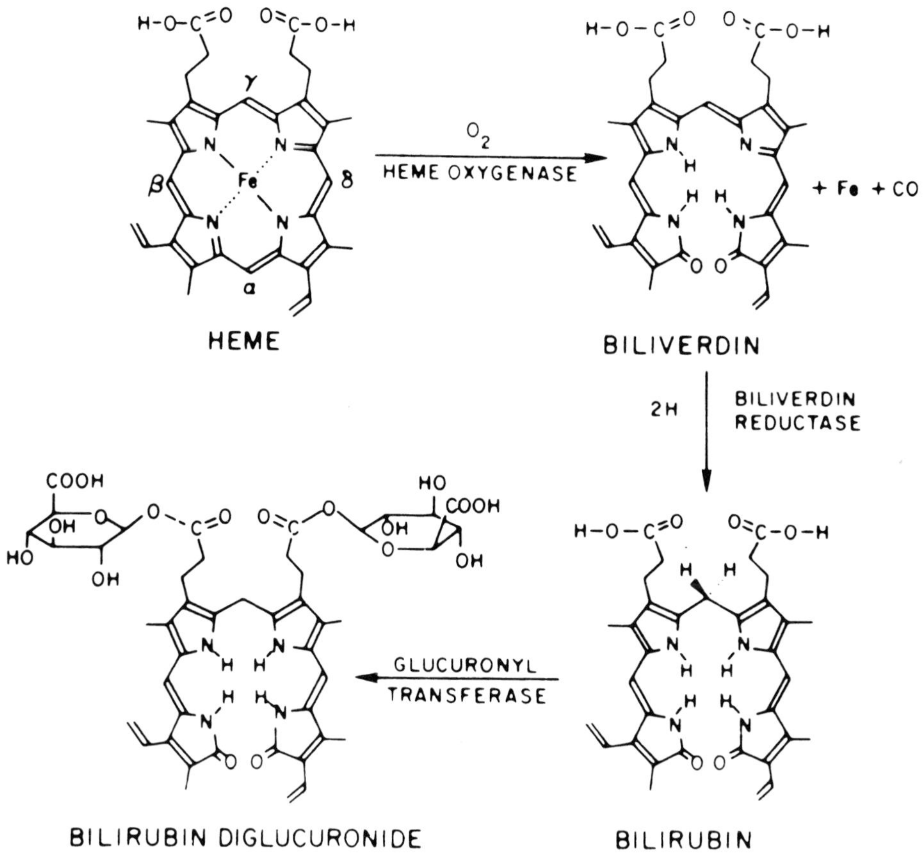

Figure 5-2 Biosynthesis of bilirubin. (From Lightner DA, McDonagh AF: Molecular mechanisms of phototherapy for neonatal jaundice. Acc Chem Res 1984;17:417–424.)

Uptake of bilirubin by the liver is efficient and rapid. When the bilirubin-albumin complex reaches the plasma membrane of the hepatocyte, bilirubin (but not albumin) is transported across the cell membrane into the hepatocyte by a carrier-mediated diffusion process.

Conjugation and Excretion of Bilirubin

In the hepatocyte, bilirubin is bound principally to ligandin and possibly other cytosolic binding proteins (see Fig. 5-1). A network of intracellular microsomes may also play an important role in the transfer of bilirubin within the cell and to the endoplasmic reticulum. There bilirubin combines enzymatically with a sugar, glucuronic acid, producing bilirubin mono- and diglucuronides. The conjugation reaction is catalyzed by a specific hepatic enzyme isoform of diphosphoglucuronate uridine diphosphate glucuronosyl transferase (UGT1A1). Both mono- and diglucuronides are more water soluble than native bilirubin and are sufficiently polar to be excreted into the bile or filtered by the kidney.

Transfer of Bilirubin into Bile and Intestinal Transport

The mono- and diglucuronides are excreted into bile by an energy-dependent process. In the adult, conjugated bilirubin is reduced by the action of colonic bacteria to urobilinogens (colorless tetrapyrroles). In a newborn infant, however, much of this conjugated bilirubin is hydrolyzed back to unconjugated bilirubin and reabsorbed into the bloodstream by way of the enterohepatic circulation. β-Glucuronidase is a small-intestinal brush border enzyme that deconjugates bilirubin in the bowel (see Fig. 5-1) and allows it to be reabsorbed into the circulation. Conjugated bilirubin does not cross the intestinal wall.

Physiologic Jaundice

Following ligation of the umbilical cord, the neonate must dispose of the bilirubin load that was previously cleared through the placenta. Because neonatal hyperbilirubinemia is an almost universal finding during the first week of life, this transient elevation of the serum bilirubin has been called *physiologic jaundice.* The total serum bilirubin (TSB) level reflects a combination of the effects of bilirubin production, conjugation, and enterohepatic circulation and the factors that affect these processes account for the bilirubinemia that occurs in virtually all newborns.

Table 5-1 summarizes the physiologic mechanisms of neonatal jaundice. Newborns produce 8 to 10 mg/kg of bilirubin per day—more than twice the rate of an adult (per kg body weight). This occurs because newborns have more circulating red blood cells (higher hematocrits), a shortened red blood cell survival (80 days versus 120 days in adults), and more early labeled bilirubin. Other mechanisms contributing to physiologic jaundice include decreased hepatic uptake of bilirubin from the plasma (developmental deficiency of the carrier protein ligandin), decreased hepatic conjugation (deficient UGT1A1 activity), and an increased enterohepatic circulation of bilirubin. Infants have fewer bacteria in the bowel and greater activity of the deconjugating enzyme β-glucuronidase. As a result, conjugated bilirubin is not converted by bacteria to urobilinogen but is hydrolyzed to unconjugated bilirubin, which is reabsorbed, thus increasing the bilirubin load on an already stressed liver (see Fig. 5-1).

Bilirubin Toxicity

Exercise 2

QUESTION

1. Which of the following statements about the pathogenesis of kernicterus are true?

   a. All bilirubin in plasma is tightly bound to albumin.

   b. Sick and low-birth-weight infants have a reduced binding capacity for bilirubin.

   c. The blood-brain barrier can be injured by hyperosmolality, hypertension, and hypercarbia allowing bilirubin to move into the central nervous system.

   d. Breastfeeding offers protection against developing kernicterus.

ANSWER

1. b and c.

Pathophysiology

The pathogenesis of kernicterus or bilirubin encephalopathy is complex and not fully elucidated. For example, bilirubin is deposited preferentially in the basal ganglia of the brain but the reasons for this are not known.

Albumin Binding and the Concept of Free Bilirubin

Bilirubin is transported in the plasma tightly, but reversibly bound to serum albumin. The portion that is unbound or loosely bound (sometimes termed *free bilirubin*) can more easily leave the intravascular space and cross the intact blood-brain barrier. Measurements of unbound bilirubin can be helpful in determining the risk of kernicterus, but currently, no test is in general use in the United States, although an automated instrument has recently been developed that measures unbound bilirubin by the peroxidase method. Because one molecule of albumin is capable of binding one

TABLE 5-1

PHYSIOLOGIC MECHANISMS OF NEONATAL JAUNDICE

Increased bilirubin load on liver cell
 Increased erythrocyte volume
 Decreased erythrocyte survival
 Increased early-labeled bilirubin
 Increased enterohepatic circulation of bilirubin
Decreased hepatic uptake of bilirubin from plasma
 Decreased ligandin
Decreased bilirubin conjugation
 Decreased uridine diphosphoglucuronosyl
 transferase activity
Defective bilirubin excretion
 Excretion impaired but not rate limiting

From Maisels MJ: Jaundice. In MacDonald MG, Seshia MMK, Mullett MD (eds): Neonatology: Pathophysiology and Management of the Newborn, 6th ed. Philadelphia, Lippincott, 2005, pp 768–846.

TABLE 5-2

SOME FACTORS THAT DECREASE THE BINDING OF BILIRUBIN TO SERUM ALBUMIN

Fatty acids: If ratio of free fatty acids to albumin exceeds 4:1. This does not occur with the usual doses of intravenous fat used in the preterm newborn.

pH: A decrease in pH might affect albumin binding. A decrease in pH also increases binding of bilirubin to brain cells.

Drugs: Drugs that can produce more than 20% increase in free bilirubin include carbenicillin, cefotetan, ceftriaxone, moxalactam, sulfamethoxazole, aminophylline.

Clinical status of the infant: Sick, preterm babies bind less bilirubin per mole of albumin.

molecule of bilirubin tightly at the primary binding site, a bilirubin-albumin molar ratio of 1 represents about 8 mg of bilirubin per gram of albumin. Thus, a well full-term infant with a serum albumin concentration of 3 to 3.5 g/dL should be able to bind, tightly, about 24 to 28 mg/dL of bilirubin (410 to 479 μmol/L). Sick and low-birth-weight infants have less effective binding capacity. In the absence of direct measurements of free bilirubin, a range of bilirubin-to-albumin ratios (in mg/g) can be used as a guide in deciding whether or not to perform an exchange transfusion, an approach that has been endorsed by the American Academy of Pediatrics (AAP) (see later discussion under Treatment).

Table 5-2 lists some of the important factors that affect the binding of bilirubin to serum albumin.

Bilirubin and the Brain

Under normal circumstances, bilirubin moves in and out of the brain, although a blood-brain barrier (BBB) exists between the brain capillary endothelium and the brain parenchyma. The BBB limits the entry of certain substances into the central nervous system. Large molecules, such as albumin, are excluded from the brain, but may enter when the BBB is damaged. Conditions that can damage the BBB include hyperosmolality, hypercarbia, hypertension, and asphyxia. Under these circumstances both unbound and albumin-bound bilirubin will enter the brain and bathe the neurons. There are substances in the brain capillary endothelial cells and in the astrocytes of the BBB that might act to limit the passage of bilirubin into the

brain. Substances such as multidrug-resistant P-glycoprotein (MDR/P-gps) and other transporters could have an important influence on helping to limit the deposition of bilirubin in the cells of the CNS.

Clinical Features of Bilirubin Encephalopathy

Terminology

Kernicterus was originally a pathologic diagnosis characterized by bilirubin staining of the brain stem nuclei and cerebellum but it has been used interchangeably with both acute and chronic *bilirubin encephalopathy*, which describes the clinical CNS findings caused by bilirubin toxicity. The AAP recommends that we use the term *acute bilirubin encephalopathy* to describe the acute manifestations of bilirubin toxicity seen in the first weeks after birth. *Kernicterus* should be reserved for the chronic and permanent clinical sequelae of bilirubin toxicity. Others have suggested the use of *bilirubin-induced neurologic dysfunction* (BIND) to describe the changes associated with acute bilirubin encephalopathy.

Acute Bilirubin Encephalopathy

The major features of acute bilirubin encephalopathy are shown in Table 5-3 and illustrated in Figure 5-3. Some 15% of infants who subsequently develop classical kernicterus mani-

TABLE 5-3

MAJOR CLINICAL FEATURES OF ACUTE BILIRUBIN ENCEPHALOPATHY

Initial Phase
Slight stupor ("lethargic," "sleepy")
Slight hypotonia, paucity of movement
Poor sucking; slightly high-pitched cry
Intermediate Phase
Moderate stupor—irritable
Tone variable—usually increased; some with retrocollis-opisthotonos
Minimal feeding; high-pitched cry
Advanced Phase
Deep stupor to coma
Tone usually increased; some with retrocollis-opisthotonos
No feeding; shrill cry

From Maisels MJ: Jaundice. In MacDonald MG, Seshia MMK, Mullett MD (eds): Neonatology: Pathophysiology and Management of the Newborn, 6th ed. Philadelphia, Lippincott, 2005, pp 768–846.

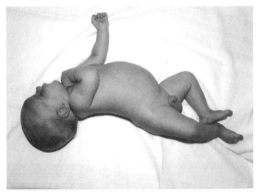

Figure 5-3 This infant presented at age 30 days with a serum bilirubin level of 30 mg/dL (513 μmol/L) secondary to the Crigler-Najjar syndrome type I. He demonstrated retrocollis and opisthotonos, signs of the intermediate to advanced stage of acute bilirubin encephalopathy. (From Maisels MJ: Jaundice. In MacDonald MG, Seshia MMK, Mullett MD [eds]: Neonatology: Pathophysiology and Management of the Newborn, 6th ed. Philadelphia, Lippincott, 2005, pp 768–846.)

fest no, or equivocal, signs of acute bilirubin encephalopathy as newborns.

Kernicterus (Chronic Bilirubin Encephalopathy)

The classic sequelae of posticteric encephalopathy are listed in Table 5-4. There is a typical temporal evolution of these changes. In the first year, these infants typically feed poorly, develop a high-pitched cry, and are hypotonic, but have increased reflexes and motor delay. The other features are often not apparent before age 1 year and sometimes not for several years. Usually these children are hypotonic for the first 6 or 7 years and become hypertonic when they reach their teens.

The hearing loss is generally most severe in the high frequencies. Recently, auditory neuropathy, or auditory dyssynchrony has been

TABLE 5-4

MAJOR CLINICAL FEATURES OF CHRONIC POSTKERNICTERIC BILIRUBIN ENCEPHALOPATHY

Extrapyramidal abnormalities, especially athetosis
Gaze abnormalities, especially of upward gaze
Auditory disturbance, especially sensorineural
    hearing loss
Intellectual deficits, but minority in mentally retarded
    range

From Maisels MJ: Jaundice. In MacDonald MG, Seshia MMK, Mullett MD (eds): Neonatology: Pathophysiology and Management of the Newborn, 6th ed. Philadelphia, Lippincott, 2005, pp 768–846.

recognized in infants with kernicterus. In this condition there is an abnormal or absent brain stem auditory evoked response (BAER) but normal inner ear function as tested by cochlear microphonic responses or otoacoustic emissions. The inner ear or cochlea is normal but the ascending auditory pathway in the nerve or brain stem is abnormal.

Diagnosis

The diagnosis of acute bilirubin encephalopathy and kernicterus can now be confirmed by magnetic resonance imaging (MRI) (Fig. 5-4). The most characteristic images are bilateral, symmetrical, high-intensity signals in the globus pallidus seen on both T_1- and T_2-weighted images.

The Relationship of Serum Bilirubin Levels to Developmental Outcome

It has not been possible to define a serum bilirubin level that is consistently associated with

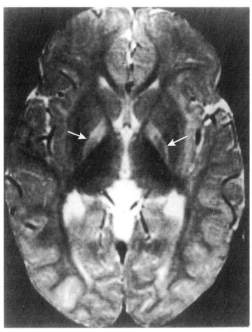

Figure 5-4 Magnetic resonance imaging scan of a 21-month-old male infant who had erythroblastosis fetalis and presented with extreme hyperbilirubinemia and clinical signs of kernicterus at age 54 hours. Note the symmetrical, abnormally high intensity signal from the area of the globus pallidus on both sides (*arrows*). (From Grobler JM, Mercer MJ: Kernicterus associated with elevated predominantly direct-reacting bilirubin. S Afr Med J 1997;87:146.)

adverse developmental outcome. Some studies have raised concerns regarding "soft signs" of neurologic dysfunction in infants exposed to moderate levels of bilirubin. Most recently, a study of 140 neonates with TSB levels at or above 25 mg/dL (428 µmol/L) found no differences between these infants and control infants in any area of neuropsychological development including detailed neurologic examinations, IQ scores, behavioral issues, and parental assessment. These data suggest that the thresholds currently recommended for the treatment of hyperbilirubinemia are both reasonable and safe (see later discussion).

Co-morbid Factors

Neurologic damage is more likely if hyperbilirubinemia is concurrent with other risk factors such as isoimmune hemolytic disease, prematurity, G6PD deficiency, asphyxia, sepsis, acidosis, and hypoalbuminemia. When these risk factors are present, more aggressive treatment of hyperbilirubinemia is appropriate (see later discussion).

Premature Infants and Low-Bilirubin Kernicterus

It is generally believed that premature infants are at greater risk of developing kernicterus or bilirubin encephalopathy than are full-term newborns exposed to similar bilirubin levels. Kernicterus with typical MRI findings was recently described in two preterm infants at 31 and 34 weeks' gestation whose TSB levels were 13.1 mg/dL (224 µmol/L) and 14.7 mg/dL (251 µmol/L), respectively. Neither of these infants was ill. In five preterm infants with gestations ranging from 25 to 29 weeks, MRI findings of kernicterus were described associated with peak TSB levels ranging from 8.7 to 11.9 mg/dL (148 to 204 µmol/L). The brain of the very low birth weight (VLBW) infant is more susceptible to damage from a number of sources and given that preterm infants have less effective albumin binding and are much more likely to be sick than are full-term infants, it makes sense to take a more aggressive approach to maintaining low bilirubin levels in this population.

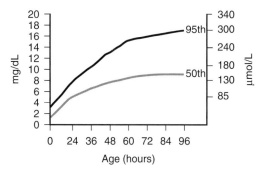

TOTAL SERUM BILIRUBIN

Figure 5-5 Smoothed curves from studies in eight different populations illustrating the expected velocity of total serum bilirubin (TSB) levels and approximate values for the 50th and 95th percentiles. (From Maisels MJ: Jaundice. In MacDonald MG, Seshia MMK, Mullett MD [eds]: Neonatology: Pathophysiology and Management of the Newborn, 6th ed. Philadelphia, Lippincott, 2005, pp 768–846.)

The Clinical Approach to the Jaundiced Newborn

Normal Serum Bilirubin Levels

Defining what represents a normal bilirubin level in the term and near term infant is challenging because TSB levels vary considerably depending on the racial composition of the population, the incidence of breastfeeding and other genetic and epidemiologic factors. Figure 5-5 provides an estimate of the natural history of neonatal jaundice in the first 96 hours after birth. These curves are derived from 8 different studies but local variation can be expected, particularly at the upper percentile limits. In our own hospital population, for example, the 95th percentile at 96 hours is a TSB of 13.1 mg/dL (224 µmol/L).

Figure 5-5 also illustrates an important point, well known but often ignored: bilirubin levels in the first few days change with every hour of the infant's life. *Thus, interpretation of what is or is not normal must be based on the relationship of the TSB to the infant's age in hours and not days.*

Case Study 1

A female infant is brought to your office at age 15 days for a routine visit and appears slightly jaundiced. She is breastfed, nursing well, thriving, and gaining weight.

Exercise 3

QUESTIONS

1. What questions would you ask the mother?
2. The infant returns to your office at age 4 weeks and is still jaundiced. What tests would you do?

ANSWERS

1. Prolonged indirect hyperbilirubinemia is very common in breastfed infants and, at 15 days, requires no additional investigations as long as you are satisfied that the infant is doing well and that there is minimal to mild jaundice. It is important to ask about the color of the urine and the stools. If the infant has cholestatic jaundice (elevation of conjugated or direct reacting bilirubin), the urine will be dark. Note that a newborn infant's urine is almost colorless and, if a mother reports that the urine is yellow, you should do a dipstick. If the dipstick is positive for bile there is bilirubin in the urine and an elevated direct reacting serum bilirubin. This requires further investigation for cholestatic jaundice. You should also ask about the color of the stools. If a breastfed infant is not having yellow mushy stools (and the stools are gray), the diagnosis of cholestatic jaundice must be considered. Note, however, that some infants with biliary artesia can still pass yellow stools. You should schedule a return visit in 1 to 2 weeks.

2. It is mandatory to obtain a total and direct reacting (or conjugated) bilirubin on any infant who is jaundiced beyond 3 weeks. If the infant's TSB is less than 5 mg/dL (86 µmol/L), a direct reacting bilirubin of more than 1 mg/dL (17 µmol/L) is abnormal. If the infant's TSB is more than 5 mg/dL (86 µmol/L), a direct reacting bilirubin of more than 20% of the total is abnormal. An elevation of direct reacting or conjugated bilirubin requires a complete evaluation for cholestatic jaundice with particular emphasis on ruling out biliary atresia.

Breastfeeding and Jaundice

An important change in the United States population has been the dramatic increase in breastfeeding at hospital discharge, from 30%

TABLE 5-5

PATHOGENESIS OF JAUNDICE ASSOCIATED WITH BREASTFEEDING

Increased enterohepatic circulation of bilirubin
  Decreased caloric intake
  Less cumulative stool output and stools contain less bilirubin (vs. formula fed infants)
  Increased intestinal fat absorption
  Less formation of urobilin in gastrointestinal tract
Mutations of the *UGT1A1* gene (Gilbert syndrome) — prolonged breast milk jaundice

From Maisels MJ: Jaundice. In MacDonald MG, Seshia MMK, Mullett MD (eds): Neonatology: Pathophysiology and Management of the Newborn, 6th ed. Philadelphia, Lippincott, 2005, pp 768–846.

---

in the 1960s to almost 70% today. In some hospitals, 85% or more of infants are breastfed.

Multiple studies have found a strong association between breastfeeding and an increased incidence of neonatal hyperbilirubinemia. The jaundice associated with breastfeeding in the first 2 to 4 days has been called "the breastfeeding jaundice syndrome" or "breastfeeding-associated jaundice." Hyperbilirubinemia that appears later (onset at 4 to 7 days and prolonged jaundice) has been called the "breast milk jaundice syndrome." There is considerable overlap between these two entities and evidence to support two distinct syndromes is meager. Prolonged indirect-reacting hyperbilirubinemia (beyond age 2 to 3 weeks) occurs in 20% to 30% of all breastfeeding infants and, in some infants, may persist for up to 3 months.

The factors that play a role in the pathophysiology of jaundice associated with breastfeeding are listed in Table 5-5.

Pathologic Causes of Jaundice

Table 5-6 lists the causes of pathologic indirect-reacting hyperbilirubinemia in the neonate.

Case Study 2

This female infant born at 38 weeks' gestation was breastfed and nursing well. At age 24 hours she was noted to be jaundiced and the TSB was 9.1 mg/dL (156 µmol/L). No further testing was done and she was discharged home with the advice to return in 24 hours for a follow-up bilirubin. At age 48 hours the TSB was 16.9 mg/dL

TABLE 5-6

CAUSES OF INDIRECT HYPERBILIRUBINEMIA IN NEWBORN INFANTS

Increased Production or Bilirubin Load on the Liver
Hemolytic disease
    Immune mediated
        Rh alloimmunization, ABO and other blood
            group incompatibilities
Heritable disorders
    Red blood cell membrane defects
        Hereditary spherocytosis, elliptocytosis,
            pyropoikilocytosis, stomatocytosis
    Red blood cell enzyme deficiencies
        Glucose-6-phosphate dehydrogenase
            deficiency* pyruvate kinase deficiency, and
            other erythrocyte enzyme deficiencies
    Hemoglobinopathies
        α-Thalassemia, β-thalassemia
    Unstable hemoglobins
        Congenital Heinz body hemolytic anemia
Other causes of increased production
    Sepsis*,[†]
    Disseminated intravascular coagulation
    Extravasation of blood—hematomas,
        pulmonary, abdominal, cerebral, or other
        occult hemorrhage
    Polycythemia
    Macrosomic infants of diabetic mothers
Increased enterohepatic circulation of bilirubin
    Breast milk jaundice
    Pyloric stenosis*
    Small or large bowel obstruction or ileus

Decreased Clearance
    Prematurity
    Glucose-6-phosphate dehydrogenase deficiency
Inborn errors of metabolism
    Crigler-Najjar syndrome, types I and II
    Gilbert syndrome
    Galactosemia[†]
    Tyrosinemia[†]
    Hypermethioninemia[†]
Metabolic
    Hypothyroidism
    Hypopituitarism[†]

---

*Decreased clearance is also part of pathogenesis.
[†]Elevation of direct-reading bilirubin also occurs.
From Maisels MJ: Jaundice. In MacDonald MG, Seshia MMK, Mullett MD (eds): Neonatology: Pathophysiology and Management of the Newborn, 6th ed. Philadelphia, Lippincott, 2005, pp 768–846.

(289 μmol/L), hemoglobin 19.5 g/dL. Home phototherapy was prescribed and a TSB the following day was 17.7 mg/dL (303 μmol/L). The following day the bilirubin level was 20.8 mg/dL (356 μmol/L). Home phototherapy was continued, breastfeeding was interrupted and the baby was given formula. Over the next 3 days the TSB slowly declined to 15.3 mg/dL (262 μmol/L), phototherapy was discontinued and breastfeeding resumed. Twenty-four hours later, however, the TSB level was 21.6 mg/dL (369 μmol/L) and

she was admitted to hospital. On admission the hemoglobin level was 12.2 mg/dL, hematocrit 34.6%. Under intensive phototherapy the TSB fell within 48 hours to 12.9 mg/dL (221 μmol/L). A peripheral smear was reviewed by the hematologists.

Exercise 4

QUESTIONS

1. Was the management of this infant at the birth hospital appropriate?

2. What was the most likely diagnosis?

3. In view of this, what additional tests would you request?

4. Was it appropriate to prescribe home phototherapy for a TSB level of 16.9 mg/dL (289 μmol/L) at age 48 hours?

5. Was it appropriate to interrupt breastfeeding and introduce formula?

6. What are the possible causes of hemolysis in this infant?

ANSWERS

1. It was appropriate to obtain a TSB level, which should be done on any infant who is jaundiced in the first 24 hours. But a TSB of 9.1 mg/dL (156 μmol/L) at 24 hours is well above the 95th percentile (Fig. 5-6; see also Fig. 5-5), so two additional actions were required: (a) an evaluation to attempt to identify the cause of the jaundice and (b) another TSB measured within 4 to 6 hours. It was inappropriate to discharge this infant with a TSB of 9.1 mg/dL (156 μmol/L) at age 24 hours.

2. By far the most likely diagnosis in an infant with a bilirubin level above the 95th percentile in the first 24 hours is some form of hemolysis. It may not always be possible to identify the exact cause of the hemolysis but the infant must be considered to have a hemolytic disease until proved otherwise.

3. Additional tests would include blood groups on the mother and infant, a direct antiglobulin test (DAT or direct Coombs' test), a reticulocyte count, and a CBC that includes evaluation of the peripheral smear. ABO hemolytic disease is the most likely diagnosis.

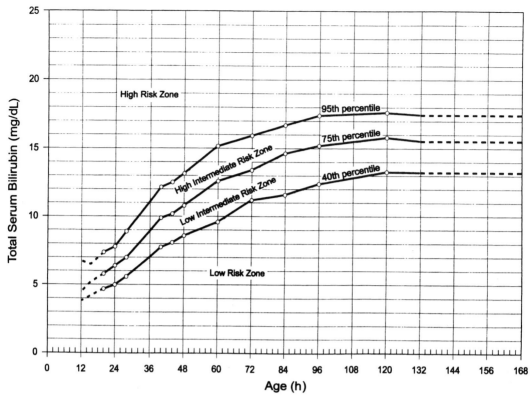

Figure 5-6 Establishing "risk zones" for hyperbilirubinemia in newborns. This nomogram is based on hour-specific bilirubin values obtained from 2840 well newborns at or above 36 weeks' gestational age with birth weight at least 2000 g or at or above 35 weeks' gestational age and a birth weight of at least 2500 g. The serum bilirubin level was obtained before discharge. The risk zone in which the value fell predicted the likelihood of a subsequent bilirubin level exceeding the 95th percentile. (From Bhutani VK, Johnson L, Sivieri EM: Predictive ability of a predischarge hour-specific serum bilirubin for subsequent significant hyperbilirubinemia in healthy-term and near-term newborns. Pediatrics 1999;103:6–14.)

4. For this age and TSB level, the AAP guidelines for phototherapy (Fig. 5-7) recommend hospitalization and intensive phototherapy.

5. In this infant the problem was clearly some kind of hemolytic process and there was no reason to interrupt breastfeeding. Once the infant was admitted and received intensive phototherapy, the TSB fell and it was obvious from the subsequent hemoglobin level of 12.2 g/dL that hemolysis was occurring.

6. Table 5-6 lists the causes of hemolysis that need to be considered. The blood types of the mother and infant were both O-Rh positive and the DAT was negative. The baby looked well and was nursing well (ruling out sepsis) and there was no bruising and no cephalhematoma. At this stage, the most likely diagnosis was one of the heritable causes of hemolysis. The first to be considered is G6PD deficiency. This infant was a female, which makes this diagnosis less likely, although female G6PD-deficient heterozygotes can certainly develop severe hyperbilirubinemia. The peripheral smear showed the features typical of congenital Heinz body hemolytic anemia (unstable hemoglobin).

ABO Hemolytic Disease

Hemolysis from ABO incompatibility is by far the most common cause of isoimmune hemolytic disease in newborn infants. In about 15% of pregnancies, an infant with blood type A or B is carried by a mother who is type O. About one third of these infants will have a positive DAT, indicating that they have anti-A or anti-B antibodies attached to the red blood cells. Of these infants, however, only 20% develop a peak TSB above 12.8 mg/dL (224 µmol/L). Consequently, although ABO-incompatible DAT-positive infants are about twice as likely as their compatible peers to have moderate hyperbiliru-

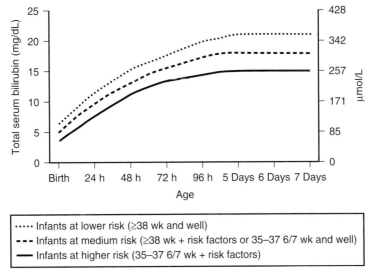

Figure 5-7 AAP guidelines for phototherapy in hospitalized infants of 35 or more weeks' gestation. Note: These guidelines are based on limited evidence and the levels shown are approximations. The guidelines refer to the use of intensive phototherapy, which should be used when the TSB exceeds the line indicated for each category. Infants are designated as "higher risk" because of the potential negative effects of the conditions listed on albumin binding of bilirubin, the blood-brain barrier, and the susceptibility of the brain cells to damage by bilirubin. "Intensive phototherapy" implies irradiance in the blue-green spectrum (wavelengths of approximately 430 to 490 nm) of at least 30 μW/cm^2/nm (measured at the infant's skin directly below the center of the phototherapy unit) and delivered to as much of the infant's surface area as possible. Note that irradiance measured below the center of the light source is much greater than that measured at the periphery. Measurements should be made with a radiometer specified by the manufacturer of the phototherapy system. If total serum bilirubin levels approach or exceed the exchange transfusion line (see Fig. 5-8), the sides of the bassinet, incubator, or warmer should be lined with aluminum foil or white material. This will increase the surface area of the infant exposed and increase the efficacy of phototherapy. If the total serum bilirubin does not decrease or continues to rise in an infant who is receiving intensive phototherapy, this strongly suggests the presence of hemolysis. Infants who receive phototherapy and have an elevated direct-reacting or conjugated bilirubin level (cholestatic jaundice) may develop the bronze-baby syndrome. (From Maisels MJ, Baltz RD, Bhutani V, et al: Management of hyperbilirubinemia in the newborn infant 35 or more weeks of gestation. Pediatrics 2004;114:297–316; reproduced with permission from Pediatrics, copyright © 2004 by the AAP.)

binemia, severe jaundice in these infants is uncommon. Nevertheless, ABO hemolytic disease can cause severe hyperbilirubinemia and kernicterus.

Diagnosing ABO Hemolytic Disease

ABO hemolytic disease is highly variable in its clinical presentation. Most infants present with a rapid rise in TSB levels within the first 24 hours, but in many, the TSB subsequently declines, often without any intervention. ABO hemolytic disease is a relatively common cause of early hyperbilirubinemia (before the infant leaves the nursery), but it is a relatively rare cause of hyperbilirubinemia in infants who have been discharged and readmitted (Table 5-7). The criteria for diagnosing ABO hemolytic disease as the cause of neonatal hyperbilirubinemia are listed in Table 5-8. Recently, it has been shown that DAT negative ABO-incompatible infants who also have Gilbert syndrome are at risk for hyperbilirubinemia. This may explain the occasional ABO-incompatible infant with a negative DAT who, nevertheless, develops early hyperbilirubinemia.

Glucose-6-Phosphate Dehydrogenase Deficiency

G6PD deficiency is the most common, clinically significant, red blood cell enzyme defect, and it affects as many as 4.5 million newborns, worldwide, each year. Although known for its prevalence in the populations of the Mediterranean, the Middle East, the Arabian Peninsula, South East Asia, and Africa, immigration and intermarriage have transformed G6PD into a global problem. Nevertheless, most pediatricians in the United States do not think of G6PD deficiency when confronted with a jaundiced infant, and they should, particularly in black infants. Although black newborns, as a group, tend to have lower TSB levels than white newborns, G6PD deficiency is found in 11% to 13% of black newborns. This means that some 32,000 to 39,000 black male G6PD-deficient hemizygous newborns are born annually in

TABLE 5-7

DISCHARGE DIAGNOSIS IN 306 INFANTS ADMITTED WITH SEVERE HYPERBILIRUBINEMIA*

Diagnosis	Number	Percentage
Hyperbilirubinemia of unknown cause or breast milk jaundice	290	94.8
Cephalhematoma or bruising	3	1.0
ABO hemolytic disease[†]	11	3.6
Anti-E hemolytic disease	1	0.3
Galactosemia	1	0.3
Sepsis	0	

*Infants were readmitted after discharge as newborns. Mean age at admission was 5 days (range, 2–17 days), and mean bilirubin level was 18.5 ± 2.8 mg/dL (range, 12.7–29.1 mg/dL).
[†]Mother was type O, infant was type A or B, direct Coombs' test was positive.
From Maisels MJ, Kring E: Risk of sepsis in newborns with severe hyperbilirubinemia. Pediatrics 1992;90:741–743.

TABLE 5-8

CRITERIA FOR DIAGNOSING ABO HEMOLYTIC DISEASE AS THE CAUSE OF NEONATAL HYPERBILIRUBINEMIA

Mother group O, infant group A or B *and*
  Positive DAT
  Jaundice appearing within 12–24 hours
  Microspherocytes on blood smear
  Negative DAT but homozygous for Gilbert syndrome

From Maisels MJ: Jaundice. In MacDonald MG, Seshia MMK, Mullett MD (eds): Neonatology: Pathophysiology and Management of the Newborn, 6th ed. Philadelphia, Lippincott, 2005, pp 768–846.

the United States. As many as 30% of infants with kernicterus in the United States have been found to be G6PD deficient.

The G6PD gene is located on the X chromosome, and hemizygous males have the full enzyme deficiency, although female heterozygotes are also at risk for hyperbilirubinemia. G6PD-deficient neonates have an increase in heme turnover, although overt evidence of hemolysis is often not present. In addition, these infants have impaired ability to conjugate bilirubin.

Management of Neonatal Hyperbilirubinemia

Case Study 3

A 36-week gestation, breastfed male infant was discharged from hospital at age 30 hours with instructions to be seen by the pediatrician when the infant was 2 weeks old. On the sixth day the mother returned to the pediatrician's office because the infant was refusing the breast and was lethargic. She reported that he had appeared increasingly jaundiced over the previous 2 days and was not nursing as well. On examination he was bright yellow and had arching of his back and a TSB level of 38.5 mg/dL (658 μmol/L). On admission, his hemoglobin was 17.5 g/dL, reticulocyte count 1%, and the peripheral smear was normal. Blood groups on the mother and baby were both A-positive. An immediate exchange transfusion was performed.

Exercise 5

QUESTIONS

1. How could this problem have been prevented?

2. Would an early follow-up have helped?

3. This infant had clinical signs of the intermediate phase of acute bilirubin encephalopathy (see Table 5-3 and Fig. 5-3). What test would confirm this diagnosis?

ANSWERS

1. This infant had two of the major risk factors for the development of severe hyperbilirubinemia (see Table 5-12)—he was only 36 weeks' gestation and was exclusively breastfed. A follow-up appointment should have been scheduled no later than 2 days after discharge.

2. The infant was 140 hours old when the TSB was 38.5 mg/dL (658 μmol/L). As the cord bilirubin level is approximately 1.5 mg/dL (26 μmol/L), he had an increase of 37 mg/dL (633 μmol/L) of bilirubin in

TABLE 5-9

ROOT CAUSES OF REPORTED CASES OF KERNICTERUS

Early discharge with failure to ensure appropriate follow-up

Failure to evaluate the measured total serum bilirubin level based on the infant's age in hours.

Failure to recognize risk factors for severe hyperbilirubinemia

Underestimating the severity of jaundice by clinical (i.e., visual) assessment

Lack of concern regarding the neurotoxic potential of bilirubin

From Maisels MJ: Jaundice. In MacDonald MG, Seshia MMK, Mullett MD (eds): Neonatology: Pathophysiology and Management of the Newborn, 6th ed. Philadelphia, Lippincott, 2005, pp 768–846.

140 hours, a rate of rise (assuming a linear increase) of 0.26 mg/dL/hour (4.4 μmol/L/hour), well above the upper limit of about 0.2 mg/dL/hour (3.4 μmol/L/hour). If he had been seen by the pediatrician within 48 hours of discharge, it is most likely that jaundice would have been noted and a bilirubin level obtained. At age 72 hours (40 hours after discharge), based on the rate of rise of the bilirubin, his TSB would have been about 20 mg/dL (344 μmol/L) and intensive phototherapy would have taken care of the problem.

3. An MRI.

We have had to change our approach to the management of neonatal jaundice because we still see kernicterus and because the hospital stay for infants is now so short. The root causes of reported cases of kernicterus are shown in Table 5-9 and the AAP has addressed this question in its 2004 clinical practice guidelines. The key elements of these guidelines are shown in Table 5-10.

TABLE 5-10

CAUSES OF PROLONGED INDIRECT HYPERBILIRUBINEMIA

Breast milk jaundice	Crigler-Najjar syndrome
Hemolytic disease	Gilbert syndrome
Hypothyroidism	Extravascular blood
Pyloric stenosis	

From Maisels MJ: Jaundice. In MacDonald MG, Seshia MMK, Mullett MD (eds): Neonatology: Pathophysiology and Management of the Newborn, 6th ed. Philadelphia, Lippincott, 2005, pp 768–846.

Visual Assessment of Jaundice

For years we have relied on identifying jaundice by blanching the skin with digital pressure to reveal the underlying color of the skin and subcutaneous tissue. Although this remains a fundamentally important clinical sign, we must recognize that it has its limitations and can be unreliable, particularly in darkly pigmented infants. The difference between a TSB level of 5 mg/dL (85 μmol/L) and 8 mg/dL (137 μmol/L) cannot be perceived by the eye, yet at 24 hours that is the difference between the 50th and the 95th percentiles (see Fig. 5-5). The potential errors associated with visual diagnosis have led some experts to recommend that all newborns should have a TSB or a transcutaneous bilirubin (TcB) level performed prior to discharge.

Measurement of Total Serum Bilirubin

The usual laboratory tests (hematocrit, CBC, reticulocyte count, and smear) are often not helpful in identifying a specific cause for hyperbilirubinemia. Nevertheless, the cause of jaundice should be sought in an infant whose TSB level is crossing percentiles or if the rate of rise exceeds 0.2 mg/dL/hour (3.4 μmol/kg/hour).

Any infant jaundiced within the first 24 hours requires a TcB or TSB measurement, and a TcB or TSB level should also be done if, at any time, the jaundice appears excessive for the infant's age. Because of the risk of error in visual assessment, particularly in darkly pigmented infants, a TcB or TSB should be measured if there is any doubt about the degree of jaundice.

Prolonged Jaundice

Infants who are jaundiced beyond age 3 weeks require measurement of a total and direct (or conjugated) bilirubin level to identify cholestasis. If the direct-reacting or conjugated bilirubin level is elevated (>1 mg/dL if TSB <5 mg/dL, or $>20\%$ of total if TSB >5 mg/dL), additional evaluation is needed for the causes of cholestasis. Infants who are jaundiced beyond 3 weeks should also have the results of the newborn thyroid and galactosemia screen checked. Table 5-10 lists the causes of prolonged indirect-reacting hyperbilirubinemia.

Preventing Hyperbilirubinemia and Kernicterus

The only primary preventive intervention available to physicians is to ensure the adequacy and success of breastfeeding. Infants who nurse frequently and effectively in the first few days are much less likely to develop hyperbilirubinemia. In many cases of severe hyperbilirubinemia in breastfed infants, poor caloric intake associated with inadequate breastfeeding appears to play an important role.

If we followed all the key elements of the AAP guidelines (Table 5-11), we would be able to prevent almost all cases of kernicterus. One of the most important recommendations in the guidelines is to perform a predischarge, systematic assessment on all infants for the risk of severe hyperbilirubinemia. These risk factors are listed in Table 5-12. Because the clinical risk factors are common while the risk of severe hyperbilirubinemia is small, individually they are of limited use as predictors of severe hyperbilirubinemia. Collectively, they are helpful. If no risk factor is present, the risk of hyperbilirubinemia is very low; the more risk factors that are present, the greater the risk of severe hyperbilirubinemia. Breastfeeding, decreasing gestation, and significant jaundice in a previous sibling are particularly important risk factors.

Predischarge Measurement of the Bilirubin Level

Infants who are clinically jaundiced in the first few days are much more likely to develop significant hyperbilirubinemia. This risk has now been quantified (see Fig. 5-6). Infants with predischarge TSB levels above the 95th percentile (high-risk zone) had a 40% risk of subsequently developing a TSB level above the 95th percentile, and those whose predischarge TSB values were in the low-risk zone (less than the 40th percentile) were at very low risk for subsequently developing significant hyperbilirubinemia. Combining a predischarge measurement of the TSB or TcB with risk factors provides the best indication of the risk, or absence of risk, that the infant will develop severe hyperbilirubinemia.

Follow-up

Identifying the infant's risk of severe hyperbilirubinemia is of little value without appropriate follow-up. The AAP guideline recommends that any infant discharged at less than 72 hours should be seen within 2 days of discharge. Infants with many risk factors might need to be seen earlier (within 24 hours of discharge), whereas those discharged with few or no risk factors could be seen after a longer interval.

Information for Parents

An essential component of ensuring the safety of a newborn is to inform parents about jaundice. The AAP has produced a parent information document entitled "Jaundice FAQs," available in four languages at www.aap.org.

TABLE 5-11

THE TEN COMMANDMENTS FOR PREVENTING AND MANAGING HYPERBILIRUBINEMIA*

1. Promote and support successful breastfeeding
2. Establish nursery protocols for the jaundiced newborn and permit nurses to obtain TSB levels without a physician's order
3. Measure the total serum bilirubin (TSB) or transcutaneous bilirubin (TcB) level on infants jaundiced in the first 24 hours
4. Recognize that visual diagnosis of jaundice is unreliable, particularly in darkly pigmented infants
5. Interpret all TSB levels according to the infant's age in hours, not days
6. Don't treat a near-term (35–38 week) infant as you would a term infant—a near-term infant is at much higher risk of hyperbilirubinemia
7. Perform a predischarge, systematic assessment on all infants for the risk of severe hyperbilirubinemia
8. Provide parents with information about newborn jaundice
9. Provide follow-up based on the time of discharge and the risk assessment
10. When indicated, treat the newborn with phototherapy or exchange transfusion

*Adapted from the American Academy of Pediatrics guidelines on hyperbilirubinemia.
Reprinted with permission from Maisels MJ: Jaundice in a newborn: How to head off an urgent situation. Contemp Pediatr 2005;22:41–54. *Contemporary Pediatrics* is a copyrighted publication of Advanstar Communications Inc. All rights reserved.

TABLE 5-12

RISK FACTORS FOR DEVELOPMENT OF SEVERE HYPERBILIRUBINEMIA IN INFANTS 35 OR MORE WEEKS OF GESTATION (IN APPROXIMATE ORDER OF IMPORTANCE)

Major Risk Factors
Predischarge total serum bilirubin (TSB) or transcutaneous bilirubin (TcB) level in the high risk zone (Fig. 5-6)
Jaundice observed in the first 24 hours
Blood group incompatibility with positive direct antiglobulin test, other known hemolytic disease (e.g., G6PD deficiency), elevated ETCOc.
Gestational age 35–36 weeks
Previous sibling received phototherapy
Cephalhematoma or significant bruising
Exclusive breastfeeding particularly if nursing is not going well and weight loss is excessive
East Asian race*

Minor Risk Factors
Predischarge TSB or TcB in the high to intermediate risk zone (see Fig. 5-6)
Gestational age 37–38 weeks
Jaundice observed before discharge
Previous sibling with jaundice
Macrosomic infant of a diabetic mother
Maternal age ≥ 25 years
Male gender

Decreased Risk
These factors are associated with decreased risk of significant jaundice, listed in order of decreasing importance.
TSB or TcB in the low risk zone (see Fig. 5-6)
Gestational age ≥ 41 weeks
Exclusive bottle feeding
Black race*
Discharge from hospital after 72 hours

*Race as defined by mother's description.
ETCOc, end tidal carbon monoxide (CO) corrected for ambient CO
From Maisels MJ, Baltz RD, Bhutani V, et al: Management of hyperbilirubinemia in the newborn infant 35 or more weeks of gestation. Pediatrics 2004;114:297–316.

Treatment

Hyperbilirubinemia can be treated in three ways: (a) exchange transfusion removes bilirubin mechanically, (b) phototherapy converts bilirubin to products that can bypass the liver's conjugating system and be excreted in the bile or in the urine without further metabolism, and (c) pharmacologic agents interfere with heme degradation and bilirubin production, accelerate the normal metabolic pathways for bilirubin clearance, or inhibit the enterohepatic circulation of bilirubin. Guidelines for the use of phototherapy and exchange transfusion in term and near-term infants are provided in Figures 5-7 and 5-8.

Phototherapy

Phototherapy works by infusing discrete photons of energy, similar to the molecules of a drug. These photons are absorbed by bilirubin molecules in the skin and subcutaneous tissue, just as drug molecules bind to a receptor. The bilirubin then undergoes photochemical reactions to form excretable isomers and break down products that can bypass the liver's conjugating system and be excreted without further metabolism. Some photochemical products are also excreted in the urine. Figure 5-9 depicts the mechanism of action of phototherapy.

Like drugs, phototherapy displays a dose-response effect, and a number of variables influence how light works to lower the TSB level. Table 5-13 shows the radiometric units used in measuring the dose of phototherapy and Tables 5-14 and 5-15 show the factors that affect the dose and efficacy of phototherapy, including type of light source, the infant's distance from the light, and the surface area exposed.

Light Sources

The light sources currently used to deliver phototherapy include fluorescent tubes, halogen lamps, light-emitting diodes (LEDs), and fiberoptic systems. Because of the optical properties of bilirubin and skin, the most effective lights are those with a wavelength predominately in the blue-green spectrum (425 to 490 nm). At these wavelengths light penetrates the skin well and is absorbed maximally by bilirubin. If fluorescent lights are used, they should be special blue fluorescent tubes (labeled F20T12/BB). Recently developed LED lights are also an effective means of providing intensive phototherapy, and fiberoptic systems are useful for providing additional phototherapy beneath the infant to increase the surface area exposed.

Using Phototherapy Effectively

Phototherapy was initially used in low-birthweight and full-term infants primarily to prevent slowly rising serum bilirubin levels from reaching levels that might require an exchange transfusion. Today, phototherapy is often used in full-term and near-term infants who have left the hospital and are readmitted on days 4 to 7 for treatment of TSB levels of 20 mg/dL

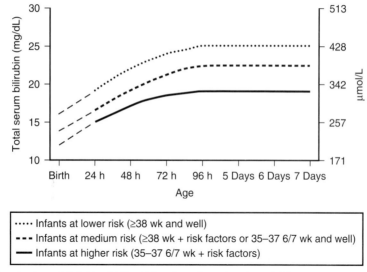

Figure 5-8 American Academy of Pediatrics (AAP) guidelines for exchange transfusion in infants 35 or more weeks' gestation. Note that these suggested levels are based on limited evidence, and the levels shown are approximations. During birth hospitalization, exchange transfusion is recommended if the total serum bilirubin (TSB) rises to these levels despite intensive phototherapy. For readmitted infants, if the TSB level is above the exchange level, repeat TSB measurement every 2 to 3 hours and consider exchange if the TSB remains above the levels indicated after intensive phototherapy for 6 hours. If the TSB is at or approaching the exchange level, send blood for immediate type and crossmatch. Blood for exchange transfusion is modified whole blood (red cells and plasma) crossmatched against the mother and compatible with the infant. (From Maisels MJ, Baltz RD, Bhutani V, et al: Management of hyperbilirubinemia in the newborn infant 35 or more weeks of gestation. Pediatrics 2004;114:297–316; reproduced with permission from Pediatrics, copyright © 2004 by the AAP.)

B:A RATIO AT WHICH EXCHANGE TRANSFUSION SHOULD BE CONSIDERED

Risk Category	TSB mg/dL/Alb, g/dL	TSB μmol/L/Alb, μmol/L
Infants ≥ 38 0/7 wk	8.0	0.94
Infants 35 0/7 to 36 6/7 wk and well, or ≥ 38 0/7 wk if higher risk or isoimmune hemolytic disease or G6PD deficiency	7.2	0.84
Infants 35 0/7 to 37 6/7 wk if higher risk, or isoimmune hemolytic disease or G6PD deficiency	6.8	0.80

These B/A ratios can be used together with, but not in lieu of, the TSB level as an additional factor in determining the need for exchange transfusion.

(342 μmol/L) or more. These infants need a full therapeutic dose of phototherapy (now termed intensive phototherapy) to get the bilirubin level down as soon as possible. Intensive phototherapy implies the use of irradiance in the 430- to 490-nm band of at least 30 μW/cm^2/nm delivered to as much of the infant's surface area as possible. To achieve this, fluorescent tubes should be placed as close to the infant as possible. This is done by having an infant in a bassinette, not an incubator, so that the fluorescent tubes can be brought to within about 10 cm of the infant. Because tungsten, halogen, or other types of spot phototherapy lamps produce considerable heat, they *should not be positioned closer to the infant than recommended by the manufacturers because of the risk of a burn.*

Maximizing Surface Exposure

Increasing the surface area exposed to phototherapy will significantly improve its efficacy. This is done by placing fiberoptic pads below the infant, or using a phototherapy device that delivers phototherapy from special blue fluorescent tubes both above and below the infant. When intensive phototherapy is appropriately applied, a decrement in the bilirubin level of 30% to 40% can be expected in the first 24

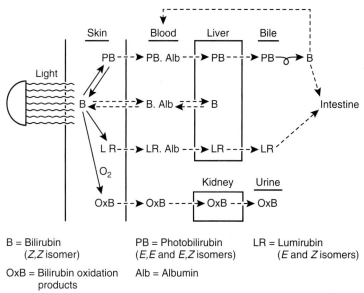

Figure 5-9 General mechanisms of phototherapy for neonatal jaundice. Chemical reactions (*solid arrows*) and transport processes (*broken arrows*) are indicated. Pigments may be bound to proteins in compartments other than blood. Some excretion of photoisomers, particularly lumirubin, in urine also occurs. (From McDonagh AF, Lightner DA: "Like a Shrivelled Blood Orange"—Bilirubin, jaundice and phototherapy. Pediatrics 1985;75:443–455; reproduced with permission from Pediatrics, copyright © 1985 by the AAP.)

TABLE 5-13

RADIOMETRIC QUANTITIES USED IN PHOTOTHERAPY

Quantity	Dimensions	Usual Units of Measure
Irradiance (radiant power incident on a surface per unit area of the surface)	W/m^2	W/cm^2
Spectral irradiance (irradiance in a certain wavelength band)	W/m^2 per nm (or W/m^2)	$\mu W/cm^2$ per nm

From Maisels MJ: Why use homeopathic doses of phototherapy? Pediatrics 1996;98:283–287; copyright © 1996 by the AAP.

---

hours, with the most significant decline occurring in the first 4 to 6 hours.

Exchange Transfusion

There has been a dramatic decline in the number of exchange transfusions performed as a result of the use of anti-D immunoglobulin to prevent Rh disease and the use of effective phototherapy. It is now possible for a pediatric resident to complete a 3-year training program without ever having performed an exchange transfusion or even witnessed one.

Pharmacologic Treatment

Pharmacologic agents such as phenobarbital and ursodeoxycholic acid improve bile flow and can help to lower bilirubin levels. Tin mesoporphyrin is a drug that will inhibit heme oxygenase and therefore the production of bilirubin (see Fig. 5-2). To date, more than 500 newborns have received tin mesoporphyrin in controlled trials, but the drug is still awaiting FDA approval. Other drugs have been used to inhibit the enterohepatic circulation of bilirubin. Most recently, a controlled trial showed that agents that inhibit β-glucuronidase

TABLE 5-14

CONTROLLING THE DOSAGE OF PHOTOTHERAPY

Factor	Technical Terminology	Rationale	Clinical Application
Type of light source	Spectrum of light (nanometers)	Blue-green spectrum is most effective at lowering total serum bilirubin (TSB); light at this wavelength penetrates skin well and is absorbed maximally by bilirubin	Use special blue fluorescent tubes or light-emitting diodes (LEDs) or another light source with output in blue-green spectrum for intensive phototherapy (PT)
Distance of light source from patient	Spectral irradiance (a function of both distance and light source) delivered to surface of infant	↑ irradiance leads to ↑ rate of decline in TSB. Standard PT units deliver 8–10 μW/cm^2/nm; intensive PT delivers $\geq$ 30 μW/cm^2/nm	If special blue fluorescent tubes are used, bring tubes as close as possible to infant to increase irradiance (do *not* do this with halogen lamps because of danger of burn); positioning special blue tubes 10–15 cm above infant will produce an irradiance of at least 35 μW/cm^2/nm
Surface area exposed	Spectral power (a function of spectral irradiance and surface area)	↑ surface area exposed leads to ↑ rate of decline in TSB	For intensive PT, expose maximum surface area of infant to PT; place lights above and fiberoptic pad or special blue fluorescent tubes* below infant; for maximum exposure, line sides of bassinet, warmer bed, or incubator with aluminum foil

*Available in the Bili-Bassinet (Olympic Medical).
From Maisels MJ: A primer on phototherapy for the jaundiced newborn. Contemp Pediatr 2005;22:38–57.
Contemporary Pediatrics is a copyrighted publication of Advanstar Communications Inc. All rights reserved.

TABLE 5-15

FACTORS THAT INFLUENCE THE EFFICACY OF PHOTOTHERAPY

Factor	Explanation	Clinical action
Dosage	See Table 5-14	See Table 5-14
Cause of jaundice	Phototherapy (PT) is likely to be less effective if jaundice is caused by hemolysis or if cholestasis is present (direct bilirubin is increased)	When hemolysis is present, start PT at a lower TSB level and use intensive PT; failure of PT suggests hemolysis is cause of the jaundice; when direct bilirubin is elevated, watch for bronze baby syndrome or blistering
TSB level at start of PT	The higher the TSB, the more rapid the decline in TSB with PT	Use intensive PT for higher TSB levels; anticipate a more rapid decrease in TSB when TSB > 20 mg/dL

From Maisels MJ: A primer on phototheray for the jaundiced newborn. Contemp Pediatr 2005;22:38–57. *Contemporary Pediatrics* is a copyrighted publication of Advanstar Communications Inc. All rights reserved.

can decrease bilirubin levels in breastfed newborns.

In infants with isoimmune hemolytic disease, the administration of intravenous immunoglobulin will significantly reduce the need for exchange transfusion.

Suggested Readings

Bhutani V, Gourley GR, Adler S, et al: Noninvasive measurement of total serum bilirubin in a multiracial predischarge newborn population to assess the risk of severe hyperbilirubinemia. Pediatrics 2000;106: e17.

Bhutani VK, Johnson LH, Maisels MJ, et al: Kernicterus: Epidemiological strategies for its prevention through systems-based approaches. J Perinatol 2004; 24: 650–662.

Bhutani VK, Johnson L, Sivieri EM: Predictive ability of a predischarge hour-specific serum bilirubin for subsequent significant hyperbilirubinemia in healthy-term and near-term newborns. Pediatrics 1999;103:6–14.

Ennever JF: Blue light, green light, white light, more light: Treatment of neonatal jaundice. Clin Perinatol 1990;17:467–481.

Gourley GR, Li Z, Kreamer BL, Kosorok MR: A controlled, randomized, double-blind trial of prophylaxis against jaundice among breastfed newborns. Pediatrics 2005;116:385–391.

Ip S, Chung M, Kulig J, et al: An evidence-based review of important issues concerning neonatal hyperbilirubinemia. Pediatrics 2004;114:e130–e153.

Kaplan M, Hammerman C: Control of hyperbilirubinemia in glucose-6-phosphate dehydrogenase–deficient newborns. Pediatrics 1999;103:536–537.

Kaplan M, Hammerman C: Severe neonatal hyperbilirubinemia: A potential complication of glucose-6-phosphate dehydrogenase deficiency. Clin Perinatol 1998;25:575–590.

Kaplan M, Hammerman C, Maisels MJ: Bilirubin genetics for the nongeneticist: Hereditary defects of neonatal bilirubin conjugation. Pediatrics 2003;111:886–893.

Kaplan M, Hammerman C, Renbaum P, et al: Gilbert's syndrome and hyperbilirubinaemia in ABO-incompatible neonates. Lancet 2000;356:652–653.

Kaplan M, Herschel M, Hammerman C, et al: Hyperbilirubinemia among African American, glucose-6-phosphate dehydrogenase–deficient neonates. Pediatrics 2004;114:e213–e219.

Kappas A: A method for interdicting the development of severe jaundice in newborns by inhibiting the production of bilirubin. Pediatrics 2004;113:119–123.

Maisels MJ: Jaundice. In MacDonald MG, Seshia MMK, Mullett MD (eds): Neonatology: Pathophysiology and Management of the Newborn. Philadelphia, Lippincott, 2005, pp 768–846.

Maisels MJ: A primer on phototherapy for the jaundiced newborn. Contemp Pediatr 2005;22:38–57.

Maisels MJ: Transcutaneous bilirubin levels in a normal newborn population ≥35 weeks gestation in the first 96 hours. Pediatrics 2006;117:1169–1173.

Maisels MJ: Why use homeopathic doses of phototherapy? Pediatrics 1996;98:283–287.

Maisels MJ, Baltz RD, Bhutani V, et al: Management of hyperbilirubinemia in the newborn infant 35 or more weeks of gestation. Pediatrics 2004;114:297–316.

Maisels MJ, Kring E: Risk of sepsis in newborns with severe hyperbilirubinemia. Pediatrics 1992;90: 741–743.

Maisels MJ, Newman TB: Jaundice in full term and near-term babies who leave the hospital within 36 hours. The pediatrician's nemesis. Clin Perinatol 1998; 25:295–302.

Maisels MJ, Newman TB: Kernicterus in otherwise healthy, breast-fed term newborns. Pediatrics 1995;96:730–733.

Maisels MJ, Ostrea EJ Jr, Touch S, et al: Evaluation of a new transcutaneous bilirubinometer. Pediatrics 2004;113:1628–1635.

Maisels MJ, Watchko JF: Neonatal Jaundice. London, Harwood Academic Publishers, 2000.

Maisels MJ, Watchko JF: Treatment of jaundice in low birthweight infants. Arch Dis Child Fetal Neonatol Ed 2003;88:F459–F463.

McDonagh AF, Lightner DA: "Like a Shrivelled Blood Orange"—Bilirubin, jaundice and phototherapy. Pediatrics 1985;75:443–455.

Newman TB, Klebanoff MA: Neonatal hyperbilirubinemia and long-term outcome: Another look at the collaborative perinatal project. Pediatrics 1993; 92:651–657.

Newman TB, Liljestrand P, Escobar GJ: Combining clinical risk factors with bilirubin levels to predict hyperbilirubinemia in newborns. Arch Pediatr Adolesc Med 2005;159:113–119.

Newman TB, Liljestrand P, Escobar GJ: Jaundice noted in the first 24 hours after birth in a managed care organization. Arch Pediatr Adolesc Med 2002; 156:1244–1250.

Newman TB, Xiong B, Gonzales VM, Escobar GJ: Prediction and prevention of extreme neonatal hyperbilirubinemia in a mature health maintenance organization. Arch Pediatr Adolesc Med 2000; 154:1140–1147.

Stevenson DK, Dennery PA, Hintz SR: Understanding newborn jaundice. J Perinatol 2001;21:S21–S24.

Stevenson DK, Vreman HJ: Carbon monoxide and bilirubin production in neonates. Pediatrics 1997; 100:252–254.

Vreman HJ, Wong RJ, Stevenson DK: Phototherapy: Current methods and future directions. Semin Perinatol 2004;28:326–333.

Watchko JF, Maisels MJ: Jaundice in low birth weight infants—Pathobiology and outcome. Arch Dis Child Fetal Neonatol Ed 2003;88:F456–F459.

Parenteral Nutrition

Gilberto R. Pereira, MD

Total parenteral nutrition (TPN) is indicated for neonates in whom enteral feedings are contraindicated or being provided in insufficient amounts. The length of time that a neonate can tolerate starvation depends on the infant's nutritional status, coexisting clinical conditions, and degree of prematurity. Neonates who are born prematurely and those who are either malnourished or small for gestational age should routinely be started on parenteral nutrition as soon as enteral feedings are being withheld or provided in insufficient amounts. This practice allows for the replenishment of their depleted nutrient stores and resumption of growth. Early commencement of parenteral nutrition solutions containing dextrose, amino acids, and calcium are recommended for use within the first 24 hours of life to critically ill and premature infants who are too sick for the initiation of enteral feedings.

Mode of Delivery

Parenteral nutrition is delivered by peripheral or central vein catheters. Peripheral vein catheters are used on patients who have adequate venous access and on those who are expected to require parenteral nutrition for relatively short periods (1 to 2 weeks). When TPN is delivered by peripheral vein, the osmolality of the infusate should not exceed 1000 mOsm/L to decrease the risk of complications resulting from fluid extravasation. Major factors contributing to the increase in osmolality of the infusate include dextrose concentrations greater than 10%, small volume

of the infusate, and high concentrations of amino acids and electrolytes. Therefore, peripheral vein TPN provides, in general, only up to 80 to 90 kcal/kg/day, even when combined with intravenous fat emulsions. A central venous catheter should be placed for nutritional support in infants who have poor venous access or in those who require fluid restriction, TPN for periods longer than 2 weeks, and energy intakes greater than those provided by a peripheral vein. Although there is an increased risk of serious infection with the use of central catheters, aseptic techniques can reduce the incidence of infection to 2% to 5%.

Composition

The composition of standard TPN solutions developed for use in neonates is presented in Table 6-1.

Energy

During parenteral nutrition, energy requirements are lower than those during enteral nutrition, because energy is neither lost in stools nor required for absorption of nutrients by the gastrointestinal tract. Energy requirements are also lower in infants receiving muscle paralysis for mechanical ventilation or heavy sedation for extracorporeal membrane oxygenation (ECMO) therapy due to their decreased physical activity. Recommended energy intakes during parenteral nutrition are 90 to 100 kcal/kg/day for full-term infants, 90 to 110 kcal/kg/day for premature

TABLE 6-1

COMPOSITION OF STANDARD TOTAL
PARENTERAL NUTRITION SOLUTIONS (Per 100 mL)

Component	Preterm	Full Term
Amino acids*	1.5/2.0/2.5/3.0[†]	1.5/2.0/2.5/3.0[†]
Dextrose*	10/15/20	10/15/20
Sodium (mEq)	4	4
Potassium (mEq)	2	2
Chloride (mEq)	4.6	4.6
Calcium (mg)	600	400
Phosphorus (mEq)	1.4	1.4
Magnesium (mEq)	0.4	0.4
Zinc (μg)	500	300
Copper (μg)	60	20
Chromium (μg)	0.17	0.17
Manganese (μg)	5	5
Selenium (μg)	3	3
Iodine (μg)	8	8
Iron (μg)[‡]	0.1	0.1
Heparin (U)[§]	50	100

*Available standard amino acid and dextrose concentrations (g/100 mL).
[†]TrophAmine or Aminosyn.
[‡]Iron is added for all infants, including premature infants, after 8 weeks of life.
[§]See text for discussion of heparin dose.

in neonates. The rationale for the routine administration of amino acids during parenteral nutrition is to provide nitrogen for protein synthesis and growth. In addition, amino acids can be oxidized as substrate for energy source. Recommended intakes of intravenous amino acids vary with the gestational age of the infant. Full-term infants require 2 to 2.5 g/kg/day, and preterm infants require 3 to 3.5 g/kg/day. Two pediatric amino acid formulations have been designed for newborn infants using as a standard the postprandial plasma amino acid levels of breastfed neonates. In comparison to others, these preparations have an increased ratio of essential to nonessential amino acids and increased concentrations of amino acids considered essential for premature infants, such as taurine, tyrosine, and cysteine. These amino acid preparations are recommended for infants up to the age of 6 months. Cysteine is considered a conditionally essential amino acid for low-birth-weight infants. Contrary to previous reports, a study by Kashyap and coworkers reported somewhat greater amino acid utilization with the supplementation of cysteine hydrochloride (121 mg/kg/day) as compared with a control group receiving TPN without cysteine supplementation. This supplementation is also beneficial in lowering the pH of the TPN solution, thus increasing the solubility of calcium and phosphorus. The fetus is known to rapidly metabolize amino acids and even to use them as an energy source. Therefore, early postnatal supplementation of amino acids along with dextrose solutions is recommended for all critically ill or premature infants who are too sick to receive enteral feedings. This early supplementation prevents the onset of the starvation response, promotes positive nitrogen balance, and improves glucose tolerance by decreasing glucose production. When amino acids are

infants, and 80 to 90 kcal/kg/day in infants who are heavily sedated or paralyzed. The nonprotein caloric contribution to the total calorie intake is usually equally distributed between dextrose and fat emulsions. Calories derived from fat emulsions generally should not exceed more than 50% of the total calorie intake.

Amino Acids

Table 6-2 displays the caloric content of various amino acid–dextrose solutions used for TPN

TABLE 6-2

CONTENT OF MIXED DEXTROSE–AMINO ACID SOLUTIONS* FOR TOTAL PARENTERAL NUTRITION IN NEONATES (kcal/mL)

Dextrose Concentration	Amino Acid Concentration (%)			
	1.5	2.0	2.5	3.0
Dextrose 10%	0.40	0.42	0.44	0.46
Dextrose 15%	0.56	0.59	0.61	0.63
Dextrose 20%	0.74	0.76	0.78	0.80

*Amino acid and dextrose concentrations as g/100 mL.

used as an energy source, the oxidation of 1 g of amino acid provides 4 kcal.

Dextrose

Carbohydrates represent the major source of energy during parenteral nutrition and should provide 35% to 55% of the total caloric intake. Fructose, sorbitol, and ethanol have all been suggested as alternative substrates in neonates receiving parenteral nutrition, but they offer no clinical advantage over dextrose, which remains the carbohydrate of choice for parenteral nutrition. Whereas dextrose concentrations in excess of 10% should not be infused through peripheral vein catheters, dextrose concentrations ranging from 20% to 30% can be safely infused through central vein catheters. Dextrose concentrations should be increased in small increments to avoid hyperglycemia, especially in small premature infants.

Glucose intolerance can also occur in premature infants receiving glucose infusion at rates not exceeding their glucose turnover rates of 6 mg/kg/minute. The use of insulin infusions under those circumstances has been shown to promote euglycemia, increase calorie intake, and enhance growth. Nevertheless, this practice is controversial owing to reports of complications of insulin infusion in preterm infants that include (1) increased lactate formation and metabolic acidosis, (2) increased CO_2 production and pulmonary elimination, and (3) increased fat deposition in liver and adipose tissue. The oxidation of 1 g of dextrose yields 3.4 kcal. A schedule for the advancement of dextrose solutions in patients receiving parenteral nutrition by peripheral and central vein catheters is presented in Table 6-3.

Fat Emulsions

Along with amino acids and dextrose, fats are an essential component of the TPN regimen. There are at least three major advantages to administering fats intravenously: They are a source of essential fatty acids, they have a high caloric density (1 g providing 11 kcal), and they have a low osmolality, which makes them suitable for peripheral vein use. Despite the great number of fat emulsions currently available in the United States, they are all derived from either soybean or safflower oil. Both types of fat emulsions have been shown to be comparably effective in correcting essential fatty acid deficiency and in sparing nitrogen catabolism in neonates. Both safflower and soybean oil emulsions contain ample amounts of linoleic acids (75% and 50%, respectively), but the concentration of linolenic acid is lower in the safflower oil emulsion than in the soybean oil emulsion (0.5% versus 9%). Furthermore, it has recently been suggested that linolenic acid is an essential fatty acid in children receiving parenteral nutrition. For that reason, it seems prudent to use soybean fat emulsions in neonates until further studies determine that minimal requirement can be met by safflower emulsions. None of the oils contained in fat emulsions commercially available in the United States contain very long

---

TABLE 6-3

SCHEDULE FOR ADVANCEMENT AND MONITORING OF PARENTERAL NUTRITION SOLUTIONS

Peripheral Line TPN
Check TPN panel, electrolytes
Day 1: $D_{10}W$, protein as required, 2 g/kg/day fat emulsion
       Check serum electrolytes, Glu, BUN, Cr, TG after 24 hr
Day 2: Increase fat emulsion to 3 g/kg/day
       Check serum TG approximately 24 hr after increase in dose

Central Line TPN
Document line placement, TPN panel, electrolytes
Day 1: $D_{10}W$, protein as required, 2 g/kg/day fat emulsion
       Check serum electrolytes, Glu, BUN, Cr, TG after 24 hr
       If the patient was on a standard peripheral TPN solution ($D_{10}W$) before placement of central line, the solution may be changed to $D_{15}W$ or $D_{20}W$ after line placement is confirmed
       Check serum electrolytes, Glu, BUN, Cr, TG after 24 hr
Day 2*: Increase to $D_{20}W$ and increase fat emulsion to 3 g/kg/day, if additional calories are needed
       Check serum electrolytes, Glu, BUN, Cr, TG after 24 hr

---

*For premature infants, use more gradual increments in dextrose (2.5–5%/day) and in lipids (0.5–1 g/kg/day).
BUN, blood urea nitrogen; C, creatinine; DW, X=% of dextrose (D) in water (W); Glu, glucose; TG, triglycerides; TPN, total parenteral nutrition.

polyunsaturated fatty acids (VLPUFA), except for a small amount present in egg phospholipids used as emulsifiers. VLPUFA are now considered conditionally essential for premature infants, due to their recognized benefit in brain and retina development. Fat emulsions are available at concentrations of 10% and 20%. The 20% emulsions contain a reduced content of phospholipids per gram of triglyceride, which had been shown to improve lipid clearance. In addition, the use of a 20% emulsion allows for a smaller infusion volume, which may be beneficial in preventing fluid overload. The 10% emulsions are clinically preferred at low fat intakes (≤ 1g/kg/day) with the intent to provide a greater amount of VLPUFA.

Minerals and Vitamins

Suggested daily intakes of minerals and vitamins are presented in Table 6-4. Higher levels of some minerals (sodium, calcium, phosphorus, zinc, copper) are recommended for premature infants. It should be emphasized, however, that intakes of calcium and phosphorus greater than those that can be safely delivered in TPN solutions are necessary to promote bone mineralization in premature infants. Osteopenia therefore remains a nonpreventable complication in neonates dependent on long-term parenteral nutrition. Clinical strategies to safely increase calcium and phosphorus concentrations in TPN

include the addition of cysteine hydrochloride or a greater intake of amino acids to the infusate. Both additives increase the solubility of calcium and phosphorus by decreasing the pH of the infusate.

The high concentration of aluminum in several additives used for the preparation of TPN solutions has been recognized as a cause of aluminum accumulation in bone and central nervous system that could potentially lead to the development of osteopenia, fractures, and encephalopathy. Infants at risk of these complications include those who are born prematurely and those who have renal insufficiency and require prolonged courses of parenteral nutrition. In 2004, the FDA published a mandate calling for a reduction in the aluminum content of TPN additives. It was recommended to decrease the total aluminum exposure of infants to less than 5 µg/kg/day. Table 6-5 describes the aluminum concentration of different additives currently used for TPN preparation.

Table 6-6 displays the daily requirements for vitamins administered intravenously to children. As shown in this table, 5 mL of multivitamin pediatric preparation added to the parenteral nutrition solution meets these requirements for children younger than 11 years of age.

Heparin

Heparin should be provided in standard TPN solutions delivered by central vein catheters at concentrations of 1 U/mL to maintain line patency. The presence of heparin in TPN solutions leads to the detachment of endothelial lipoprotein lipases, resulting in faster lipolysis, and enhanced release of free fatty acids. Heparin is provided at a lower dose (0.5 U/mL) in TPN solutions prepared for premature infants to

TABLE 6-4

INTRAVENOUS ELECTROLYTE AND MINERAL REQUIREMENTS

Component	Requirement
Phosphorus	0.25–0.5 mEq/kg/day
Sodium	2–4 mEq/kg/day
Potassium	2–4 mEq/kg/day
Chloride	2–3 mEq/kg/day
Magnesium	0.25–0.5 mEq/kg/day
Calcium	10–40 mg/kg/day
Phosphorus	0.4–0.8 mM/kg/day
Zinc	
$\leq$2.5 kg	500 µg/kg/day
>2.5 kg	300 µg/kg/day
Copper	
$\leq$2.5 kg	60 µg/kg/day
>2.5 kg	20 µg/kg/day
Chromium	0.14–0.2 µg/kg/day
Manganese	2–10 µg/kg/day
Selenium	3 µg/kg/day
Iodine	5 µg/kg/day
Iron	0.1–0.2 mg/kg/day

TABLE 6-5

ALUMINUM CONTENT OF TPN ADDITIVES

Additive	Al Content
Potassium phosphate	62,000 µg/L
Potassium acetate	25,000 µg/L
Sodium acetate	25,000 µg/L
Magnesium sulfate	12,500 µg/L
Sodium phosphate	12,500 µg/L
Zinc, copper, manganese	2,500 µg/L
Chromium (plastic), KCl, NaCl	100 µg/L
MVI pediatric	42 µg/L
Dextrose	25 µg/L

INTRAVENOUS VITAMIN RECOMMENDATIONS

| Vitamin | Recommended Daily Intake | |
	Children < 11 yr	MVI Pediatric (per 5 mL)
Vitamin A (retinol) (IU)	2000–3000	2300
Vitamin D (IU)	400	400
Vitamin E (α-tocopherol) (IU)	7–10	7
Ascorbic acid (mg)	40	80
Folate (μg)	100–300	140
Niacin (mg)	9–16	17
Riboflavin (mg)	0.8–1.2	1.4
Thiamine (mg)	0.7–1.3	1.2
Vitamin B_6 (mg)	0.6–1.2	1.0
Vitamin B_{12} (mg)	1.0–2.0	1.0
Pantothenic acid (mg)	5.0	5.0
Biotin (μg)	20	20
Vitamin K (mg)	0.1	0.2

prevent marked elevation in serum free fatty acids. In patients with severe hyperbilirubinemia, free fatty acids may compete with bilirubin for albumin binding sites, causing bilirubin displacement.

Case Study 1

Baby E, a 10-day-old, 2000-g premature infant, suddenly developed feeding intolerance with vomiting, abdominal distention, and grossly bloody stools. The abdominal x-ray showed mild generalized bowel dilation but no other abnormalities. Because of the clinical suspicion of necrotizing enterocolitis, feedings were stopped, antibiotics were started, and plans were made to start parenteral nutrition.

Exercise 1

QUESTIONS

Select the one best answer to each of the following questions about the clinical use and composition of parenteral nutrition solutions for neonates.

1. Which of the following parenteral nutrition regimens would you select to start parenteral nutrition in this infant? (Assume an infusion rate of 100 mL/kg/day [excluding fat emulsions] administered via a peripheral vein catheter.)
   a. Amino acids 2%, dextrose 10%, and fat emulsion 20%, providing 2 g/kg/day
   b. Amino acids 2%, dextrose 12.5%, and fat emulsion 20%, providing 3 g/kg/day
   c. Amino acids 2.5%, dextrose 12.5%, and fat emulsion 20%, providing 2 g/kg/day
   d. Amino acids 2%, dextrose 15%, and fat emulsion 10%, providing 0.5 g/kg/day

2. Which of the four TPN regimens described in question 1 will provide baby E with an energy intake of 83.5 kcal/kg/day?

ANSWERS

1. a. This TPN regimen is the most appropriate because it satisfies initial amino acid requirements (2 g/kg/day) and maintains the dextrose concentration at 10%. It is not advisable to infuse more than 10% dextrose through a peripheral vein.

2. b. This regimen provides 8 kcal/kg from amino acids, 42.5 kcal/kg from dextrose, and 33 kcal/kg from fat, for a total of 83.5 kcal/kg/day.

On the second day of parenteral nutrition, baby E has a serum glucose concentration of 100 mg/dL, a serum albumin level of 1.9 g/dL, and a serum triglyceride level of 75 mg/dL.

QUESTION

3. Which of the following four TPN regimens would you select for administration by peripheral vein catheter at this time? (Assume a fluid rate of 100 mL/kg/day, excluding fat emulsion.)
   a. Amino acids 2%, dextrose 10%, and 20% fat emulsion (providing 3 g/kg/day)
   b. Amino acids 2.5%, dextrose 12.5%, and 20% fat emulsion (providing 3 g/kg/day)
   c. Amino acids 3%, dextrose 10%, and 20% fat emulsion (providing 3 g/kg/day)
   d. Amino acids 3.5%, dextrose 10%, and 20% fat emulsion (providing 2 g/kg/day)

ANSWER

3. c. This regimen is correct because it provides a greater amino acid intake (3 g/kg/day) in the presence of low serum albumin levels, it

maintains dextrose at a 10% concentration, and it enhances the intake of fat emulsion (serum triglycerides are normal).

On the third day of parenteral nutrition, baby E becomes lethargic and apneic. Marked abdominal wall redness and generalized abdominal distention are observed. The abdominal radiograph demonstrates signs of pneumatosis intestinalis and pneumoperitoneum. In the operating room, 20 cm of necrosed distal ileum with two perforations are resected, and a central line is placed for parenteral nutrition.

QUESTION

4. Which of the following four TPN regimens would you choose to start parenteral nutrition through a central vein? (Assume a rate of fluid administration of 150 mL/kg/day and the following laboratory values: serum glucose 138 mg/dL, serum triglycerides 375 mg/dL, serum albumin 1.5 g/dL, and normal serum electrolytes.)

   a. Amino acids 3%, dextrose 15%, and 1 g/kg/day of a 10% fat emulsion
   b. Amino acids 4%, dextrose 20%, and 1 g/kg/day of a 10% fat emulsion
   c. Amino acids 3%, dextrose 25%, and 2 g/kg/day of a 20% fat cmulsion
   d. Amino acids 3.5%, dextrose 10%, and 3 g/kg/day of a 20% fat emulsion

ANSWER

4. a. This regimen provides increased quantities of amino acids (4.5 g/kg/day, which is appropriate given the low serum albumin concentration), an increased dextrose concentration (15% dextrose; the serum glucose concentration is normal), and a limited dose of fat emulsion (serum triglycerides are slightly elevated).

On the following day baby E received a dose of furosemide, which caused the serum sodium to drop from 136 to 128 mmol/L and the serum potassium to decrease from 4.5 to 3 mmol/L.

QUESTION

5. What additives could be used for correction of these electrolyte abnormalities with the purpose of reducing potential aluminum accumulation?

   a. Sodium acetate and potassium phosphate
   b. Sodium chloride and potassium chloride
   c. Sodium phosphate and potassium phosphate
   d. Sodium acetate and potassium phosphate

ANSWER

5. b. Sodium chloride and potassium chloride are the additives with the lowest levels of aluminum contamination and should be preferably used for the correction of hyponatremia and hypokalemia.

On the seventh day of parenteral nutrition, baby E weighs 2100 g. During the preceding 3 days, baby E received a daily energy intake of 144 kcal/kg/day and gained weight at an average rate of 35 g/day.

QUESTION

6. Which of the four parenteral nutrition regimens below would you select to reduce the total energy intake to approximately 120 kcal/kg/day? (Assume that the dose of intravenous fat emulsion is maintained at 2 g/kg/day.)

   a. Amino acids 3%, dextrose 20%, fluid rate 122 mL/kg/day
   b. Amino acids 2%, dextrose 20%, fluid rate 100 mL/kg/day
   c. Amino acids 3%, dextrose 20%, fluid rate 150 mL/kg/day
   d. Amino acids 3%, dextrose 10%, fluid rate 100 mL/kg/day

ANSWER

6. a. This regimen provides 119.6 kcal/kg/day, which should be adequate to permit acceptable growth.

Monitoring

Before the initiation of TPN, the physician should assess the infant's nutritional status and growth parameters and obtain baseline laboratory chemical values. This so-called TPN panel includes serum electrolytes (sodium, potassium, chloride, carbon dioxide, magnesium, calcium, and phosphorus), serum total protein, albumin, blood urea nitrogen, creatinine, triglycerides, and liver function studies. A 2-day advancement in the TPN regimen is recommended for most patients to maximize nutritional rehabilitation. A schedule for advancement and initial monitoring of peripheral and central parenteral nutrition solutions is summarized in Table 6-3.

The following procedures should routinely be performed during the course of TPN:

- Strict daily measurements of intake and output and urine specific gravity and dipstick determinations for urine glucose should be obtained each shift by the patient's nurse. Bedside glucose determinations should be obtained whenever glycosuria is detected.

- Daily weight determinations and weekly measurements of length and head circumference should be obtained and plotted on available growth charts for neonates.

- The TPN panel should be repeated daily while the parenteral nutrition regimen is being advanced and weekly thereafter. Additional biochemical tests may need to be obtained when specific nutritional deficiencies are suspected (e.g., zinc, copper, selenium, vitamins).

- Central line dressings should be changed at least twice a week by trained personnel using aseptic technique. The catheter site should be inspected for signs of swelling, redness, or discharge. If a discharge is present, the material should be sent for Gram stain and culture. An antiseptic solution (e.g., povidone-iodine) should be applied to the catheter site before replacement of the dressing.

- Sepsis is a constant threat in all infants receiving TPN via a central vein. In babies with suspected sepsis, blood cultures should be obtained from the central line and from a peripheral vein. Central lines inserted to administer parenteral nutrition should be used solely for the delivery of these solutions to minimize the risk of infection.

- To prevent hypertriglyceridemia, lipid emulsions should be administered over prolonged periods (preferably over 24 hours). When serum triglyceride levels exceed 500 mg/dL, lipid emulsions should be discontinued and the level repeated 24 hours later. If the triglyceride level is still elevated, other causes

of hypertriglyceridemia should be investigated. Possible adverse effects of fat emulsions on platelet number and host defenses are not thought to be clinically significant with the use of currently available formulations at recommended doses.

Complications

Metabolic Complications

These complications can be identified by the routine biochemical monitoring of patients receiving parenteral nutrition solutions. The most common metabolic complications of parenteral nutrition in neonates include the following.

Hypoglycemia. This complication may occur when TPN solutions are discontinued abruptly and can be prevented or treated by immediate re-initiation of intravenous fluid solutions with appropriate concentrations of dextrose.

Hyperglycemia. This complication is relatively common in preterm infants and in patients with proven sepsis or surgical stress. When hyperglycemia occurs, the dextrose concentration in the infusate, or the rate of dextrose infusion, should be decreased. The rate of lipid infusion may also be a contributing factor to the incidence of hyperglycemia and small reductions in the dose of lipids can often counter this problem. Small premature infants who develop persistent hyperglycemia (serum glucose levels > 150 mg/dL) during the course of TPN should receive insulin along with the TPN solution.

Cholestatic Jaundice. This common complication is related to the long-term administration of parenteral nutrition in neonates. It is especially common in premature infants. Cholestasis is usually observed after the second week of parenteral nutrition and is characterized by an elevation of total and direct serum bilirubin values (5 to 10 mg/dL and 2.5 to 5 mg/dL, respectively). Although the cause is still unclear, several factors have been associated with the development of cholestasis, including (1) lack of enteral feedings, resulting in decreased bile flow, altered bowel flora, decreased bile acid pool size, and increased ratio of lithocholic to taurocholic acid; (2) direct liver toxicity from the amino acid solution; (3) direct liver toxicity from the hypertonic dextrose concentrations; (4) bacterial sepsis associated with the use of central lines; and (5) production of hepatotoxic bile acids. Although the majority of patients affected by this complication exhibit transient elevations of conjugated bilirubin and liver enzymes, some infants in whom parenteral nutrition cannot be discontinued develop progressive liver disease, leading to cirrhosis. Should the results of liver function studies show deterioration, one should attempt to advance enteral feeding and discontinue parenteral nutrition. If parenteral nutrition cannot be discontinued, high dextrose and protein concentrations should be avoided. In addition, ursodeoxycholic acid (15 to 30 mg/kg/day) may be beneficial in patients with TPN-related cholestasis. Copper and manganese should be removed from TPN solutions because these trace elements are excreted from the body primarily by the liver. Serial monitoring of serum copper and manganese is indicated to determine further supplementation.

Hyperammonemia. This complication is a rare problem with use of modern crystalline parenteral amino acid solutions, but it should be investigated in neonates who unexpectedly become lethargic or comatose or have other signs of liver toxicity.

Metabolic Acidosis. Acidosis is frequently observed in premature infants receiving amino acid solutions. Premature infants are predisposed to this complication because of impaired renal acidification mechanisms. The severity of the metabolic acidosis is related to the daily intake of amino acids, the degree of prematurity, and the postnatal age of the infant. Thus, metabolic acidosis may be corrected or prevented by the addition of sodium acetate to the TPN solution.

Osteopenia. This complication is usually seen in premature neonates who require parenteral nutrition solutions for prolonged periods. Osteopenia is believed to be secondary to the inability of TPN solutions to deliver the amounts of calcium and phosphorus required for proper mineralization of the skeleton in growing premature infants. The intravenous administration of vitamin D does not prevent the occurrence of osteopenia in patients receiving parenteral nutrition. The solubility of calcium and phosphorous salts in TPN solutions can be improved by providing a high amino acid intake and supplementation with cysteine hydrochloride. These measures allow

for a greater (but still inadequate) intake of calcium and phosphorus without the risk of precipitation in TPN solutions. Other contributing factors to the development of osteopenia include the prolonged use of postnatal steroids and diuretics for the treatment of chronic lung disease.

Hyperlipemia. Abnormally high serum concentrations of triglycerides, free fatty acids, or cholesterol result from the infant's inability to metabolize infused fats. Serial determinations of serum triglycerides are commonly used to monitor lipid infusions during parenteral nutrition. Fasting serum triglyceride levels in excess of 250 mg/dL and serum triglyceride levels in excess of 500 mg/dL during lipid infusions are indicative of significant hyperlipemia and mandate a reduction in the lipid dose or a temporary elimination of lipid from the TPN regimen. The presence of in-line heparin (0.5 to 1 U/mL) improves triglyceride clearance by stimulating the release of lipoprotein lipase from the capillary walls.

Alterations in Pulmonary Function. This complication can occur in premature infants with respiratory distress syndrome during the first week of life and in older infants with diffuse pulmonary disease. The administration of fat emulsions should be temporarily discontinued in patients who exhibit a deterioration of pulmonary function (as evidenced by a change in oxygenation) during the administration of fat emulsions.

Bilirubin Displacement. An elevation in the serum concentration of free fatty acids results from the hydrolysis of infused fat emulsions. In jaundiced infants, elevated levels of free fatty acids may compete with bilirubin for albumin binding and therefore increase the risk of kernicterus by increasing the serum level of free bilirubin. In jaundiced premature infants born at less than 30 weeks' gestation who require phototherapy, the maximal rate of fat infusion should be 1 g/kg/day; jaundiced premature infants born at greater than 30 weeks' gestation can receive up to 2 g/kg/day. If an infant requires an exchange transfusion for the treatment of hyperbilirubinemia, the fat infusion should be discontinued.

Complications Resulting from the Method of Delivery

These complications are usually associated with placement or use of central vein catheters for the delivery of TPN solutions. The incidence of central vein catheter complications ranges from 4% to 9.2%. These complications include pneumothorax, pneumomediastinum, arterial puncture, hemorrhage, cardiac arrhythmia, superior vena cava syndrome, chylothorax, and pericardial tamponade. Broken catheters at the site of connection with the plastic TPN tubing are not infrequent in patients who require placement of a Broviac catheter for long-term parenteral nutrition. Patients receiving parenteral nutrition by peripheral vein catheters are at risk for skin slough in the event of accidental infiltration of TPN solutions. Therefore, the dextrose concentration in TPN solutions administered by peripheral vein catheters should not exceed 10%.

Infectious Complications

The reported incidence of sepsis in neonates receiving parenteral nutrition varies from 21% to 45%. However, in recent years, the incidence of sepsis has plummeted (to 2% to 10%) because of the broader acceptance of aseptic techniques. Predisposing factors for the development of sepsis in neonates receiving parenteral nutrition include the adverse effects of prematurity and malnutrition on the immune system and the contamination of the central catheter by skin pathogens at the insertion site. In addition, both parenteral nutrition solutions and fat emulsions can easily become contaminated during the preparation process, as they are known to support the growth of staphylococcal and candidal species, as well as other gram-negative organisms. The most common organisms causing sepsis in patients receiving parenteral nutrition include coagulase-positive and -negative staphylococci, *Streptococcus viridans*, *Escherichia coli*, *Pseudomonas* spp., *Klebsiella* spp., and *Candida albicans*. Aseptic preparation of TPN solutions by trained pharmacists working with automated systems precludes handling and minimizes the risk of contamination. The risk of infection is further decreased if the central vein catheter is not used for the administration of blood products or medications, blood sampling, or monitoring of central venous pressure. Sepsis must be ruled out in any patient receiving TPN by a central vein catheter who develops fever or other signs of infection. When sepsis is suspected, blood cultures should be obtained from the central line and peripheral vein catheters. The central vein catheter should be promptly removed in patients with catheter-related sepsis due to *Staphylococcus aureus* or candidiasis. For other pathogens, central catheters should be removed only if cultures remain positive after 95 hours of treatment for *Staphylococcus epidermidis* and after 48 hours of appropriate antibiotic therapy administered through the central line.

The next set of questions are designed to assess your knowledge of the kinds of monitoring required for infants receiving TPN and the complications associated with its use. (Note that more than one answer may be correct.)

Exercise 2

QUESTIONS

1. Which of these complications have been associated with the prolonged use of parenteral nutrition in premature infants?

   a. Increased serum conjugated bilirubin

   b. Candidiasis

   c. Osteopenia

   d. Vitamin D deficiency

2. Routine clinical and laboratory monitoring of neonates during the first week of parenteral nutrition therapy should include which of the following measurements?

   a. Daily weight

   b. Daily fluid intake and output

   c. Daily blood glucose

   d. Daily urine specific gravity

3. Which of the complications of TPN listed below has not been associated with the use of fat emulsions in premature infants?

   a. Bilirubin displacement

   b. Hypertriglyceridemia

   c. Cholestatic jaundice

   d. Impaired respiratory function

4. A 1200-g premature infant who is receiving TPN through a central vein catheter develops catheter-related sepsis with *Staphylococcus epidermidis*. How should this infant be managed?

   a. Continue parenteral nutrition.

   b. Initiate antibiotic therapy through the central catheter.

c. Remove the central catheter.

d. Initiate antibiotic therapy through a peripheral venous line.

5. An infant receiving TPN by central vein catheter at the right atrium suddenly develops cardiorespiratory arrest and severe hypotension with very narrow pulse pressure. The chest radiograph shows severe cardiomegaly suggestive of pericardial effusion. The heart sounds are distant, and cardiac tamponade is suspected. A pericardial tap is emergently performed yielding 35 mL of milky yellow fluid containing 800 mg/dL of glucose, and 187 mg/dL of protein and 780 mg/dL of triglycerides. The patient improves dramatically. How would you continue further management?

a. Keep the central line at the same location and infuse TPN solutions of lower osmolality

b. Remove the central line immediately and start peripheral TPN

c. Repeat the chest radiograph and monitor TPN panel

d. Obtain blood cultures from a peripheral vein and from the central line and start antibiotic therapy for a minimum of 48 hours, pending culture results

6. An infant with severe short bowel syndrome from surgical necrotizing enterocolitis develops progressive cholestatic jaundice during the third month of TPN. What measures should be initiated for the treatment of this complication?

a. Attempt to increase the amount of enteral feedings

b. Avoid excessive intake of protein and glucose in TPN

c. Start supplementation of ursodiol to enteral feedings

d. Additional supplementation of copper and manganese to TPN

ANSWERS

1. a, b, and c. Vitamin D deficiency should not occur in infants receiving TPN because multivitamin preparations contain ample amounts of vitamin D.

2. a, b, and d. Blood glucose levels should not be measured on a daily basis, except when glycosuria occurs or glucose test strip values are elevated.

3. c. The use of intravenous fat emulsions is the only factor that has not been associated with the development of cholestatic jaundice.

4. a and b. *S. epidermidis* sepsis can usually be treated successfully by administering antibiotics through the central line. The central line should be removed only if blood cultures from the central line remain positive, despite antibiotic therapy.

5. b, c, and d. The central line should be immediately removed and peripheral TPN started along with antibiotics. Close biochemical monitoring should be performed to ensure tolerance to peripheral TPN solutions.

6. a, b, and c. TPN cholestasis is treated by increasing the intake of enteral feedings and by decreasing the intake of TPN as tolerated. In addition, ursodeoxycholic acid can be administered with enteral feedings. Copper and manganese should be removed from TPN solutions and not given as additional supplements. Serial monitoring of serum copper and manganese should be performed to determine the need to re-initiate supplementation.

Suggested Readings

American Medical Association, Department of Foods and Nutrition: Multivitamin preparations for parenteral use—A statement by the Nutrition Advisory Group. J Parent Ent Nutr 1979;3:258.

Cornblath M, Wybright SH, Baens GS: Studies on carbohydrate metabolism in the newborn infant. VII. Tests on carbohydrate tolerance in premature infants. Pediatrics 1963;32:1007.

Dhainreddy R, Hamosh M, Sivasubramanian KN, et al: Post-heparin lipolytic activity and intralipid clearance in very low birthweight infants. J Pediatr 1981;98:617.

Filer RM, Takada Y, Carreras T, et al: Serum intralipid levels in neonates during parenteral nutrition: The relation to gestational age. Pediatr Surg 1980;15:1405.

Gillis J, Jones G, Penchaz P: Delivery of vitamins A, D, and E in parenteral nutrition solutions. J Parent Ent Nutr 1983;7:11.

Heird WC, Dell RB, Driscoll JN Jr, et al: Metabolic acidosis resulting from intravenous alimentation mixtures containing synthetic amino acids. N Engl J Med 1972;287:943.

Heird WC, Hay W, Helms RA, et al: Pediatric parenteral amino acid mixture in low birthweight infants. Pediatrics 1988;81:41.

Holman RT, Johnson SB, Hatch TF: A case of human linolenic acid deficiency involving neurological abnormalities. Am J Clin Nutr 1982;35:617.

Karpen SJ: Update on the etiologies and management of neonatal cholestatsis. Clin Perinatol 2002;29(1):159–194.

Kashyap S, Abildskov A, Heird C: Cysteine supplementation of very low-birthweight infants receiving parenteral nutrition. Pediatr Res 1992;31:290A.

Kaye R, Williams ML, Barbero G: A comparative study of the metabolism of glucose and fructose in infants. Am J Dis Child 1957;93:85.

Pereira GR, Fox WW, Stanley CA, et al: Decreased oxygenation and hyperlipemia during intravenous fat infusions in premature infants. Pediatrics 1980;66:26.

Pereira G, Glassman M: Parenteral nutrition in the neonate. In Rombeau J, Caldwell M (eds): Parenteral Nutrition, Vol 2. Philadelphia, WB Saunders, 1986, pp 702–720.

Pereira GR, Sherman MS, DiGiacomo J, et al: Hyperalimentation induced cholestasis: Increased incidence and severity in premature infants. Am J Dis Child 1981;135:842.

Pereira GR, Yudkoff M, Moskowitz S: Effect of intralipid therapy on nitrogen retention in premature infants. J Parent Ent Nutr 1981;4:112.

Shennan AT, Bryan MH, Angel A: The effect of gestational age on Intralipid tolerance in newborn infants. J Pediatr 1977;91:134.

Stahl GE, Spear ML, Hamosh M, et al: The intravenous administration of lipid emulsions in premature infants. Clin Perinatol 1986;13:133.

U.S. Food and Drug Adminstration: Aluminum in large and small volume parenterals used in total parenteral nutrition. Federal Register 2002;67(228):70691–70692.

Van den Berghe G, Hers HG: Dangers of intravenous fructose and sorbitol. Acta Pediatr Belg 1978;31:115.

Veleisis RA, Inwood R, Hunt CR: Prospective controlled study of parenteral nutrition associated cholestatic jaundice: Effect of protein uptake. Pediatrics 1980;996:893.

Winters RW, Heird WC, Dell RB, et al: Plasma amino acids in infants receiving parenteral nutrition. In Green HL, Holliday MA, Munro HN (eds): Clinical Nutrition Update. Chicago, American Medical Association Publishing, 1977, pp 147–157.

Zlotkin SH, Bryan MH, Anderson GH: Cysteine supplementation to cysteine-free intravenous feeding regimens in newborn infants. Am J Clin Nutr 1981;34:914.

Zlotkin SH, Buchanan BE: Meeting zinc and copper intake requirements in the parenterally fed preterm and full-term infant. J Pediatr 1983;103:441.

Enteral Nutrition in the High-Risk Neonate

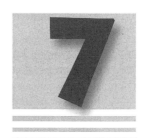

Brenda B. Poindexter, MD, MS

Evidence is increasingly accumulating that nutritional inadequacies in the early neonatal period can have both short- and long-term consequences; thus, provision of adequate nutritional support to the high-risk premature neonate remains a significant clinical challenge. Among extremely low birth weight (ELBW) infants (birth weight < 1000 g), postnatal growth failure remains a nearly universal complication of neonatal intensive care. This chapter contains exercises designed to help those who care for premature neonates review enteral nutrient requirements, identify some of the inherent difficulties in providing adequate nutrition, and recognize and identify contributing factors to and the consequences of growth failure in infants born prematurely. In addition, areas in which further research is needed to determine optimal nutritional support to improve outcomes in this population are emphasized.

Classification of Intrauterine Growth

Case Study 1

AL and ML are twin boys delivered at 26 weeks' gestation to a 36-year-old primigravida whose pregnancy was complicated by twin gestation and twin-twin transfusion syndrome status–post laser ablation. Delivery was via emergent cesarean section for breech presentation and variable fetal heart rate pattern with decelerations in twin A.

Anthropometric parameters of the infants at birth were as follows:
Twin A: weight 800 g; length 32 cm; head circumference 23.5 cm
Twin M: weight 860 g; length 34.5 cm; head circumference 24 cm

Exercise 1

QUESTION

1. Mrs. L asks if her infants weigh more or less than you would have expected for twins born at 26 weeks. Which of the following is the best answer to her question?

   a. Both infants are small for gestational age (SGA).

   b. Both infants are appropriate for gestational age (AGA).

   c. Twin M is large for gestational age (LGA).

   d. Given the 60-g difference in birth weight, the twins are considered discordant.

ANSWER

1. b. Although intrauterine growth restriction is more frequent in multiple gestations, both infants are appropriate for gestational age based on the reference for fetal growth reported by Alexander. Small for gestational age is a term used to describe an infant whose weight is less than a specified cutoff, usually less than the 10th percentile for a given gestational age. Identification of

infants who are small for gestational age at the time of birth may suggest a genetic syndrome or chromosomal abnormality, metabolic disorder, or infectious etiology. Infants who are small for gestational age are at increased risk of neonatal morbidity and neurodevelopmental delay, particularly if head growth is also compromised. In addition, the incidence of postnatal growth failure is significantly greater among SGA infants than AGA infants. At 18 to 22 months' corrected age, significantly more children born SGA than AGA will be below the 10th percentile for weight, length, and head circumference.

The medical student on rounds is somewhat surprised that an infant who weighs less than 1000 g at birth is not automatically considered to have experienced intrauterine growth restriction. He asks what percentage of very low birth weight (VLBW) infants (birth weight < 1500 g) are actually small for gestational age at the time of birth.

QUESTION

2. Which of the following answers best represents the percentage of VLBW infants who are SGA at birth?

   a. 90%

   b. 74%

   c. 22%

   d. 10%

ANSWER

2. *c*. It is important to recognize that not all premature infants are small for gestational age at birth. Depending on which fetal growth curve is used, the prevalence of SGA infants is quite variable. Large multicenter studies have reported that 22% of VLBW and 17% of ELBW infants are small for gestational age at birth. The percentage of SGA infants tends to be disproportionately higher among infants 30 to 32 weeks' gestation when VLBW cohorts are evaluated.

Postnatal Growth Failure

A number of growth charts are available for assessment of postnatal growth. Similar to the intrauterine definition of small for gestational age, postnatal growth failure is typically defined as body weight less than the 10th percentile for completed weeks of gestation according to the reference data reported by Alexander. Once the corrected age of the infant reaches term, the growth standards published by the National Center for Health Statistics (NCHS) can be used.

As discussed in the previous exercise, approximately 22% of VLBW infants are classified as small for gestational age at the time of birth. However, at 36 weeks' corrected age, 97% of the VLBW and 99% of the ELBW cohort followed by the NICHD Neonatal Research Network between 1995 and 1996 had weight less than the 10th percentile. Although more recent data from 1999–2001 show a modest improvement, the incidence of postnatal growth failure in ELBW infants remains approximately 90%.

Exercise 2

QUESTION

1. Which of the following neonatal factors are associated with postnatal growth failure in ELBW infants?

   a. Duration of mechanical ventilation

   b. Exposure to postnatal steroids

   c. Grade III/IV intracranial hemorrhage

   d. Necrotizing enterocolitis (NEC)

   e. All of the above

ANSWER

1. e. All of these factors are associated with postnatal growth failure in ELBW infants.

   Although the risk of postnatal growth failure is inversely related to birth weight and gestational age, there are also many neonatal factors associated with poor in-hospital growth of premature infants, including duration of mechanical ventilation, use of postnatal steroids, severe intracranial hemorrhage/periventricular leukomalacia, and necrotizing enterocolitis (NEC). Many of the morbidities that are associated with slow growth velocity, such as NEC, also affect the provision of nutritional support and the utilization of nutrients supplied.

Benefits of Human Milk

Case Study 2

The attending obstetrician requests a prenatal consult for a 22-year-old primigravida who has presented at 24 weeks' estimated gestational age with premature labor, rupture of membranes, and imminent delivery. After discussing the morbidity and mortality risks associated with extreme prematurity, you encourage the mother to consider expressing human milk for her premature baby.

Exercise 3

QUESTION

1. Which of the following statements regarding provision of human milk to premature infants should be included in your discussion?

    a. Human milk offers protection against infection in premature infants.

    b. Premature infants who receive their mother's milk may have a lower incidence of necrotizing enterocolitis.

    c. Premature infants who receive human milk demonstrate improved developmental outcomes compared with formula-fed premature infants.

ANSWER

1. All of the above statements are true.

   The recent policy statement issued by the American Academy of Pediatrics Section on Breastfeeding states that "hospitals and physicians should recommend human milk for premature and other high-risk infants either by direct breastfeeding and/or using the mother's own expressed milk." It is important to recognize that many mothers who deliver prematurely will choose to express milk for their infant once they are properly informed of the numerous benefits. For many mothers with a critically ill infant, expressing breast milk provides a means to make a contribution in a situation in which they otherwise have very little control.

   Several studies have demonstrated the immunologic benefits of human milk for premature infants, including higher concentrations of secretory IgA, lysozyme, lactoferrin, and inter-

feron in preterm human milk. Compared to their exclusively formula-fed counterparts, VLBW infants who receive human milk have decreased rates of infection. In addition, recent observational data in ELBW infants suggests a dose-response relationship between human milk intake in the first 14 days of life and decreased risk of late-onset sepsis. Although conflicting data exist, human milk may also decrease the risk of necrotizing enterocolitis in premature infants.

Banked Human Milk

Case Study 2 *Continued*

After observing your conversation with the mother, the nurse practitioner in the NICU asks your opinion regarding the use of banked human milk if the infant's mother is unable to maintain an adequate milk supply.

Exercise 4

QUESTION

1. Which of the following statements are true based on currently available evidence?

    a. Most donors to milk banks are mothers who delivered at term.

    b. Premature infants who receive donor milk demonstrate similar rates of weight gain as those who are fed premature formula.

    c. Banked donor milk confers all the same immunologic benefits as mother's own milk.

ANSWER

1. Only the first statement is true.

   Human milk banks usually obtain milk from donors who delivered term infants; consequently, the protein content of donor milk is usually less than that obtained from women who have delivered prematurely. A randomized trial of donor human milk versus preterm formula as a substitute for the mother's own milk in the feeding of extremely premature infants found lesser rates of weight gain in infants fed donor milk; a substantial number of infants in this study were switched to premature formula because of poor weight gain. Future studies are needed to more clearly define the potential role of banked human milk in infants whose mothers are unable to provide their own milk.

Nutrient Considerations

Current recommendations for nutrient intake in premature infants are primarily based on the goal of approximating growth and nutrient accretion rates of the fetus at the same postmenstrual age. However, this standard is not universally accepted and recommendations for extremely low birth weight infants have, for the most part, been extrapolated from studies in larger premature infants. What is clear is that neither term infant formula nor unfortified human milk is an appropriate standard by which to calculate the nutrient requirements of premature infants.

Formulas for use in premature infants were developed in the early 1980s. The rationale for having a different nutrient profile came from the observation by many investigators that the growth of premature infants was improved when protein and minerals were added to term formula and human milk.

The Life Sciences Research Office (LSRO) of the American Society for Nutritional Sciences (ASNS) published a report in 2002 outlining the nutrient requirements for preterm infant formulas. This expert panel reviewed nutrient requirements for premature infants receiving infant formula and evaluated how these requirements differed from those of formulas designed for term infants. However, owing to limited data available in infants weighing less than 750 g, the panel determined that the needs for the smallest premature neonates remain unknown.

Composition of Premature Formulas

Case Study 3

EG is an 1150-g female who was delivered at 28 weeks' estimated gestational age to a 34-year-old gravida 3, para 2 woman whose pregnancy was complicated by the diagnosis of stage III breast cancer. The mother of the infant is scheduled to begin intensive chemotherapy shortly after delivery. EG's mother asks what types of formulas are available for premature infants, knowing that

she will not be able to provide expressed human milk for her daughter.

Exercise 5

QUESTION

1. Which of the following statements regarding premature infant formulas are true?

   a. Like human milk, lactose is the exclusive source of carbohydrate in premature infant formulas such as Enfamil Premature or Similac Special Care.

   b. In contrast to formulas designed for term infants, premature infant formulas supply 40% to 50% of the total lipid content as medium chain triglycerides.

   c. The protein composition of premature infant formulas is predominantly casein based.

   d. The protein content of premature infant formulas is similar to fortified human milk.

   e. The calcium and phosphorus content of premature infant formulas is lower than that of term formula.

ANSWER

1. Statements b and d are true; the remaining statements are false.

Lactose is the only source of carbohydrate in both term and preterm human milk. The carbohydrate content of premature infant formulas, on the other hand, is a blend of 40% to 50% lactose and 50% to 60% glucose polymers (such as corn syrup solids). Premature infants have low levels of intestinal lactase activity; consequently, the reduced lactose content of premature formulas theoretically enhances digestion. Glucose polymers are easily digested by α-glucosidase enzymes (sucrase, isomaltase, maltase, glucoamylase); these enzymes, in contrast to lactase, are abundant in the small intestine of premature infants and approximate adult levels much sooner.

Human milk supplies approximately 50% of total calories from fat. Premature infant formulas contain medium-chain triglycerides (MCT) in order to compensate for low levels of intestinal lipase and bile salts in premature infants. In addition, most formulas are now supplemented with docosahexanoic acid (DHA) and arachido-nic acid (ARA), long-chain polyunsaturated fatty acids found in human milk and thought to be important for brain and retinal development.

The protein content of premature infant formulas is higher than term formulas (3 g/100 kcal versus 2.0 to 2.1 g/100 kcal). Protein requirements are higher in growing premature infants than their term counter-parts. Patterned after human milk, premature infant formulas are whey-predominant. Soy-based formulas are not routinely recommended for the premature infant as they contain signif-icantly less phosphorus and may result in met-abolic bone disease; in addition, the phytates in soy formulas can interfere with iron absorption. The nutrient composition of standard prema-ture infant formulas is shown in Table 7-1.

Mrs. L (see Case Study 1) has decided to express human milk for her twins.

QUESTION

2. Compared to premature formula (with iron), which of the following applies to premature human milk?

   a. Higher in protein content

   b. Lower in iron content

   c. Higher in calcium content

   d. Higher in vitamins A and D content

ANSWER

2. Only response b is correct. Although pre-mature human milk is higher in protein

content than term human milk, the protein content of premature formulas is much higher. The iron supplied by human milk has a high bioavailability; however, the iron content of both term and preterm human milk is low. Premature formulas with iron provide approximately 2 mg/kg/day ele-mental iron when the infant is receiving 120 kcal/kg from enteral feeds. The use of low-iron formulas is not warranted in premature infants. Compared to premature formula, premature human milk is lower in calcium, phosphorus, zinc, vitamin A, vitamin D, and folic acid.

Initiation of Enteral Feeds

Case Study 4

HR is a 4-day-old former 780-g 27 weeks' estimated gestational age black female who was delivered via cesarean section because of worsening maternal preeclampsia. The infant required intubation and a total of three doses of exogenous surfactant for respiratory distress syndrome; she subsequently weaned to low ventilatory support and less than 30% oxygen. Upon admission to the NICU, 3 g/kg/day of intravenous amino acids were immediately initiated; total parenteral nutrition is now providing 3.5 g/kg/day amino acids, 4 g/kg/day lipid, and 12 g/kg/day carbohydrate (total of 95 kcal/kg/day). A three-dose course of indomethacin for IVH prophylaxis was completed last evening. There are umbilical arterial and venous lines in place. HR's mother is expressing milk for her. On

TABLE 7-1		
NUTRIENT COMPOSITION OF STANDARD PREMATURE FORMULAS		
Nutrient (per 100 kcal)	**Similac Special Care Advance (24 kcal/fl oz)**	**Enfamil Premature Lipil (24 kcal/fl oz)**
Protein, g	3	3
Fat, g	5.43	5.1
Linoleic acid, mg	700	810
DHA, mg	14	17
ARA, mg	22	34
Carbohydrate, g	10.3	11
Calcium, mg	180	165
Phosphorus, mg	100	83
Iron,* mg	1.8	1.8
Zinc, mg	1.5	1.5
Vitamin A, IU	1250	1250
Vitamin D, IU	150	240

*Values shown are for iron-fortified product.
ARA, arachidonic acid; DHA, docosahexanoic acid.

rounds, the baby's nurse inquires as to when the patient will start to receive enteral feeds.

Exercise 6

QUESTION

1. Which of the statements reflect an evidence-based decision related to the initiation of enteral feeds in this infant?

  a. Parenteral nutrition is supplying the infant with all necessary nutrients; enteral feeding should be delayed until the infant is no longer at risk of developing NEC.

  b. Feedings cannot be initiated until both umbilical lines are removed.

  c. Feedings can be initiated using half-strength human milk or premature formula at 40 to 60 mL/kg/d.

  d. Trophic or minimal enteral feeds (10–20 mL/kg/d) with full-strength expressed human milk should be initiated today.

ANSWER

1. The best response is d. Although the infant is receiving a reasonable intake from parenteral nutrition, there are known benefits of minimal enteral feeds in premature neonates.

Minimal Enteral Nutrition

Minimal enteral feeds, also known as trophic feeds, are typically defined as low-volume feeds that do not provide sufficient calories to support somatic growth but rather help to promote maturation of the structure and function of the premature intestinal tract. Several clinical studies have demonstrated reductions in the number of days to achieve full enteral feeding, total number of days that enteral feeds are withheld, and days of hospital stay. If available, full-strength expressed human milk should be given. There is no evidence to suggest that use of diluted formula is an effective strategy to decrease the risk of necrotizing enterocolitis.

Advancement of Enteral Feeds

Even under the best of circumstances, it takes a substantial amount of time to achieve full enteral feeds in premature neonates. Among ELBW infants cared for at participating centers of the NICHD Neonatal Research Network, the mean age at which full enteral feeds (defined as ≥110 kcal/kg/day) were achieved was as long as 35 days. Small retrospective studies have suggested an increased risk of NEC if feeds are advanced rapidly. Prospective, randomized clinical trials have not demonstrated a relationship between rate of feeding advancement and NEC. However, a more recent single-center study demonstrated a reduced incidence of NEC among infants who received prolonged small feedings (20 mL/kg/day for 10 days) as compared to a group whose feedings were advanced by 20 mL/kg/day. Based on currently available evidence, providing minimal volume feeds for some period of time seems reasonable; the rate of advancement thereafter has not been adequately studied, although the most common approach is to advance by 15 to 20 mL/kg/day. Regardless of the approach, parenteral nutrition should be maintained until enteral nutrition supplies a minimum of 80 kcal/kg/day.

Fortification of Human Milk

Case Study 5

Twin A tolerates advancement of enteral feeds by 20 mL/kg/day. Parenteral nutrition is discontinued once he is receiving 120 mL/kg/day. At 16 days of age, he is receiving 150 mL/kg/day of his mother's milk. After regaining his birth weight at 6 days of age, the infant has gained approximately 10 g/day.

Exercise 7

QUESTIONS

1. Which of the following alterations should be made to his feeding regimen?

  a. Add additional source of carbohydrate, such as Polycose, to increase caloric density.

  b. Fortify with a commercial human milk fortifier (HMF).

  c. Change to premature infant formula.

d. No changes are required; weight gain is adequate for a premature infant.

2. Which of the following nutrients do human milk fortifiers supply?

a. Protein, primarily whey based

b. A balanced source of calories from protein, carbohydrate, and lipid

c. Calcium and phosphorus

d. Sodium, zinc, and vitamins

e. All of the above

ANSWERS

1. The correct response is b. Human milk fortifiers should be used in premature infants with birth weight less than 1500 g, and should be considered in those with birth weight less than 2000 g. Owing to concerns related to the osmolality and tolerance of human milk fortifier, a reasonable approach is to delay the addition of fortifier until the infant is approaching full volume feeds.

2. e. All the responses are correct.

The nutrient composition of human milk and human milk with fortifiers added is shown in Table 7-2. Although human milk is considered to be the optimal source of primary nutrition for premature infants, human milk does not completely meet the nutritional needs of premature infants. Milk expressed from mothers who have delivered prematurely does contain higher concentrations of protein and electrolytes than does milk expressed from mothers who deliver at term. However, the amount of protein and sodium gradually declines over the first several weeks and approximates that of term milk. When using a standard HMF, supplementation with a multivitamin preparation is not indicated. Infants who take volumes greater than 360 mL/day (15 fortifier packets) will receive intakes of some vitamins in excess of 200% of amounts recommended for premature infants; in these cases alternate methods of fortification should be discussed with a neonatal dietitian. Depending on which HMF product is used, an iron supplement may also be indicated in order to achieve the recommended intake of 2 to 4 mg/kg/day of elemental iron.

Consequences of Postnatal Growth Failure

Case Study 6

EG is a former 25-week 780-g preterm infant who is now 11 weeks old. At the time of birth, her weight, length, and head circumference were all at the 50th percentile for gestational age. She regained her birth weight at 10 days of age and achieved full enteral feeds at 26 days of age. At 36 weeks' corrected age (CA), both her weight and weight-length ratio are less than the 10th percentile.

TABLE 7-2

NUTRIENT COMPOSITION OF HUMAN MILK (HM) AND HUMAN MILK FORTIFIERS (HMF)

Nutrient (per 100 kcal)	Human Milk Term	Human Milk Preterm	Similac HMF (1 packet, 25 mL HM)	Enfamil HMF (1 packet, 25 mL HM)	Similac Natural Care (50:50 HM)
Protein, g	1.5	2.1	2.97	3.12	2.6
Calcium, mg	45	37	175	145	132
Phosphorus, mg	22.6	19	98	77	72
Iron, mg	0.06	0.18	0.58	1.93	0.28
Zinc, mg	0.38	0.51	1.7	1.3	1.1
Vitamin A, IU	319	581	1246	1652	949
Vitamin D, IU	3	3	151	187	84
Folic acid, μg	12	5	32	35	23
Osmolality	286	290	385	350	280

Exercise 8

QUESTION

1. Which of the following statements regarding her growth are true?

    a. Although EG is SGA at 36 weeks' CA, she will more than likely experience "catch-up" growth and be AGA when she is 18 months CA.

    b. EG's growth has been suboptimal, but this will not affect her neurodevelopmental outcome.

ANSWER

1. Neither statement is true.

    In general, once an extremely premature infant regains birth weight, the rate of weight gain typically follows the rate of intrauterine growth. However, at 36 weeks' corrected age, the vast majority of these infants remain less than the 10th percentile according to the reference data for fetal growth. The obvious question is whether failure to grow in the NICU is associated with longer-term growth failure or neurodevelopmental deficits. At 18 to 22 months' chronological age, 40% of ELBW infants still weigh less than the 10th percentile. As the rate of in-hospital weight gain of ELBW infants increases, the incidence of cerebral palsy, Bayley Mental Developmental Index (MDI) and Psychomotor Developmental Index (PDI) less than 70, abnormal neurologic examination, neurodevelopmental impairment, and need for rehospitalization decreases. The unacceptably high incidence of postnatal growth failure underscores the urgent need to improve outcomes and reduce complications in VLBW infants with nutritional practices.

Postdischarge Nutrition

Case Study 7

TE is a former 29-week premature infant whose clinical course was complicated by mild RDS. He received two doses of surfactant and was mechanically ventilated for less than 72 hours. He weaned from nasal cannula oxygen to room air at 32 weeks' corrected gestational age. He has had no episodes of apnea or bradycardia for 3 to 4 weeks. He is now 37 weeks' corrected gestational age and is taking all feeds orally with 24 kcal/oz premature formula and has been demonstrating excellent weight gain. TE's mother is no longer expressing human milk. The social worker informs you that TE will qualify for assistance from WIC.

Exercise 9

QUESTION

1. Which formula would be most appropriate for TE's discharge needs?

    a. Standard term formula (20 kcal/oz) such as Enfamil Lipil with iron

    b. Standard premature formula (24 kcal/oz) such as Similac Special Care Advance

    c. Elemental formula such as Enfamil Pregestimil

    d. Transitional premature formula (22 kcal/oz) such as Enfacare Lipil or Similac NeoSure Advance.

ANSWER

1. The correct response is d. In order to maintain optimal growth following hospital discharge, premature infants are likely to benefit from a nutrient-enriched formula or ongoing fortification of human milk.

    Table 7-3 provides the nutrient composition of preterm discharge formulas. These formulas typically supply 22 kcal/oz and contain nutrient

TABLE 7-3

NUTRIENT COMPOSITION OF PRETERM DISCHARGE FORMULAS

Nutrient (per 100 kcal)	Similac NeoSure Advance (22 kcal/fl oz)	Enfamil EnfaCare Lipil (22kcal/fl oz)
Protein, g	2.8	2.8
Fat, g	5.5	5.3
Linoleic acid, mg	750	950
DHA, mg	8.3	17
ARA, mg	22	34
Carbohydrate, g	10.1	10.4
Calcium, mg	105	120
Phosphorus, mg	62	66
Iron, mg	1.8	1.8
Zinc, mg	1.2	1.25
Vitamin A, IU	460	450
Vitamin D, IU	70	80
Folic acid, µg	25	26

ARA, arachidonic acid; DHA, docosahexaenoic acid.

TABLE 7-4

FORTIFICATION OF HUMAN MILK FOR HOME USE

Caloric Density	Amount of Formula Powder*	Amount of Human Milk
24 kcal/oz	1 level teaspoon	60 mL
	1 level scoop	300 mL
27 kcal/oz	1 level scoop	160 mL
30 kcal/oz	1 level scoop	120 mL

*Formula powders for use with this recipe include Similac NeoSure Advance, Enfamil EnfaCare Lipil, Similac Advance, and Enfamil Lipil; use unpacked scoops and use only the scoop that comes in the original can.

levels in between those of premature and term infant formulas. In most cases, feeding a nutrient-enriched formula after discharge should be continued until the premature infant reaches 12 months' corrected age. Commercial human milk fortifiers (HMF) are typically recommended for in-hospital use only. If needed to maintain growth, formula powder can be used as outlined in Table 7-4 to increase the caloric density of human milk. This strategy may be particularly helpful in the infant who is transitioning to the breast for the majority of feeds.

Future studies are needed to more clearly define the nutrient requirements of extremely low birth weight infants during their initial hospitalization as well as the postdischarge period thereafter in order to minimize complications and optimize growth and neurodevelopment. The optimal rate of catch-up growth for this high-risk population has yet to be defined.

Suggested Readings

Alexander G, Himes J, Kaufman R, et al: A United States national reference for fetal growth. Obstet Gynecol 1996;87(2):163–168.

American Academy of Pediatrics Section on Breastfeeding: Breastfeeding and the Use of Human Milk. Pediatrics 2005;115(2):496–506.

Berry MA, Abrahamowicz M, Usher RH: Factors associated with growth of extremely premature infants during initial hospitalization. Pediatrics 1997;100(4):640–646.

Berseth CL, Bisquera JA, Paje VU: Prolonging small feeding volumes early in life decreases the incidence of necrotizing enterocolitis in very low birth weight infants. Pediatrics 2003;111(3):529–534.

Carver JD: Nutrition for preterm infants after hospital discharge. Adv Pediatr 2005;52:23–47.

Clark RH, Wagner CL, Merritt RJ, et al: Nutrition in the neonatal intensive care unit: How do we reduce the incidence of extrauterine growth restriction? J Perinatol 2003;23(4):337–344.

Dusick AM, Poindexter BB, Ehrenkranz RA, Lemons JA: Growth failure in the preterm infant: Can we catch up? Semin Perinatol 2003;27(4):302–310.

Ehrenkranz RA, Younes N, Lemons JA, et al: Longitudinal growth of hospitalized very low birth weight infants. Pediatrics 1999;104(2 Pt 1):280–289.

Ehrenkranz R, Dusick A, Vohr B, et al: Growth in the NICU influences neurodevelopmental and growth outcomes of extremely low birth weight infants. Pediatrics 2006;117:1253–1261.

Hamill PVV, Drizd TA, Johnson CL, et al: Physical growth: National Center for Health Statistics percentiles. Am J Ciln Nutr 1979;32:607–629.

Hay WWJr, Lucas A, Heird WC, et al: Workshop summary: Nutrition of the extremely low birth weight infant. Pediatrics 1999;104(6):1360–1368.

Hylander MA, Strobino DM, Dhanireddy R: Human milk feedings and infection among very low birth weight infants. Pediatrics 1998;102(3):E38.

Klein CJ: Nutrient requirements for preterm infant formulas. J Nutr 2002;132:1395S–1577S.

Lemons JA, Bauer CR, Oh W, et al: Very low birth weight outcomes of the National Institute of Child Health and Human Development Neonatal Research Network, January 1995 through December 1996. NICHHD Neonatal Research Network. Pediatrics 2001;107(1):E1.

Lucas A, Cole TJ: Breast milk and neonatal necrotising enterocolitis. Lancet 1990;336(8730):1519–1523.

Lucas A, Morley R, Cole TJ: Randomised trial of early diet in preterm babies and later intelligence quotient. BMJ 1998;317(7171):1481–1487.

Meinzen-Derr J, Poindexter BB, Donovan EF, et al: The role of human milk feedings in risk of late-onset sepsis. Pediatr Res 2004;55:393A.

Olsen I, Meinzen-Derr J, Lawson M, Morrow A: Unexpectedly high SGA rates by gestational age in VLBW cohort. PAS 2005;57:2569.

Poindexter BB, Ehrenkranz RA, Stoll BJ, et al: Parenteral glutamine supplementation does not reduce the risk of mortality or late-onset sepsis in extremely low birth weight infants. Pediatrics 2004;113(5):1209–1215.

Rodriguez NA, Miracle DJ, Meier PP: Sharing the science on human milk feedings with mothers of very-low-birth-weight infants. J Obstet Gynecol Neonatal Nurs 2005;34(1):109–119.

Schanler RJ, Lau C, Hurst NM, Smith EO: Randomized trial of donor human milk versus preterm formula as substitutes for mothers' own milk in the feeding of extremely premature infants. Pediatrics 2005;116(2):400–406.

Schanler RJ, Shulman RJ, Lau C: Feeding strategies for premature infants: Beneficial outcomes of feeding fortified human milk versus preterm formula. Pediatrics 1999;103(6 Pt 1):1150–1157.

Tyson JE, Kennedy KA: Trophic feedings for parenterally fed infants. Cochrane Database Syst Rev 2005(3):CD000504.

Wilson DC, Cairns P, Halliday HL, et al: Randomised controlled trial of an aggressive nutritional regimen in sick very low birthweight infants. Arch Dis Child Fetal Neonatal Ed 1997;77(1):F4–F1.

Anemia in the Newborn Infant

Robin K. Ohls, MD

During the newborn period red blood cell (RBC) indices vary remarkably from indices of children and adults. Determining the etiology of anemia in an infant becomes a challenge, requiring expert knowledge of both normal and abnormal blood values. Anemia is defined as an inability of the circulating RBCs (erythrocytes) to meet the oxygen demands of the tissues. In this sense, many of the conditions affecting newborn erythropoiesis represent early alterations from "normal" values, but do not represent true anemia. It is important to discover the etiology of an infant's altered hemoglobin concentrations or RBC indices to prevent a future anemic state, when an erythrocyte transfusion might be required. Thus, it is critical to gather information beyond the hemoglobin or hematocrit in order to define a pathologic state.

Anemia can occur at various times in the neonatal period, and is the result of one (or a combination) of three main causes: hemorrhage of RBCs (either internal or external to the body), increased destruction of RBCs (hemolysis), or inadequate production of RBCs. Severe anemia presenting in the first hours of life likely is due to acute hemorrhage or significant hemolysis due to isoimmunization. Anemia presenting after the first day or two of life can be due to various reasons, including new or continued hemorrhage, immune-mediated hemolysis, or nonimmune hemolysis. The clinician's task is to prevent a further drop in RBC concentration and, if possible, to treat the anemia appropriately.

Fetal Erythropoiesis and Adaptation to Extrauterine Life

Erythropoiesis in utero is controlled by erythroid growth factors produced solely by the fetus. Erythropoietin (Epo) is the primary regulator of erythropoiesis in adults and appears to be the controlling factor for fetal erythropoiesis. Epo does not cross the placenta in humans, and stimulation of maternal Epo production does not result in stimulation of fetal RBC production.[1] Moreover, suppression of maternal erythropoiesis by hypertransfusion does not suppress fetal erythropoiesis.[2]

Both hypoxia and anemia stimulate erythropoiesis by stimulating mRNA transcription and Epo protein production.[3] The liver is the primary source of Epo production in fetal life, both in humans and sheep; however, the fetal kidney can produce Epo in lesser amounts during the second and third trimesters.[4,5] It is not known what factors regulate the switch of Epo production from the liver to the kidney.

Epo concentrations in the fetus gradually increase until birth.[6,7] Epo concentrations measured in infants of laboring and nonlaboring mothers[8] may reflect hypoxic stress during delivery. An increase in nucleated red blood cells (NRBCs) and Epo concentrations may be associated with chronic in utero hypoxia, but acute hypoxia (<24 hours) may be associated with elevated Epo concentrations alone. Serum Epo concentrations at birth normally range from 5 to 100 mU/mL. Epo concentrations in healthy adults range from 0 to 25 mU/mL, while serum

Epo concentrations in anemic, nonuremic adults range from 300 to 400 mU/mL.[9]

Red Blood Cell Indices in the Fetus and Neonate

Red Blood Cell Concentrations and Hematocrit. Red blood cell indices vary during gestation and continue to do so through the first year of life. Table 8-1 shows changes in RBC indices during gestation. Circulating RBC concentrations gradually increase during the second and third trimesters. At term, RBC concentrations range from 5.0 to 5.5 $\times$ $10^6/\mu L$. The RBC value generally reflects the hemoglobin and hematocrit, and is useful in determining the absolute reticulocyte count, or ARC (RBC concentration $\times$ % reticulocytes = ARC).

Parallel to increasing RBC concentrations, hematocrits increase from 30% to 40% during the second trimester, and continue to increase over the latter part of the third trimester. Term hematocrits range from 50% to 63%, with some variability due to delayed clamping of the umbilical cord.[10,11] Values are also dependent on the sampling site. Capillary hematocrits may measure 9 to 12 hematocrit points higher than venous samples.

Hemoglobin. Hemoglobin concentrations gradually rise during gestation. At 10 weeks' gestation, the average hemoglobin is approximately 9 g/dL. By 22 to 24 weeks' gestation, fetal hemoglobin values reach approximately 12 g/dL, and by 30 weeks the hemoglobin concentrations are 13 to 14 g/dL.[12] Premature male infants reach term cord hemoglobin values earlier than females, possibly due to the erythropoietic effects of testosterone.[13] Hemoglobin concentrations are relatively constant over the last 6 to 8 weeks of gestation, and at term the average hemoglobin concentration is approximately 16 to 17 g/dL. At birth there may be a 1 to 2 g/dL rise in hemoglobin as a result of transfusion of placental blood at delivery. An increase in the concentration of hemoglobin within the first 2 hours of postnatal life occurs in most infants and is due to a decrease in plasma volume. By 8 to 12 hours of life, the hemoglobin concentration achieves a relatively constant level. Similar to the hematocrit, capillary hemoglobin concentrations may measure 3 to 4 g/dL higher than venous samples.

In term infants, improved oxygenation after birth results in significantly decreased erythrocyte production, reflecting a natural adaptation to the extrauterine environment. Table 8-2 illustrates RBC indices over the first 2 weeks of life. The continued decline of the hemoglobin concentrations over the next several weeks results from (1) decreased RBC production; (2) a shortened life span of the fetal erythrocyte; and (3) plasma dilution and an increase in blood volume related to growth. The nadir of hemoglobin concentration in full-term infants is seen at approximately 8 weeks with an average hemoglobin concentration of 11.2 g/dL. This value gradually rises so that by 6 months the average term infant has a hemoglobin concentration of 12.1 g/dL. Table 8-3 shows changes in RBC indices over the first 6 months of life.

The average decline in the hemoglobin of preterm infants weighing less than 1500 g is significantly different from that of term infants. This is due in part to phlebotomy losses that often occur, as well as the effects of transfusions on endogenous erythropoiesis. Such infants reach a nadir of hemoglobin that averages 8 g/dL at 4 to 8 weeks of age. Table 8-4 demonstrates relationships between birth weight, chronologic age, and hemoglobin in preterm infants.

The changes in RBC indices mentioned here do not always apply to infants born small for gestational age, as placental insufficiency and secondary polycythemia occur commonly.[14,15] Infants of diabetic mothers, infants of mothers who smoke, and infants born at higher altitudes also tend to have higher hemoglobin concentrations at birth.[16-18]

Mean Cell Volume. The size of the RBC gradually decreases during development. The mean cell volume (MCV) is greater than 180 fL in the embryo, falls to 130 to 140 fL by midgestation, and decreases to 115 fL by the end of pregnancy.[18] By 1 year of age, the MCV reaches an average of 82 fL. Figure 8-1 demonstrates the changes in MCV observed from 28 weeks' gestation through the first months of life. Curiously, the MCV of preterm infants declines quickly after birth, and the postpartum changes in MCV appear to be related to chronological age rather than postconceptional age.

Mean Corpuscular Hemoglobin Concentration. The mean corpuscular hemoglobin concentration (MCHC) remains relatively constant from

TABLE 8-1

MEAN RED BLOOD CELL (RBC) VALUES DURING GESTATION

Age (Wk)	Hemoglobin (g/dL)	Hema-tocrit (%)	RBCs (×10⁶/mL)	Mean Cell Volume (fL)	Mean Corpuscular Hemoglobin (pg)	Mean Corpuscular Hemoglobin Concentration (g/dL)	Nucleated RBCs (% of RBCs)	Reticulocytes (%)	Diameter (U)
12	8.0–10.0	33	1.5	180	60	34	5.0–8.0	40	10.5
16	10.0	35	2.0	140	45	33	2.0–4.0	10–25	9.5
20	11.0	37	2.5	135	44	33	1.0	10–20	9.0
24	14.0	40	3.5	128	38	31	1.0	5–10	8.8
28	14.5	45	4.0	120	40	31	0.5	5–10	8.7
34	15.0	47	4.4	118	38	32	0.2	3–10	8.3

U, microns.
Modified from Oski FA: Normal blood values in the newborn period. In Oski FA, Naiman JL (eds): Hematologic Problems in the Newborn, 3rd ed. Philadelphia, WB Saunders, 1982, p 4.

TABLE 8-2

NORMAL HEMATOLOGIC VALUES DURING THE FIRST 2 WEEKS OF LIFE IN THE TERM INFANT*

Value	Cord Blood	Day 1	Day 3	Day 7	Day 14
Hemoglobin (g/dL)	16.8	18.4	17.8	17.0	16.8
Hematocrit (%)	53.0	58.0	55.0	54.0	52.0
Red blood cells ($\times 10^6$/mm^3)	5.25	5.8	5.6	5.2	5.1
Mean cell volume (fL)	107	108	99.0	98.0	96.0
Mean corpuscular hemoglobin (pg)	34	35	33	32.5	31.5
Mean corpuscular hemoglobin concentration (g/dL)	31.7	32.5	33	33	33
Reticulocytes (%)	3–7	3–7	1–3	0–1	0–1
Nucleated red blood cells (mm^3)	500	200	0–5	0	0
Platelets (1000/mm^3)	290	192	213	248	252

*During the first 2 weeks of life, a venous hemoglobin less than 13 g/dL or a capillary hemoglobin less than 14.5 g/dL should be regarded as anemia.
Modified from Oski FA, Naiman JL: Hematologic Problems in the Newborn, 2nd ed. Philadelphia, WB Saunders, 1972, p 12.

TABLE 8-3

POSTNATAL CHANGES IN HEMOGLOBIN AND RED BLOOD CELL (RBC) INDICES IN TERM INFANTS

RBC Parameters	Age of Infants								
	Days			Weeks		Months			
	1	3	7	2	4	2	3	4	6
Hemoglobin (g/dL)									
$\bar{x}$	19.4	18.6	18.7	17.6	13.9	11.2	11.4	12.0	12.1
±2 SD	17.2	16.5	16.5	13.9	10.6	9.3	9.5	10.7	10.4
(N)	(78)	(66)	(78)	(275)	(272)	(271)	(73)	(123)	(114)
Mean cell volume (fL)									
$\bar{x}$	114	110	108	106	101	95	88	84	77
±2 SD	101–128	104–116	102–114	88–125	90–112	83–107	78–98	74–95	67–87
(N)	(78)	(66)	(78)	(275)	(272)	(271)	(73)	(123)	(114)
Mean corpuscular hemoglobin (pg)									
$\bar{x}$	36.6	36.7	36.2	33.6	32.5	30.4	30.4	28.1	26.4
(N)	(59)	(47)	(66)	(232)	(240)	(241)	(60)	(123)	(114)
Mean corpuscular hemoglobin concentration (g/dL)									
$\bar{x}$	33.0	33.1	33.9	31.7	32.1	32.0	34.6	33.3	34.2
(N)	(78)	(66)	(78)	(275)	(272)	(271)	(73)	(123)	(114)

Modified from Guest GM, Brown EW: Erythrocytes and hemoglobin of the blood in infancy and childhood. III. Factors in variability, statistical studies. Am J Dis Child 1957;93:486–509; Saarinen UM, Siimes MA: Developmental changes in red blood cell counts and indices of infants after exclusion of iron deficiency by laboratory criteria and continuous iron supplementation. J Pediatr 1978;92:412–416; Matoth Y, Zaizov R, Varsano I: Postnatal changes in some red cell parameters. Acta Paediatr Scand 1971;60:317–323.

TABLE 8-4

SERIAL HEMOGLOBIN VALUES IN LOW-BIRTH-WEIGHT INFANTS

Birth Weight (g)	Age (Wk)				
	2	4	6	8	10
800–1000	16.0 (14.8–17.2)	10.0 (6.8–13.2)	8.7 (7.0–10.2)	8.0 (7.1–9.8)	8.0 (6.9–10.2)
1001–1200	16.4 (14.1–18.7)	12.8 (7.8–15.3)	10.5 (7.2–12.3)	9.1 (7.8–10.4)	8.5 (7.0–10.0)
1201–1400	16.2 (13.6–18.8)	13.4 (8.8–16.2)	10.9 (8.5–13.3)	9.9 (8.0–11.8)	9.8 (8.4–11.3)
1401–1500	15.6 (13.4–17.8)	11.7 (9.7–13.7)	10.5 (9.1–11.9)	9.8 (8.4–12.0)	9.9 (8.4–11.4)
1501–2000	15.6 (13.5–17.7)	11.0 (9.6–14.0)	9.6 (8.8–11.5)	9.8 (8.4–12.1)	10.0 (8.6–11.8)

Modified from Williams ML, Shott RJ, O'Neal PL, et al: Dietary iron and fat in vitamin E deficiency anemia of infancy. N Engl J Med 1975;292:877.

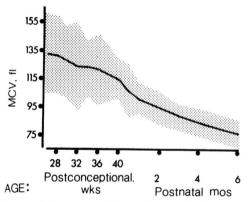

Figure 8-1 Developmental changes in mean cell volume (MCV) from cord measurements in premature infants to 38 postconceptional weeks and term infants to 6 months postnatal age. Line and hatched areas represent mean and ±2 SD of combined means and pooled variances. (From Zaizov R, Matoth Y: Red cell values on the first postnatal day during the last 16 weeks of gestation. Am J Hematol 1976;1:275–278; Saarinen UM: Need for iron supplementation in infants on prolonged breast feeding. J Pediatr 1978;93:177–180; Matoth Y, Azizov R, Varsano I: Postnatal changes in some red cell parameters. Acta Paediatr Scand 1971;60:317–323.)

birth to adulthood.[18] MCHC ranges between 31 and 33 g/dL during the newborn period. Increases in MCHC reflect distortions of RBC volume that cause compression of hemoglobin into a smaller space. Disorders such as hereditary spherocytosis, ABO incompatibility, or microangiopathic hemolytic anemia, will show elevated MCHCs, as the surface area of the RBC decreases while the hemoglobin concentration remains stable.

Red Blood Cell Distribution Width. The RBC distribution width (RDW) reflects the variation in RBC size. A more heterogeneous RBC population will be reflected by a larger RDW. Because immature cells are larger than older RBCs, an infant with active erythropoiesis will have an elevated RDW. Infants who are frequently transfused will have lower RDWs.

Reticulocyte Count. Active erythropoiesis occurs in utero, and reticulocyte counts are elevated at birth. Infants born at term generally have reticulocyte counts in the range of 3% to 7% (ARC 150,000 to 400,000 cells/μL). Infants born prematurely will have higher reticulocyte counts, generally between 6% and 10%.[19] Erythropoiesis decreases significantly after birth, with a concomitant decrease of the reticulocyte count to 1% by 1 week of life. Reticulocyte counts will

increase following the physiologic nadir (around 4 to 8 weeks of life) when erythropoiesis becomes active.

Shape and Deformability. Just as there is much variation in the size of newborn red blood cells, there is much variation in shape. Irregularly shaped cells are present in much greater numbers in the peripheral blood of newborn infants as compared with those of adults.[19] Target cells, acanthocytes, puckered immature erythrocytes, and other irregular projections may normally be found (Fig. 8-2). In normal adults, only 2.6% of erythrocytes appear to have surface pits or craters varying in size from 0.2 to 0.5 μm in diameter.[20] In contrast, pits can be found in almost half of the erythrocytes of preterm infants, and in a quarter of the erythrocytes of term infants.

RBC deformability is principally governed by three factors: the surface area/volume relationship of the red blood cell, the viscosity of the cytoplasm of the cell, and intrinsic RBC membrane rigidity. The deformability of erythrocytes is important for several reasons. First, RBC deformability appears to be an important determinant of RBC life span in vivo. The removal of a red blood cell from the circulation is thought to be a consequence of declining deformability, making the RBC susceptible to sequestration in the spleen and other organs where it must negotiate extraordinarily narrow passages. Second, RBC deformability directly influences blood flow in the peripheral circulation. Third, whole blood viscosity is affected by RBC deformability, which in turn affects peripheral vascular resistance and cardiac workload.

The densest neonatal red blood cells (representing the oldest cells in the circulation) lose more volume than adult red blood cells, have a higher mean corpuscular hemoglobin concentration, and are less deformable than the oldest red blood cells seen in adults. This suggests that there is an accelerated decrease in deformability of aging red blood cells related to a more pronounced increase in the MCHC, which is the principal determinant of the internal viscosity of the red blood cell. Neonatal RBC membranes deform more to a given shear force than do adult RBC membranes, resulting in greater susceptibility of neonatal cell membranes to fragmentation.[21] These mechanical properties may lead to accelerated membrane loss and a decreased lifespan.

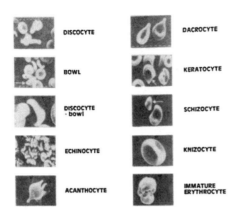

THE ERYTHROCYTE DIFFERENTIAL COUNT
(Median and 5% to 95% range)

Cell Type	Premature Infant	Term Infant	Normal Adult
Discocyte	39.5 (18-57)	43 (18-62)	78 (42-94)
Bowl	29.0 (13-53)	40 (14-58)	18 (4-50)
Discocyte-Bowl	3.0 (0-10)	2 (0-5)	2 (0-4)
Spherocyte	0.0 (0-3)	0 (0-1)	0 (0-0)
Echinocyte	5.5 (1-23)	1 (0-4)	0 (0-3)
Acanthocyte	0.0 (0-2)	1 (0-2)	0 (0-1)
Dacrocyte	1.0 (0-5)	1 (0-3)	0 (0-1)
Keratocyte	3.0 (0-7)	2 (0-5)	0 (0-1)
Schizocyte	2.0 (0-5)	0 (0-2)	0 (0-1)
Knizocyte	3.0 (0-11)	3 (0-8)	1 (0-5)
Immature erythrocyte	1.0 (0-6)	0 (0-2)	0 (0-0)

Figure 8-2 The variety of morphologic abnormalities of the erythrocyte observed in premature infants, term infants, and normal adults. (Photomicrographs courtesy of and figure adapted from Zipursky A, Brown E, Brown A, et al: The erythrocyte differential count in newborn infants. Am J Pediatr Hematol Oncol 1983;5:48–49. Adapted with permission of Raven Press, Ltd.)

TABLE 8-5

CAUSES OF HEMORRHAGE IN THE PERINATAL PERIOD

Prior to Delivery
Chronic or acute twin-to-twin transfusion syndrome
Chronic or acute fetal-maternal hemorrhage
Hemorrhage into amniotic fluid following
 periumbilical blood sampling (PUBS)
Traumatic amniocentesis
Maternal trauma
Trauma following external cephalic version

During Delivery
Placental abruption
Placenta previa
Vasa previa
Trauma or incision of placenta during cesarean
 section
Ruptured normal or abnormal (varices, aneurysms)
 umbilical cord
Cord or placental hematoma
Velamentous insertion of the cord
Nuchal cord

During or Following Delivery
Subgaleal hemorrhage
Cephalhematoma
Intraventricular/intracranial hemorrhage
 (prematurity, trauma, isoimmune
 thrombocytopenia)
Hemorrhage associated with disseminated
 intravascular coagulation/sepsis
Organ trauma (liver, spleen, adrenal, renal)
Pulmonary hemorrhage
Iatrogenic blood loss (phlebotomy, central line
 accidents, arterial line accidents)

Hemorrhage

Hemorrhage is a common cause of anemia in neonates. Blood loss can occur prior to birth or during delivery, can be associated with maternal hemorrhage or obstetric accidents, or can be due to internal hemorrhage or recurrent phlebotomy losses after birth. Maternal factors that increase the incidence of hemorrhage include third trimester bleeding with placenta previa, placental abruption, vasa previa, emergency cesarean section, twin gestation, amniocentesis, and percutaneous umbilical blood sampling (PUBS).

The clinical manifestations of hemorrhage at birth depend on the extent and duration of blood loss. When significant acute blood loss has occurred, the infant will be limp, pale, unresponsive, and require immediate volume expansion and (likely) a rapid transfusion. Although the hemoglobin may be in the normal range initially, or may be low, it will fall within 6 to 8 hours after birth. Internal hemorrhage should be suspected when a newborn who is 24 to 48 hours old has evidence of hypovolemic shock without signs of external blood loss.

As many as one fourth of newborns admitted to newborn intensive care units experience a decrease in their RBC volume due to hemorrhage.[22] The blood loss may equal 50% to 100% of the total blood volume following a severe hemorrhage. Hemorrhagic anemia in the newborn period can be divided temporally into three general categories (Table 8-5): prenatal hemorrhage from the fetus into the maternal circulation or into a twin; hemorrhage due to obstetric accidents of the placenta or cord around the time of delivery; and postnatal hemorrhage due to trauma, sepsis/disseminated intravascular coagulation (DIC), or phlebotomy loss. Severe hemorrhage will produce pallor and shock, and should be recognized immediately in order to prevent significant organ damage or death.

Blood Volume

The placenta and umbilical cord contain 75 to 125 mL of blood at term, or approximately a quarter to a third of the fetal blood volume.[23] Umbilical arteries constrict shortly after birth, but the umbilical vein remains dilated, and blood flows in the direction of gravity. Infants held below the level of the placenta can receive half of the placental blood volume (30 to 50 mL) in 1 minute. Conversely, infants held above the placenta can lose 20 to 30 mL of blood back into the placenta per minute.[24] The blood volume of infants with early cord clamping averages 72 mL/kg, but the volume of infants with delayed cord clamping averages 93 mL/kg.[25] The neonatal blood volume can be 50% higher in infants who experience delayed cord clamping than in infants who have their cord clamped immediately after birth.

Preterm infants have slightly larger blood volumes (89 to 105 mL/kg) due to an increased plasma volume. At 30 weeks' gestation, half of the approximately 120 mL/kg total blood volume of the fetoplacental circulation is in the fetus.[26] Preterm infants commonly experience rapid cord clamping resulting in a decreased blood volume. This occurs in part because of the urgency in initiating resuscitative measures in some preterm infants.

Case Study 1

Baby boy B is a newborn term infant born to a 22-year-old, AB positive, antibody screen negative, gravida 2 para 2 Hispanic mother via repeat cesarean section at 38 weeks' gestation. The infant required "blow-by" oxygen and positive pressure ventilation for 30 seconds before spontaneous respirations occurred. Apgar scores were 6 at 1 minute and 7 at 5 minutes. Birth weight was 2710 g. On physical examination, heart rate was 178 bpm, respiratory rate 64, temperature 36.9°C, and blood pressure 58/34 mm Hg. The infant was pale, not jaundiced, and in moderate respiratory distress. Oxygen saturation on 35% inspired oxygen by oxygen hood was 98%. The cardiac examination reveals a 2/6 systolic ejection murmur over the lower left sternal border, a liver edge 3.5 cm below the right costal margin, and decreased pulses. The rest of the physical examination is completely normal.

Exercise 1

QUESTIONS

1. Which of the following diagnoses would be consistent with this clinical picture?
   a. Perinatal hypoxic injury
   b. Septic shock
   c. Acute hemorrhage
   d. Congenital heart disease
   e. All of the above

2. What is the first step in management of this infant?
   a. Transfuse with 10 mL/kg type O negative packed RBCs
   b. Obtain a blood gas analysis for acid-base and ventilation status
   c. Intubate and provide 100% oxygen
   d. Administer prostaglandins
   e. Begin phototherapy

ANSWERS

1. e. All of these diagnoses may present in similar fashion in the immediate newborn period as a pale infant with respiratory distress.

2. b. Determining the infant's ability to ventilate and the adequacy of overall circulation via acid-base status will be the most helpful of these choices in providing rapid, appropriate care. An immediate transfusion is not indicated without knowing the infant's circulatory status. Intubation may be required if the infant is not ventilating adequately. Administering prostaglandins prior to further evaluations is not recommended. Phototherapy is not indicated at this time until a bilirubin determination is made or knowledge of hemolytic disease is obtained.

A spun hematocrit is determined to be 16% and the complete blood count (CBC) demonstrated a hematocrit of 14.8%, hemoglobin 5.0 g/dL, MCV 94 fL, MCHC 32 g/dL, RDW 21%. The capillary blood gas shows the following: pH 7.10, Pco_2 32 mm Hg, Po_2 41 mm Hg, bicarbonate 8, base deficit 16. Further maternal information is gathered. The mother had noted decreased fetal movement during the last 2 days prior to birth. External monitoring prior to cesarean section showed a sinusoidal pattern. There *was no evidence of abruption or trauma to the placenta or cord.*

QUESTION

3. Which of the following maternal laboratory tests would be helpful?

    a. Repeat antibody screen

    b. Maternal CBC and RBC indices

    c. Kleihauer-Betke (KB) test

    d. Group B streptococcus (GBS) status

    e. Maternal liver function tests

ANSWER

3. c. A Kleihauer-Betke test to search for evidence of fetal hemorrhage into the maternal circulation would be the most helpful in determining the cause of this infant's anemia. In this case, the KB test was positive for fetal cells in the maternal circulation. This infant's anemia was the result of chronic, severe fetomaternal hemorrhage.

Fetomaternal Hemorrhage

Maternal and fetal circulating cells may, at varying times, cross the placental barrier. Fetal contamination of the maternal circulation can occur prior to delivery. Although 50% to 75% of pregnancies are associated with some degree of fetomaternal hemorrhage (FMH), the volumes of fetal transplacental transfer are relatively small, usually on the order of 0.01 to 0.1 mL. About 1 pregnancy in 400 is associated with a fetal transplacental bleed of 30 mL or greater, and about 1 pregnancy in 2000 is associated with a fetal transplacental hemorrhage of 100 mL or more.[27]

Given the frequency of FMH, it is understandable why mothers can become sensitized to fetal blood. The overall risk of Rh immunization occurring in an Rh-incompatible pregnancy is 16% if the fetus is Rh positive, ABO compatible with its mother. This risk decreases to 1.5% if the fetus is Rh positive, ABO incompatible. Fetal transfer of cells to the mother occurs during abortions as well (about a 2% incidence of such transfer with spontaneous abortion and a 4% to 5% rate if abortion is induced).[28]

Because fetal hemoglobin is resistant to acid elution, cells containing fetal hemoglobin (hemoglobin F) can be distinguished from cells

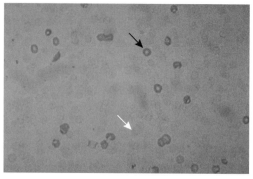

Figure 8-3 Kleihauer-Betke (KB) stain of maternal blood. Dark cells (*black arrow*) contain fetal hemoglobin, and clear or "ghost" cells (*white arrow*) contain adult hemoglobin.

containing adult hemoglobin (hemoglobin A). The Kleihauer-Betke (KB) stain of peripheral maternal blood utilizes this characteristic of fetal hemoglobin to detect fetal cells in the maternal circulation.[29] Peripheral smears of maternal blood stained in this fashion will reveal "ghost-like" cells of maternal origin (previously containing adult hemoglobin), and pink fetal cells, still containing fetal hemoglobin that has resisted elution (Fig. 8-3). Results from mothers with increased fetal hemoglobin synthesis (i.e., sickle cell disease, thalassemia, and hereditary persistence of fetal hemoglobin) are less reliable owing to increased maternal hemoglobin F, and other measures should be taken to detect FMH in these cases. Diagnosis of FMH may also be missed when the mother and infant are ABO incompatible. In these cases the fetal cells are rapidly cleared from the maternal circulation by maternal anti-A or anti-B antibodies. An example of how to estimate fetal blood loss based on the results of a KB stain follows:

Example. *Information to gather:* maternal weight, maternal hematocrit, infant weight, KB stain results.

Normal values: average maternal blood volume is 75 mL/kg at term (normal adult blood volume = 60 mL/kg); average fetal-placental blood volume is 120 mL/kg at term.

You are given a KB stain result of 2%. This means that 2% of the RBCs on the mother's peripheral smear contain fetal blood. If the mother weighs 80 kg and her hematocrit is 35%, then her RBC volume can be calculated as:

$$80 \text{ kg (weight)} \times 0.35 \text{ (hematocrit)}$$
$$\times 75 \text{ mL/kg (blood volume)}$$
$$= 2100 \text{ mL (RBC volume)}$$

If 2% of this RBC volume is fetal, then the estimated fetal RBC mass transferred into the maternal circulation is:

$$2100 \text{ mL} \times 0.02 = 42 \text{ mL}$$

If the infant weighs 3 kg and had a prehemorrhage hematocrit of 45%, then the fetoplacental RBC volume can be calculated as:

$$3 \text{ kg} \times 0.45 \times 120 \text{ mL/kg} = 162 \text{ mL}$$

The infant would therefore have hemorrhaged 42 of 162 mL, or 26% of its RBC volume into the maternal circulation. This would be considered a moderate fetomaternal hemorrhage. The infant would likely exhibit signs of volume loss if the hemorrhage occurred acutely.

Severe FMH occurs in 1 in 1000 deliveries, and has been associated with decreased fetal movements and a fetal sinusoidal heart rate (SHR) pattern.[30] Low neonatal RBC volumes are associated with a maternal history of vaginal bleeding, placenta previa or abruption, nonelective cesarean section, and deliveries associated with cord compression. Significant FMH has been described following trauma, and fetal hemorrhage into the placenta has been associated with placental chorioangioma.[31]

Infants in whom a significant hemorrhage is suspected need rapid evaluation and treatment. The infant with massive hemorrhage will present with pallor and tachypnea, but generally without an oxygen requirement. Hemoglobin concentrations can be extremely low at birth, between 4 and 6 g/dL.[32] A significant metabolic acidosis is often present as a result of hypoperfusion.

Other causes of pallor in the newborn period do occur, and can be ruled out once the infant is stable. Infants with asphyxia and infants with chronic anemia due to hemolysis can also present with pallor. These diagnoses can be distinguished from acute hemorrhage based on differences in clinical signs and symptoms (Table 8-6). The clinical picture with chronic blood loss is usually mild, and infants respond to conservative therapy with iron alone. Asphyxiated infants will be pale, floppy, and may have poor peripheral circulation. The hemoglobin concentration will be stable, but may decrease if DIC and internal bleeding occur.

Twin-to-Twin Transfusion Syndrome

Twin-to-twin transfusion syndrome (TTS) is a complication of monochorionic twin gestations, occurring in 5% to 30% of these pregnancies.[33] The perinatal mortality rate can be as high as 70% to 100%, depending on severity and timing of presentation.

Acute TTS generally results in twins of similar size, but with hemoglobin concentrations that vary by more than 5 g/dL. In the chronic form of TTS, one twin becomes progressively anemic and growth retarded, while the recipient twin becomes polycythemic, macrosomic, and sometimes hypertensive. Both infants can develop hydrops fetalis; the donor twin becomes

---

TABLE 8-6

DIFFERENTIAL DIAGNOSIS OF THE PALE NEWBORN

Affected Organ System	Asphyxia	Severe Acute Hemorrhage	Hemolysis
Neurologic	Abnormal transition period, hypotonic, decreased arousal state, seizures in first days of life	Normal or hyperalert/hyperirritable ("catecholamine response")	Normal
Respiratory	Respiratory distress, O_2 requirement	Tachypnea, no O_2 requirement	Normal
Cardiovascular	Normal to bradycardia	Tachycardia, hypotension	May vary from normal to presence of congestive heart failure and hydrops, depending on degree of anemia
Hematologic	Hematocrit/hemoglobin remains stable over time; may develop thrombocytopenia and disseminated intravascular coagulopathy from hypoxic injury to marrow	Drop in hematocrit/hemoglobin	Anemic from birth, hepatosplenomegaly, jaundice, positive Coombs' test

hydropic from profound anemia, while the recipient twin becomes hydropic from congestive heart failure and hypervolemia. Because of significant differences in blood volume, renal blood flow, and urine output, the donor twin experiences oligohydramnios, while the recipient twin experiences polyhydramnios.

The diagnosis of chronic TTS can be made by serial prenatal ultrasound studies measuring cardiomegaly, discordant amniotic fluid production, fetal growth discrepancy of more than 20%, and hemoglobin concentration differences greater than 5 g/dL between infants. After birth the donor twin often requires transfusions, and can also experience neutropenia, hydrops from severe anemia, growth restriction, congestive heart failure, and hypoglycemia. The recipient twin is often sicker, and can suffer from hypertrophic cardiomyopathy, congestive heart failure, polycythemia, hyperviscosity, respiratory difficulties, hypocalcemia, and hypoglycemia. The risk of antenatally acquired neurologic cerebral lesions is 20% to 30% in both twins,[33] and the incidence of neurologic morbidities following the intrauterine death of one of the fetuses averages 20% to 25%. Morbidities include multiple cerebral infarctions, hypoperfusion syndromes from hypotension, and periventricular leukomalacia. Long-term neurologic follow-up is indicated for all TTS survivors.

Consensus is lacking on the ideal treatment for TTS. Treatment consists of close monitoring, and may include reduction amniocenteses to decrease uterine stretch and prolong the pregnancy, selective feticide, laser ablatement of bridging vessels, or septostomy.[34–38] In a randomized study comparing amnioreduction versus septostomy, investigators reported similar rates of at least one twin surviving (78% for amnioreduction and 80% for septostomy); however, those women randomized to septostomy were more likely to require only one procedure (46% versus 64% with reduction).[39] Another study compared laser ablation with amnioreduction[40] in mothers randomized before 26 weeks' gestation. The study was concluded early due to a significant benefit in the laser group. Infants in the laser group had a 76% survival rate of at least one twin at 28 days, compared to a 56% survival rate in the amnioreduction group. Infants in the laser group had a lower incidence of cystic periventricular leukomalacia (6% versus 14%, $P = 0.02$) and were more likely to be free of neurologic complications at 6 months of age (52% versus 31%, $P = 0.003$).

Obstetric Accidents

Obstetric accidents occur infrequently, but can be a significant cause of blood loss. Obstetric complications include placenta previa and placental abruption, incision or tearing of the placenta during cesarean section, and cord avulsion of normal or abnormal umbilical cords. In addition, newborns may experience significant blood loss back into the placenta (fetoplacental hemorrhage). Moreover, placental anomalies (including multilobed placenta and placental chorioangiomas) may be a source of hemorrhage during the perinatal period.

Placental Abruption and Placenta Previa. Placental abruption involves premature separation of the placenta from the uterus, and occurs in 3 to 6 per 1000 live births. Severe fetal growth restriction, prolonged rupture of membranes, chorioamnionitis, hypertension (chronic or pregnancy-induced), cigarette smoking, advanced maternal age, and male fetal gender are potential risk factors for placental abruption. The incidence increases with decreasing gestation, and mortality rate ranges 0.8 to 2 per 1000 births,[41] which equates to 15% to 20% of deliveries in which significant abruption occurs.

Placenta previa occurs when part or all of the placenta overlies the cervical os. Women with a history of a previous cesarean birth and increased parity are at increased risk of having a pregnancy complicated by placenta previa.[42] In addition, current cigarette smoking is associated with a two- to fourfold increased risk of placenta previa.[43]

Infants born following placental abruption may be anemic, but may also present with signs of hypoxia or anoxia. In these infants it is important to monitor changes in hematocrit and neurologic signs.

The need for postnatal transfusions in the infant is generally associated with the volume of maternal hemorrhage. Whenever there is evidence of placental abruption, placenta previa, or unusual vaginal bleeding, the infant's hemoglobin should be measured at birth and again at 12 to 24 hours. A KB stain should also be performed on maternal blood to determine if fetomaternal hemorrhage occurred. Monitoring mothers with a history of second or third trimester bleeding with Doppler flow ultrasound may decrease the incidence of anemia and fetal loss by anticipating fetal hemorrhage associated with placental abnormalities.[44]

Cord Rupture and Hematomas of the Cord.

Excess traction on an abnormally formed or shortened umbilical cord can result in cord rupture, usually occurring on the fetal side. Abnormalities in cord formation include cord aneurysms, varices, and cysts. Cord infections can increase the risk for rupture by weakening the cord. Infants born precipitously may also be at increased risk for hemorrhage due to a ruptured cord.

Subamniotic hematomas can occur when chorionic vessels rupture near the cord insertion. Most subamniotic hematomas are the result of excessive traction on a normal or shortened umbilical cord, and are not noted until after delivery. Hematomas of the cord occur infrequently (1 in 5000 to 6000 deliveries), but can also be a cause of fetal blood loss, and may be associated with significant risk of perinatal death.[45] Intrauterine death may occur due to compression of the umbilical vein and arteries by the hematoma. Cord hematomas can result from trauma due to PUBS, and can also be associated with high maternal alpha-fetoprotein levels. Hematomas of the cord can be accurately diagnosed in utero by ultrasound and differentiated from other lesions of the placenta and cord.[46] The lesion can be associated with poor fetal growth and FMH.

Velamentous Insertion.

Velamentous insertion of the umbilical cord occurs in approximately 0.5% to 2% of pregnancies. In velamentous insertion the umbilical cord enters the membranes distant from the placenta. Blood vessels are, therefore, unprotected by Wharton's jelly and are more likely to tear. Rupture of anomalous vessels in the absence of traction or trauma can occur even if the cord itself attaches centrally or paracentrally. The fetal mortality rate remains very high in this condition, because detection by routine ultrasound is rare. Eddleman and coworkers noted that targeted sonographic examination of the placental site of umbilical cord insertion could reveal abnormal placental cord insertions, but distinguishing the specific type of abnormal insertion would likely require the use of ultrasound.[47]

Vasa Previa.

Prenatal diagnosis of vasa previa (anomalous vessels overlying the internal os of the cervix) can be detected with transvaginal color Doppler, and should be suspected in any case of antepartum or intrapartum hemorrhage. Although uncommon (1 in 3000 deliveries), the perinatal death rate is high, ranging from 33% to 100% when undetected before delivery. Infants are often stillborn.[48]

Fetoplacental Hemorrhage.

Blood loss into the placenta is a common cause of anemia in neonates. As mentioned previously, a large residual volume of blood remains in the placenta, and blood will continue to flow in the direction of gravity after birth. Fetoplacental hemorrhage can occur when the infant is held above the placenta after birth, and for this reason infants born by cesarean section have smaller blood volumes than those born vaginally.[49] In addition, infants can lose 10% to 20% of their total blood volume when born with a tight nuchal cord.[50] Tight nuchal cords allow blood to be pumped through umbilical arteries while constricting flow through the umbilical vein.

Birth Trauma

Subgaleal Hemorrhage

Blood loss into the subgaleal space can occur during difficult deliveries requiring instrument assistance, such as face presentation, occiput posterior presentations, and shoulder dystocias. Subgaleal hematomas are potentially life-threatening events, and must be recognized as early as possible to prevent significant morbidity or death. These hematomas occur when emissary or "bridging" veins are torn. Blood accumulates into a large potential space between the galea aponeurotica (the epicranial aponeurosis) and the periosteum of the skull. The subgaleal space extends from the orbital ridge to the base of the skull, and can easily accommodate greater than 85 mL/kg of blood, or an infant's entire blood volume.

Subgaleal hematomas may form because of preexisting risk factors (such as coagulopathy or asphyxia), but vacuum extraction itself predisposes an infant toward subgaleal bleeding. The presence of a ballotable fluid collection in dependent regions of the infant's head, coupled with signs of hypovolemia in a neonate should raise the possibility of subgaleal bleeding. Treatment of symptomatic infants requires restoration of blood volume and control of bleeding. Exsanguination due to subgaleal hemorrhage has been reported, and the mortality rate is high if the hemorrhage goes unrecognized. A formula predicting the volume of blood loss has been developed: for every 1 cm increase in head circumference, 38 mL of blood has been lost.[51]

Limiting the frequency and duration of vacuum assistance in high-risk infants may decrease the incidence of subgaleal hematomas. In a study of 134 infants undergoing vacuum extraction, 28 had scalp trauma, and only 1 infant had subgaleal, subdural, and subarachnoid hemorrhage.[52] The duration of vacuum application is thought to be the best predictor of scalp injury, followed by duration of second stage of labor and paramedian cup placement. In another study, of those infants with reported subgaleal hemorrhages, 80% to 90% had some history of vacuum or instrument-assisted delivery.[53] It is important to remember that delivery by cesarean section does not preclude the use of vacuum or forceps, and significant hemorrhage can still occur via this route of delivery.

Intracranial Hemorrhage

Infants born prematurely are at risk for intraventricular hemorrhage (IVH), and the risk increases with decreasing gestation. Other risk factors for IVH include duration of painful labor, duration of antibiotic therapy, and maternal age.[54] The incidence and severity of intraventricular hemorrhage and periventricular leukomalacia increase in women with premature rupture of membranes and preterm labor, especially if infection is present.[55]

Infants with IVH may be asymptomatic, or may develop signs such as apnea and bradycardia, lethargy, seizures, hypoglycemia, acidosis, anemia, or a bulging fontanel. The volume of blood loss may be as great at 10% to 15% of the total blood volume. Treatment consists of supportive care, including maintaining adequate intravascular volume and oxygen delivery, supporting oxygenation and ventilation, and maintaining blood glucose concentrations. An erythrocyte transfusion may be indicated in severely affected preterm infants.

Infants with alloimmune thrombocytopenia are also at increased risk for intracranial hemorrhage. Alloimmune thrombocytopenia results from platelet-antigen incompatibility between the mother and fetus, and occurs in 1 to 2 per 1000 live births.[56] Infants present with unexplained neonatal thrombocytopenia. From 10% to 20% of newborns with platelet alloimmunization will have intracranial hemorrhages, of which half occur in utero. The risk for intracranial hemorrhage is increased in newborns with an affected sibling who had an antenatal intracranial hemorrhage, and the second affected newborn generally has more severe disease than the first. Treatment includes platelet transfusions and intravenous immunoglobulin (IVIG). Treatment of fetal thrombocytopenia includes maternal IVIG administration, maternal steroid administration, and fetal platelet transfusions.[57]

Infants born to mothers using cocaine are at risk for anemia due to abruption and intracranial hemorrhage. Prenatal cocaine exposure increases the risk of maternal hypertension, placental abruption, and spontaneous abortion. The fetus is at risk for intrauterine growth restriction, intracranial hemorrhage, and fetal edema.[58]

Internal Hemorrhage

Anemia appearing after the first 24 hours of life in an infant without jaundice may result from internal hemorrhage. In addition to birth trauma causing visible hemorrhages such as cephalhematomas, excessive bruising, and subgaleal hemorrhages, internal hemorrhage can occur following a traumatic delivery. Breech deliveries may be associated with renal, adrenal, or splenic hemorrhage into the retroperitoneal space. Delivery of large infants, such as infants born to diabetic mothers, may also result in organ damage and hemorrhage. Infants with overwhelming sepsis may develop disseminated intravascular coagulation (DIC) and hemorrhage into liver, adrenal glands, and lungs.

Adrenal Hemorrhage. Adrenal hemorrhage may result in anemia, but may also result in circulatory collapse due to the loss of organ function. The reported incidence of adrenal hemorrhage is 1.7 per 1000 births.[59] Adrenal hemorrhage can be caused by trauma, but infectious causes of DIC and hemorrhage have also been reported. Adrenal hemorrhage can also affect surrounding organs, resulting in intestinal obstruction and kidney dysfunction. Diagnosis can be made using ultrasonography, whereby calcifications or cystic masses are noted. Adrenal hemorrhage can be distinguished from renal vein thrombosis by ultrasound. In addition, infants with renal vein thrombosis may have gross or microscopic hematuria, and may also develop renal failure and hypertension.

Hepatic, Splenic, and Other Soft Tissue Hemorrhages. Hepatic or splenic rupture can result from birth trauma or from distention caused by extramedullary hematopoiesis, such as that seen in erythroblastosis fetalis. Abdominal distention and discoloration, scrotal swelling, and pallor are clinical signs of splenic rupture, but may also be seen with adrenal hemorrhage or hepatic rupture. Other less common causes of hemorrhage in the newborn include hemangiomas of the gastrointestinal tract,[60] vascular malformations of the skin, and hemorrhage into soft tumors such as giant sacrococcygeal teratomas.

Disseminated Intravascular Coagulation/Sepsis. Hemorrhage associated with overwhelming sepsis can occur due to DIC and consumption of clotting factors in the neonate. Infections caused by group B streptococcus (GBS), *Escherichia coli*, and other organisms can progress to septic shock and DIC. Viral pathogens such as cytomegalovirus (CMV), herpes simplex virus, and others may cause a hemolytic anemia, but may also be a cause of overwhelming sepsis and DIC.

Hemorrhage due to Abnormal Clotting Mechanisms or Iatrogenic Causes. Infants may develop a hemorrhagic anemia due to abnormalities in hemostasis. Male infants with factor VIII and IX deficiencies may bleed excessively following circumcision, and infants with factor XIII deficiency may have continual oozing of blood from the umbilical stump. These infants require further evaluation of their bleeding.

Infants with central umbilical lines are at risk for external hemorrhage from accidental blood loss. Lines should be constantly monitored to make sure that connections do not become displaced, as exsanguination can occur. Preterm infants can also develop anemia due to excessive phlebotomy losses. Losses during the first few weeks of hospitalization can equal or exceed 10% of the infant's total blood volume per day. Blood removed for laboratory tests should be recorded on the infant's flowsheet, and every effort should be made to limit blood sampling.

Diagnosis and Management of Hemorrhage

The diagnosis of hemorrhage in the newborn can at times be difficult. Infants can present with a spectrum of clinical characteristics, depending on the degree of hypovolemia and anemia, and depending on the timing of blood loss. Table 8-7 describes the differences seen in acute versus chronic blood loss. Infants with

TABLE 8-7

ACUTE VERSUS CHRONIC BLOOD LOSS IN THE NEONATE

Parameters	Acute Blood Loss	Chronic Blood Loss
Clinical characteristics		
General appearance	Pale, hyperalert, "stunned" gaze	Pale, normal neurologic examination
Cardiovascular	Tachycardic, weak pulses, low blood pressure	Normal, rarely may have congestive heart failure with hepatomegaly, normal or increased blood pressure
Respiratory	Tachypneic, no oxygen requirement	Normal, rarely may be tachypneic with an oxygen requirement if congestive heart failure is present
Hematologic		
Hemoglobin	May be normal, drops over 24 hours	Low at birth
Morphology	Macrocytic normochromic (normal)	Microcytic hypochromic anemia
Iron	Normal iron at birth	Low iron at birth
Course	Promptly treat hypovolemia, may need rapid volume expansion to prevent shock, disseminated intravascular coagulation, and death	Usually uneventful hospital course, may need treatment for congestive heart failure and hydrops
Treatment	Volume expansion with isotonic fluid and packed red blood cells, fresh frozen plasma, and platelets; iron therapy later; Epo therapy may be appropriate to enhance erythropoiesis	Initiate iron therapy; packed red blood cell transfusion rarely needed; Epo therapy may be appropriate to enhance erythropoiesis

acute hemorrhage will be pale and tachycardic. They may be neurologically normal, hyperalert, or may appear lethargic. Infants who present with hypotension have generally experienced significant blood loss, and are at risk for shock and death. Infants are often tachypneic, but do not improve with oxygen administration. The tachypnea results from the metabolic acidosis seen with underperfusion. Hemoglobin concentrations may initially be normal, and then drop in the first 6 to 8 hours of life. Iron stores are normal at birth, and the RBC morphology shows typical normochromic, macrocytic newborn cells.

Rapid resuscitative measures can be life-saving for infants with a significant acute hemorrhage. The ABCs of newborn resuscitation are followed, which include drying, suctioning the mouth and nose, stimulating the infant, and administering oxygen. In a newborn with extreme pallor, further resuscitative measures are required to establish rapid intravenous access. A 5 or 8 French umbilical catheter (or orogastric tube if an umbilical catheter is not available) should be inserted into the umbilical vein until blood return is present (generally 4 to 6 cm). A sample of blood is sent for hemoglobin determination, blood type, and cross-match. Volume resuscitation with available fluid, generally normal saline, is given as a 20 mL/kg bolus. The volume can be given even if the cause of the pallor has not yet been determined, because some infants present with both anemia and asphyxia (such as infants born following placental abruption). Infants with acute blood loss will often show dramatic improvement, while those with ongoing internal hemorrhage, DIC, subgaleal hemorrhage, or asphyxia may remain limp and unresponsive.

Once the diagnosis of hypovolemia due to acute blood loss has been established, a repeat bolus should be given. If available, type O negative packed RBCs should be infused rapidly. Infants with acute blood loss (unlike those with chronic blood loss) have lost platelets and plasma clotting factors along with the loss of RBCs. Further resuscitative measures should therefore include evaluation of the infant's bleeding status and replacement with fresh frozen plasma and platelets as needed.

Infants who are anemic at birth from chronic blood loss may be asymptomatic. Their hemoglobin concentration will be low, and the peripheral smear often reveals microcytic, hypochromic cells indicating iron deficiency. Infants with significant chronic blood loss (such as the donor twin in TTS) may present in congestive heart failure and hydrops. Therapy includes supporting cardiac function with pressors and diuretics as needed, performing pleurocenteses if significant effusions are present in order to improve lung expansion, and maintaining oxygen delivery to tissues.

Iron therapy is indicated for both groups of infants. Infants suffering acute blood loss will receive iron in the form of transfused blood, but generally the replacement does not equal the amount of iron lost. Infants who have experienced chronic blood loss are iron deficient at birth, and replacement therapy should start immediately at 6 mg/kg/day of ferrous sulfate. The administration of Epo to enhance erythropoiesis may be appropriate for some of these infants, especially those born prematurely.

Hemolysis

Hemolytic anemia is commonly seen in the newborn period, and can be caused by a variety of factors both intrinsic and extrinsic to the red blood cell. Regardless of etiology, the fundamental characteristic of all hemolytic anemias is a reduction in the lifespan of red blood cells. The average lifespan for a neonatal red blood cell is 60 to 90 days, approximately one half to two thirds that of an adult red blood cell. Remarkably shorter RBC lifespans (35 to 50 days) are found with increasing prematurity. The shortened RBC lifespan of the preterm and term neonate may be explained by some of the characteristics specific to newborn red blood cells. These include a rapid decline in intracellular enzyme activity and ATP, loss of membrane surface area, decreased levels of intracellular carnitine, and increased mechanical fragility and susceptibility to peroxidation.[21,61–63]

Hemolysis in the newborn period is most commonly marked by jaundice, and may also be associated with hepatosplenomegaly. Some of the more common causes of hemolysis in the newborn period are listed in Table 8-8. Hemolysis can be classified into three general categories: immune-mediated hemolysis, congenital defects of the RBC, and acquired defects of the RBC.

TABLE 8-8

CAUSES OF HEMOLYSIS IN THE NEWBORN PERIOD

Immune-mediated
Rh incompatibility (anti-D antibody)
ABO incompatibility
Minor blood group incompatibility: c, C, e, G, Fya
  (Duffy), Kell group, Jka, MNS, Vw
Drug-induced (penicillin, alpha-methyldopa,
  cephalothin)
Maternal autoimmune hemolytic anemia

Infection
Bacterial sepsis (*Escherichia coli*, group B
  streptococcus)
Parvovirus B-19 (can present with hydrops fetalis)
Congenital syphilis
Congenital malaria
Congenital TORCH infections (toxoplasmosis,
  cytomegalovirus, rubella, disseminated herpes)
Other congenital viral infections

Disseminated Intravascular Coagulation

Hereditary Erythrocyte Membrane Disorders
Spherocytosis
Elliptocytosis
Stomatocytosis
Pyropoikilocytosis
Other membrane disorders

Congenital Erythrocyte Enzyme Defects
Glucose-6-phosphate dehydrogenase (G6PD)
  deficiency
Pyruvate kinase (PK) deficiency
Hexokinase deficiency
Glucose phosphate isomerase deficiency
Pyrimidine 5'-nucleotidase deficiency

Hemoglobin Defects
Alpha-thalassemia syndromes
Gamma-thalassemia syndromes
Alpha and gamma chain structural anomalies

Macro- and Microangiopathic Hemolysis
Cavernous hemangiomas
Arteriovenous malformations
Renal artery stenosis or thrombosis
Other large vessel thrombi
Severe coarctation of the aorta
Severe valvular stenoses

Other Causes
Galactosemia
Lysosomal storage diseases
Prolonged metabolic acidosis from metabolic disease
  (amino acid and organic acid disorders)
Transfusion reactions
TAR (thrombocytopenia–absent radius) syndrome
Drug-induced hemolysis (valproic acid)

Case Study 2

Baby girl A is a preterm AGA (appropriate for gestational age) infant born to a 30-year-old gravida 3 now para 3 mother via spontaneous vaginal delivery at 34 {4/7} weeks' gestation, following preterm premature rupture of membranes. The mother received intrapartum antibiotics. Apgar scores were 7 at 1 minute and 9 at 5 minutes. Birth weight was 2240 g. A complete blood count with differential showed an hematocrit of 41%, hemoglobin 13.9 g/dL, RBC 3.9 × 10⁶/μL, MCV 110 fL, MCHC 35.8 g/dL, RDW 16.8%, nucleated red blood cells (NRBCs) 12/100 white blood cells (WBCs). The peripheral smear was remarkable for moderate spherocytosis, poikilocytosis, and anisocytosis. On physical examination the following morning, the heart rate is 152 bpm, the respiratory rate is 40 and unlabored, the temperature is 36.9°C, and the blood pressure is 63/40 mm Hg. The infant is pink, slightly jaundiced, and in no distress. She has a normal cardiac examination, no hepatosplenomegaly, and is normal neurologically. She appears to be 34 weeks by examination. A total bilirubin obtained at 24 hours of life is 14.2 mg/dL with a direct component of 0.3 mg/dL. A repeat spun hematocrit is 38%.

Exercise 2

QUESTIONS

1. True or false: The RBC indices are normal for a preterm newborn.

2. Which of the general categories of hemorrhage, hemolysis, or hypoproliferative disorder would be most likely, and which would be least likely?

3. Which of the following laboratory values would be helpful?

   a. Coombs' test

   b. Maternal blood type

   c. Maternal antibody screening test

   d. Osmotic fragility test

   e. b and c

   f. a, b, and c

ANSWERS

1. False. The hematocrit is below average for a 34-week gestation infant, the MCHC is elevated, and the RDW is increased.

2. Hemolysis is most likely, given the rapid elevation in bilirubin and the mild decrease in hematocrit. A hypoproliferative disorder would be least likely, given the elevated RDW, which reflects a wide range of blood cell sizes and thus new RBC production.

3. f. Maternal blood type, antibody screening test, and a direct Coombs' test on neonatal blood will assist in the diagnosis of hemolytic disease. The presence of spherocytes on the peripheral smear may be due to immune-mediated hemolysis or may represent congenital spherocytosis. However, an osmotic fragility test would not be performed until the presence or absence of immune-mediated hemolysis is determined, and until the infant reaches a period without significant active hemolysis. In this case, the mother was type O positive, antibody screening test negative, and the infant was type A positive, direct Coombs' test positive. This infant has one of the most common diagnoses for hemolytic disease: ABO incompatibility resulting in immune-mediated hemolysis, elevated bilirubin, and a decrease in hematocrit.

Isoimmune Hemolytic Anemias

RBC antigens in the ABO, MN, Rh, Kell, Duffy, and Vel systems are well developed in early intrauterine life.[64] They are easily demonstrated in the fifth to seventh gestational weeks and remain constant through the remainder of intrauterine development. A and B antigens are present early in utero, but antibody production occurs much later.[65] By 30 to 34 weeks' gestation, however, about 50% of infants will have some measurable anti-A or anti-B antibodies. The fetal production of such antibodies is not related to maternal ABO blood type. Intrauterine exposure to gram-negative organisms whose antigens are chemically related to those of blood groups A and B is a potent stimulus for the development of these antibodies.

Rh and ABO Isoimmunization

Isoimmunization due to maternal anti-D antibody is one of the most common forms of immune-mediated hemolysis. Severe hemolysis can lead to hydrops and fetal demise. With the development of RhoGAM the incidence of severe Rh hemolytic disease has decreased dramatically.

In fetuses severely affected with Rh hemolytic disease, ultrasound-guided intravascular intrauterine transfusions can treat anemia and reverse hydrops. Infants with Rh hemolytic disease often have an early (congenital) anemia due to hemolysis, and can develop a "late" (age 1 to 3 months) anemia due to diminished erythrocyte production.

Isoimmunization due to ABO incompatibility is a common cause of hemolytic disease in the newborn period. ABO incompatibility represents a spectrum of hemolytic disease in newborns, ranging from infants with little or no evidence of erythrocyte sensitization but evidence of hemolysis, to infants with severe hemolytic disease in which erythrocyte sensitization is markedly present. ABO incompatibility can occur during a first pregnancy, as well as during subsequent pregnancies. Unlike Rh disease, there is no way to predict severity for ABO incompatibility in subsequent pregnancies. Table 8-9 compares the laboratory and clinical aspects of Rh isoimmune hemolytic anemia and ABO isoimmune hemolytic anemia.

Other Isoimmune Anemias

Fetuses with anemia secondary to anti-Kell antibodies have lower reticulocyte counts and total serum bilirubin levels than do fetuses affected by anti-D antibodies. The level of hemolysis caused by anti-Kell antibodies is less than that caused by anti-D antibodies, but fetal erythropoiesis appears blunted, suggesting that Kell sensitization results in suppression of fetal erythropoiesis as well as hemolysis. Fetuses with anti-Kell hemolytic anemia may therefore benefit from fetal blood sampling rather than amniotic fluid analyses, which might underestimate the degree of anemia.[66]

Extremely high titers of anti-C antibody have been associated with neonatal hemolysis, but routine screening of titers is not warranted, because antibody titers do not accurately reflect the severity of hemolytic disease.[67] In a recent study the following frequencies of specific isoimmunization were identified: anti-D, 18.4%; anti-E, 14%; anti-c, 5.8%; anti-C, 4.7%; Kell group, 22%; anti-MNS, 4.7%; anti-Fya (Duffy), 5.4%; and anti-Jka, 1.5%. The study concluded that anti-D was still a common antibody causing hemolysis in the newborn, despite the use of RhoGAM.[68]

Rhesus and Kell antigen status can be determined by DNA studies, and molecular biology techniques such as polymerase chain reaction (PCR) have been used recently to determine fetal blood type.[69]

TABLE 8-9

COMPARISON OF Rh AND ABO INCOMPATIBILITY

	Rh	**ABO**
Blood group setup		
Mother	Negative	O
Infant	Positive	A or B
Type of antibody	Incomplete (IgG)	Immune (IgG)
Clinical aspects		
Occurrence in firstborn	5%	40%–50%
Predictable severity in	Usually	No
subsequent pregnancies		
Stillbirth or hydrops	Frequent	Rare
Severe anemia	Frequent	Rare
Degree of jaundice	+++	+
Hepatosplenomegaly	+++	+
Laboratory findings		
Direct Coombs' test (infant)	+	(+) or O
Maternal antibodies	Always present	Not clear-cut
Spherocytes	0	+
Treatment		
Need for antenatal measures	Yes	No
Value of phototherapy	Limited	Great
Exchange transfusion		
Frequency	Approx. 67%	Approx. 1%
Donor blood type	Rh-negative	Rh same as infant
	Group-specific, when possible	Group O only
Incidence of late anemia	Common	Rare

Modified from Naiman JL: Erythroblastosis fetalis. In Oski FA, Naiman JL (eds): Hematologic Problems in the Newborn, 3rd ed. Philadelphia, WB Saunders, 1982, p 333.

Congenital Erythrocyte Defects

Congenital defects of the RBC include enzymatic defects, membrane defects, and defects of hemoglobin synthesis. Enzyme defects such as glucose-6-phosphate dehydrogenase (G6PD) deficiency, pyruvate kinase deficiency, hexokinase deficiency, and glucose phosphate isomerase deficiency may present with hemolytic anemia in the first week of life.

Membrane defects such as hereditary spherocytosis, hereditary elliptocytosis, and other hereditary disorders of the RBC cytoskeleton may also cause hemolysis in the newborn period. Neonatal RBC membranes deform more to a given shear force than do adult RBC membranes, resulting in greater susceptibility of neonatal cells to yield and fragment. These mechanical properties lead to accelerated membrane loss and a decreased RBC lifespan in normal newborns. The RBCs of infants with membrane abnormalities have even shorter lifespans.

Hereditary spherocytosis is a congenital defect in membrane deformability caused by various defects in erythrocyte membrane proteins such as spectrin, ankyrin, band 3, and protein 4.2. A diagnosis of hereditary spherocytosis is made by determining the RBC osmotic fragility. Neonatal RBCs have an increased osmotic resistance when compared to adults. When an osmotic fragility test is obtained in a neonate, neonatal reference values should be used. In addition, erythrocytes in other hemolytic states such as ABO incompatibility may demonstrate a similar abnormality in osmotic fragility; therefore, further testing may be necessary to distinguish these two disorders. The increased osmotic fragility of hereditary spherocytosis (but not ABO incompatibility) can be reduced by the addition of glucose.

Disorders of hemoglobin synthesis can also lead to increased hemolysis. α-Thalassemia trait is an important diagnosis to make in the newborn period. This abnormality of α-chain production is common in black and Asian populations. These newborns may benefit from an initial evaluation of their RBC indices to look for microcytosis, in order to detect the presence of the α-thalassemia trait. Because the differential diagnosis of microcytosis at this age is limited, the newborn period is the best time to establish the diagnosis. Beyond a few months of life, iron deficiency becomes a more common cause of microcytosis. Hemoglobin electrophoresis in the α-thalassemia trait is normal, although some studies have reported minor increases in hemoglobin Bart's (2% to 8%) that is transiently present in neonates and detectable in many newborn screening laboratories.[70] Molecular biologic techniques are being evaluated, but it remains easiest to make this diagnosis by the observation of a low MCV (<95 fL) in the newborn period.

The α-thalassemia syndromes are gene deletion disorders, involving up to four genes. Four genes are necessary to make the total complement of α-globin. Twenty-eight percent of black children and adults lack a single gene. This condition is known as the silent carrier state of α-thalassemia. The silent carrier state is not detectable by any routine laboratory study. A two-gene deletion state, seen in about 3% of black Americans, is known as the α-thalassemia trait. A three-gene deletion disorder is known as hemoglobin H disease. Hemoglobin H disease results in the production of large quantities of γ-chains (compared to α-globin chains) leading to the formation of Bart's hemoglobin. The four-gene deletion state causes hydrops fetalis and is incompatible with life.

Unlike α-thalassemia, β-thalassemia trait does not produce abnormalities in RBC indices at birth because β-globin chain production is not sufficiently developed in comparison to γ-globin chain production. Structural β-globin chain defects (such as sickle cell anemia) do not normally present at birth. β-Thalassemia trait can be diagnosed in the older infant or child by an elevation of hemoglobin A_2 or hemoglobin F on electrophoresis assays.

Case Study 3

Baby E is a term male infant born to a 30-year-old gravida 1 mother. The pregnancy was uncomplicated, and delivery occurred vaginally with low forceps and a nuchal cord at delivery. Apgar scores were 7 and 9, and the infant was transitioned in the nursery. He was noted to be pale and tachycardic and exhibited diminished pulses.
A glucose determination and a spun hematocrit were ordered. The glucose was 89, and the spun hematocrit was 44%.

Exercise 3

QUESTIONS

1. Which of the following diagnoses are possible?
   a. Twin-to-twin transfusion syndrome
   b. Acute fetomaternal hemorrhage
   c. Erythroblastosis fetalis
   d. Autotransfusion into the placenta
   e. b and d

2. What test would differentiate fetomaternal hemorrhage from autotransfusion into the placenta?
   a. KB test on cord blood
   b. MCV
   c. KB test on maternal blood
   d. Elevated bilirubin

ANSWERS

1. e. Both of these causes of acute hemorrhage could result in the presentation of this infant.

2. c. A maternal KB test would be positive with FMH, negative with autotransfusion. In this case, the differential diagnosis includes those disorders capable of causing pallor in the immediate newborn period. More careful questioning of the obstetrician indicates that the infant had a tight nuchal cord at the time of delivery. Infants with tight nuchal cords can develop hypovolemia during labor and delivery because of compression of the umbilical vein and inhibition of blood flow from the placenta to the infant. The umbilical arteries, in contrast, are not readily compressible because of their differing anatomy and more rigid structure.

   Blood is delivered through the umbilical arteries under much higher systolic and diastolic pressures than through the umbilical vein. During deliveries in which cord compression occurs, an infant can lose a significant amount of blood through the umbilical arteries into the placenta, at the same time demonstrating poor venous return (from the umbilical vein). These infants will appear pale with thready pulses and a tachycardia. The hemoglobin concentration will initially be normal because a fall in hemoglobin concentration can only result from reexpansion of the plasma volume (either from fluids given intravenously or from the transfer of fluid from the extravascular space). Because the hemoglobin level itself is unremarkable, it does not help in differentiating the cause of the pallor. In this situation it is important to recognize that the infant's clinical signs and symptoms are consistent with hypovolemic shock.

Acquired RBC Defects

Infection, drugs, and toxins may cause acquired hemolytic anemias. In addition, vascular pathology such as arteriovenous malformations, cavernous hemangiomas, and vascular thromboses can result in a hemolytic process.

Infection and DIC

Infants with viral or bacterial sepsis can develop a hemolytic anemia. Sepsis due to bacteria such as group B streptococcus (GBS) and *E. coli* may result in hemolysis, DIC, and hemorrhage. Infants are often jaundiced and have hepatosplenomegaly, although the degree of hyperbilirubinemia does not always correlate with the degree of anemia. Infants may have an elevated direct bilirubin as well due to cholestasis or hepatitis. Some bacteria such as *E. coli* will produce hemolytic endotoxins, which result in increased RBC destruction, often associated with a microangiopathic process.

Congenital viral infections due to CMV, toxoplasmosis, rubella, and herpes simplex may also be associated with a hemolytic anemia, and are a cause of nonimmune hydrops. Table 8-10 reviews some of the more common causes of nonimmune hydrops. Congenital syphilis may present with hemolytic anemia despite negative testing in the mother. Initial negative screening for syphilis may be seen despite overwhelming infection, a condition termed the "prozone effect."[71] The prozone effect occurs because a higher than optimal amount of antibody in the tested sera prevents the flocculation reaction seen in positive reagin test results. Nontreponemal testing should be repeated using diluted serum to diagnose syphilis in women with initial negative syphilis serologic results, especially if their infant is born with nonimmune hydrops.[72]

Fetal and neonatal infection with parvovirus B19 can cause severe anemia, hydrops, and fetal demise.[73] The infant generally presents with a hypoplastic anemia,[74] but hemolysis can occur as well. The virus replicates primarily in erythroid progenitor cells. Thus, in infants with an underlying hemolytic disorder, infection with parvovirus B19 can result in aplastic anemia. In utero transfusions for hydropic fetuses have been investigated, but are not successful in all patients. Treatment with IVIG during aplastic crises leads to resolution of the anemia.

Other infections associated with neonatal anemia include malaria and the human immunodeficiency virus (HIV). Congenital malaria may occur in endemic urban areas where imported cases of malaria are increasing. Congenital HIV infection can be asymptomatic in newborns. Infants born to mothers on zidovudine (AZT) may have a hypoplastic anemia due to side effects of the drug.[75]

Other Causes of Acquired Hemolysis

Some maternal drugs can lead to hemolysis. Maternal ingestion of valproic acid has been reported to cause hemolytic disease in a breast-fed newborn.[76] Mothers exposed to some oxidizing agents may induce hemolysis in their fetus with G6PD deficiency, and infants with G6PD deficiency are at risk for increased hemolysis when exposed to oxidizing agents such as sulfonamides, antimalarials, naphthalene, and henna.[77] Other unusual causes of hemolytic disease in the newborn include metabolic diseases such as galactosemia, lysosomal storage diseases, and some amino acid disorders. In addition, prolonged metabolic acidosis, transfusion reactions, thrombocytopenia–absent radius (TAR) syndrome, and osteopetrosis[78] can all present with hemolytic anemia in the newborn. Finally, macro- and microangiopathic hemolytic anemias can occur with vascular malformations such as severe coarctation of the aorta, arteriovenous malformations, large vessel thromboses, and cavernous hemangiomas.

Case Study 4

Baby girl D is a newborn infant born at 34 weeks' gestation to a 29-year-old gravida 5, now para 4 mother. Initial CBC shows hematocrit 28%, hemoglobin 9.1 g/dL, MCV 102 fL, MCHC 33 g/dL, RDW 11%, and

TABLE 8-10

NONIMMUNE HYDROPS FETALIS: CAUSES AND ASSOCIATIONS

Hematologic
 Homozygous α-thalassemia
 Chronic fetomaternal transfusion
 Twin-to-twin transfusion (recipient or donor)
 Multiple gestation with "parasitic" fetus

Cardiovascular
 Severe congenital heart disease (atrial septal defect,
  ventricular septal defect, hypoplastic left side of
  the heart, pulmonary valve insufficiency, Ebstein's
  subaortic stenosis)
 Premature closure of foramen ovale
 Myocarditis
 Large arteriovenous malformation
 Tachyarrhythmias: paroxysmal supraventricular
  tachycardia, atrial flutter
 Bradyarrhythmias: heart block
 Fibroelastosis

Pulmonary
 Cystic adenomatoid malformation of lung
 Pulmonary lymphangiectasia
 Pulmonary hypoplasia (diaphragmatic hernia)

Renal
 Congenital nephrosis
 Renal vein thrombosis

Intrauterine infections
 Syphilis

Intrauterine infections—cont'd
 Toxoplasmosis
 Cytomegalovirus
 Leptospirosis
 Chagas disease
 Congenital hepatitis

Congenital anomalies
 Achondroplasia
 E trisomy
 Multiple anomalies
 Turner syndrome

Miscellaneous
 Meconium peritonitis
 Fetal neuroblastomatosis
 Dysmaturity
 Tuberous sclerosis
 Storage disease
 Small bowel volvulus

Placental
 Umbilical vein thrombosis
 Chorionic vein thrombosis
 Chorioangioma

Maternal
 Diabetes mellitus
 Toxemia

Idiopathic

From Etchers PC, Lemons JA: Nonimmune hydrops. Pediatrics 1979;64:326.

peripheral smear shows moderate polychromasia. On examination the infant appears pale and in moderate respiratory distress. The heart rate is 170 bpm, respiratory rate is 65, and the blood pressure is 44/33 mm Hg. Cardiac examination is significant for quiet heart sounds, a 2/6 systolic murmur, and equal pulses. Lung sounds are slightly diminished bilaterally. Abdomen is slightly protuberant, with a spleen palpable 1 cm below the left costal margin, and a liver palpable 2 cm below the right costal margin.

Exercise 4

QUESTIONS

1. Which of the following statements are true?
 a. This infant has nonimmune hydrops fetalis.
 b. This infant has immune-mediated hydrops fetalis.
 c. This infant has evidence of hydrops fetalis.
 d. Rh hemolytic disease is a common cause of immune-mediated hydrops.
 e. Tachyarrhythmia can be a cause of nonimmune hydrops fetalis.

2. Maternal workup for infection would include which of the following?
 a. IgG and IgM for CMV
 b. PCR for parvovirus B19
 c. Cervical cultures for GBS
 d. Rapid plasma reagin and rubella screen
 e. Sputum for respiratory syncytial virus and influenza

ANSWERS

1. c, d, and e are true. The infant has signs consistent with hydrops fetalis, but the etiology could be immune-mediated or nonimmune-mediated. Rh hemolytic disease and tachyarrhythmias can both cause hydrops, although through different mechanisms. Maternal blood type was AB positive and antibody screen negative. Infant was O negative and direct Coombs' test negative. The mother had an ultrasound at 18 weeks that was consistent with dates, and showed a healthy fetus. She had had a non-specific "flu-like" illness at the beginning of the third trimester, but was otherwise without medical problems.

2. a, b, and d. CMV, syphilis, rubella, and parvovirus are all known causes of non-immune hydrops. In this case, PCR was positive for parvovirus in maternal serum. This infant has a low RDW and no hepatosplenomegaly, reflecting the hypoproliferative state seen with in utero infection.

Case Study 5

Baby boy M is a term, large for gestation male born to a 32-year-old gravida 1 white mother with gestational diabetes. The delivery required vacuum assistance for the last 15 minutes prior to birth. The infant was pale and gasping at birth, and had a significant caput succedaneum. He received routine drying, stimulation, and some "blow-by" oxygen. Apgar scores were 7 at 1 minute and 8 at 5 minutes. His respirations are 70, heart rate is 180 bpm, and blood pressure is 55/29 mm Hg. He is taken to the newborn nursery. Birth weight is 3965 g and oxygen saturation on room air is 95%. At 80 minutes of life his respirations are 65, his heart rate is 190 bpm, and blood pressure is 44/22 mm Hg. He is pale, not jaundiced, and appears in distress. The cardiac examination is significant for tachycardia; pulses are weak but symmetrical, and the abdominal examination is normal.

Exercise 5

QUESTIONS

Are the following statements true or false?

1. During the transition period, the respiratory rate should decrease over the first hour of life.

2. During the transition period, the heart rate should increase over the first hour of life.

3. During the transition period, the blood pressure should remain stable or increase over the first hour of life.

4. This infant shows clinical signs of acute hemorrhage.

ANSWERS

1. True. The respiratory rate should decrease during the first hour of life.

2. False. The heart rate should decrease during the first hour of life.

3. True. The blood pressure should be maintained or increase during the first hours of life.

4. True. The infant is tachycardic, tachypneic, and hypotensive, reflecting acute blood loss.

A CBC is obtained which shows a hematocrit of 28%, hemoglobin 9.7 g/dL, MCV 105 fL, MCHC 32.5 g/dL, RDW 13.2%, NRBCs 8/100 WBCs, and platelets 89,000/μL. Baby M is quickly transferred to the newborn intensive care unit where an umbilical venous catheter is placed and 20 mL/kg of normal saline are rapidly administered. A blood gas is obtained which shows pH 7.22, P_{CO_2} 36 mm Hg, P_{O_2} 87 mm Hg, bicarbonate 12, and base deficit 14.

QUESTION

5. What additional studies would be helpful in the ongoing care of this infant?

    a. Chemistry panel

    b. Liver function studies

    c. Coagulation studies

    d. Head CT

    e. Abdominal ultrasound

ANSWERS

5. c. This infant shows evidence of significant acute blood loss and hypovolemic shock due to a subgaleal hemorrhage. Table 8-6 provides a differential diagnosis for pallor in the neonate. Any cause of acute prepartum or intrapartum hemorrhage can present with a similar clinical picture and should be distin-guishable from the causes of chronic blood loss. Because subgaleal hemorrhages can result in the infant's entire blood volume accumulating in the subgaleal space, this potentially life-threatening event must be recognized immediately so that the shock and possible ensuing DIC can be treated effectively.

Impaired Erythrocyte Production

Impaired erythrocyte production can result for a variety of reasons. Lack of an appropriate or suffi-cient marrow environment for growth, as seen in osteopetrosis, can cause decreased RBC produc-tion. Lack of specific substrates or their carriers, such as iron, folate, vitamin B_{12}, or transcobalamin II deficiency, can lead to deficient production. Lack of specific RBC growth factor activity, such as decreased Epo production seen in anemia of prematurity or abnormalities in Epo receptors seen in Diamond-Blackfan syndrome, can also lead to a hypoproliferative anemia.

Nutritional Deficiencies Causing Anemia

With the exception of iron deficiency anemia in newborns with prolonged hemorrhage, hypoproliferative anemias due to nutritional deficiencies rarely present in term newborns. In preterm infants, however, nutritional deficiency anemias do occur, although they generally do not become evident until after the first weeks of life. Deficiencies of iron, folate, vitamin B_{12}, vitamin E, and copper have been described, and can lead to varying degrees of anemia.[79]

Iron. Iron deficiency anemia can occur at various times during the newborn period in both term and preterm infants. Following chronic FMH or TTS, term and preterm infants can present with iron deficiency anemia manifested by hypochromic, microcytic RBCs and a low hematocrit. Because 75% to 80% of the total body iron is stored in hemoglobin, infants born with decreased RBC volumes have decreased iron stores. Preterm infants will develop an iron-deficient state even more rapidly, given their relatively smaller total blood volumes and greater phlebotomy losses. As blood cells are destroyed, the iron from hemoglobin is recycled, becoming available for future erythropoiesis. Without adequate initial RBC volumes, the iron for new hemoglobin production is lacking, and iron deficiency anemia ensues. Thus, the initial hemoglobin concentration has a significant impact on the ability of preterm infants to maintain normal hematologic indices during growth.

The use of parenteral iron in preterm infants is still being investigated. Past concerns about parenteral iron administration included increased risk of infection, increased risk of oxidation, and systemic reactions to intravenous preparations. Friel and coworkers[80] evaluated the use of iron dextran added to the total parenteral nutrition (TPN) of 14 very low birth weight (VLBW) infants and noted that despite parenteral doses of 200 to 250 µg/kg/day (with

a total enteral plus parenteral iron intake of 400 µg/kg/day), infants remained in negative iron balance during the course of study. They noted no adverse effects, and recommended an iron intake of 1000 µg/kg/day supplemented in TPN. Pollak and colleagues evaluated the oxidative stress associated with IV administration by measuring plasma malondialdehyde (MDA) and *o*-tyrosine concentrations after a 2-hour infusion of 2 mg/kg iron sucrose.[81] They noted an increase of MDA just after the infusion was complete, which resolved 2 hours later, and there were no differences in overall iron or oxidative indices between infants receiving oral iron and those receiving parenteral iron. The authors recommended that parenteral iron administration occur over at least 2 hours' duration to minimize oxidative stress.

The use of Epo to prevent and treat anemia in preterm infants has added a new level of complexity in determining the iron requirements of preterm infants. Numerous studies of preterm infants receiving Epo have shown evidence of iron deficiency when iron supplementation is not adequate. Iron has been administered both parenterally and enterally in published studies. Oral iron supplementation has ranged from 2 to 40 mg/kg/day in clinical studies. No evidence of hemolysis was noted in either of the two Epo trials in which the greatest amounts of supplemental iron were used.[82,83] Infants receiving Epo are likely at greater risk for iron deficiency than they are at risk for iron overload and increased oxidant stress. However, no studies to date have directly evaluated iron requirements in preterm infants receiving Epo. Further evaluation is required to determine the optimal dose and route of administration of iron in preterm infants.

Vitamin E. Vitamin E is an antioxidant, inhibiting peroxidation of polyunsaturated fatty acids (PUFAs) present in the lipid bilayer of all cell membranes. Because vitamin E is transferred across the placenta to the greatest degree in the last trimester, preterm infants are born with lower stores than term infants.[79] Unlike other nutritional deficiency anemias, vitamin E deficiency does not result in a hypoproliferative anemia, but rather a hemolytic anemia. Vitamin E deficiency anemia in preterm infants was first described in the 1960s and 1970s.[84] Early preterm infant formulas containing high concentrations of PUFAs and low vitamin E caused increased hemolysis and anemia. Studies in the mid-1970s showed that when preterm infants were fed diets high in PUFAs and given iron supplementation, their hemolytic anemia worsened.[85,86] The anemia resolved with vitamin E administration. Vitamin E–deficient hemolytic anemia has largely disappeared owing to improvements in preterm infant formulas containing lower concentrations of PUFAs and adequate vitamin E supplementation.

Infants with severe fat malabsorption require greater vitamin E supplementation. In addition, vitamin E requirements are likely increased in preterm infants receiving increased iron supplementation, because iron promotes oxidation of cellular membranes and also inhibits intestinal absorption of vitamin E. Preterm infants receiving Epo require greater iron supplementation, and should therefore receive vitamin E supplementation as well. The optimal dose of vitamin E in preterm infants receiving Epo has not been determined, but oral doses in recent studies ranged from 15 to 25 IU/day. The use of higher doses of vitamin E (50 IU/day) has not provided increased benefit to preterm infants 32 weeks' gestation or less.[87]

Folate. Folate is stored in the fetal liver late in gestation, and infants can become deficient if born prematurely.[79] Infants fed diets low in folate, those with malabsorption, and infants receiving goat's milk or milk that has been boiled are at risk for becoming folate deficient. RBC folate concentrations represent total body folate stores, while serum folate concentrations reflect recent folate intake. Both serum and RBC folate concentrations are greater in preterm and term infants than in adults. RBC folate concentrations decrease rapidly after birth, and are generally lower than adult concentrations by 1 to 3 months of life. Folate deficiency results in a megaloblastic anemia, with MCVs generally greater than 110 fL. Preterm infants with lower folate stores need supplementation in situations in which erythropoiesis is increased, such as infants with hemolytic anemia, or infants receiving Epo. General requirements for term and preterm infants are 25 to 50 µg orally per day.

Vitamin B$_{12}$. Vitamin B$_{12}$ (or cobalamin) must be obtained through dietary intake because only microorganisms are able to synthesize the compound. Vitamin B$_{12}$ is actively transported across the placenta and stored in the fetal liver. Vitamin B$_{12}$ deficiency is rare in preterm

infants, but can sometimes be seen in breast-fed infants of vegetarian mothers who are vitamin B$_{12}$ deficient, or in infants with gastrointestinal abnormalities such as short gut syndrome, necrotizing enterocolitis (NEC), or post-NEC stenoses.[79] The hematologic characteristics of vitamin B$_{12}$ deficiency anemia are similar to those seen in folate deficiency anemia. Erythroid hyperplasia and a decreased myeloid to erythroid ratio (M:E) is present in the range of 2:1 to 1:1. Megaloblastic proerythroblasts have a shortened survival, and remaining cells have an increased MCV. Reticulocytosis occurs rapidly following supplementation with vitamin B$_{12}$.

Copper. Copper deficiency anemia may occur in some specific situations in which supplemental copper is not given: low-birth-weight premature infants fed milk only, protracted total parenteral nutrition without trace mineral supplements, and chronic diarrhea with severe malnutrition. Severe neutropenia generally precedes the onset of a sideroblastic, hypochromic anemia. Serum iron concentrations are usually low, but iron therapy is ineffective in resolving the anemia. The diagnosis is established by low serum copper concentrations, the presence of fractures or periosteal reaction on radiographs, and a dramatic reticulocytosis in response to copper therapy. The recommended intake of copper for term infants is 0.4 to 0.6 mg/day.

Case Study 6

Baby girl E is a 32-day-old former 900-g infant born at 27 weeks' gestation to a 17-year-old gravida 1 now para 1 mother with preterm labor and premature rupture of membranes. The initial hematocrit was 42%, and the rest of the CBC and RBC indices were within normal limits. The infant received 14 days of mechanical ventilation and is currently on nasal cannula oxygen. She is receiving full gavage feedings. Her spun hematocrit today is 24%.

A central CBC shows hematocrit 22%, hemoglobin 7.4 g/dL, MCV 92 fL, MCHC 33.0 g/dL, RDW 12.8%, NRBCs 0/100 WBCs. An uncorrected reticulocyte count is 1.0%, with an absolute reticulocyte count of 30,000 cells/µL. The peripheral smear shows mild anisocytosis and poikilocytosis.

Exercise 6

QUESTIONS

Are the following statements true or false?

1. This anemia can be rapidly corrected with iron supplementation.
2. This disorder is rare in preterm infants.
3. The RBC indices show active erythropoiesis.
4. This anemia results from inadequate production of erythropoietin.

ANSWERS

1. False.
2. False.
3. False.
4. True.

This neonate has the most common anemia seen in preterm infants, the anemia of prematurity. This normocytic, normochromic, hypoproliferative anemia affects preterm infants born before 32 weeks' gestation, and involves inadequate Epo production despite signs of anemia. Clinical studies administering recombinant Epo to preterm infants to treat the anemia of prematurity have resulted in reduced transfusion requirements. Preterm, otherwise healthy infants receiving 200 to 400 units/kg three times per week will increase their reticulocyte counts within 3 to 7 days, and will generally maintain or increase hematocrits by 7 to 14 days. Supplemental iron (6 mg/kg/day) is important to provide optimal substrate for new red blood cell production.

Congenital Anemias

Congenital syndromes may primarily diminish or inhibit RBC production, or may secondarily alter the RBC mass through chronic blood loss or hemolysis. Table 8-11 presents some genetic disorders associated with anemia in the newborn.

Diamond-Blackfan Syndrome

Diamond-Blackfan anemia (DBA) consists of a group of congenital pure red blood cell aplasias diagnosed generally within the first year of life. The syndrome represents a phenotypic expression of multiple genotypic abnormalities affecting erythropoiesis.[88] Up to 25% of patients are anemic at birth. Hydrops fetalis associated with severe anemia has been reported, but is rare. The majority of cases are sporadic, but 10% to 15% of cases are familial, and more cases of autosomal dominant (AD) inheritance have recently been reported.[89-91]

Physical abnormalities are present in about one third of DBA patients. Abnormalities include short stature, triphalangeal or duplicated thumbs, cleft palate, ocular anomalies, short or webbed neck, and congenital heart disease. Patients can be profoundly anemic and reticulocytopenic, but other cell lineages are normal in number and function. The bone marrow reflects hypoproliferative erythropoiesis, showing a very low number of erythropoietic precursors and a reduction of erythroid progenitor cells. Proliferation and differentiation of the other lineages are normal. Most DBA patients have elevated Epo concentrations; however, the very high Epo levels are usually not proportionate to the level of anemia. Erythroid progenitors from some DBA patients show a defective or incomplete response to other erythropoietic growth factors, such as interleukin 3 (IL-3), IL-6, or stem cell factor.[92] Some patients exhibit a significant response in vitro to stem cell factor and IL-9.[93,94]

Many patients respond clinically to corticosteroids, and some develop hematologic remissions (both spontaneous and following corticosteroid therapy). Patients who do not respond to corticosteroids and those who have to discontinue treatment because of side effects must rely on chronic transfusions. New treatment strategies are being investigated that involve the administration of growth factors such as IL-3, granulocytic-monocytic colony-stimulating factor (GM-CSF), and stem cell factor.[95] Successful bone marrow transplantation has been performed in some individuals,[96] suggesting a normal marrow microenvironment in those patients.

Congenital Dyserythropoietic Anemia

Congenital dyserythropoietic anemia (CDA) is a rare disorder marked by ineffective erythropoiesis, megaloblastic anemia, and characteristic abnormalities of the nuclear membrane and cytoplasm seen on electron microscopy. Both autosomal dominant (AD) and autosomal recessive (AR) inheritance patterns have been reported. Three types of congenital dyserythropoietic

TABLE 8-11

GENETIC DISORDERS ASSOCIATED WITH ANEMIA

Syndrome	Genetic Characteristics	Hematologic Phenotype
Diamond-Blackfan syndrome	Autosomal recessive (AR); sporadic mutations and autosomal dominant (AD) inheritance have been described	Steroid-responsive hypoplastic anemia, often macrocytic after 5 months of age
Fanconi pancytopenia	AR, thought to be due to abnormalities in multiple genes (at least five genetic subtypes have been identified)	Steroid-responsive hypoplastic anemia, reticulocytopenia, some macrocytic red blood cells (RBCs), shortened RBC lifespan: cells are hypersensitive to DNA cross-linking agents
Aase syndrome	AR, possible AD	Steroid-responsive hypoplastic anemia that improves with age
Pearson's syndrome	Mitochondrial DNA abnormalities, X-linked or AR	Hypoplastic sideroblastic anemia unresponsive to pyridoxine
Lethal osteopetrosis	AR, due to defective resorption of immature bone	Hypoplastic anemia due to marrow compression
Congenital dyserythropoietic anemias (CDA)	AR	Type I: megaloblastoid erythroid hyperplasia and nuclear chromitin bridges between cells. Type II: erythroblastic multinuclearity and positive acidified serum test results (HEMPAS). Type III: erythroblastic multinuclearity and macrocytosis.
Peutz-Jeghers	AD	Iron deficiency anemia from chronic blood loss
Dyskeratosis congenita	X-linked recessive, locus on Xq28, some cases with AD inheritance	Hypoplastic anemia usually presenting between 5 and 15 years of age
X-linked α-thalassemia/ mental retardation (ATR-X and ATR-16) syndromes	ATR-X: X-linked recessive, mapped to Xq13.3 ATR-16: mapped to 16p13.3, deletions of α-globin locus	ATR-X: hpochromic, microcytic anemia; mild form of hemoglobin H disease. ATR-16: more significant hemogobin H disease and anemia are present
Thrombocytopenia–absent radius (TAR) syndrome	AR	Hemorrhagic anemia, possibly hypoplastic anemia as well
Osler hemorrhagic telangiectasia syndrome	AD, mapped to 9q33–34	Hemorrhagic anemia

anemia have been described. Type I CDA shows megaloblastoid erythroid hyperplasia and nuclear chromatin bridges between cells. Type II CDA is the most common form, characterized by erythroblastic multinuclearity and positive acidified serum test results (HEMPAS anemia). Type III CDA is marked by erythroblastic multinuclearity and macrocytosis.

CDA can present in the newborn period with megaloblastic anemia, early jaundice, hepatosplenomegaly, and intrauterine growth restriction. Infants with type 1 CDA may have bony abnormalities and syndactyly.[97] Fetuses with hydrops fetalis and CDA have been reported.[98] Although rare, this disorder should be included in the differential diagnosis of newborns with anemia, jaundice, and hepatosplenomegaly. In a recent study half of the patients with CDA I presented in the neonatal period, although macrocytosis did not become

evident until later in the course of disease.[97] Treatment for this disorder consists of supportive therapy and close observation for side effects of chronic transfusions. Splenectomy in some patients with severe anemia has been helpful.

Aase Syndrome

Aase syndrome is another congenital hypoplastic anemia syndrome involving marrow and skeletal anomalies. The syndrome is characterized by hypoplastic anemia and abnormally digitalized thumbs, and may also be associated with growth failure. Bony abnormalities have been reported in these patients as well. Similar to DBA, bone marrow cultures reveal decreased production of erythropoietic precursors. The inheritance pattern is thought to be comparable to that seen in DBA, in that both AD and AR conditions have been reported.[98]

Osteopetrosis

Osteopetrosis is a rare autosomal recessive disorder characterized by defects in osteoclastic function, resulting in a decreased bone marrow space.[99] Developmental delay, ocular involvement, and neurodegenerative findings occur in association with hypoplastic anemia, although patients may also present with hemolytic anemia. Longitudinal studies in the United States and Europe have shown variability in outcome, although the survival rate beyond 5 to 6 years is less than 30%.

Fanconi's Anemia

Fanconi's anemia (FA) is an autosomal recessive disorder characterized by marrow failure and congenital anomalies, including abnormalities in skin pigmentation, gastrointestinal anomalies, renal anomalies, and upper limb anomalies.[100] Approximately one third of patients have no obvious congenital anomalies. Most patients present in early childhood, but newborns with FA have been reported, usually when obvious congenital anomalies are present.[101] Patients generally have a steroid-responsive hypoplastic anemia, reticulocytopenia, macrocytic RBCs on peripheral smear, and shortened RBC lifespan. Epo concentrations are usually elevated, and hemoglobin F production is increased. A significant percentage of patients will develop myelodysplastic syndrome or acute myelogenous leukemia later in life. Treatment of FA is similar to that for DBA, and marrow transplantation has been successful.

Pearson's Syndrome

Pearson's marrow-pancreas syndrome is a disorder involving the hematopoietic system, exocrine pancreas, liver, and kidneys.[102] Patients present in infancy with macrocytic anemia, which is sometimes associated with neutropenia and thrombocytopenia. Marrows have normal cellularity, but other abnormalities including vacuolization of erythroid and myeloid precursors, hemosiderosis, and ringed sideroblasts are present. The anemia is unresponsive to pyridoxine supplementation. Bone marrow transplantation has not been reported in these patients, and the disorder is considered fatal.

The Anemia of Prematurity

In preterm infants, adaptive mechanisms to the extrauterine environment are incomplete. Epo concentrations in anemic preterm infants are still significantly lower than those found in adults, given the degree of their anemia.[103] This normocytic, normochromic anemia, termed the *anemia of prematurity*, commonly affects infants of 32 weeks' gestation or less. The anemia of prematurity is "nutritionally insensitive" and, therefore, is not responsive to the addition of iron, folate, or vitamin E. Some infants may be asymptomatic, but others demonstrate signs of anemia, which are alleviated by transfusion. These signs include tachycardia, increased episodes of apnea and bradycardia, poor weight gain, an increased oxygen requirement, and elevated serum lactate concentrations that decrease following transfusion.[104–106]

Infants with the anemia of prematurity have a decreased ability to increase serum Epo concentrations, despite diminished "available oxygen" to tissues and the appearance of signs of anemia.[103,107] However, marrow erythroid progenitors are highly sensitive to Epo,[108] and concentrations of other erythropoietic growth factors responsible for erythrocyte production appear to be normal.[109]

The molecular and cellular mechanisms responsible for the anemia of prematurity remain undefined. Possible explanations include the transition from fetal to adult hemoglobin, shortened erythrocyte survival, and hemodilution associated with a rapidly increasing body mass. It is unknown whether preterm infants rely on Epo produced by the liver (the source of Epo in utero), or that produced by the kidney, or a combination of the two. The anemia of prematurity likely involves a delay in shifting the anatomic site of Epo production from the liver to peritubular cells in the kidney.

Clinical trials published in the last 15 years evaluating Epo administration to preterm infants to prevent or treat the anemia of prematurity have reported a variety of results. Initial studies utilized adult doses and reported little or no effect. Pharmacokinetic studies indicated that neonates have a larger volume of distribution and a more rapid elimination of Epo necessitating the use of higher doses than those required for adults.[110] Recent controlled studies using higher doses of Epo (600 to 1200 units/kg/week, divided into 3 to 5 doses) have reported decreased transfusion requirements.[111]

It could be argued that given the risks of transfusions, such as transmission of hepatitis, CMV, and HIV, as well as the possible development of graft-versus-host disease, treatment of anemic neonates using recombinant Epo might be cost effective. It is likely that Epo administration, in combination with instituting more rigorous and standardized transfusion criteria and diminishing the volume of blood lost through phlebotomy, will have the greatest impact in decreasing transfusion requirements in term and preterm infants. Regardless of treatment strategy, a critical understanding of the physiologic influences affecting oxygen delivery in term and preterm infants is required before altering the hematocrit, either through the administration of an erythrocyte transfusion or the administration of Epo.

Guidelines for Erythrocyte Transfusions

Guidelines for administering an erythrocyte transfusion differ in term and preterm infants, and depend on the etiology and duration of blood loss. Regardless of etiology, an infant should never be transfused based on hemoglobin alone. Factors such as heart rate, blood pressure, oxygen requirements, neurologic status, metabolic status, and hemoglobin concentration should all be considered in order to determine the immediate need for erythrocytes.

Indications for transfusions in preterm infants have been gradually changing in the past decade, primarily due to clinical studies of Epo administration in this population. The impact of instituting strict transfusion guidelines has been as great as the impact of decreasing phlebotomy losses or beginning Epo therapy. This is most beneficial to preterm infants in a practical sense, because it can be implemented in newborn intensive care units throughout the world, without additional cost and without obtaining new medications. An example of specific transfusion criteria for preterm infants is presented in Table 8-12.

Caregivers will need to determine their group's level of comfort in following specific transfusion criteria; however, general guidelines can still be used. Phlebotomy losses should be minimized to the greatest extent possible without compromising patient care. Hemoglobin or hematocrit values should be determined

---

TABLE 8-12

TRANSFUSION GUIDELINES FOR PRETERM INFANTS

Hematocrit/ hemoglobin*	Ventilator Requirements and/or Symptoms	Transfusion Volume
Hct ≤ 30/Hgb ≤ 10:	Infants requiring **moderate or significant mechanical ventilation** (MAP >8 cm H_2O and F_{IO_2} >40%)	15 mL/kg PRBCs over 2–4 hours
Hct ≤ 27/Hgb ≤ 9	Infants requiring **minimal mechanical ventilation** (any mechanical ventilation, or CPAP > 6 cm H_2O and F_{IO_2} ≤ 40%)	15 mL/kg PRBCs over 2–4 hours
Hct ≤ 24/Hgb ≤ 8	Infants on supplemental oxygen who are **not requiring mechanical ventilation,** and **one or more** of the following is present: • ≥24 hours of tachycardia (HR > 180) or tachypnea (RR > 80) • An increased oxygen requirement from the previous 48 hours • An elevated lactate concentration (≥2.5 mEq/L) • Weight gain <10 g/kg/day over the previous 4 days while receiving ≥110 kcal/kg/day • An increase in the episodes of apnea and bradycardia (>9 episodes in a 24-hour period or ≥2 episodes in 24 hours requiring bag-mask ventilation) while receiving therapeutic doses of methylxanthines • Undergoing significant surgery	20 mL/kg PRBCs over 2–4 hours (divide into two 10 mL/kg volumes if fluid sensitive)
Hct ≤ 20/Hgb ≤ 7	Infants **without any symptoms** and an absolute reticulocyte count < 100,000 cells/μL (RBC × %uncorrected reticulocytes).	20 mL/kg PRBCs over 2–4 hours (divide into two 10 mL/kg volumes if fluid sensitive)

*Hematocrit (Hct) values in %; hemoglobin (Hgb) values in g/dL.
CPAP, continuous positive airway pressure; MAP, mean airway pressure; PRBCs, packed red blood cells.

at birth, and then followed at 1- to 2-week intervals during hospitalization (less frequently as the infant grows older). During the first week of life, replacing the volume of blood lost with an alternative isotonic colloid or crystalloid may benefit extremely low birth weight infants in maintaining adequate intravascular volume. This can be especially important when daily phlebotomy losses exceed 10% of the infant's total blood volume. Finally, optimizing nutrition and ensuring adequate vitamin and mineral supplements (including iron) will improve RBC production and decrease RBC destruction, whether or not the infant is receiving Epo.

Two recent studies evaluating specific transfusion strategies have reported conflicting results. Bell and colleagues randomized 100 preterm infants to a liberal versus restrictive transfusion strategy.[112] Those investigators reported an increase in serious intraventricular hemorrhage (IVH) and periventricular leukomalacia (PVL) in infants randomized to a lower transfusion threshold. (Any grade IVH: 17/51 in the liberal transfusion group versus 14/49 in the restrictive transfusion group; grade 3 or 4 IVH: 8/51 liberal versus 5/49 restrictive; PVL: 0/51 liberal versus 4/49 restrictive.) A more recent multicenter study by Kirpalani and colleagues (the PINT study) randomized 451 infants to low or high threshold hemoglobin strategies.[113] Infants in the low threshold group (hemoglobins were allowed to drop lower before transfusion) did not have an increase in neurologic morbidities (12.6% with brain injury in the low threshold group compared to 16% in the high threshold group). Further investigation is needed to determine a more accurate measure for transfusion thresholds in term and preterm infants.

Differential Diagnosis of Anemia

The diagnosis of anemia in the newborn period often requires rapid investigation and laboratory evaluation. Infants presenting in shock from their anemia have most likely suffered massive hemorrhage, and patient stabilization is of utmost importance to avoid organ damage and death. The ABCs of newborn resuscitation should be followed. Initial steps include stabilizing the infant's airway, administering oxygen if needed, and determining the infant's cardiovascular and intravascular volume status.

Immediate volume expansion should begin with normal saline when acute hemorrhage is suspected, followed by 5% albumin or available colloid. An immediate transfusion of type O, Rh negative packed RBCs is needed in the first hour if massive hemorrhage has occurred, and repeat transfusions of cross-matched packed RBCs may be necessary.

Once the infant is stable, information can be gathered to help determine the cause of anemia. One example of a diagnostic approach to anemia is shown in Figure 8-4. Information should first be gathered from the maternal chart. Any family history of anemia, bleeding, "low blood" counts, transfusions, jaundice, or unusual hematologic indices should be noted. Ethnicity of both parents should be obtained, as some inherited disorders (for example G6PD deficiency and thalassemias) are more prevalent in specific ethnic groups.

A thorough maternal history should be obtained, and should include information on vaginal bleeding, trauma, infection or exposure to infected individuals, and any prescribed or illicit drug use during the pregnancy. Exposure to substances that increase oxidative stress and hemolysis in G6PD-deficient mothers include naphthalene (mothballs) and fava beans. The maternal use of cocaine or crack prior to delivery increases the potential for placental abruption, fetal infarction, and postinfarction hemorrhage. Important maternal laboratory values to record include blood type and antibody screen and maternal hepatitis, and syphilis and rubella status.

Information regarding labor and delivery can sometimes be difficult to obtain, especially if the route of delivery was not anticipated (such as an emergent cesarean section for fetal distress). The length of labor, vaginal bleeding, evidence of placenta previa, vasa previa, or placental abruption, and route of delivery should be noted. Information regarding the placenta (cord hematoma, cord rupture, chorioangioma, velamentous insertion of the cord) should be gathered, and the placenta examined if possible. The use of forceps, vacuum, or other manipulations should be noted. It is important to document the presence of multiple gestations, especially those associated with discordant growth.

The timing of presentation of anemia is important to note. Infants with significant acute blood loss before or during delivery may be anemic and hypovolemic at birth, but infants with chronic fetomaternal hemorrhage,

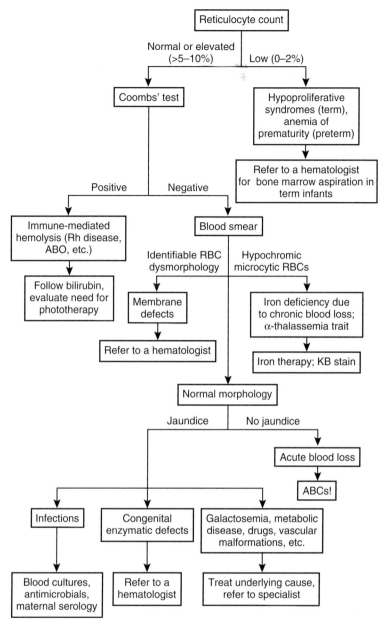

Figure 8-4 Diagnostic approach to neonatal anemia. KB stain, Kleihauer-Betke stain; RBC, red blood cell.

TTS, or hemolysis from isoimmunization may not be symptomatic for 24 to 48 hours. Similarly, infants with internal trauma and hemorrhage (adrenal, renal, splenic, or hepatic) may not become symptomatic for 48 to 72 hours, then may rapidly decompensate. The initial laboratory evaluation of the anemic infant includes a complete blood count with RBC indices and peripheral smear, a reticulocyte count, a direct Coombs' test, and a bilirubin determination if jaundice is evident. In addition, a Kleihauer-Betke stain of maternal blood is helpful in iden-

tifying fetal cells in the maternal circulation. With minimal laboratory tests, a thorough history, and a physical examination, most causes of anemia in the newborn period can be determined.

Anemic infants with low reticulocyte counts (less than 2%) in the first day or two of life have evidence of decreased erythropoiesis. Although the peripheral smear may present clues to the diagnosis, in most cases a bone marrow aspiration is required to diagnose hypoproliferative anemias presenting in the newborn period.

These anemias include Diamond-Blackfan syndrome, Aase syndrome, Pearson's syndrome, osteopetrosis, congenital dyserythropoietic anemia, and transcobalamin II deficiency.

Anemic infants with elevated reticulocyte counts (>7% to 10%) have evidence of stimulated erythropoiesis; their anemia is often due to hemolysis or hemorrhage. A positive Coombs' test is further evidence for immune-mediated hemolysis. A blood type should be obtained on the infant, and maternal serum evaluated for antibodies. A negative Coombs' test (or matching blood types) does not completely rule out immune-mediated hemolysis, and minor blood group incompatibilities should be considered.

A negative Coombs' test associated with jaundice is common in nonimmune hemolytic anemias, and further workup is required to determine a specific cause. Infants may have normal or elevated reticulocyte counts, and may not present with symptomatic anemia at birth. The major causes of hemolysis in the newborn period are listed in Table 8-8. Abnormalities in RBC morphology such as spherocytosis and elliptocytosis can be determined by evaluating the peripheral smear. The presence of microcytic, hypochromic anemia can be evidence for iron deficiency anemia caused by chronic fetomaternal hemorrhage or TTS. The obstetric history should be evaluated and the maternal blood screened with a KB stain for fetal hemoglobin. Anemias with an MCV less than 95 fL are associated with specific hemoglobinopathies, such as α-thalassemia trait. Further workup includes electrophoresis mobility assays for hemoglobin determination.

Infants with normocytic, normochromic RBCs will need further evaluation. If jaundice is not present, then acute blood loss due to a perinatal hemorrhage should be suspected. The obstetric history should be reviewed and the infant evaluated for evidence of internal hemorrhage, sepsis, and DIC. Infants may present simply with pallor, or may be in shock. Infants with continued active bleeding should be evaluated for deficiencies in clotting factors, such as factor 8 or factor 9 deficiency.

Intrinsic RBC defects may present with hemolytic anemia and jaundice in the first days to weeks of life. RBC enzyme deficiencies such as G6PD, pyruvate kinase, and hexokinase deficiencies may lead to increased hemolysis. Male infants of Mediterranean or Asian descent are at increased risk for G6PD deficiency.

Both bacterial and viral infections can cause hemolytic anemia in the newborn period, and can also cause marrow suppression if present for some time prior to delivery. Hepatosplenomegaly, jaundice, and DIC can result from viral or bacterial sepsis. Appropriate antibiotic therapy should be instituted when these symptoms are present, and continued until the cause is determined, or until it becomes clear that the infant does not have a bacterial infection. Congenital infections caused by toxoplasma, CMV, herpes simplex virus, and parvovirus can all be associated with varying degrees of anemia. Hydrops fetalis may be present in cases of in utero infection, and may be severe enough to result in fetal demise.

If a cause for hemolytic anemia has not been determined, other unusual causes of hemolytic disease in the newborn should be evaluated. Such causes include galactosemia, lysosomal storage diseases, and amino acid disorders. In addition, prolonged metabolic acidosis, transfusion reactions, thrombocytopenia–absent radius (TAR) syndrome, and osteopetrosis can all present with hemolytic anemia in the newborn. Finally, macro- and microangiopathic hemolytic anemias can occur with vascular malformations such as coarctation, hemangiomas, and large vessel thromboses.

A working knowledge of the various therapies is required in order to determine the best treatment strategy for each infant. Would the infant benefit from specific growth factors, such as stem cell factor, interleukin 3, GM-CSF, or Epo? Is nutritional support with iron, vitamin E, folate, or vitamin B_{12} required? Will repeated erythrocyte transfusions be required and, therefore, increase risk for iron overload? Are steroids or IVIG indicated? Will a bone marrow transplant give the infant the best chance for long-term survival? Although a few infants with anemia presenting in the newborn period go undiagnosed despite vigorous evaluation, most newborn anemias can be diagnosed and treated successfully.

References

1. Matoth Y, Zaizov R: Regulation of erythropoiesis in the fetal rat. Proceedings of the Tel Aviv University Conference on Erythropoiesis, Petah Tikva, Israel. New York, Academic Press, 1970, p 24.
2. Jacobsen LO, et al: The effect of transfusion-induced polycythemia in the mother of the fetus. Blood 1959;4:694.

3. Peschle C, Marone G, Genovese A, et al: Erythropoietin production by the liver in fetal-neonatal life. Life Sci 1975;17:1325.

4. Davis LE, Widness JA, Brace RA: Renal and placental secretion of erythropoietin during anemia or hypoxia in the ovine fetus. Am J Obstet Gynecol 2003;189:1764–1770.

5. Ohls RK: Erythropoietin and hypoxia inducible factor-1 expression in the mid-trimester human fetus. Acta Paediatr Suppl 2002;91(438):27–30.

6. Meberg A: Hemoglobin concentration and erythropoietin levels inappropriate in small for gestational age infants. Scand J Haematol 1980;24:162.

7. Thomas RM, Canning CE, Cotes PM, et al: Erythropoietin in cord blood hemoglobin and the regulation of fetal erythropoiesis. Br J Obstet Gynaecol 1983;90:795.

8. Widness JA, Clemons GK, Garcia JF, et al: Increased immunoreactive erythropoietin in cord blood after labor. Am J Obstet Gynecol 1984;148:194.

9. Erslev AJ, Wilson J, Caro J: Erythropoietin titers in anemic, nonuremic patients. J Lab Clin Med 1987; 109:429–433.

10. Usher R, Shepherd M, et al: The blood volume of a newborn infant and placental transfusion. Acta Paediatr Scand 1963;52:497.

11. Oettinger L Jr, Mills WB: Simultaneous capillary and venous hemoglobin determinations in newborn infants. J Pediatr 1949;35:362.

12. Forestier F, Daffos F, Catherine N, et al: Developmental hematopoiesis in normal human fetal blood. Blood 1991;77:2360–2363.

13. Zanjani ED, Banisadre M: Hormonal stimulation of erythropoietin production and erythropoiesis in anephric sheep fetuses. J Clin Invest 1979;64:1181.

14. Humbert JR, Abelson H, Hathaway WE, et al: Polycythemia in small for gestational age infants. J Pediatr 1969;75:812.

15. Hakanson DO, Oh W: Hyperviscosity in the small for gestational age infant. Pediatr Res 1977;11:472A.

16. Moore LG, Newberry MA, Freeby GM, Crnic LS: Increased incidence of neonatal hyperbilirubinemia at 3100 m in Colorado. Am J Dis Child 1984; 138:158.

17. Bureau MA, Shapcott D, Berthiaume Y, et al: Maternal cigarette smoking and fetal oxygen transport: A study of P_{50}, 2,3-diphosphoglycerate, total hemoglobin, hematocrit, and type F hemoglobin in fetal blood. Pediatrics 1983;72:22.

18. Matoth Y, Zaizov R, Varsano I, et al: Postnatal changes in some red cell parameters. Acta Paediatr Scand 1971;60:317.

19. Zipursky A, Brown E, Palko J, et al: The erythrocyte differential count in newborn infants. Am J Pediatr Hematol Oncol 1983;5:45.

20. Holyrode CP, Oski FA, Gardner FH, et al: The "pocked" erythrocyte. N Engl J Med 1969;281:516.

21. Bohler T, Leo A, Stadler A, et al: Mechanical fragility of erythrocyte membrane in neonates and adults. Pediatr Res 1992;32:92–96.

22. Faxelius G, Raye J, Gutberlet R, et al: Red cell volume measurements and acute blood loss in high-risk newborn infants. J Pediatr 1977;90:273–281.

23. Oski FA: The erythrocyte and its disorders. In Oski FA, Nathan DG (eds): Hematology of Infancy and Childhood. Philadelphia, WB Saunders, 1993, pp 18–43.

24. Oh W, Lind J: Venous and capillary hematocrit in newborn infants and placental transfusion. Acta Paediatr Scand 1966;55:38.

25. Linderkamp O, Nelle M, Kraus M, Zilow EP: The effect of early and late cord-clamping on blood viscosity and other hemorheological parameters in full-term neonates. Acta Paediatr 1992;81:745–750.

26. Wardrop CA, Holland BM: The roles and vital importance of placental blood to the newborn infant. J Perinat Med 1995;23:139–143.

27. Scott JR, Warenski JC: Tests to detect and quantitate fetal maternal bleeding. Clin Obstet Gynecol 1982;25:277.

28. Bowman JM: Maternal blood group immunization. In Eden RD, Boehm FH (eds): Assessment and Care of the Fetus. Physiologic, Clinical and Medicolegal Principles. Norwalk, CT, Appleton & Lange, 1989, pp 749–772.

29. Kleihauer E, Brown H, Betke K: Demonstration of fetal hemoglobin in the erythrocytes of the blood of a newborn. Klin Wochenschr 1957;35:637.

30. Kosasa TS, Ebesugawa I, Nakayama RT, et al: Massive fetomaternal hemorrhage preceded by decreased fetal movement and a nonreactive fetal heart rate pattern. Obstet Gynecol 1993;82:711–714.

31. Stiller AG, Skafish PR: Placental chorioangioma: A rare cause of fetomaternal transfusion with maternal hemolysis and fetal distress. Obstet Gynecol 1986;67(2):296–298.

32. Kosasa TS, Ebesugawa I, Nakayama RT, et al: Massive fetomaternal hemorrhage preceded by decreased fetal movement and a nonreactive fetal heart rate pattern. Obstet Gynecol 1993;82:711–714.

33. Lopriore E, Vandenbussche FP, Tiersma ES, et al: Twin-to-twin transfusion syndrome: New perspectives. J Pediatr 1995;127:675–680.

34. Dennis LG, Winkler CL: Twin-to-twin transfusion syndrome: Aggressive therapeutic amniocentesis. Am J Obstet Gynecol 1997;177(2):342–347.

35. Dommergues M, Mandelbrot L, Delezoide AL, et al: Twin-to-twin transfusion syndrome: Selective feticide by embolization of the hydropic fetus. Fetal Diagn Ther 1995;10(1):26–31.

36. De Lia JE, Kuhlmann RS, Harstad TW, et al: Fetoscopic laser ablation of placental vessels in severe previable twin-twin transfusion syndrome. Am J Obstet Gynecol 1995;172(4 Pt 1):1202–1208.

37. Ville Y, Hyett J, Hecher K, et al: Preliminary experience with endoscopic laser surgery for severe twin-twin transfusion syndrome. N Engl J Med 1995;332(4):224–227.

38. Van Heteren CF, Nijhuis JG, Semmekrot BA, et al: Risk for surviving twin after fetal death of co-twin in twin-twin transfusion syndrome. Obstet Gynecol 1998;92(2):215–219.

39. Moise KJ Jr, Dorman K, Lamvu G, et al: A randomized trial of amnioreduction versus septostomy in the treatment of twin-twin transfusion syndrome. Am J Obstet Gynecol 2005;193(3):701–707.

40. Senat MV, Deprest J, Boulvain M, et al: Endoscopic laser surgery versus serial amnioreduction for severe twin-to-twin transfusion syndrome. N Engl J Med 2004;351(2):136–144.

41. Rasmussen S, Irgens LM, Bergsjo P, et al: Perinatal mortality and case fatality after placental abruption in Norway 1967–1991. Acta Obstet Gynecol Scand 1996;75(3):229–234.

42. McMahon MJ, Li R, Schenck AP, et al: Previous cesarean birth. A risk factor for placenta previa? J Reprod Med 1997;42(7):409–412.

43. Chelmow D, Andrew DE, Baker ER: Maternal cigarette smoking and placenta previa. Obstet Gynecol 1996;87(5 Pt 1):703–706.

44. McMahon MJ, Li R, Schenck AP, et al: Previous cesarean birth. A risk factor for placenta previa? J Reprod Med 1997;42(7):409–412.

45. Schreier R, Brown S: Hematoma of the umbilical cord: Report of a case. Obstet Gynecol 1962; 20:798.

46. Deans A, Jauniaux E: Prenatal diagnosis and outcome of subamniotic hematomas. Ultrasound Obstet Gynecol 1998;11:319–323.

47. Eddleman KA, Lockwood CJ, Berkowitz GS, et al: Clinical significance and sonographic diagnosis of velamentous umbilical cord insertion. Am J Perinatol 1992;9:123–126.

48. Chen KH, Konchak P: Use of transvaginal color Doppler ultrasound to diagnose vasa previa. J Am Osteopath Assoc 1998;98(2):116–117.

49. Kleinberg F, Phibbs R, Dong L: Lack of placenta to infant transfusion with delayed cord clamping after cesarian section delivery. Pediatr Res 1973;7:403.

50. Cashore WJ, Usher RH: Hypovolemia resulting from a tight nuchal cord at birth. Pediatr Res 1973; 7:399.

51. Robinson RJ, Rossiter MA: Massive subaponeurotic haemorrhage in babies of African origin. Arch Dis Child 1968;43:684.

52. Teng FY, Sayre JW: Vacuum extraction: Does duration predict scalp injury? Obstet Gynecol 1997;89 (2):281–285.

53. Chadwick LM, Pemberton PJ, Kurinczuk JJ: Neonatal subgaleal haematoma: Associated risk factors, complications and outcome. J Paediatr Child Health 1996;32(3):228–232.

54. Thorp JA, Poskin MF, McKenzie DR, et al: Perinatal factors predicting severe intracranial hemorrhage. Am J Perinatol 1997;14:631–636.

55. Verma U, Tejani N, Klein S, et al: Obstetric antecedents of intraventricular hemorrhage and periventricular leukomalacia in the low-birth-weight neonate. Am J Obstet Gynecol 1997;176:275–281.

56. Bussel JB, Zabusky MR, Berkowitz RL, et al: Fetal alloimmune thrombocytopenia. N Engl J Med 1997;337(1):22–26.

57. Bussel JB: Immune thrombocytopenia in pregnancy: Autoimmune and alloimmune. J Reprod Immunol 1997;37(1):35–61.

58. Church MW, Crossland WJ, Holmes PA, et al: Effects of prenatal cocaine on hearing, vision, growth, and behavior. Ann NY Acad Sci 1998;846:12–28.

59. Felc Z: Ultrasound in screening for neonatal adrenal hemorrhage. Am J Perinatol 1995;12(5): 363–366.

60. Nagaya M, Kato J, Niimi N, et al: Isolated cavernous hemangioma of the stomach in a neonate. J Pediatr Surg 1998;33(4):653–654.

61. Komazawa M, Oski FA: Biochemical characteristics of "young" and "old" erythrocytes of the newborn infant. J Pediatr 1975;87:102–106.

62. Schmidt-Sommerfield E, Penn D: Carnitine and total parenteral nutrition of the neonate. Biol Neonate 1990;58:81–88.

63. Bracci R, Martini G, Buonocore G, et al: Changes in erythrocyte properties during the first hours of life: Electron spin resonance of reacting sulfhydryl groups. Pediatr Res 1988;24:391–395.

64. Toivanen B, Hirvonen T: Iso- and heteroagglutinins in human fetal and neonatal sera. Scand J Haematol 1969;6:42.

65. Thomaidis T, Agathopoulos A, Matsaniotis N, et al: Natural isohemagglutinin production by the fetus. J Pediatr 1969;74:39.

66. Weiner CP, Widness JA: Decreased fetal erythropoiesis and hemolysis in Kell hemolytic anemia. Am J Obstet Gynecol 1996;174:547–551.

67. Van Dijk BA, Dooren MC, Overbeeke MA: Red cell antibodies in pregnancy: There is no "critical titre." Transfus Med 1995;5(3):199–202.

68. Geifman-Holtzman O, Wojtowycz M, Kosmos E, et al: Female alloimmunization with antibodies known to cause hemolytic disease. Obstet Gynecol 1997;89: 272–275.

69. Lipitz S, Many A, Mitrani-Rosenbaum S, et al: Obstetric outcome after RhD and Kell testing. Hum Reprod 1998;13(6):1472–1475.

70. Miller ST, Desai N, Pass KA, Rao SP: A fast hemoglobin variant on newborn screening is associated with alpha-thalassemia trait. Clin Pediatr 1997;36:75–78.

71. Levine Z, Sherer DM, Jacobs A, et al: Nonimmune hydrops fetalis due to congenital syphilis associated with negative intrapartum maternal serology screening. Am J Perinatol 1998;15(4):233–236.

72. Berkowitz K, Baxi L, Fox HE: False-negative syphilis screening: The prozone phenomenon, nonimmune hydrops, and diagnosis of syphilis during pregnancy. Am J Obstet Gynecol 1990;163(3):975–977.

73. Vogel H, Kornman M, Ledet SC, et al: Congenital parvovirus infection. Pediatr Pathol Lab Med 1997;17(6):903–912.

74. Brown KE, Young NS: Parvovirus B19 infection and hematopoiesis. Blood Rev 1995;9(3):176–182.

75. Ferrazin A, De Maria A, Gotta C, et al: Zidovudine therapy of HIV-1 infection during pregnancy: Assessment of the effect on the newborns. J Acquir Immune Defic Syndr 1993;6(4):376–379.

76. Stahl MM, Neiderud J, Vinge E: Thrombocytopenic purpura and anemia in a breast-fed infant whose mother was treated with valproic acid. J Pediatr 1997;130:1001–1003.

77. Zinkham WH, Oski FA: Henna: A potential cause of oxidative hemolysis and neonatal hyperbilirubinemia. Pediatrics 1996;97:707–709.

78. Gerritsen EJ, Vossen JM, van Loo IH, et al: Autosomal recessive osteopetrosis: Variability of findings at diagnosis and during the natural course. Pediatrics 1994;93(2):247–253.

79. Gallagher PG, Ehrenkranz RA: Nutritional anemias in infancy. Clin Perinatol 1995;22:671–692.

80. Friel AK, Andrews WL, Hall MS, et al: Intravenous iron administration to very-low-birth-weight newborns receiving total and partial parenteral nutrition. J Parenteral Enteral Nutr 1995;19: 114–118.

81. Pollak A, Hayde M, Hayn M, et al: Effect of intravenous iron supplementation on erythropoiesis in erythropoietin-treated premature infants. Pediatrics 2001;107(1):78–85.

82. Carnielli V, Montini G, Da Riol R, et al: Effect of high doses of human recombinant erythropoietin on the need for blood transfusions in preterm infants. J Pediatr 1992;121:98–102.

83. Bechensteen AG, Hågå P, Halvorsen S, et al: Erythropoietin, protein, and iron supplementation and the prevention of anaemia of prematurity. Arch Dis Child 1993;69:19–23.

84. Oski FA, Barness LA: Vitamin E deficiency: A previously unrecognized cause of hemolytic anemia in premature infants. J Pediatr 1967;79:569.

85. Williams ME, Shott RJ, Oski FA: Role of dietary iron and fat on vitamin E deficiency anemia of infancy. N Engl J Med 1975;292:887.

86. Melhorn DK, Gross S: Vitamin E dependent anemia in the preterm infant: Effects of large doses of medicinal iron. J Pediatr 1971;79:569.

87. Pathak A, Roth P, Piscitelli J, Johnson L: Effects of vitamin E supplementation during erythropoietin treatment of the anaemia of prematurity. Arch Dis Child Fetal Neonatal Ed 2003;88(4):F324–328.

88. Diamond LK, Wang WC, Alter BP: Congenital hypoplastic anemia. Adv Pediatr 1976;22:349–378.

89. Rogers BB, Bloom SL, Buchanan GR: Autosomal dominantly inherited Diamond-Blackfan anemia resulting in nonimmune hydrops. Obstet Gynecol 1997;89(5 Pt 2):805–807.

90. McLennan AC, Chitty LS, Rissik J, et al: Prenatal diagnosis of Blackfan-Diamond syndrome: Case report and review of the literature. Prenat Diagn 1996;16(4): 349–353.

91. Gojic V, van't Veer-Korthof ET, Bosch LJ, et al: Congenital hypoplastic anemia: Another example of autosomal dominant transmission. Am J Med Genet 1994;50(1):87–89.

92. Ohls RK, Liechty KW, Schibler KR, et al: Assessment of stem cell factor as a candidate defect for Diamond-Blackfan anemia in a Utah kindred. Pediatr Res 1992;31(4):144A.

93. Abkowitz JL, Sabo KM, Nakamoto B, et al: Diamond-blackfan anemia: In vitro response of erythroid progenitors to the ligand for c-kit. Blood 1991;78(9): 2198–2202.

94. Dianzani I, Garelli E, Crescenzio N, et al: Diamond-Blackfan anemia: Expansion of erythroid progenitors in vitro by IL-9, but exclusion of a significant pathogenetic role for the IL-9 gene and the hematopoietic gene cluster on chromosome 5q. Exp Hematol 1997;25(12):1270–1277.

95. Sieff C, Guinan E: In vitro enhancement of erythropoiesis by steel factor in Diamond-Blackfan anemia and treatment of other congenital cytopenias with recombinant interleukin 3/granulocyte-macrophage colony stimulating factor. Stem Cells (Dayt) 1993;11:113–122.

96. Dianzani I, Garelli E, Ramenghi U: Diamond-Blackfan anemia: A congenital defect in erythropoiesis. Haematologica 1996;81(6):560–572.

97. Shalev H, Tamary H, Shaft D, et al: Neonatal manifestations of congenital dyserythropoietic anemia type I. J Pediatr 1997;131(1 Pt 1):95–97.

98. Cantu-Rajnoldi A, Zanella A, Conter U, et al: A severe transfusion-dependent congenital dyserythropoietic anaemia presenting as hydrops fetalis. Br J Haematol 1997;96(3):530–533.

99. Charles JM, Key LL: Developmental spectrum of children with congenital osteopetrosis. J Pediatr 1998;132(2):371–374.

100. Alter BP: Fanconi's anaemia and its variability. Br J Haematol 1993;85(1):9–14.

101. Perel Y, Butenandt O, Carrere A, et al: Oesophageal atresia, VACTERL association: Fanconi's anaemia related spectrum of anomalies. Arch Dis Child 1998;78(4):375–376.

102. Pearson HA, Lobel JS, Kocoshis SA, et al: A new syndrome of refractory sideroblastic anemia with vacuolization of marrow precursors and exocrine pancreatic dysfunction. J Pediatr 1979;95(6):976–984.

103. Brown MS, Garcia JF, Phibbs RH, et al: Decreased response of plasma immunoreactive erythropoietin to "available oxygen" in anemia of prematurity. J Pediatr 1984;105:793–798.

104. Ross MP, Christensen RD, Rothstein G, et al: A randomized trial to develop criteria for administering erythrocyte transfusions to anemic preterm infants 1 to 3 months of age. J Perinatol 1989; 9:246–253.

105. Bifano EM, Smith F, Borer J: Relationship between determinants of oxygen delivery and respiratory abnormalities in preterm infants with anemia. J Pediatr 1992;120:292–296.

106. Izraeli S, Ben-Sira L, Harell D, et al: Lactac acid as a predictor for erythrocyte transfusion in healthy preterm infants with the anemia of prematurity. J Pediatr 1993;122:629–631.

107. Keyes WG, Donohue PK, Spivak JL, et al: Assessing the need for transfusion of premature infants and the role of hematocrit, clinical signs, and erythropoietin level. Pediatrics 1989;84:412–417.

108. Rhondeau SM, Christensen RD, Ross MP, et al: Responsiveness to recombinant human erythropoietin of marrow erythroid progenitors from infants with the "anemia of prematurity." J Pediatr 1988;112:935–940.

109. Ohls RK, Liechty KW, Turner MC, et al: Erythroid "burst promoting activity" in the serum of patients with the anemia of prematurity. J Pediatr 1990; 116:786–789.

110. Ohls RK, Veerman MW, Christensen RD: Pharmacokinetics and effectiveness of recombinant erythropoietin administered to preterm infants by continuous infusion in parenteral nutrition solution. J Pediatr 1996;128:518–523.

111. Ohls RK: Erythropoietin to prevent and treat the anemia of prematurity. Curr Opin Pediatr 1999; 11:108–114.

112. Bell EF, Strauss RG, Widness JA, et al: Liberal versus restrictive guidelines for red blood cell transfusion in preterm infants. Pediatrics 2005; 115:1685.

113. Kirpalani H, Whyte R, Andersen C, et al The Premature Infants in Need of Transfusion Study (PINT): A randomized trial of a low versus high transfusion threshold for extremely low birth weight infants. J Pediatr 2006;149:301–307.

Respiratory Distress Syndrome

Colin J. Morley, MA, MD

Preterm birth and respiratory distress syndrome (RDS) are the greatest causes of neonatal morbidity and death in our society. The infants at greatest risk represent about 1.5% of births. They need resuscitation at birth and respiratory assistance during their first weeks of postnatal life because their lungs are immature. Ventilating these infants injures their lungs, causing lung tissue inflammation, and increases the possibility of bronchopulmonary dysplasia (BPD). BPD can be fatal and has long-term implications for respiratory health and brain development. Very preterm infants require prolonged intensive care, usually spending weeks in hospital. Of the survivors, approximately 50% are rehospitalized in their first year of life for serious respiratory disease. This represents a huge cost to the community.

Case Study 1

You are asked to provide counsel to a mother who is in early labor at 26 weeks of gestation.

Exercise 1

QUESTIONS

1. What information would you like to know about her that might alter your management of the baby and why do you need to know it?

2. How are you going to talk to the mother about what might happen to her and the baby?

3. What preparations will you make so that you can care for this baby?

ANSWERS

1. a. How far advanced is the labor and how soon is she likely to deliver? This gives you some idea of whether you are going to have to manage the baby soon or you have time to discuss, plan, and prepare.

   b. What is the cause of the premature labor and what were the precipitating factors? This will help you prepare for a baby who may have hemorrhage or infection. Many women have a spontaneous labor or cervical incompetence and there is no obvious precipitating cause.

   c. Has an antenatal ultrasound been done? This shows whether there are any congenital abnormalities and the estimated fetal weight and percentile of the baby, and whether it has been growing normally.

   d. Has a vaginal swab been done for group B streptococcus (GBS)? All very premature babies are treated with antibiotics soon after birth because of the risk of unknown infection. However, if the mother was GBS positive, that finding would mean the obstetrician and the pediatrician would give antibiotics to the mother and baby. Many obstetricians would treat a mother in preterm labor with antibiotics because of the possibility that infection had precipitated the labor.

e. Has there been rupture of the membranes? If so, how long ago, and how much fluid is present? Prolonged rupture of the membranes (>18 hours) increases the chance of neonatal infection. Prolonged rupture of the membranes with very little or no liquor for days or weeks increases the chance that the baby will have small, noncompliant lungs.

f. Is this a multiple or singleton pregnancy? About 25% of preterm labors are related to multiple pregnancy; advance knowledge will help you be prepared.

g. How many previous pregnancies has the mother had, and what has been the outcome? It is important to know whether she has had previous fetal deaths, premature babies, or neonatal deaths. This will alter your counseling and possibly treatment of the baby. The number of previous children may alter her ideas about this baby's care.

h. Has she had any social, medical, or obstetric problems during pregnancy? The social or religious history may have some influence on the parents' thoughts about how they want their baby treated. The mother may be in a supportive relationship or may be completely alone. The mother's medical problems may mean she is being treated with drugs that might affect the baby or alter the way she is able to care for the baby after birth. Her obstetric problems may alter her treatment by the obstetricians or the type of delivery; for example, she may have toxemia or a placenta previa.

i. Has the obstetrician treated her with betamethasone, and if so when was it started and how many doses were given? Giving the mother a full course of betamethasone, two doses of 12 mg, 12 hours apart, and if possible 48 hours before delivery reduces the severity of the baby's neonatal problems and increases chances of survival.

j. Has she been treated with tocolytics? If at all possible, the premature labor must be stopped, or inhibited, to give time for the betamethasone to work. Gaining even a few extra days in utero benefits the baby at this gestation.

k. What other drugs has the obstetrician used? Sedating or antihypertensive drugs may affect the baby after birth.

l. What mode of delivery is anticipated? Unless this is a precipitate delivery, most very premature babies are born in better condition, less bruised, and asphyxiated if they are delivered by cesarean section.

m. What is her blood group? Are there any blood group antibodies? This is core information for diagnosing and managing jaundice after birth.

n. Is her hepatitis B and HIV status known? If the mother is hepatitis B positive, the baby will need appropriate prophylaxis. If the mother is HIV positive, then she will probably be delivered by cesarean section. The baby will need appropriate treatment after birth.

2. a. Try to talk to the mother and her partner together. This means they both hear the same thing, and this allows them to support each other.

b. Have plenty of time to talk to the parents. If possible, this conversation should not be rushed. You need time to talk to the parents and learn about them. They need to get to know you, and gain confidence that you will look after them and their baby with respect and that you will provide the best care you can. Assure them that you will respect their wishes in the care of their baby.

c. Ask them what they know about very premature babies and get a feel for their level of understanding. Some parents may have had a previous very premature baby and will be quite knowledgeable. Others may be ignorant and fearful about what is going to happen. Some may have firm views about the baby's treatment, and others may be indecisive.

d. Inform them about the delivery, resuscitation, postnatal management, possible neonatal problems, and the possible outcomes for their baby. It is best if you have a leaflet or booklet about the care and outcomes for premature babies of different ages that you can use to inform the parents but also to ensure that all the staff say similar things. Some facts that you might like to give them are shown in Table 9-1.

3. a. Inform the neonatal intensive care unit (NICU) about a possible admission. One of

TABLE 9-1

FACTS ABOUT OUTCOMES OF VERY PRETERM BABIES (<28 WEEKS' GESTATION)

Mode of delivery	60% cesarean section
Birth weight range	680 g to 1230 g (1 pound 8 oz to 2 pounds 12 oz)
Chance of survival after delivery	90% survive if delivered alive
Need for respiratory support	100%
Chance of a serious brain hemorrhage	15%
Chance of retinopathy needing treatment	5%
Chance of necrotizing enterocolitis	10%
Chance of serious infection	50%
Need for a blood transfusion	80%
Duration of ventilator support (range)	0 to 50 days
Duration of CPAP support (range)	0 to 65 days
Gestation at discharge	Term
Duration of baby's stay in hospital	95 days
Chance of serious disability	10%
Chance of moderate disability	10%

the key elements of caring for very premature babies is to be prepared.

b. Ensure you will have two doctors and an experienced nurse at the delivery. There are a number of things that need to be done quickly, and it is good to have experienced hands available.

c. Ensure that you have equipment at the delivery to:

 I. Ventilate the baby with PEEP.

 II. Give CPAP (continuous positive airway pressure) through a face mask and nasal prongs

 III. Give blended oxygen, warmed and humidified if possible.

 IV. Measure the oxygen saturation (Spo$_2$) and heart rate from the right hand.

 V. Keep the infant warm under a radiant heater with appropriate covering (plastic wrap) and blankets.

 VI. Put in an umbilical venous catheter.

d. Transport the infant to the NICU while giving appropriate respiratory support, and monitor temperature control.

Case Study 2

You are asked to see a baby on the postnatal ward who was born at 37 weeks of gestation by elective cesarean section because of maternal diabetes. The infant is now 2 hours old and the nurse is concerned the baby might have RDS.

Exercise 2

QUESTIONS

1. How would you assess this baby's respiratory status?

2. If this baby has signs of respiratory difficulty and is admitted to the nursery, what is the differential diagnosis?

ANSWERS

1. a. Ask whether there was any antenatal history of a congenital abnormality of the respiratory system, or ruptured membranes. This is to ensure you do not miss an abnormality in the lungs.

 b. Ask whether mother had a vaginal swab for GBS before delivery? Was the mother treated with antibiotics before or during delivery? GBS septicemia/pneumonia can present at this age, and it is more likely if the mother is GBS positive. It is less likely with elective cesarean delivery but does occur. Treat the baby on the suspicion of GBS.

 c. Undress and examine the baby to ascertain the following:

  I. The degree of retractions at the lower costal border. This is the surest sign of respiratory difficulty. If the baby exhibits retractions, admission to the nursery for investigation is necessary. Normal babies breathe so shallowly you can hardly see the chest move.

  II. The oxygen saturation (measured from the right hand) and whether the baby needs to be treated with oxygen (Spo_2 less than 93%). Any baby of this age who has a low oxygen concentration must be considered to be unwell and admitted to the nursery for investigation.

    III. The respiratory rate. If an increased rate is obvious and faster than about 60/minute, the baby needs to be evaluated.

  d. Any of these signs warrants admission to the nursery for further investigation, especially arterial blood gases, a chest x-ray, and tests for infection.

2. a. Hyaline membrane disease (HMD), also called neonatal respiratory distress syndrome (RDS)

  b. Bacterial infection

  c. Wet lung syndrome, transient tachypnea

  d. Pneumothorax

  e. Diaphragmatic hernia

  f. Aspiration

  g. Upper airway obstruction

  h. Cyanotic heart disease

  i. Intrathoracic space-occupying lesion

  j. Metabolic acidosis

Signs of Respiratory Illness in Neonates

When examining a newborn the doctor has to recognize and understand the importance of the signs of respiratory distress. Doctors are alerted to the fact that a newborn has a respiratory problem when some or all of the following physical signs are present (absence of these signs means the baby does not have significant respiratory disease):

Cyanosis. Cyanosis is the need for oxygen treatment to maintain an oxygen saturation (Spo_2, measured by pulse oximetry in the right hand) greater than 90%. The need for oxygen treatment may not be due only to respiratory disease; it may be due to cyanotic congenital heart disease or persistent pulmonary hypertension (PPHN). However, in neonates, respiratory illness is common and cyanotic heart disease and PPHN are rare, so it is assumed that a baby

who requires oxygen treatment has a respiratory disease until proved otherwise. Hypoxia in a baby with respiratory difficulty is due to either a lack of surface area in the lung for adequate oxygen exchange or a right-to-left shunt of blood from the venous side to the systemic side without passing through aerated areas of the lung. Babies who have respiratory disease will have one or another of the following signs.

Retraction. Retraction, or indrawing of the lower part of the sternum and chest wall, occurs in babies with respiratory disease because that is where the diaphragm is attached to the chest wall. Retractions are due to the increased diaphragmatic contraction needed to draw gas into the chest. This may be because the lungs are stiff with disease (e.g., slow clearance of lung fluid, RDS pneumonia) or because the lungs are compressed by a space-occupying lesion or pleural effusion. Retractions of the chest wall may also occur because there is obstruction to the upper airway making it difficult for the baby to draw gas into the chest during inspiration. The chest wall distorts because in the premature baby the ribs and sternum are cartilaginous and more compliant than in later life. *Retraction is one of the most important signs.*

Grunting. Grunting during expiration is heard in infants who have a compromised lung volume, often due to RDS, excess lung fluid, or pneumonia. Grunting represents an attempt by the infant to increase intrathoracic pressure, and thereby open atelectatic alveoli and maintain lung volume. In the first phase of "grunting" respiration, the infant inhales, closes the glottis, contracts the abdominal muscles, and thereby increases the intrathoracic pressure. During a short exhalation the closed larynx relaxes slightly and the gas is expelled under pressure, causing the grunting sound. The infant then inhales quickly so that the inspiratory time is shorter than in babies who are breathing normally. Grunting babies do not always have a respiratory problem but may have other serious illnesses, such as septicemia or meningitis.

Tachypnea. Tachypnea, or rapid respiration, is defined as a respiratory rate of more than 60 breaths a minute. Tachypnea is significant when associated with retraction of the chest wall. Alone, it is not very useful because normal babies can breathe quickly for a short time following birth. Babies with respiratory difficulty breathe fast by altering their inspiratory and expiratory pattern from a short inspiration and long expiration to inspiration and expiration of almost equal length. Shortening the expiratory time is one of the baby's mechanisms for reducing atelectasis and preserving lung volume.

Causes of Neonatal Respiratory Distress

Respiratory distress can be due to a variety of different diseases. Therefore, the differential diagnosis has to be considered before coming to conclusions about the diagnosis and treatment. This section discusses some of the main causes of respiratory distress.

Hyaline Membrane Disease. Hyaline membrane disease (HMD), also called respiratory distress syndrome, occurs predominantly in very premature babies and the incidence increases in inverse proportion to gestational age. Most babies born at less than 29 weeks of gestation will have RDS, and only a small proportion born at 36 weeks' postconceptual age and older will have this disorder. It is the most common respiratory diagnosis in very premature infants. It is a serious condition that can cause death if not treated properly.

RDS is acute injury of a structurally immature lung. Part of the problem is due to a surfactant deficit (both quantitative and qualitative). Surfactant functions to lower surface tension of the air-liquid interface to facilitate lung expansion and also to form a stable surface monolayer that holds the alveoli open during expiration. If the surfactant does not function normally, it becomes more difficult for the baby to expand the lungs and prevent atelectasis.

RDS has a classic chest x-ray appearance of generalized fine granular opacities throughout both lungs (Fig. 9-1). These opacities may be so dense that it may be difficult to clearly see the borders of the lungs, heart, and liver. The airways show up against this background as an air bronchogram. In a ventilated baby the lungs may not appear as opaque because the ventilator is supporting lung volume.

Infection. Infection is most often a bacterial pneumonia and associated septicemia, which

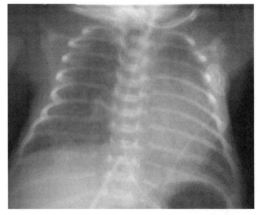

Figure 9-1 Chest x-ray of respiratory distress syndrome in an unventilated baby.

may be caused by a wide variety of gram-positive (e.g., group B streptococcus) and gram-negative organisms (e.g., *Escherichia coli*). Initially, it mimics RDS, and without early antibiotic treatment, these infants soon deteriorate and may die. The chest x-ray appearance is similar to that of RDS (see Fig. 9-1). Infection can occur at any gestational age, but the clinician must be most suspicious in more mature infants who have been well after birth and then develop respiratory difficulty in the next few hours. The threat of overwhelming infection is the reason all babies with RDS must be treated early with antibiotics.

Wet Lung Syndrome. Wet lung syndrome or transient tachypnea (TTN) mainly occurs after elective cesarean section in near-term infants. It is due to a delay in clearing lung fluid. There is about as much fluid in the lung before birth as the lung volume (functional residual capacity, FRC) after birth. Lung fluid is continuously secreted in utero. During labor, secretion stops and the fluid is cleared from the lungs by adrenergic stimuli. TTN is most common in infants who have not experienced the stress of labor (i.e., cesarean delivery), and is rare after vaginal birth. This condition is diagnosed by the chest x-ray appearance of streaky lines radiating out from the lung hila (Fig. 9-2).

Clinically these infants appear to have mild RDS because they rarely need more than 30% oxygen, infrequently require treatment with CPAP or ventilation, and recover in 48 to 96 hours.

Slow clearance of lung fluid can also contribute to RDS, and premature infants are especially

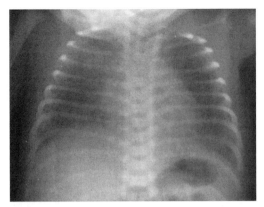

Figure 9-2 Chest x-ray of a baby with a wet lung syndrome.

susceptible because their ability to clear lung fluids is limited, even after vaginal delivery.

Pneumothorax. A pneumothorax can occur soon after birth in spontaneously breathing babies or babies who are resuscitated and given respiratory support. When a pneumothorax occurs, inspired gas collects inside the plural cavity and compresses the lung. It can be unilateral or bilateral. A pneumothorax can be accurately diagnosed only from a chest x-ray (Fig. 9-3). In many cases the side of the chest with the pneumothorax does not move as well as the other side and may appear to be rather prominent. Usually it glows when that side of the chest is transilluminated. A pneumothorax must be considered in all infants with respiratory difficulty, particularly if there is a sudden deterioration in their respiratory status. It is commonest in babies on respiratory support.

Pulmonary Interstitial Emphysema. In pulmonary interstitial emphysema (PIE), gas tracks into the lung interstitial tissue, but outside the airways. It occurs in babies who have a respiratory disease and are receiving ventilatory support. It can be diagnosed only from a chest x-ray, which will show small linear cystic areas in line with the respiratory vascular bundles (Fig. 9-4). These areas are commonly seen throughout one or both lungs.

Diaphragmatic Hernia. A diaphragmatic hernia is a congenital defect in the diaphragm. During fetal life bowel enters the thorax, compresses the lung, and interferes with lung development. Many diaphragmatic hernias are now diagnosed antenatally; therefore, neonatologists are currently alerted before birth. However, if there has been no antenatal diagnosis, then babies with a diaphragmatic hernia present with respiratory problems soon after birth. Although subtle signs such as a scaphoid abdomen and an asymmetrical chest may be recognized, the diagnosis is made by chest x-ray (Fig. 9-5). Diaphragmatic hernias occur most commonly on the left but are occasionally seen on the right side. The x-ray shows bowel and often stomach on the left side of the chest with no obvious diaphragm on that side and a shift of the mediastinum to the right.

Persistent Pulmonary Hypertension of the Newborn. A high pulmonary blood pressure is normal in the fetus. After birth the pulmonary

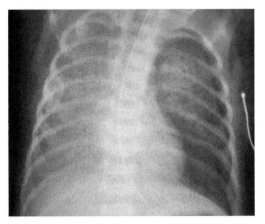

Figure 9-3 Chest x-ray of a baby with a left-sided pneumothorax.

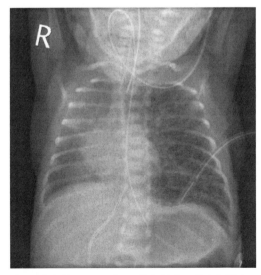

Figure 9-4 Chest x-ray of a ventilated baby with left-sided pulmonary interstitial emphysema and an intercostal drain in situ.

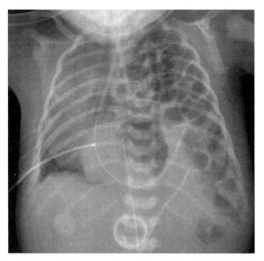

Figure 9-5 Chest x-ray of a ventilated baby with a left-sided diaphragmatic hernia.

artery pressure falls rapidly as the lungs expand. In idiopathic persistent pulmonary hypertension of the newborn (PPHN) the pulmonary artery pressure is high, so a large proportion of the blood from the right ventricle bypasses the lungs through the foramen ovale and the ductus arteriosus and then enters the aorta, resulting in hypoxia. In its primary form, these babies often present with hypoxia but with little lung disease. They need a high inspiratory oxygen concentration (FiO_2), often up to 1.0, and have a respiratory illness picture that does not match the degree of hypoxia. The diagnosis is made from a combination of chest-x-ray showing minimal lung disease with oligemic lungs (Fig. 9-6) and an echocardiogram showing evicence of pulmonary hypertension. PPHN can occur secondary to many lung diseases; especially those associated with early hypoxia.

Hypoplastic Lungs. Fetal lung development depends upon distention of the lung by amniotic fluid under pressure. This pressure stimulates lung growth, and without it the lung does not develop properly. In infants with pulmonary hypoplasia, there is usually a history of premature rupture of the membranes, and antenatal ultrasound examinations show very little liquor around the baby for days or weeks. Babies with hypoplastic lungs present with lung disease that may mimic severe RDS. Hypoplastic lungs also occur if the baby has no kidney function and therefore little amniotic fluid. This is a difficult diagnosis to confirm clinically because it overlaps with severe RDS (Fig. 9-7).

Aspiration. Aspiration of meconium or blood causes severe inflammation and obstruction of the airways and respiratory distress. It is diagnosed based on the history, the presence of meconium or blood in endotracheal aspirates, and the chest x-ray, which shows patchy areas of collapse and overinflation (Fig. 9-8).

Upper Airway Obstruction. Partial obstruction of the upper airway (nose, pharynx, or trachea) increases inspiratory difficulty for the baby. This results in chest wall and suprasternal retractions. Babies with upper airway problems usually do not have other symptoms, and the chest x-ray is frequently normal.

Cyanotic Heart Disease. Babies with heart disease causing cyanosis may present in the first day or two of life with a low SpO_2, which is not influenced very much by altering the FiO_2. They also have little or no lung disease, so they may have no retractions, grunting, or tachypnea

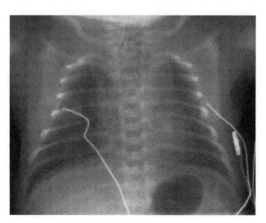

Figure 9-6 A chest x-ray of a ventilated baby with pulmonary hypertension and mild lung disease.

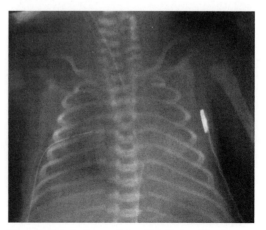

Figure 9-7 A chest x-ray of a ventilated baby with pulmonary hypoplasia with a chest drain on the right.

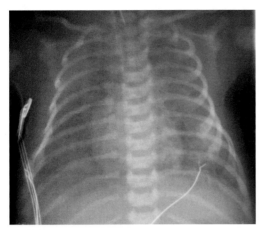

Figure 9-8 A chest x-ray of a ventilated baby showing meconium aspiration syndrome.

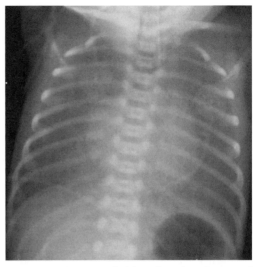

Figure 9-10 Chest x-ray of a baby with esophageal atresia and tracheoesophageal fistula.

and a chest x-ray with normal aeration (Fig. 9-9). Cardiac conditions causing cyanosis are diagnosed by echocardiography.

Tracheoesophageal Fistula or Esophageal Atresia. Tracheoesophageal fistula or esophageal atresia causes lung disease if secretions or milk is aspirated into the lungs. There is often a history of polyhydramnios, and many are detected by antenatal ultrasound examination. Postnatally, the diagnosis is made from a chest x-ray appearance showing the esophagus ending in a blind pouch in the middle of the chest. This can be visualized on chest x-ray by passing a tube through the mouth into the esophagus (Fig. 9-10).

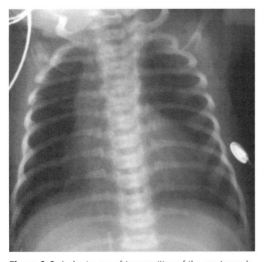

Figure 9-9 A chest x-ray of transposition of the great vessels with intact ventricular septal defect.

Metabolic Acidosis. Severe metabolic acidosis may cause a baby to breathe deeply. This happens because the baby is trying to produce a respiratory alkalosis (low $Paco_2$) to compensate for the metabolic acidosis. The baby may look as though it has respiratory difficulty. The diagnosis is made on history, blood gas analysis demonstrating metabolic acidosis and a low $Paco_2$, and often a normal chest x-ray.

Factors in the Development of Respiratory Distress Syndrome

RDS is a lung disease caused by immaturity, inadequate surfactant, and acute lung injury. It is the most common lung disease of premature infants.

Case Study 3

You attend the delivery of a baby who is being delivered at 26 weeks' gestation.

Exercise 3

QUESTION

1. What are you going to do to minimize the severity of the baby's subsequent lung disease?

ANSWER

1. a. Resuscitate very gently and hand-ventilate only if necessary with a low tidal volume/pressure.

   b. Give CPAP or PEEP (positive end-expiratory pressure) during any respiratory support.

   c. Treat with air and only give oxygen if the baby is slow to respond.

   d. Measure the heart rate and Sp_{O_2} with an oximeter on the right hand.

   e. Keep warm from birth.

   f. Give surfactant as early as possible if intubated.

   g. Give only enough 10% dextrose to maintain the blood glucose in a normal range, and prevent dehydration.

   h. Maintain a normal blood pressure.

   i. Withhold feedings.

Lung Development

The viability of an infant who has been born very prematurely is directly related to the degree of lung maturation at birth. An understanding of the different stages of lung development is useful in understanding the pathophysiology of RDS and neonatal chronic lung disease.

Classically, lung development occurs in four sequential stages: embryonic, pseudoglandular, canalicular, and alveolar. Although each stage of development was once thought to occur during a specific period of fetal life, in reality, each stage blends into the next with considerable individual variation.

The human lung initially develops as an endodermal outgrowth of the ventral aspect of the primitive foregut during the fourth week following conception. This marks the beginning of the embryonic stage. By 6 weeks, all the segmental bronchi have formed. During the pseudoglandular stage (5 to 17 weeks), these bronchi give rise (via dichotomous branching) to the terminal bronchioles. At the conclusion of this period, all major elements of the lung have formed except those directly involved with gas exchange.

The canalicular period (16 to 25 weeks) is characterized by the continued enlargement and division of the peripheral airways. By this stage, the terminal bronchioles have divided into respiratory bronchioles and alveolar ducts. Simultaneously, lung tissue becomes highly vascularized, and capillaries become intimately associated with the epithelium to form the future alveolar-capillary unit. Throughout this stage, the terminal airspaces are lined by simple cuboidal epithelium. By 22 to 24 weeks' gestation, the alveolar epithelium thins and starts to differentiate into type I and type II alveolar epithelial cells. Type II cells are responsible for surfactant synthesis and secretion. Surfactant-containing lamellar bodies appear in type II cells by approximately 24 weeks' gestation. Toward the end of this stage some thin-walled terminal saccules develop. As infants at this gestation can survive with respiratory support, thin-walled terminal saccules can be sufficient for gas exchange to occur. The alveolar stage is 24 weeks to term. Early in this stage the terminal air sacs are transformed into primitive, relatively thick-walled alveoli; type I alveolar cells attenuate to an extremely thin squamous epithelial layer, and surfactant is produced. As gestation advances, surfactant is produced in increasing amounts and the lipid and protein composition matures. After birth, the primitive alveoli enlarge and increase in number. These processes of subdivision, growth, and hypertrophy continue until approximately the eighth year of life.

In infants who develop acute (RDS) and chronic (bronchopulmonary dysplasia [BPD]) lung injury, damaged portions of the lung may become fibrotic, but undamaged areas have the potential to grow normally, providing the child with adequate surface area for gas exchange. However, with infants born at the limits of viability, an arrest of alveolar development may occur and the lung may lose its ability to develop normally. This may be the reason almost all very immature infants develop chronic lung disease.

The Role of Surfactant

Mature surfactant is a complex mixture mainly consisting of phospholipids and specific apoproteins. It is synthesized in the alveolar type 2 cells and packaged into lamellar bodies. In response to adrenergic stimulation, labor, and alveolar distention, the lamellar bodies are secreted onto the alveolar surface where the surfactant spreads over the whole of the inside of the lung. Surfactant spreads easily and rapidly over the inside of the lung because it is an oily liquid with an equilibrium surface tension about one third that of the aqueous fluid on the lung surface. The properties of surfactant are primarily due to the phospholipid, dipalmitoylphosphatidylcholine (DPPC). The apoproteins have important roles in surfactant spreading, homeostasis, and host defense.

Surfactant is a unique fluid because when the layer is laterally compressed it changes its physical nature from liquid to semisolid. This is important for its function.

Surfactant functions as follows:

1. It forms a protective oily layer on the surface of the lung to reduce the surface tension and facilitate lung expansion with a lower pressure. It also reduces damage to the underlying epithelium during repeated expansion and contraction.

2. It lowers surface tension and aids fluid clearance from the alveolar surface into the interstitium.

3. It stabilizes the alveolar surface during expiration so that end-expiratory volume is maintained. It facilitates the development and maintenance of the functional residual capacity, improves compliance, and prevents atelectasis.

4. It maintains the patency of the small airways, preventing their collapse during expiration.

5. It works as an antimicrobial agent.

Surfactant does not function properly in babies born very prematurely, because it is inadequate both in quantity and quality. As a result, the lungs do not fully expand. When the alveoli collapse during expiration (atelectasis) the surface epithelium becomes damaged and proteins leak onto the air-liquid interface, forming the hyaline membranes.

Surfactant Treatment

References about surfactant trials and treatment are largely derived from reviews[1,2] and the Cochrane Database of Systematic Reviews.[3–8]

Types of Surfactant

The animal-derived surfactants currently used are surfactant TA, Survanta, Infasurf, Alveofact, BLES, and Curosurf. Although derived from animal lungs, they are highly engineered. Surfactant TA and Survanta are extracts of

bovine lung mince with DPPC, tripalmitin, and palmitic acid added to improve the surface properties. Infasurf, Alveofact, and BLES are bovine lung washes subjected to chloroform/methanol extraction. Curosurf is porcine lung mince submitted to chloroform/methanol extraction and then purified by liquid-gel chromatography.

The synthetic surfactants are Exosurf (made from DPPC, hexadecanol, and tyloxapol) and Pumactant (Alec) (made from DPPC 70% and phosphatidylglycerol 30%). Neither of these are being marketed in Europe or the United States any longer. Two synthetic surfactants are currently under development: KL4 (sinapultide) and rSPC (Venticute).

Should we use an animal-derived or synthetic surfactant? The old synthetic surfactants are no longer marketed in Europe, the United States, and Australasia, so the choice is easy; only animal-derived surfactants can be used. The Cochrane Review of 11 randomized clinical trials with about 3600 infants shows that, in general, infants treated with animal-derived surfactants have fewer pneumothoraces and a slightly reduced mortality rate compared to infants treated with synthetic surfactants (Table 9-2).[4]

Clinical Trials of Surfactant Therapy

When considering the data from the randomized clinical trials (RCTs) of surfactant therapy one needs to be cautious about whether the

TABLE 9-2

OUTCOMES OF ANIMAL SURFACTANT EXTRACT VERSUS SYNTHETIC SURFACTANT FOR VERY PREMATURE INFANTS

Outcome	Odds Ratio (95% CI)
Pneumothorax	0.63 (0.53, 0.75)
Patent ductus arteriosus	0.96 (0.91, 1.08)
Sepsis	1.00 (0.90, 1.12)
Intraventricular hemorrhage	1.09 (1.00, 1.19)
Severe intraventricular hemorrhage	1.08 (0.92, 1.28)
Retinopathy of prematurity	0.95 (0.88, 1.01)
Oxygen at 28 days	1.02 (0.93, 1.11)
Bronchopulmonary dysplasia	1.01 (0.90, 1.12)
Death	0.87 (0.76, 0.98)
Bronchopulmonary dysplasia or death	0.95 (0.90, 1.01)

Soll RF, Blanco F: Natural surfactant extract vs synthetic surfactant for neonatal respiratory distress syndrome. Cochrane Database Syst Rev 2001;(2):CD000144.

results are still applicable. The trials were largely done in the 1980s when there were fewer very premature babies than are cared for now. In most trials the use of antenatal steroids was very low, on average about 30%. The use of antenatal steroids has a profound effect on RDS and its complications, and therefore, may alter the effects of surfactant treatment. The increased use of antenatal steroids will lead to fewer babies with surfactant deficiency and RDS and alter the benefit/risk ratio of surfactant treatment.

Most trials enrolled selected groups of babies and often excluded babies with complicating problems. The results may not be entirely applicable to those babies who are now considered candidates for surfactant treatment. One trial, the randomized European multicenter trial of Curosurf[9] only enrolled ventilated babies with weights between 700 g and 2000 g who received surfactant treatment between 2 and 15 hours when they had an F_{IO_2} greater than 0.6 and no complicating diseases. This only represents about 10% of babies with RDS and so the results should not be extrapolated to all babies with RDS. The American trial of Survanta[10] only enrolled babies between 3 and 6 hours after birth with weights between 750 g and 1750 g, who had RDS, were ventilated with an F_{IO_2} greater than 0.4 to maintain a Pa_{O_2} above 80 mm Hg, had a normal blood pressure, a blood glucose above 2.1 mmol/L, and no seizures.

Many trials emphasize only short-term outcomes, such as a fall in F_{IO_2} or airway pressure in the first few hours after treatment. Although interesting, these findings are relatively unimportant compared with the effects on survival and long-term outcome.

Effects of Surfactant Treatment

The main acute effect of surfactant is improvement in oxygenation. Many trials show a reduction in mean airway pressure. The magnitude of the effects and rapidity of onset vary depending on the type of trial and surfactant. Many trials also report an improvement in the chest x-ray. Table 9-3 shows the main effects of surfactant therapy on major outcomes in a meta-analysis of the 35 RCTs of surfactant versus placebo.[1] There was no significant effect on bronchopulmonary dysplasia, brain hemorrhages, retinopathy of prematurity, or hospital length of stay (see Table 9-3).

Adverse Effects. Administering surfactant can cause potentially serious problems, including transient hypoxia and bradycardia, acute airway obstruction, and transient falls in blood pressure and cerebral blood flow. Because surfactant treatment can acutely destabilize a baby, only experienced clinicians should administer it. There is a small increased risk of pulmonary hemorrhage in babies treated with animal-derived surfactants. As yet there is no evidence of any long-term adverse effects of using surfactant from animal sources.

Effects on Extremely Premature Infants. Is surfactant treat-ment as effective in micropremature infants as in relatively mature preterm babies? The data that are available suggest that surfactant treatment for babies as small as 500 g reduces complications.

Long-Term Effects. What are the long-term effects of surfactant treatment? There are several follow-up studies of treatment with different surfactants. They all show that the neurodevelopmental outcome for the surviving babies is similar to that for control infants. Therefore, surfactant saves lives without increasing the rate of handicaps.

Indications for Surfactant Treatment

Should we use surfactant prohylactically or treat established RDS? Prophylactic treatment

TABLE 9-3

EFFECTS OF SURFACTANT THERAPY ON MAJOR OUTCOMES

Outcome	Surfactant Therapy	Control Group	Odds Ratio	NNT
Pneumothorax	12.9%	24.3%	0.53	9
Pulmonary interstitial emphysema	17.9%	30.3%	0.59	8
Mortality rate in hospital	19.8%	25.9%	0.76	16
28-day mortality rate	13.6%	19.3%	0.70	18

NNT, number of infants needed to treat to prevent one adverse outcome.
Morley CJ, Davis PG: Surfactant treatment for premature lung disorders: A review of best practices in 2002. Paediatr Respir Rev 2004;5(Suppl A):S299–S304.

with surfactant means giving it within 10 minutes of birth. This aids initial lung expansion and may reduce lung damage. However, reserving treatment for babies with established disease will reduce the cost of surfactant and expose fewer infants to any risk of the therapy.

Rescue treatment with surfactant means giving it when the baby has established RDS. This may be too late to prevent some of the damage. One of the frustrations of rescue surfactant treatment is that there are no consistent criteria for when it should be used.

The evidence is strongly in favor of using surfactant as early as possible and preferably in the delivery unit. The beneficial effect of prophylactic animal-derived surfactant on mortality rate (compared with rescue treatment) is highly significant (odds ratio of 0.62). This is similar to the benefit of antenatal steroids (OR of 0.60).[11] However, there are no trials comparing prophylactic with early treatment. Early surfactant therapy (within 2 hours of birth) is more effective than administration when RDS is already established. Therefore, surfactant should be administered to intubated babies soon after intubation, otherwise it is given as soon after birth as feasible.

Dosage and Delivery of Surfactant

How many doses of surfactant should be used? Most babies respond well to one dose. However, others respond initially and then their respiratory condition deteriorates. This may be because the surfactant can be inactivated after it has been instilled in the lung. It seems appropriate to give further doses to such babies. RCTs of animal-derived surfactant have compared a single dose with multiple doses for the treatment of established RDS. Multiple doses were associated with a reduction in the incidence of pneumothorax. Little difference was shown in other clinical outcomes. There is little data to encourage the use of more than two doses.

Should the dose of surfactant be related to the size of the baby? Several manufacturers recommend that the dose be adjusted for the size of the baby. This seems obvious, but there is no good data to support the idea. In addition, there is very little data about the optimal dose to use. Approximately 100 mg/kg seems to be as effective as larger doses.

Criteria for Redosing. The criteria for giving repeated doses of surfactant are not clear. In one study re-treatment of ventilated infants at an FIO_2 above 0.3 was compared with an FIO_2 above 0.4 at a mean airway pressure of greater than 7 cm H_2O. There were no differences in the main clinical outcomes. The time interval for redosing has not been established. Pragmatically, many people use an interval of 12 hours and an FIO_2 above 0.4.

Administering Surfactant. There are a number of different techniques for giving surfactant treatment.

1. A bolus into the trachea is easy, seems to work well for small volume surfactants, but can destabilize the baby.

2. Several bolus doses over a few minutes are needed if large volumes of surfactant are used.

3. Moving the baby to different positions while the small boluses are given does not improve the effect of the surfactant, and therefore, is not necessary.

4. Administering surfactant through a side port on the endotracheal tube connector may work well and has the advantage of the endotracheal tube not being disconnected from the ventilator. Therefore, no lung volume is lost before the surfactant is given.

5. Surfactant may be administered through a dual lumen endotracheal tube. This seems to work well, but most babies are not intubated with these tubes, and it is not appropriate to reintubate a very premature baby to give surfactant.

6. Slow infusion of surfactant using a fine catheter inserted in the trachea does not seem to work as well as bolus installation.

Intubation for Surfactant Treatment. Should stable babies treated with nasal CPAP from birth be intubated to give surfactant? The research is in progress, and no firm recommendations can be made at this time. Alternative strategies that have been advocated include (a) prophylactic CPAP from birth with intubation and surfactant administration if the baby has worsening RDS (e.g., an increasing carbon dioxide level and oxygen requirement) and (b) intubation of a baby treated with CPAP followed by surfactant administration and early extubation.

The RCTs of surfactant versus placebo only enrolled ventilated babies and not babies who were being treated with nasal CPAP. The babies were not specifically intubated to give the surfactant and so the results cannot be extrapolated to babies treated with nasal CPAP.

Although there are trials of intubating babies treated with surfactant and then extubating them to CPAP, the results cannot easily be extrapolated to all babies. In the study by Verder and associates,[12] the small number enrolled were relatively mature with gestational ages up to 35 weeks. Moreover, the age at entry was about 12 hours, which is relatively late for surfactant treatment. The intubation rate in the group treated with CPAP alone was 85%. This is very high for babies of this gestation and much higher than the rate reported by others using CPAP from birth. The rate of intubation in the surfactant-treated group at 43% was no better than the rate found by other groups when CPAP was used alone. In 1999 Verder and associates[13] investigated early versus late intubation and surfactant treatment. The enrollment criteria were so selective that it is difficult to extrapolate the results to all babies on CPAP.

There are problems with intubating a stable baby on nasal CPAP. It will destabilize the baby and will lead to deterioration, albeit transiently in most cases. If the baby is treated with muscle-relaxing drugs for intubation, this will interfere with spontaneous ventilation for many hours and slow the baby's extubation to CPAP. Treating babies on CPAP with surfactant is not a simple procedure and its use should not be recommended until there is more supporting data.

There is good evidence that even very premature babies can be successfully treated with nasal CPAP without surfactant.[14] This may be in part because positive end-expiratory pressure conserves surfactant and improves lung volume.

Prevention of Respiratory Distress Syndrome

The incidence of RDS is inversely related to gestational age. Therefore, to prevent RDS, we must prevent prematurity. Unfortunately, despite many years of research there has been little progress in preventing preterm labor, although tocolytic therapy can delay delivery in some cases for several days.[15] As the delivery of very premature babies is associated with RDS and its comorbidities, it is very important that such babies are not delivered unless absolutely necessary. Increasing gestation by even a few days can be very beneficial in reducing the severity of RDS. The best use of tocolysis is to delay labor for at least 48 hours to allow administration of glucocorticoids.

Antenatal Steroids

Antenatal administration of 24 mg of betamethasone to women expected to give birth preterm is associated with a significant reduction in mortality rate (odds ratio 0.60, 95% CI 0.48 to 0.75), respiratory distress syndrome (odds ratio 0.53, 95% CI 0.44 to 0.63), and intraventricular hemorrhage in preterm infants.[11] These benefits extend to a broad range of gestational ages and are not limited by gender or race. No adverse consequences of prophylactic corticosteroids for threatened preterm birth have been identified. There is not enough evidence to evaluate the use of repeated doses of corticosteroids in women who remain undelivered but who are at continued risk of preterm birth. This is the subject of ongoing trials.

Careful Resuscitation of Very Premature Infants

The very premature baby has several potential problems that may contribute to RDS if not carefully managed during the first few minutes of resuscitation.

Very premature babies have difficulty with lung expansion due to a number of physiologic immaturities:

1. An immature lung structure with air sacs with unformed septae rather than alveoli
2. Immature respiratory muscles and a very compliant thoracic wall that is not able to adequately expand the stiff lungs or stabilize lung volume very well during expiration
3. Unaerated lungs at birth, filled with lung fluid with a volume close to the postnatal functional residual capacity (FRC) (about 20 to 30 mL/kg)

During lung expansion and the struggle to breathe deeply the lungs are easily damaged. The epithelial cells become necrotic and proteinaceous fluid leaks into the airspace of the lung.[16] The resulting hyaline membranes cover the airway surface, reduce lung compliance, and interfere with surfactant function.[17]

Controlling Tidal Volume

Very premature babies need careful assistance with establishing breathing and lung volume soon after birth without damaging the lungs in the process. Excessive tidal volumes are a major contributor to lung injury.[18] When ventilation is required during neonatal resuscitation, the appropriate tidal volume is rarely measured and has to be judged by eye. It should be sufficient to just produce visible chest wall movement. If the chest is seen to move any more, the tidal volume is likely to be too high. Large tidal volumes are associated with overventilation and hypocarbia. Hypocarbia has been associated with increased lung damage.[19] As hypocarbia can occur during resuscitation,[20] this is another reason why it is important to take great care with preventing excessive tidal volumes. If possible, tidal volumes should be measured and controlled during resuscitation.

Avoiding Repeated Alveolar Collapse and Expansion

Another problem during the early phase of lung stabilization is repeated expansion and collapse of the peripheral airways which causes excessive shearing and injury of the airway surface (atelectotrauma).[21] This can be reduced by using a positive distending pressure (CPAP or PEEP) during the initial inflations from a resuscitation device. The use of PEEP improves oxygenation during resuscitation (without increasing the carbon dioxide level[22]) due to the establishment of a surface area for oxygen absorption.[23]

Considering the Inspired Gas

Very premature babies are commonly resuscitated with 100% oxygen. This is damaging to the lungs. There is increasing evidence that most babies can be resuscitated with air, including premature babies,[24] and this may be beneficial in reducing early lung injury. The oxygen used is dry and cold. Although there is no direct evidence that this may contribute to early lung damage, it seems reasonable for the gas to be warmed and humidified during the resuscitation of very premature infants.

Temperature Control

Maintaining the baby's body temperature during resuscitation is important. Hypothermia has been associated with increased mortality and morbidity rates.[25] Early hypothermia can be prevented in very premature infants with the use of polyethylene wraps immediately after birth and during resuscitation.[26] This is an easy and effective intervention, which may reduce the severity of RDS.

Infection, Asphyxia, and Acidosis

Infection, asphyxia, and acidosis all make these problems worse by damaging the endothelium and interfering with surfactant function.

Case Study 4

A baby of 28 weeks' gestation is admitted to the NICU with RDS.

Exercise 4

QUESTION

1. How are you going to decide on the most suitable respiratory management for this baby?

ANSWER

1. a. Assess the respiratory signs.
   b. Do arterial blood gases to determine the severity of the lung disease.
   c. Do a chest x-ray to determine the diagnosis.
   d. Start with the simplest treatment and observe the effect closely.

Management of Respiratory Distress Syndrome

Early Nursery Management

When a baby with respiratory difficulty is admitted to the nursery there are several things that need to be done within the first hour.

Oxygenation. A baby's oxygen levels are quickly measured using pulse oximetry with the probe placed on the right hand to measure preductal blood. The F_{IO_2} is then adjusted to achieve an optimal Sp_{O_2}. Ideas about the most appropriate Sp_{O_2} are changing, although there is still no firm evidence for the exact target range. An Sp_{O_2} target of 88% to 92% steers a good course between the competing problems of hyperoxia-induced lung injury, and retinopathy of prematurity *and* hypoxia, cerebral injury, and anaerobic metabolism.

Surfactant. All intubated very premature babies should be treated with surfactant as soon as possible after intubation, preferably during resuscitation in the delivery unit.[5] If surfactant is not given just after birth, it must be given as soon as possible in the nursery. During surfactant instillation the baby's condition may deteriorate and increased ventilatory support may be needed for a while. Careful monitoring is required during and after surfactant instillation. There are reports that many very premature babies can be managed with CPAP and without intubation and surfactant.[27–32] Furthermore, there is no good evidence that stable babies treated with CPAP need to be intubated and treated with surfactant.

Dextrose. Premature babies may become hypoglycemic soon after birth. This can exacerbate the severity of RDS. An intravenous infusion of 10% dextrose must be started as soon as practical in the first hour after birth.

Arterial Blood Gas Measurements. Understanding and assessing arterial blood gases is essential in providing optimal care of a baby with RDS. Unless the baby has mild RDS, as assessed by the low F_{IO_2} and minimal dyspnea, then an arterial line should be inserted, as soon as possible, to enable the easy and repeated measurement of arterial blood gases. A baby with RDS will require several accurate blood gases in the hours and days after birth. In this situation an arterial line is optimal for the baby and the care providers. At this stage, capillary blood gases can be misleading and venous blood gases should never be used to assess the respiratory function of the baby.

Chest X-ray. An anteroposterior chest x-ray should be done as early as possible to exclude other diagnoses and to confirm the respiratory diagnosis. If umbilical arterial and venous lines have been used, then the x-ray should include the abdomen to show their position.

Infection Control. Infection must be suspected in all babies presenting with RDS because it cannot easily be excluded, even in babies born by cesarean section without obvious rupture of the membranes. Infection at this age usually causes septicemia and can be life-threatening if antibiotics are not given quickly. Blood cultures and blood tests for indicators of infection should be taken and if indicated, intravenous antibiotics are given that will be effective against the common perinatally acquired bacteria.

Respiratory Treatment

The majority of babies with RDS require respiratory support. There are three modes of respiratory management for babies with respiratory difficulties: (1) oxygen into the incubator, head box, or nasal cannulae, (2) CPAP, and (3) endotracheal intubation and ventilation. One of the first decisions in the care of a baby with RDS is to decide which of these treatments to use.

Oxygen

Babies with RDS need oxygen treatment to maintain their Pa_{O_2} in a normal range: Pa_{O_2} 50 to 80 mm Hg or Sp_{O_2} 89% to 92%. Oxygen can be given without any other respiratory support and low concentrations can be delivered into the incubator. If the baby needs more than about 25% oxygen, it is easier to give oxygen as a low flow through small binasal cannulae. In this way, the baby can be handled and the incubator doors opened without interfering with the treatment.

Nasal Continuous Positive Airway Pressure

For many years nasal CPAP was primarily used to support mature babies with RDS only when they were several hours old. It is now well recognized that it can be used as a primary means of respiratory support for very premature babies from birth. Using CPAP very soon after birth reduces the number of babies who require ventilation.[27] CPAP has the following beneficial effects[33]:

1. Helps establish and maintain the FRC

2. Improves oxygenation

3. Conserves surfactant

4. Decreases upper and lower airway resistance

5. Improves the compliance of stiff lungs

6. Regularizes and slows the respiratory rate

7. Reduces apnea

8. Reduces lung injury and inflammation

9. Reduces energy expenditure

A baby with RDS for whom intubation and ventilation are being considered may improve when treated with nasal CPAP instead.

Nasal CPAP is indicated in the following situations:

1. In the delivery room during stabilization of babies who have started breathing but are at risk of RDS. This helps to establish and maintain lung volume.

2. A baby who is being treated with oxygen, but is obviously breathing hard with retraction of the lower chest wall, tachypnea, and grunting during expiration. This baby is struggling to maintain lung volume and needs help before becoming fatigued.

3. A very premature baby with intermittent apnea and bradycardia. This is not necessarily a baby with RDS, but it is one of the common indications for CPAP.

To use nasal CPAP effectively requires attention to the following details:

1. Short binasal prongs are more effective at delivering CPAP than a single nasal prong or a nasopharyngeal tube.[34,35]

2. The prongs should be as wide as possible to fill the nostrils; otherwise, some of the applied pressure is immediately lost in the leak around the prongs. Skilled nursing care is required to ensure the nostrils, and particularly the nasal septum, are not damaged by the prongs.

3. The prongs must be fixed to the head and face in such a way that they do not move and damage the nostrils.

4. The CPAP pressure can be provided satisfactorily with a number of different pressure-generating devices. There is no good evidence that one system is more effective than another.

5. The baby must be positioned so that breathing is most effective:

a. The neck is slightly extended just enough to open the airway.

b. The baby is positioned prone with the hips and knees slightly flexed.

c. The nostrils should be cleared of secretions, but cautiously, because frequent deep suctioning can cause damage.

6. The pressure should be at least 5 cm H_2O and may need to be increased if the F_{IO_2} is high and the chest x-ray shows atelectatic lungs.

Some babies treated with nasal CPAP whose respiratory status is deteriorating may be effectively supported with nasal intermittent ventilation (IMV).[36]

Case Study 5

A baby of 26 weeks' gestation is being treated with nasal CPAP. The baby is retracting hard, receiving 55% oxygen, and an arterial blood gas shows a pH of 7.27, $Paco_2$ 58 mm Hg, Pao_2 50 mm Hg, and base deficit of −5. The chest x-ray shows lungs with a reticulogranular pattern and air bronchograms but no other pathology.

Exercise 5

QUESTION

1. How are you going to optimize this baby's respiratory management?

ANSWER

1. Before deciding to intubate and ventilate, several steps can be taken to assist the baby's ventilation:

a. Make sure the CPAP prongs are in the nose.

b. Make sure the prongs fit the nostrils well and are not too small.

c. Lay the baby prone, with the knees drawn up.

d. Extend the neck slightly to open the airway.

e. Minimize handling.

f. Put the CPAP pressure up to 8 or 10 cm H_2O.

g. Repeat the blood gas after the baby has been quiet and stable for 30 minutes.

h. If there was no improvement, add nasal IMV.

If the infant's condition deteriorates (i.e., apnea occurs, the $F_{IO_2} > 0.60$, the $Pa_{CO_2} > 60$ mm Hg), then intubate, ventilate, and give surfactant.

Mechanical Ventilation and Intubation

Intubation and ventilation of very premature babies with respiratory difficulty soon after birth was once considered mandatory. However, it has become apparent that even very premature babies with RDS can often be supported with CPAP without ventilation.

There are no absolute guidelines about when to ventilate a baby with RDS. It is often a matter of clinical judgment and local policy, considering the infant's gestational age, and other factors. The following criteria should be considered:

1. *Apnea.* Apnea unresponsive to short-term stimulation or hand ventilation is an absolute indication for ventilation.

2. *A high and rising* Pa_{CO_2}. Pa_{CO_2} that has risen above 60 mm Hg (~8 kPa) is a reliable sign of respiratory failure. However, this judgment should not be made on the first blood gas measurement, unless the baby is obviously very ill, because many babies improve over the first hour or two with careful and gentle management that includes appropriate positioning and, if possible, nasal CPAP.

3. *A high and rising* F_{IO_2}. A high and rising F_{IO_2} despite treatment with nasal CPAP is a strong indication for mechanical ventilation. There is little consensus about the F_{IO_2} value that should be used to determine the need for intubation. To a certain degree, the F_{IO_2} does not matter if the Pa_{O_2} can be maintained. However, a high F_{IO_2} is a sign of low lung volume and is a good indicator of severe RDS. Furthermore, oxygen is toxic at high levels, and the higher the F_{IO_2}, the more likely it will injure the lungs. Pragmatically, an F_{IO_2} of 0.60 or higher is an indication for ventilation in a very premature infant.

4. *The criteria for ventilation may vary depending on the size of the baby.* Babies born at less than 26 weeks' gestation are more likely to need earlier ventilator support because of their extreme immaturity. More mature babies, near term, are stronger, and ventilation should not be used unless absolutely necessary.

Several aspects of mechanical ventilation need to be adjusted to optimize blood gases and lung volumes and to minimize lung injury.

Oxygenation

1. Oxygenation can be improved by increasing the F_{IO_2}. However, the higher the F_{IO_2}, the greater the chance this will cause lung injury because high levels of oxygen are toxic to the epithelium. Therefore, other techniques as described later in the chapter should be used to reduce the F_{IO_2}.

2. Oxygenation is not dependent on the movement of gas in and out of the lungs. It only requires oxygen to enter the lungs and an appropriate surface area for diffusion.

3. Adequate oxygenation depends on ensuring the lungs are expanded with a good surface area for gas exchange. Oxygenation is closely related to the PEEP used. This is most important for maintaining end-expiratory lung volume in stiff lungs with RDS. The level of PEEP should range between 5 and 10 cm H_2O. There is no easy guide for optimal PEEP level. The pressure should be increased when a high F_{IO_2} is being used or when the chest x-ray shows low volume lungs.

4. Altering peak inspiratory pressure and expiratory times will change the mean airway pressure, and have some effect on oxygenation, but adjusting these is not as effective as changing the PEEP.

5. In a *normal* lung the use of excessive PEEP may worsen oxygenation by compressing the alveolar capillaries. However, there is no evidence that this is a problem in babies ventilated for the treatment of RDS.

6. Oxygenation is dependent on the lungs being appropriately perfused with blood. Inadequate oxygenation may be related to a low blood pressure or pulmonary hypertension. Therefore, to ensure optimal pulmonary perfusion and oxygenation the mean blood pressure must be kept in an appropriate range for the baby's gestational age

(about equivalent to the gestational age in weeks) with intravenous fluid or inotrope infusions.

7. Pulmonary hypertension with right-to-left shunting of venous blood past the lungs is best recognized by the need for a high F_{IO_2} to obtain a satisfactory Pa_{O_2}, yet the Pa_{CO_2} is relatively easily controlled. In primary pulmonary hypertension, the chest x-ray shows lungs with a normal volume and reduced vascular markings. Pulmonary hypertension with right-to-left shunting can also occur in infants with RDS.

8. In neonatal pulmonary hypertension, treatment with nitric oxide inhalation at 10 ppm often improves pulmonary blood flow. However, the benefits and safety of nitric oxide in preterm infants are controversial.

9. Not infrequently, oxygenation will deteriorate when ventilator pressure is increased. This is because the increased airway pressure overdistends the lung and interferes with pulmonary blood flow. A clue to this complication is that oxygenation improves when the baby is transiently disconnected from the ventilator.

Controlling the Blood Level of Carbon Dioxide

1. Carbon dioxide control is primarily related to moving gas in and out of the lung. This is done by altering the tidal volume and the ventilator rate.

2. The tidal volume is determined by the applied peak inspiratory ventilator pressure. Although neonatologists often talk of neonatal ventilation in terms of the applied pressures, these terms are just a proxy for the tidal volume entering the lung. Most modern neonatal ventilators measure and display the tidal volume so this can now be easily targeted. The guiding principle is that tidal volume during ventilation should be close to the normal range for spontaneously breathing babies, and as small as possible. Large tidal volumes can damage the lungs very quickly.[37] The appropriate tidal volume for ventilated spontaneously breathing babies is around 4 to 5 mL/kg.

3. The ventilator rate should be adequate to ensure the Pa_{CO_2} is in the normal range. Most babies are ventilated while spontaneously breathing. They breathe at a rate between 50 and 90 breaths per minute.

Modern ventilators can synchronize with each inspiration to assist the baby's own respiratory efforts. This is called the patient-triggered mode of ventilation. This means that the baby triggers inflations and controls the ventilator rate and to some extent the minute volume. With triggered ventilation, the back-up rate should be set about 10/minute below the baby's spontaneous rate. The product of ventilator rate and tidal volume is the minute volume. The normal minute volume is approximately 200 to 300 mL/kg/minute.

4. Careful control of the Pa_{CO_2} is very important during neonatal ventilation. Overventilation causes hypocarbia ($Pa_{CO_2} < 30$ mm Hg) and is strongly associated with chronic lung disease and adverse neurodevelopmental outcomes. Hypercarbia ($Pa_{CO_2} > 60$ mm Hg) may also be damaging because it can cause a respiratory acidosis and increase cerebral perfusion. The normal Pa_{CO_2} range for a baby with RDS is about 45 to 60 mm Hg.

Controlling Neonatal Ventilation

1. *Blood gases.* Neonatal ventilation, in particular Pa_{CO_2} and pH, are controlled by assessing frequent measurements of blood gases. The frequency depends on the stability of ventilation. In the acute phase of RDS, when the baby's lung function is changing, blood gases should be measured every 4 hours and no more than 30 minutes after a change in ventilator settings. Transcutaneous measurements of CO_2 can be very useful, give quick feedback about changes in CO_2, and reduce the number of blood gas measurements needed.

2. *Tidal volume, or peak inflating pressure, and ventilator rate.* The Pa_{CO_2} is primarily controlled by altering the tidal volume, or peak inflating pressure, with a ventilator rate set around 60/minute. If the Pa_{CO_2} is too high or too low, the tidal volume (or peak inflating pressure) is altered a little (0.5 mL/kg or 2 cm H_2O), and the Pa_{CO_2} is rechecked in about 30 minutes. The Pa_{CO_2} is loosely related to the minute volume and so it can be increased or decreased by altering ventilator rate. However, because ventilated babies are spontaneously breathing and triggering the ventilator, altering the set rate may have little effect on the delivered minute volume.

3. *PEEP.* Controlling the PEEP depends on clinical assessment, chest x-ray appearance, and F_{IO_2}. PEEP can be increased to open the lungs if the F_{IO_2} is high and the chest x-ray shows the lungs to be underinflated. The appropriate levels of PEEP have not been determined.

4. *Muscle-relaxing drugs.* There is no evidence that the use of muscle-relaxing drugs improves the outcome for babies with RDS. In fact, their use reduces venous return, causes edema, increases ventilator pressure required, and prolongs ventilation. They should only be used when babies are very difficult to ventilate and *fighting* the ventilation.

Modes of Ventilation

1. *Assist control* (A/C). In this mode, the ventilator is triggered by the baby's inspiration. It then inflates the baby in synchrony with each spontaneous inspiration. This means that every breath the baby makes is supported by inflation. This is the appropriate mode to use when the baby requires full ventilatory support. This can be very useful in the treatment of RDS.

2. *Synchronized intermittent ventilation* (SIMV). In this mode the ventilator is triggered by the baby's inspiration to inflate in synchrony with only a set number of spontaneous inspirations. This means that only those breaths are supported by ventilator inflation. Any other breaths are not supported and the baby has to inspire through the endotracheal tube. This increases the work of breathing and can lead to exhaustion. This mode can be used when the baby is weaning from ventilator support, although it has not been shown to be superior to other modes of ventilation or weaning.

3. *Volume-targeted ventilation.* This mode targets the delivery of a set tidal volume and reduces the proportion of high or low tidal volumes. As both of these may be disadvantageous to a baby with RDS, this mode can reduce the incidence of volutrauma to the lungs.

4. *High-frequency ventilation.* This mode of ventilation is used when "conventional" ventilation is unable to ensure satisfactory gas exchange without using a high peak pressure ($\geq$30 cm H_2O). The use of high-frequency ventilation has not been shown to have long-term benefits.

Weaning from Ventilation. The longer the baby is intubated and ventilated, the more likely chronic lung disease will develop. It is therefore important to wean babies from the ventilator and extubate them as soon as possible.

The F_{IO_2} is reduced to maintain appropriate Pa_{O_2} and Sp_{O_2}. The peak inflating pressure (or tidal volume) is reduced to maintain the Pa_{CO_2} in the normal range.

When the F_{IO_2} and the peak inspiratory pressure have been reduced to approximately 0.40 and 16 cm H_2O, respectively, the RDS is improving, and if the baby is breathing adequately, it may be possible to extubate the baby.

Some people advocate slowly reducing the ventilator rate using the SIMV mode so that the baby has more spontaneous and less supported breaths. One problem with this strategy is that the unsupported breaths are made through the endotracheal tube, and for these breaths the infant receives only endotracheal CPAP. This increases the work of breathing that the baby has to do and becomes significant if the ventilator rate is reduced below about 30/minute. Many babies can be extubated directly from assist control ventilation when the F_{IO_2} and peak inspiratory pressure are low. Similarly, babies can be extubated from SIMV at a rate of 30/minute.

To help decide whether a baby is likely to breathe adequately after extubation, the ventilator can be switched to endotracheal CPAP for approximately 3 minutes, to see how well the heart rate, Sp_{O_2}, and respiratory pattern are maintained. A baby who maintains the Sp_{O_2} and heart rate on ETCPAP has a high chance of successful extubation. A baby who becomes bradycardic or hypoxic during this time is unlikely to breathe well after extubation.

Most premature babies should be treated with methylxanthines, caffeine, or theophylline before extubation. This increases the chance of successful extubation.[38] Similarly, most premature babies should be extubated to nasal CPAP rather than to spontaneous breathing. This has been shown to reduce the incidence of reintubation.[39]

Case Study 6

A baby of 26 weeks' gestation who is 24 hours old and treated with mechanical ventilation starts to have an increasing oxygen requirement and a blood gas shows the Pa_{CO_2} is rising.

Exercise 6

QUESTIONS

1. What is the differential diagnosis of this problem?
2. What investigations would you do?

ANSWERS

1. a. The endotracheal tube has become displaced either too high or too low.
   b. The baby has developed an air leak, either a pneumothorax or PIE.
   c. The baby has become infected.
2. a. Transillumination of the chest.
   b. Chest x-ray.
   c. Blood cultures and tests for infection.

Case Study 7

A 7-day-old baby of 26 weeks' gestation is being ventilated in the assist/control mode with a peak inspiratory pressure of 12 cm H_2O, a PEEP of 5 cm H_2O, an FIO_2 of 0.25, and a ventilator rate of 30 per minute. The arterial blood gas measurement shows a pH of 7.34, a $Paco_2$ of 38 mm Hg, Pao_2 of 70 mm Hg, and base excess of 0.

Exercise 7

QUESTIONS

1. How would you interpret these data?
2. What management strategies should now be considered?

ANSWERS

1. This baby's lung disease has improved. The baby may be ready for extubation.
2. Give caffeine or theophylline in a loading dose. See if the baby can maintain breathing, Spo_2 and heart rate on endotracheal CPAP for a few minutes. If so, extubate to nasal CPAP.

Complications

There are several serious complications of RDS.

Pneumothorax

A pneumothorax can occur in babies who are breathing hard or receiving respiratory support. A tension pneumothorax is one of the most common causes of an acute deterioration in a baby with RDS. This is manifested by an increased FIO_2 and a rising $Paco_2$ and increased ventilatory pressures. Occasionally the infant presents with apnea.

The diagnosis is made when a pneumothorax is seen on an anteroposterior chest x-ray (see Fig. 9-3). Occasionally, the appearance of the pneumothorax is not very obvious because the gas is anterior and with the baby lying supine the stiff lung appears to fill the whole chest. One of the best signs is an obvious clear demarcation around the heart, diaphragm, or mediastinum. These boundaries are normally slightly blurred in a baby with RDS. Transillumination of the chest with a bright light in darkened surroundings usually shows the hemithorax glowing. Although this is a useful test in an emergency, it is not completely reliable, and so a chest x-ray should always be obtained to confirm the diagnosis.

The treatment of a pneumothorax is an intercostal drain, placed under strict sterile conditions, with the distal tubing underwater in a sealed bottle with suction applied to the outlet. The insertion site should be the fourth or fifth intercostal space in the anterior axillary line but away from the breast bud. The baby should be on its back with the affected side elevated so the body is at approximately 45 degrees to the mattress. The drain is then inserted from the posterior lateral aspect. This ensures the drain passes anteriorly rather than posteriorly and therefore drains the air at the front of the chest. A small hole is made in the chest wall, just above a rib, and then enlarged appropriately with small artery forceps. These forceps are then used to carefully introduce the catheter. A trocar should not be used because this increases the chance of perforating the lung. Local and systemic analgesia should always be provided.

Pulmonary Interstitial Emphysema

This complication mostly occurs in ventilated very premature babies. It can be a serious problem and may cause the death of the baby if not treated promptly and effectively. In PIE, gas tracks into the interstitial tissues and compresses the airways. It commonly occurs throughout one or both lungs and probably comes from a tear in the hilum where the gas is forced into the tissues. It may cause a serious deterioration in the respiratory and clinical status of the baby. The diagnosis is made from the AP chest x-ray (see Fig. 9-4).

There are two important aspects to the treatment of PIE.

1. Reduce the ventilator pressure, even if the F_{IO_2} must be increased or the Pa_{CO_2} rises as a consequence. However, do not compromise the baby's clinical and physiologic stability.

2. Lay the baby with the affected side down and with the back at right angles to the mattress. The affected lung is dependent and slowly loses the PIE. This is one of the best ways of treating PIE. If both lungs are affected, lay the baby so the worst lung is dependent. This treatment may lead to complete collapse of the dependent lung. This is a transient problem and, with repositioning, the lung usually reinflates without PIE. High-frequency ventilation may occasionally be needed when the PIE is extensive.

Mechanical Complications

Endotracheal Tube Inserted Too Far Down. If the endotracheal tube (ETT) is inserted too far or slips down after insertion, it will enter the right main bronchus and the left lung and right upper lobe will not be ventilated. The diagnosis is made from a chest x-ray, and treatment is to withdraw the endotracheal tube to the appropriate level.

Accidental Extubation. Accidental extubation of a ventilated very premature baby is a serious problem because the baby's condition will deteriorate quickly. It can be prevented by initially securing the ETT so that it does not come loose. Extubation can sometimes be difficult to differentiate from other causes of a rapid deterioration. There are several ways to make the diagnosis.

1. One of the quickest, most accurate and effective techniques is to have a continuous display of the flow wave of gas entering and leaving the endotracheal tube. This shows the pattern during inspiration and expiration. If the ETT becomes dislodged, then the flow pattern immediately changes so that there is flow down the ETT but not back up.[40]

2. Placing a carbon dioxide detector on the distal end of the ETT will quickly show whether CO_2-containing gas is coming out of the ETT. This is rapid and very sensitive.[41]

3. *Auscultation* can be helpful but may be confusing because the sound of the gas entering the pharynx can sound like gas entering the lungs in a small baby.

4. A complete *lack of chest wall movement* suggests no ventilation. However, if the ETT has slipped into the esophagus, the stomach may be inflated by the ventilator, and this can cause some abdominal movement, which may be confused with ventilation.

5. *A chest x-ray* will show the ETT in the pharynx, but if the ETT has slipped into the upper esophagus, this can be confusing.

6. Inspection of the larynx with a laryngoscope is invasive but is the only way to determine the position of the endotracheal tube if other methods are not available.

Methods 3 to 6 are less accurate than the first two methods.

Periventricular Hemorrhage

Periventricular hemorrhage (PVH) is strongly associated with the presence and severity of RDS.[42] The fragile blood vessels in the germinal matrix below the ventricular lining, instability of blood flow, and ischemia in this area are the main mechanisms behind PVH.[43] PVH is also associated with hypocarbia, and it should be avoided.[44,45] Intraventricular hemorrhage (IVH) is often not clinically obvious and can be diagnosed only from a cranial ultrasound. There is no treatment for IVH once it has occurred.

Subglottic Stenosis

Subglottic stenosis is a rare complication that only occurs in infants who have been intubated and ventilated for a long period. It is manifested by retractions and stridor that increases in severity in the hours following extubation. The diagnosis is made using laryngoscopy and bronchoscopy. The exact cause is unknown, but it is associated with the number of times the baby has been intubated.[46]

Initial treatment is supportive:

1. Use of nasal CPAP to distend the upper airways and relax the larynx
2. A short course of dexamethasone for 36 hours before extubation to reduce edema
3. Inhaled racemic epinephrine after extubation

Frequently, the obstruction improves with supportive treatment after extubation. If the stenosis is severe, and gas exchange is deteriorating, then reintubation is mandatory. Laryngeal surgery or tracheostomy is often required in these cases.

Chronic Lung Disease

Neonatal chronic lung disease (CLD) is a major complication of RDS, particularly in very premature babies; it affects about 80% of babies born at less than 24 weeks and 50% of infants born at less than 28 weeks. Chronic lung disease is defined by a need for oxygen or positive pressure at 36 weeks' postconceptual age.[47]

CLD is associated with an arrest of lung vascular and alveolar development due to early lung inflammation from oxygen inhalation and mechanical ventilation. It is exacerbated by infection. Clinically these infants require prolonged intensive care and respiratory support. Some are discharged home receiving oxygen treatment. CLD is associated with an increase in early death and later neurodevelopmental problems. Prevention is important, although in the most immature babies some CLD is almost inevitable.

The following factors should be considered to reduce the incidence and severity of CLD:

1. Avoid intubation and ventilation by using CPAP soon after birth
2. Reduce the time of intubation and ventilation
3. Reduce F_{IO_2} by using CPAP or PEEP to maintain lung volume and reduce atelectotrauma
4. Target the lowest possible tidal volume (no more than 6 mL/kg); try to reduce the peak inflating pressure even if this results in mild hypercarbia
5. Target an Sp_{O_2} of less than 95%
6. Undertake all measures to prevent infection

The key to management of chronic lung disease is patience. Most babies will slowly improve even if they have been very ill. There are a number of interventions (for example, diuretics) that improve clinical symptoms, but they do not affect long-term outcomes.

Death

A baby with RDS can die from respiratory failure or one of the complications. This is now uncommon with antenatal steroid treatment to the mother, postnatal surfactant therapy, and good techniques of respiratory support. However, it still occurs in some extremely premature infants or if the disease is not managed appropriately.

References

1. Morley C, Davis P: Surfactant treatment for premature lung disorders: A review of best practices in 2002. Paediatr Respir Rev 2004;5(Suppl A):S299–S304.
2. Suresh GK, Soll RF: Overview of surfactant replacement trials. J Perinatol 2005;25(Suppl 2):S40–S44.
3. Stevens TP, Blennow M, Soll RF: Early surfactant administration with brief ventilation vs selective surfactant and continued mechanical ventilation for preterm infants with or at risk for respiratory distress syndrome. Cochrane Database Syst Rev 2004;(3):CD003063.
4. Soll RF, Blanco F: Natural surfactant extract versus synthetic surfactant for neonatal respiratory distress syndrome. Cochrane Database Syst Rev 2001;(2):CD000144.
5. Soll RF, Morley CJ: Prophylactic versus selective use of surfactant in preventing morbidity and mortality in preterm infants. Cochrane Database Syst Rev 2001;(2):CD000510.
6. Soll RF: Multiple versus single dose natural surfactant extract for severe neonatal respiratory distress syndrome. Cochrane Database Syst Rev 2000;(2):CD000141.
7. Soll RF: Prophylactic natural surfactant extract for preventing morbidity and mortality in preterm infants. Cochrane Database Syst Rev 2000;(2):CD000511.
8. Soll RF: Prophylactic synthetic surfactant for preventing morbidity and mortality in preterm infants. Cochrane Database Syst Rev 2000;(2):CD001079.
9. Collaborative European Multicentre Study Group: Surfactant replacement therapy for severe neonatal respiratory distress syndrome: An international randomized clinical trial. Pediatrics 1988;82(5):683–691.
10. Horbar JD, Soll RF, Sutherland JM, et al: A multicenter randomized, placebo-controlled trial of surfactant therapy for respiratory distress syndrome. N Engl J Med 1989;320(15):959–965.

11. Crowley P: Prophylactic corticosteroids for preterm birth. Cochrane Database Syst Rev 2000;(2): CD000065.

12. Verder H, Robertson B, Griesen G, et al: Surfactant therapy and nasal continuous positive airway pressure for newborns with respiratory distress syndrome. N Engl J Med 1994;331:1051–1055.

13. Verder H, Albertsen P, Ebbesen F, et al: Nasal continuous positive airway pressure and early surfactant therapy for respiratory distress syndrome in newborns of less than 30 weeks' gestation. Pediatrics 1999;103(2):e24.

14. De Paoli AG, Morley C, Davis PG: Nasal CPAP for neonates: What do we know in 2003? Arch Dis Child Fetal Neonatal Ed 2003;88(3):F168–F172.

15. King JF, Flenady V, Papatsonis D, et al: Calcium channel blockers for inhibiting preterm labour: A systematic review of the evidence and a protocol for administration of nifedipine. Aust N Z J Obstet Gynaecol 2003;43(3):192–198.

16. Gandy G, Jacobson W, Gairdner D: Hyaline membrane disease I. cellular changes. Arch Dis Child 1970;45:289–310.

17. Seeger W, Stohr G, Wolf HRD, Heuhof H: Alteration of surfactant function due to protein leakage: Special interaction with fibrin monomer. J Appl Physiol 1985;58:326–338.

18. Bjorklund L, Ingimarsson J, Curstedt T, et al: Manual ventilation with a few large breaths at birth compromises the therapeutic effect of subsequent surfactant replacement in immature lambs. Ped Res 1997;42(3):348–355.

19. Garland JS, Buck RK, Allred EN, Leviton A: Hypocarbia before surfactant therapy appears to increase bronchopulmonary dysplasia risk in infants with respiratory distress syndrome. Arch Pediatr Adolesc Med 1995;149:617–622.

20. Tracy M, Downe L, Holberton J: How safe is intermittent positive pressure ventilation in preterm babies ventilated from delivery to newborn intensive care unit? Arch Dis Child Fetal Neonatal Ed 2004;89(1):F84–F87.

21. Attar MA, Donn SM: Mechanisms of ventilator-induced lung injury in premature infants. Semin Neonatol 2002;7(5):353–360.

22. Probyn ME, Hooper SB, Dargaville PA, et al: Positive end expiratory pressure during resuscitation of premature lambs rapidly improves blood gases without adversely affecting arterial pressure. Pediatr Res 2004;56(2):198–204.

23. Thome U, Topfer A, Schaller P, Pohlandt F: The effect of positive end expiratory pressure, peak inspiratory pressure, and inspiratory time on functional residual capacity in mechanically ventilated preterm infants. Eur J Pediatr 1998;157(10):831–837.

24. Saugstad OD, Ramji S, Vento M: Resuscitation of depressed newborn infants with ambient air or pure oxygen: A meta-analysis. Biol Neonate 2005;87 (1):27–34.

25. Herting E, Speer CP, Harms K, et al: Factors influencing morbidity and mortality in infants with severe respiratory distress syndrome treated with single or multiple doses of a natural porcine surfactant. Biol Neonate 1992;61(Suppl 1):26–30.

26. McCall EM, Alderdice FA, Halliday HL, et al: Interventions to prevent hypothermia at birth in preterm and/or low birthweight babies. Cochrane Database Syst Rev 2005;(1):CD004210.

27. Avery ME, Tooley WH, Keller JB, et al: Is chronic lung disease in low birth weight infants preventable? A survey of eight centers. Pediatrics 1987;79 (1):26–30.

28. Lindner W, Vossbeck S, Hummler H, Pohlandt F: Delivery room management of extremely low birth weight infants: Spontaneous breathing or intubation? Pediatrics 1999;103(5 Pt 1):961–967.

29. Van Marter LJ, Allred EN, Pagano M, et al: Do clinical markers of barotrauma and oxygen toxicity explain interhospital variation in rates of chronic lung disease? Pediatrics 2000;105(6):1194–1201.

30. Sun S: Minimising the use of assisted ventilation to reduce the risk of chronic lung disease: A tried and tested management. Paediatr Respir Rev 2004;5 (Suppl A):S353–S356.

31. Tooley J, Dyke M: Randomized study of nasal continuous positive airway pressure in the preterm infant with respiratory distress syndrome. Acta Paediatr 2003;92(10):1170–1174.

32. Aly H, Massaro AN, Patel K, El Mohandes AA: Is it safer to intubate premature infants in the delivery room? Pediatrics 2005;115(6):1660–1665.

33. Morley CJ: Continuous distending pressure. Arch Dis Child Fetal Neonatal Ed 1999;81:F152–F156.

34. Davis PG, Davies M, Faber B: A randomised controlled trial of two methods of delivery nasal continuous positive airway pressure after extubation to infants weighing less than 1000g: Binasal (Hudson) versus single nasal prongs. Arch Dis Child Fetal Neonatal Ed 2001;85:F82–F85.

35. De Paoli AG, Davis PG, Faber B, Morley CJ: Devices and pressure sources for administration of nasal continuous positive airway pressure (NCPAP) in preterm neonates. Cochrane Database Syst Rev 2002;(4):CD002977.

36. Davis PG, Lemyre B, De Paoli AG: Nasal intermittent positive pressure ventilation (NIPPV) versus nasal continuous positive airway pressure (NCPAP) for preterm neonates after extubation. Cochrane Database Syst Rev 2004;(3):CD003212.

37. Bjorklund LJ, Curstedt T, Ingimarsson J, et al: Lung injury caused by neonatal resuscitation of immature lambs—Relation of volume of lung inflations. Ped Res 1996;39:326A.

38. Henderson-Smart DJ, Davis PG: Prophylactic methylxanthines for extubation in preterm infants. Cochrane Database Syst Rev 2003;(1):CD000139.

39. Davis PG, Henderson-Smart DJ: Nasal continuous positive airways pressure immediately after extubation for preventing morbidity in preterm infants. Cochrane Database Syst Rev 2003;(2):CD000143.

40. Lilley CD, Stewart M, Morley CJ: Respiratory function monitoring during neonatal emergency transport. Arch Dis Child Fetal Neonatal Ed 2005;90 (1):F82–F83.

41. Aziz HF, Martin JB, Moore JJ: The pediatric disposable end-tidal carbon dioxide detector role in endotracheal intubation in newborns. J Perinatol 1999; 19(2):110–113.

42. Vergani P, Patane L, Doria P, et al: Risk factors for neonatal intraventricular haemorrhage in spontaneous prematurity at 32 weeks gestation or less. Placenta 2000;21(4):402–407.

43. Whitelaw A: Intraventricular haemorrhage and posthaemorrhagic hydrocephalus: Pathogenesis, prevention and future interventions. Semin Neonatol 2001;6(2):135–146.

44. Dammann O, Allred EN, Kuban KC, et al: Hypocarbia during the first 24 postnatal hours and white matter echolucencies in newborns < or = 28 weeks gestation. Pediatr Res 2001;49(3):388–393.

45. Erickson SJ, Grauaug A, Gurrin L, Swaminathan M: Hypocarbia in the ventilated preterm infant and its effect on intraventricular haemorrhage and bronchopulmonary dysplasia. J Paediatr Child Health 2002;38(6):560–562.

46. Sherman JM, Lowitt S, Stephenson C, Ironson G: Factors influencing acquired subglottic stenosis in infants. J Pediatr 1986;109(2):322–327.

47. Jobe AH, Ikegami M: Prevention of bronchopulmonary dysplasia. Curr Opin Pediatr 2001;13: 124–129.

Principles of Mechanical Ventilation

Steven M. Donn, MD, and
Matthew E. Abrams, MD

Mechanical ventilation is used to provide partial or total assistance to the newborn with respiratory compromise or failure. It can support pulmonary gas exchange and the work of breathing when pulmonary, neurologic, or systemic conditions prevent this from happening normally.

Respiratory support (beyond simple supplemental oxygen) ranges from the most minimally invasive, continuous positive airway pressure (CPAP), to the most invasive, extracorporeal membrane oxygenation (ECMO). In between are conventional (tidal) and high-frequency (nontidal) ventilation. Although the application of intermittent positive pressure ventilation through nasal prongs has received recent attention, this chapter will focus on the principles of conventional mechanical ventilation (CMV) and high-frequency ventilation (HFV), which includes high-frequency jet ventilation (HFJV) and high-frequency oscillatory ventilation (HFOV).

Mechanisms of Respiratory Failure

Respiratory failure results when there is inadequate pulmonary gas exchange to provide sufficient oxygenation of the blood and removal of carbon dioxide, usually referred to as alveolar hypoventilation.[1] Respiratory failure is usually subclassified based on whether its cause is extrinsic (extrapulmonary) or intrinsic (pulmonary). Examples of these are listed in Table 10-1. Infants may have more than one mechanism, such as a premature infant with severe respiratory distress syndrome complicated by apnea.

Extrinsic respiratory failure generally occurs because there is a limitation of gas flow into or out of the lung. This can result, for example, from a compression of the airways or from inadequate respiratory drive.

Intrinsic respiratory failure results from pathology related to lung parenchyma (such as pneumonia) or pulmonary vasculature (such as persistent pulmonary hypertension of the

TABLE 10-1
CAUSES OF NEONATAL RESPIRATORY FAILURE

Extrapulmonary (Extrinsic)
Neurologic
   Central (e.g., brain stem injury)
   Peripheral (e.g., phrenic nerve palsy)
Drug-induced (e.g., hypermagnesemia)
Airway malformation or obstruction
   (e.g., tracheal stenosis)
Right-to-left shunting (e.g., persistent pulmonary
   hypertension of the newborn)
Altered oxygen-carrying capacity
   (e.g., methemoglobinemia)
Cyanotic congenital heart disease
Inadequate inspired oxygen (e.g., high altitude)

Pulmonary (Intrinsic)
Lung malformations (e.g., CCAM)
Diminished surface area (e.g., pulmonary hypoplasia)
Surfactant deficiency (e.g., respiratory distress
   syndrome)
Inflammation
   Pneumonia
   Meconium aspiration
Air leaks
   Pneumothorax
   Pulmonary interstitial emphysema
Edema (e.g., congestive heart failure)
Diffusion abnormalities (e.g., alveolar capillary
   dysplasia)
Chronic lung disease

CCAM, congenital cystic adenomatoid malformation.

newborn, PPHN). Parenchymal lung disease may impede gas exchange at the alveolar-capillary level. Increased pulmonary vascular resistance may restrict pulmonary blood flow and result in ventilation/perfusion mismatch (often referred to as intrapulmonary shunting) and extrapulmonary shunting through the foramen ovale and patent ductus arteriosus.

Case Study 1

An 800-g 25-week male baby is born by cesarean delivery because of worsening maternal preeclampsia. The baby has severe respiratory distress syndrome (RDS) in the delivery room requiring intubation. You administer surfactant and bring the baby to the neonatal intensive care unit (NICU). Assume that you decide to place this baby on a conventional ventilator (tidal ventilation).

Exercise 1

QUESTIONS

1. What mode on the ventilator would you choose and why?
   a. Time-cycled pressure-limited assist control
   b. Volume-targeted ventilation
   c. Time-cycled pressure-limited synchronized intermittent mandatory ventilation (SIMV)
   d. Pressure control ventilation

2. How would you choose your initial ventilator settings?
   a. Place the baby on the ventilator on an arbitrary setting and wait for a blood gas
   b. Place the baby on the ventilator and adjust the settings to meet goal tidal volumes, minute ventilation, and oxygenation
   c. Manually ventilate the baby with a bag and manometer and see what kind of pressures are required for adequate air exchange and chest wall movement

3. What should be the initial tidal volume goal in this baby with RDS?
   a. 4 to 7 mL/kg
   b. 6 to 8 mL/kg
   c. 8 to 10 mL/kg

ANSWERS

1. a, b, or d. The choice of mode of ventilation depends on a number of factors, including which ventilator is at one's disposal, level of experience and comfort with particular modes, goals of mechanical ventilation, and the disease state. The best available evidence does not clearly define one brand of ventilator or one mode of ventilation as clearly being superior. Different companies use different names for similar modes of ventilation, which makes it all the more confusing. What is important is an understanding of the underlying principles, the factors that affect oxygenation and ventilation, and a vision of what one is trying to accomplish with mechanical ventilation. However, SIMV is not a good mode for a baby with acute respiratory dysfunction, as spontaneous breaths are supported only by positive end-expiratory pressure (PEEP). If SIMV is chosen, pressure support should be added to overcome the imposed work of breathing.

2. b, c. This begins to get into the art of mechanical ventilation. Choosing the initial ventilator settings should be done with some specific goals in mind. The target tidal volumes (discussed later in this chapter) will depend both on the disease state and a desire to avoid overinflation and excessive volume (volutrauma). Choosing the initial ventilator settings should be based on specific ventilation and oxygenation goals, paying particular attention to mean airway pressure, tidal volume, and minute ventilation. Although different manufacturers may have different names for different modes of ventilation, the basic settings are similar (discussed later). Many ventilators also incorporate real-time pulmonary graphics, such as pressure/volume and flow/volume loops, which assist in choosing or modifying the settings. Adjusting the ventilator depends on a thorough understanding of the relationship between the ventilator variables and the patient.

3. a. Based on the best available evidence, the goal tidal volume for an infant of this size should be in the 4 to 7 mL/kg range. This seems to be the most optimal range to avoid lung injury while providing adequate ventilation.

Ventilator Variables

Oxygen Concentration. The fraction of inspired oxygen (F_{IO_2}) refers to the percentage of oxygen in the gas delivered to the patient. It ranges from 21% (room air) to 100% (pure oxygen). A blender, either external to the ventilator or within it, is used to adjust the concentration. Oxygen is warmed and humidified by an external device before it reaches the airway. The temperature of the delivered gas can be manipulated to prevent excessive condensation in the ventilator circuit or endotracheal tube.

Pressure. The peak inspiratory pressure (PIP) refers to the highest pressure delivered during inspiration. It is set during pressure-targeted ventilation and is variable during volume-targeted ventilation. The baseline pressure is the lowest pressure reached during expiration, and if it is above zero, it is referred to as positive end-expiratory pressure. The mean airway pressure (mean Paw or MAP) is the average pressure delivered to the airway; it is not a set variable except during high-frequency oscillatory ventilation (HFOV) but is usually displayed on a data screen or digital monitor.

Volume. Tidal volume is set during volume-targeted ventilation, and pressure is allowed to vary. During pressure-targeted ventilation, tidal volume is displayed on machines capable of measuring it, and some devices display inspired and expired tidal volumes and calculate minute ventilation.

Flow. Flow is the time rate of volume delivery. During continuous flow ventilation, the patient has a source of fresh gas flowing through the ventilator circuit (bias flow) from which to breathe. Flow rate is usually set by the clinician. It should be high enough so that the desired PIP is reached during inspiration but not so high that it might cause turbulence, inadvertent PEEP, and gas trapping. If it is set too low, it may result in air hunger and increased work of breathing for the patient. Inappropriate flow has been referred to as rheotrauma.[2] Some ventilatory modalities use variable inspiratory flow, proportional to patient effort (see later discussion), and others use a demand flow system, in which the patient must "open" a valve to initiate inspiratory flow.

Rate. For intermittent mandatory ventilation (IMV) and synchronized intermittent manda-

tory ventilation (SIMV), the clinician chooses the frequency of mandatory breaths to be delivered to the patient, irrespective of spontaneous breaths. For assist/control (A/C) ventilation, the clinician chooses the control rate, which is a true back-up rate. This determines the minimum number of breaths the baby will receive in the event of apnea or inadequate patient effort.

Cycle. The respiratory cycle consists of inspiratory and expiratory phases. During inspiration, gas flows into the airway under positive pressure. During expiration, gas flows passively from the airway, dependent on the elastic recoil of the lungs, except during HFOV, when exhalation is active, with gas being withdrawn from the airway by the oscillator. Between inspiration and expiration, and between expiration and inspiration, there is a zero flow state. The cycling mechanism is the way in which the switchover from inspiration to expiration and expiration to inspiration occurs.[3] Most ventilatory modes use time as the cycling mechanism, and thus distinct inspiratory and expiratory times (and inspiratory/expiratory ratios) can be selected. Cycling can also be accomplished by changes in airway flow (inspiration ends when airway flow declines to a preselected percentage of peak flow) or by changes in inspired volume (however, true volume cycling does not occur if uncuffed endotracheal tubes are used; see later discussion).[4]

Mode. The clinician selects the mode of ventilation. The available modes vary from one ventilator to the next. They include IMV, SIMV, A/C ventilation, and pressure support ventilation (PSV). Newer ventilators also offer hybrid modes, such as SIMV/PSV.

Assist Sensitivity. For ventilators offering patient-triggered ventilation, assist sensitivity refers to the triggering threshold, usually in liters per minute (LPM) for flow triggers and cm H_2O for pressure triggers. The lower the assist sensitivity, the easier it is for the patient to trigger the ventilator.

Rise Time. This feature, available on some ventilators, modifies the slope of the inspiratory pressure waveform. It is a semiquantitative variable, for which "1" may represent the steepest (most aggressive) slope, "3" or "4" may represent an intermediate slope, and "7" may represent the gentlest slope. If set too low (steep), pressure overshoot may occur, and if set too high, there may be inadequate hysteresis and lung inflation.[5] This is demonstrated in Figure 10-1.

Case Study 2

A 1250-g 30-week infant is born by vaginal delivery after progression of preterm labor and is placed on a ventilator and given surfactant. Initial ventilator settings are PIP 16, PEEP 4, rate 40, and inspiratory time of 0.3 second. Oxygen saturations are in the mid-80s on 50% oxygen, and the chest x-ray shows low lung volume.

Exercise 2

QUESTION

1. What is the best way to improve oxygenation in this patient?

   a. Increase peak inspiratory pressure by 1

   b. Increase positive end-expiratory pressure by 1

   c. Increase the inspiratory time by 0.1 second

   d. Increase the ventilator rate

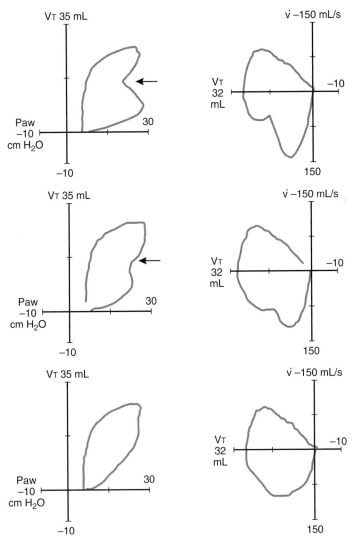

Figure 10-1 Effect of rise time on pressure-volume relationship. **A**, Rise time of 1 produces the steepest slope of the inspiratory pressure waveform and results in significant pressure overshoot (*arrow*). **B**, A more moderate setting, 3, results in less overshoot but is still too high. **C**, The gentlest setting, 7, results in a normal degree of hysteresis.

ANSWER

1. b. Given the foregoing findings, increasing the PEEP is the safest and most effective way to improve oxygenation in this patient. Although all of the preceding measures will increase the mean airway pressure, increasing the PEEP by 1 would be the most effective, as discussed in the next section.

   Adjusting settings on a ventilator requires a familiarity with the machine and the patient. For example, the initial chest x-ray may demonstrate low lung volumes, but by the time you review the chest x-ray and go see the patient again the oxygen saturations are likely to have improved. Never respond to the findings on a chest radiograph or a blood gas analysis without first examining the patient. Even if the results of a blood gas analysis are "good," it does not mean that the ventilator settings are ideal or that the pressure should not be weaned.

Oxygenation

The primary determinants of oxygenation are the fraction of inspired oxygen (F_{IO_2}) and the mean airway pressure. Increasing the amount of oxygen delivered to the alveoli may help to overcome diffusion gradients and improve the delivery of oxygen to the capillary blood. Raising the mean airway pressure recruits collapsed alveoli, thus increasing the pulmonary surface area available for gas exchange. However, excessive pressure may be detrimental, contributing to hyperinflation, dead space ventilation, and increased pulmonary vascular resistance, which can impair venous return, cardiac output, and pulmonary blood flow.

There are several ways to increase mean airway pressure. Raising the PEEP has a direct 1:1 relationship to increases in the mean airway pressure. Thus, a 1.0 cm H_2O increase in PEEP raises the mean airway pressure by 1.0 cm H_2O. Increasing the PIP will also increase the mean airway pressure but not in a 1:1 relationship. Increasing the inspiratory time will raise the mean pressure by increasing the duration of positive pressure. Increasing the ventilator rate may also have a small impact on increasing the mean airway pressures by decreasing time spent in expiration. Mean airway pressure during HFOV is set directly and represents a static inflation value.

Because the mean airway pressure is represented by the area under the curve of the pressure waveform for the entire respiratory cycle, maneuvers that increase the area under the curve increase the mean. These effects are represented in Figure 10-2.

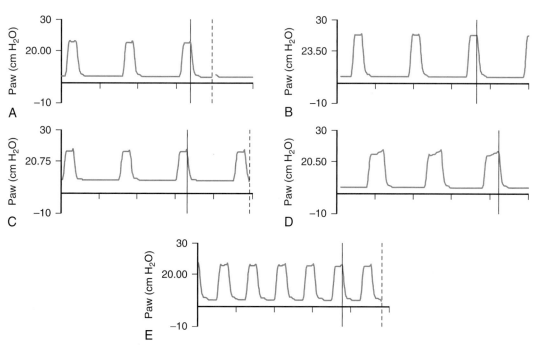

Figure 10-2 Changes that affect mean airway pressure, shown here as the area under the pressure waveform. **A,** Initial settings, peak pressure 20 cm H_2O, end-expiratory pressure 3 cm H_2O, inspiratory time 0.25 second. **B,** Peak pressure increased to 24 cm H_2O. **C,** End-expiratory pressure increased to 6 cm H_2O. **D,** Inspiratory time increased to 0.4 second. **E,** Rate increased.

Ventilation

Case Study 3

You are on day 1 of your NICU rotation and are assigned to care for a baby requiring mechanical ventilation. The first thing that you ask your senior resident is how to adjust the ventilator if the baby exhibits abnormal gas exchange. Almost on cue, a nurse approaches you to show you the results of a blood gas analysis and you observe that the carbon dioxide tension is 75 torr.

Exercise 3

QUESTION

1. After your full assessment of the baby, including a physical examination, reviewing the chest radiograph, and observing the ventilator graphics, what setting could you adjust to lower the carbon dioxide level?

   a. Increase the PEEP

   b. Increase the inspiratory time

   c. Increase the ventilator rate

   d. Increase the PIP

   e. Increase the tidal volume

ANSWER

1. c, d, e. Increasing the ventilator rate, PIP, and tidal volume should all result in improved ventilation. Again, making proper ventilator changes requires a review of all aspects of respiratory management. Sometimes, it is appropriate to make no changes at all in the ventilator settings but to suction the endotracheal tube or reposition the infant. Always make sure that when the carbon dioxide level is elevated the problem is not related to a mechanical problem, such as plugging of the endotracheal tube with mucus, inadvertent extubation, kinking of the endotracheal tube, crying or agitation, stacking, or air leak.

Ventilation refers to the removal of carbon dioxide. Carbon dioxide removal during CMV can be calculated as the product of the frequency and the delivered volume of gas ($f \times V_T$). Thus, maneuvers that increase either the ventilator rate or the tidal volume will increase CO_2 removal. V_T is reflected by the difference between the PIP and PEEP, referred to as amplitude, or ΔP. Amplitude may be increased by raising the PIP, lowering the PEEP, or doing both. During HFV, CO_2 removal is proportional to $f \times (V_T)^2$ and small changes in amplitude can have a profound effect on ventilation. With HFOV, amplitude is adjusted directly, whereas it is controlled the same way during HFJV as it is during CMV by adjusting to the difference between PIP and PEEP.

Ventilation is also affected by the expiratory time (Te), because the lung needs sufficient time to empty after being filled. This is determined by the respiratory time constant, the product of resistance and compliance. Generally, a length of time equal to three time constants is necessary to achieve 95% emptying.[6] Failure to appreciate this may result in gas trapping and inadvertent PEEP, increasing the risk of pulmonary air leaks. Gas trapping occurs when inspiratory flow begins before expiratory flow has been completed (Fig. 10–3).

Modes of Ventilation

Modes describe the way in which mechanical ventilators deliver positive pressure. There are four major modes of ventilation used in newborns: IMV, SIMV, A/CV, and PSV.[7]

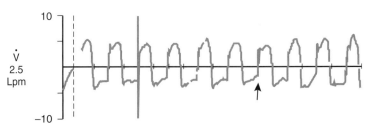

Figure 10-3 Flow waveform demonstrating gas trapping. Note that the expiratory portion of the waveform (the area below the baseline) never returns to the baseline before the subsequent breath begins (*arrow*). Lpm, liters per minute.

IMV has been used for more than three decades to treat newborns with respiratory failure. The most common application is time-cycled, pressure-limited IMV, in which the clinician chooses a pressure limit, cycle time, and ventilator rate, and regular mechanical breaths are delivered to the baby. In between these breaths, the baby may breathe spontaneously from the fresh gas flowing continuously through the ventilator circuit, but these breaths are supported only by PEEP and may be ineffective if pulmonary compliance or patient effort is low. Moreover, the baby's spontaneous effort may be asynchronous with the mechanical breaths, and the delivered tidal volumes may fluctuate widely. When the infant is inhaling while the ventilator is in the inspiratory phase, tidal volumes will be larger than if the infant is trying to exhale against incoming positive pressure. Asynchronous ventilation can result in inefficient gas exchange, increased work of breathing, and a higher need for sedatives,[8] and has been associated with an increased risk of intraventricular hemorrhage.[9] Achieving synchrony during IMV can be challenging and may require the use of sedatives, higher ventilator rates or pressures (to "capture" the infant), or even the use of skeletal muscle relaxants in refractory cases.

SIMV attempts to synchronize the onset of the mandatory breaths with the onset of spontaneous breaths, and is thus a form of patient-triggered ventilation (PTV). Again, the clinician chooses the mandatory breath rate and the baby is free to breathe spontaneously. However, when the ventilator is ready to cycle, it will wait for a few milliseconds before and after its "scheduled" onset of inspiration, waiting for patient effort. If this occurs, the ventilator will cycle in response to the patient "trigger," and inspiratory synchrony is achieved. The trigger signal is a measure of spontaneous effort, most commonly a change in airway pressure or flow, although changes in abdominal or thoracic impedance have also been used.[10] As in IMV, spontaneous breaths that do not trigger mechanical breaths are supported only by PEEP.

A/C ventilation was introduced into widespread neonatal use in the mid-1990s. In this mode of ventilation, every spontaneous breath that exceeds the trigger threshold results in the delivery of a mechanical breath synchronized to the onset of respiration.[8] The baby thus controls the rate of ventilator cycling, provided that spontaneous breathing exceeds the control rate. In this mode there is a mandatory minimum set rate. Synchrony can be enhanced even further if flow cycling is used rather than time cycling. With flow cycling, a change in airway flow is used not only to trigger inspiration, but to trigger expiration as well. It does this by arbitrarily terminating inspiration when inspiratory flow has declined to a small fraction—but not zero—of peak inspiratory flow. This is indicative of the patient's nearing the end of his/her own inspiratory phase.[11] It is also a safeguard against inversion of the inspiratory/expiratory ratio if the infant becomes tachypneic, because inspiration will end at a percentage of peak flow, rather than after a preset time. In the latter case, the faster the infant breathes, the shorter the expiratory time. Additionally, flow cycling affords the infant the chance to set the cycle time and rate.

PSV may be used to overcome the shortcomings of unsupported spontaneous breathing during SIMV.[12] It is a "spontaneous" mode applied to spontaneous breaths to provide an inspiratory pressure "boost" to overcome the increased work of breathing created by both the underlying disease process and the imposed work of breathing created by the narrow lumen endotracheal tube, ventilator circuit, and demand valve of the ventilator. PSV is pressure- and time-limited and flow-cycled. It can be adjusted to provide a fully supported (e.g., full tidal volume) breath, referred to as PS_{max}, or a partially supported breath during weaning. PS_{min} represents the minimal amount of pressure needed to overcome the imposed work of breathing, estimated to be about 4 mL/kg in term infants. If PSV is used, it is reasonable to use a low SIMV rate. If PSV is successful, the synchrony developed between baby and ventilator will not be interrupted by the mandatory breaths.

Case Study 4

A 2.5-kg 34-week infant with RDS is being weaned from ventilator support after receiving surfactant. He is on a time-cycled assist-control mode. The carbon dioxide tension is 38 torr, the tidal volume is 7 mL/kg, PIP is 18, PEEP is 5, inspiratory time is 0.3 second, and the rate is 20.

Exercise 4

QUESTION

1. What would be the next step to wean this infant from support?

   a. Decrease the rate

   b. Decrease the PIP

   c. Decrease the PEEP

   d. Decrease the inspiratory time

ANSWER

1. b. The best choice would be to decrease the peak inspiratory pressure. Because the baby is being managed in the assist control mode, weaning the ventilator rate will not affect ventilation as long as the baby is breathing above the control rate. Decreasing the PEEP will increase the ΔP and increase ventilation. Decreasing the inspiratory time will allow more time for exhalation and result in increased ventilation.

Pressure-Targeted Ventilation

In pressure-targeted ventilation, the inspiratory pressure is set by the clinician, usually by adjusting a pressure limit. The mechanical breaths will not exceed this limit. However, the delivered tidal volume will depend on the patient's compliance and to a lesser extent on resistance. At the same pressure, more tidal volume will be delivered at a higher compliance than at a lower one. This has important clinical implications. For instance, compliance generally improves after exogenous surfactant treatment. If the inspiratory pressure is not decreased, tidal volume delivery will increase, and thus the probability of lung injury will increase.

Three major ventilatory modalities utilize pressure targeted ventilation: time- or flow-cycled, pressure-limited ventilation; pressure control ventilation; and pressure support ventilation.

Time- or flow-cycled, pressure-limited ventilation has been described previously. Its major advantage is its ease of use. Delivered breaths are all at the same pressure. Pressure-limited ventilation may be used in IMV, SIMV, and A/C ventilation modes.

Pressure control (PC) ventilation is a newer pressure-targeted modality.[5] In PC ventilation,

the inspiratory time is usually fixed; that is, it is time-cycled. Inspiratory flow is rapid and is variable, depending upon the patient's inspiratory effort. The harder the baby "pulls," the greater is the flow rate. PC also has a rapidly rising pressure waveform. Its theoretical advantage is that this quickly pressurizes the ventilator circuit and delivers gas flow to the baby, enhancing diffusion and alveolar inflation. Most ventilators offering PC also have an adjustable rise time, which affects the slope of the inspiratory pressure waveform. If the rise time, a qualitative parameter, is set too low, there will be inadequate hysteresis on the pressure-volume loop. If it is set too high, pressure overshoot may occur, as demonstrated in Figure 10-1. Pressure control may benefit babies who have high airway resistance because of the more rapid flow rate during inspiration. It can also be delivered as IMV, SIMV, or A/C ventilation.

Pressure support was described earlier. It, too, is pressure-targeted, and is time-limited and flow-cycled. Tidal volume delivery depends upon patient compliance.

Table 10-2 lists the differences and the similarities among these three modalities.

Volume-Targeted Ventilation

In contrast to pressure-targeted ventilation, volume-targeted ventilation enables the clinician to choose a desired volume of gas to be delivered and allows the pressure required to deliver this volume to vary. For safety reasons, pressure may be limited. Because cuffed endotracheal tubes are not used in newborns, the term "volume-cycled" should not be applied to this form of ventilation, since there is almost always a degree of gas leak around the endotracheal tube. It is preferable to think of this as "volume-targeted," "volume-limited," or "volume-controlled" ventilation. A

TABLE 10-2

A COMPARISON OF PRESSURE-TARGETED MODALITIES

Parameter	Pressure-Limited	Pressure Control	Pressure Support
Flow	Fixed	Variable	Variable
Cycle	Time or flow	Time or flow	Flow
Limit	Pressure	Pressure	Pressure

unique feature of volume-targeted ventilation is its auto-weaning capability. As compliance improves, the pressure required to deliver an equivalent volume of gas decreases, and the ventilator automatically responds by weaning the pressure. Conversely, a decrease in compliance results in an automatic increase in pressure to deliver the desired tidal volume.

Clinicians using volume-targeted ventilation should choose a device that measures the tidal volume at the proximal airway.[13] When the lungs are stiff, there may be considerable compression of gas volume within the ventilator circuit, and it is critical to know exactly how much volume is being delivered to the patient. In addition, clinicians need to be aware of the minimal tidal volume the machine is capable of delivering to avoid overinflation (Fig. 10-4) in extremely low–birth-weight babies.

During volume-targeted ventilation, inspiratory time is a function of the flow rate. The faster the flow rate, the shorter the inspiratory time. This needs to be checked each time there is a change in ventilator parameters. Volume-targeted ventilation also differs from pressure-targeted ventilation by delivering flow in a "square waveform" and pressure in a "shark's fin waveform," resulting in a slower ramping of pressure and the delivery of maximal volume at the end of inspiration (Fig. 10-5). Newer devices allow the optional use of a decelerating flow waveform.

Volume-targeted ventilation may be applied in IMV, SIMV, and A/C ventilation, and may be combined in SIMV with PSV. Recent advances have enabled hybrid forms of ventilation, such as Pressure Regulated Volume Control and Volume Guarantee, in which a targeted volume is delivered after sequential breath averaging, and Volume Assured Pressure Support, in which

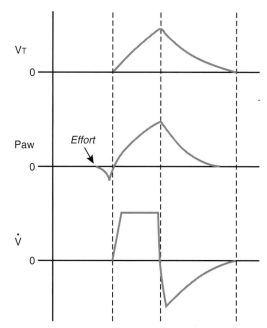

Figure 10-5 Characteristics of volume-targeted ventilation. On the top is the volume waveform. Note that peak volume delivery occurs at the end of inspiration. In the middle is the "shark's fin" pressure waveform. On the bottom is the "square" flow waveform, which differs from the more sinusoidal pattern in pressure-targeted ventilation.

a targeted volume is delivered within a single breath by transitioning a pressure-targeted breath to a volume-targeted breath by extending flow in inspiration, and increasing pressure, if necessary.

High-Frequency Ventilation

Case Study 5

An 820-g 25-week gestation infant with RDS is currently being supported with high-frequency

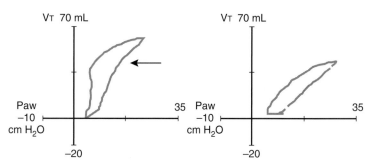

Figure 10-4 Pressure-volume loops. On the left, there is hyperinflation. Note the change in slope at the upper end of the inflation limb (*arrow*). On the right is a normal loop.

oscillatory ventilation with a mean Paw of 8, amplitude of 10, and frequency of 12 Hz. The carbon dioxide tension is 75 torr on a recent blood gas analysis.

Exercise 5

QUESTION

1. Which of the following would improve ventilation and lower the carbon dioxide level?

   a. Increase the amplitude

   b. Increase the rate

   c. Decrease the rate

ANSWER

1. a, c. Increasing the amplitude or decreasing the rate will probably result in improved ventilation, although adjusting the amplitude is usually the preferred choice. Although it may be counterintuitive, increasing the frequency may further attenuate gas flow and therefore decrease patient ventilation (see the following discussion).

High-frequency ventilation delivers extremely small tidal volumes (less than anatomic dead space) at extremely rapid rates.[14] The two major forms of HFV are HFJV[15] and HFOV.[16] HFJV uses a pulsatile, high-velocity flow to deliver gas, but it involves passive exhalation. HFOV uses a piston-driven diaphragm, which delivers gas to the airway and also actively withdraws it (active exhalation). Tidal volumes are larger during HFJV, and ventilator rates are faster during HFOV, typically 8 to 15 Hz. HFJV has been shown to be superior to conventional ventilation in the management of air leaks,[17] but HFOV may result in chronic lung disease less often than conventional SIMV.[18]

The principles of management are similar to CMV; mean airway pressure determines oxygenation, amplitude determines ventilation. HFJV is applied in tandem with a conventional ventilator to provide PEEP and sigh breaths, whereas HFOV (in the United States) is used alone. During HFV most clinicians choose to keep the ventilator frequency constant and adjust other parameters to affect carbon dioxide removal. Weaning from HFV tends to be a personal preference. Some clinicians will extubate a baby

directly from HFV, and others prefer to transition to CMV first.

QUESTION

2. How should initial oscillator settings for this infant be selected and why?

   a. Arbitrarily choose some settings and wait for a blood gas analysis

   b. Place the baby on the oscillator and adjust the settings until there is good "chest wiggle" (up and down motion of the chest) and oxygen saturations are within the target range

ANSWER

2. b. There are some strategies to be considered when choosing the initial ventilator settings. It may depend upon one's familiarity with the device and whether it is used as a rescue therapy or a primary mode of ventilation. Of course, it will also depend upon the disease state. If a baby is given surfactant in the delivery room and then placed on the oscillator, the settings will likely be initially lower than in the baby who is initially placed on the oscillator and then given surfactant. It is crucial, however, that once the baby is placed on the oscillator, the clinician does not leave the bedside, particularly if the baby has recently received surfactant. There can be a rapid improvement in compliance over only a few minutes. Utilization of noninvasive monitoring methods, such as pulse oximetry and transcutaneous carbon dioxide monitoring, are useful to make frequent necessary adjustments. The physical examination is also important in assessing the settings on the oscillator. Assessment of "chest wiggle" takes experience but allows for some fine tuning of the settings. Many clinicians will obtain a chest radiograph 30 to 60 minutes after initially placing the baby on the oscillator to assess lung expansion. It may be useful to obtain a follow-up film 2 to 3 hours later to reassess expansion. Many clinicians will obtain a chest radiograph every 6 to 8 hours while a baby is on the oscillator to further monitor lung expansion. Proper use of the oscillator depends on integrating the findings of the physical examination, chest radiograph, and blood gas analysis.

Matching Strategy with Pathophysiology

Although considerable controversy still exists over the "best" ventilator mode or modality, the major changes brought about by the new technology enable the clinician to "customize" management for the individual patient and to develop strategies that match specific pathophysiologic states. This is an important element in maximizing outcomes and minimizing complications. The following brief review of the major respiratory disorders afflicting the newborn will illustrate this.

Respiratory Distress Syndrome. RDS is the primary respiratory disorder of the preterm infant.[19] Its pathophysiology is related to both anatomic and biochemical abnormalities of the immature lung. The more premature the baby, the greater these problems are. Anatomic problems result from decreased alveolarization, underdeveloped airways, and in extreme cases, an increased distance from the terminal breathing unit to the adjacent capillary. The biochemical abnormality is the absence or reduction of pulmonary surfactant, leading to an increase in alveolar surface tension and a tendency toward progressive atelectasis. RDS has been referred to as a low lung volume disease.

Although the advent of exogenous surfactant therapy has radically altered the disease process, infants with severe disease are generally treated with mechanical ventilation.[20] The infant with RDS, at least prior to surfactant administration, has diminished pulmonary compliance and increased resistance. Ventilatory strategies should be designed to achieve normal inflation and lung volumes and to overcome the tendency of alveoli to collapse. Use of sufficient PEEP to overcome the need for high opening pressure, and adequate PIP to ensure reasonable tidal volumes (4 to 6 mL/kg in infants < 1500 g and 5 to 7 mL/kg in infants > 1500 g) is suggested. Careful attention must be paid to rapid changes in compliance after surfactant administration. These changes may be manifested by increases in chest excursions, higher delivered tidal volumes, hyperinflation on radiography, or hypocapnia on blood gas analysis.

The incidence of pulmonary air leaks (pneumothorax and pulmonary interstitial emphysema) has been markedly reduced in the exogenous surfactant era, but they still occur, more so with extreme prematurity. Therefore, avoidance of gas trapping, inadvertent PEEP, and prolonged inspiratory times are all warranted in this population. Treatment of air leaks may be facilitated by HFV, especially for pulmonary interstitial emphysema.

Meconium Aspiration Syndrome. Intrauterine passage of meconium occurs in about 30% of term infants and in up to 40% of post-term infants. It may be aspirated prior to birth or during/after delivery and can lead to significant pulmonary disease.[21] Meconium contains bile salts, which inactivate surfactant. It can also cause airway obstruction, leading to gas trapping, hyperinflation, and air leaks. It may progress to chemical pneumonitis, with resultant ventilation/perfusion mismatch, and ultimately persistent pulmonary hypertension of the newborn (see later discussion). It may even interfere with gas diffusion at the alveolar level. Because of the tendency for gas trapping and hyperinflation, meconium aspiration syndrome (MAS) should be thought of as a high lung volume disease.

Ventilatory management is directed at maintaining reasonable gas exchange without contributing to the risks of hyperinflation, gas trapping, and air leaks. This involves the use of shorter inspiratory times, slower ventilator rates, and lower flow rates. Monitoring pulmonary waveforms for evidence of gas trapping, and observing pulmonary mechanics for evidence of hyperinflation are strongly recommended. Even greater care is necessary if the disease is patchy and nonhomogeneous.

Persistent Pulmonary Hypertension of the Newborn. PPHN is generally a disorder of the term infant. It is a condition characterized by maintenance of elevated pulmonary vascular resistance, leading to right-to-left shunting of blood, profound hypoxemia, and metabolic acidosis. PPHN may occur as a primary process, believed to result from excessive muscularization of the pulmonary arterioles, or it may be secondary to a number of processes that affect either lung parenchyma (such as pneumonia or asphyxia), pulmonary vasculature (such as chronic hypoxia), or both (such as congenital diaphragmatic hernia or pulmonary hypoplasia).[22]

The pathophysiology of the disorder centers around abnormally elevated pulmonary vascular resistance (PVR) and suprasystemic pulmonary arterial pressure. This causes shunting of blood away from the lung, creating a venous admixture, ultimately resulting in profound hypoxemia. This may lead to acidosis, further constricting pulmonary vessels and impairing myocardial contractility, systemic blood pressure, and pulmonary blood flow. Thus, a vicious circle is established.

For several decades, the management of PPHN was highly controversial. Two strategies evolved. The first, deliberate hyperventilation, sought to take advantage of the pulmonary vasodilating effects of hyperoxia, hypocapnia, and extreme alkalosis.[23] The second, referred to as "conservative ventilation," sought to minimize the contributory effects of high intrathoracic pressure to increased PVR, and it promoted the acceptance of marginal gas exchange until remodeling of the pulmonary vasculature had been accomplished.[24] Unfortunately, no direct randomized controlled trials were ever performed, and ventilator management tended to be based on personal preferences.

The introduction of inhaled nitric oxide (iNO), a selective pulmonary vasodilator, has significantly altered the approach to PPHN. iNO has been shown to be effective in reversing the hypoxemic respiratory failure associated with PPHN. It is administered directly into the inspiratory limb of the ventilator circuit and delivered to the alveolus, where it diffuses into the capillaries and results in vascular relaxation. iNO has also been shown to work best when the lungs are optimally inflated, often using HFOV.[25,26]

Whatever strategy is adopted, care must be taken to avoid situations that contribute to increased PVR, including high peak and mean airway pressures, overdistention of the lung, and inadvertent PEEP, especially if rapid ventilator rates are used and there is inadequate time for lung emptying. In addition, weaning needs to be accomplished very slowly; small changes in F_{IO_2} or Pa_{CO_2} can have profound effects on Pa_{O_2}. In addition, clinicians need to recognize "transition disease," usually around the fourth postnatal day, when pulmonary vasoreactivity begins to diminish, and the effects of hyperoxia, hyperventilation, and alkalosis are less apparent.

Case Study 6

A 4-day-old near-term infant with meconium aspiration syndrome complicated by PPHN has an echocardiogram that shows worsening pulmonary hypertension. The baby is receiving iNO (20 ppm), *100% oxygen, and HFOV. Oxygen saturation and Pa_{O_2} values have actually improved over the last 12 hours.*

Exercise 6

QUESTION

1. What is a likely cause for the interpretation of worsening PPHN by echocardiogram?
   a. The PPHN is getting worse.
   b. There is overdistention of the lungs on HFOV.
   c. The baby is developing sepsis.

ANSWER

1. b. Although the baby could be developing sepsis or the PPHN could be getting worse, the clinical course is inconsistent with those interpretations. Oxygenation has actually seemed to improve by the noninvasive measures. The use of echocardiogram to assess pulmonary hypertension must be done with caution. Echocardiograms can identify whether there is evidence of increased pulmonary vascular resistance, but it is up to the clinician to find the cause. Hyperinflation of the lungs from excessive HFOV can increase pulmonary vascular resistance, worsen oxygenation, and decrease cardiac output (as noted in this case).

Chronic Lung Disease or Bronchopulmonary Dysplasia. Chronic lung disease (CLD), or bronchopulmonary dysplasia (BPD), is a disorder affecting newborns that have undergone mechanical ventilation. Clinical BPD was originally attributed to the combined effects of exposure to high concentrations of oxygen and positive pressure ventilation over time.[27] Affected infants displayed the histopathologic changes of inflammation, fibrosis, and vascular smooth muscle hypertrophy, with radiographic findings of alternating areas of hyperinflation and atelectasis, producing the "honeycomb" lung appearance.[28] Infants with CLD—so-called "new BPD"—are likely to be much more premature and not exposed to as severe a degree of mechanical ventilation. Radiographs show a hazy to granular pattern with diminished lung volumes, and histopathologic examination of the lungs shows much less inflammation and fibrosis.[29]

BPD is thought to result from a combination of factors. Infants with BPD are delivered before adequate alveolarization of the lung has occurred, and this process is further interrupted by an entity referred to as ventilator-induced lung injury (VILI). VILI is multifactorial, and is related to barotrauma (excessive pressure), volutrauma (excessive volume), atelectotrauma (damage resulting from the continuous opening and closing of lung units), biotrauma (injury resulting from infection and inflammation),[30] and rheotrauma (abnormal airway gas flow; excessive flow causes turbulence, gas trapping, and inadvertent PEEP, and inadequate flow causes air hunger and increased work of breathing).[2]

CLD has been defined in many different ways, most centering around a prolonged oxygen dependency. Infants who require mechanical ventilation are often difficult to manage. First, it must be recognized that CLD affects not only lung parenchyma but also the airways. Thus, airway resistance may be significantly elevated. If so, a modality offering variable inspiratory flow, such as pressure control or pressure support, may be beneficial.[31] Second, the expectation for the degree of gas exchange needs to be revised from that during RDS. Tolerance of a higher $Paco_2$ (and perhaps a slightly lower Pao_2) and careful attention to other complications such as pulmonary edema and cor pulmonale may help guide ventilator management. The clinician must remember that the lungs of these babies are still undergoing alveolarization and the damaging effects of mechanical ventilation must be minimized.

Weaning and Extubation

Weaning is the process by which the work of breathing is transferred from the mechanical ventilator to the patient. Before being ready for extubation, a baby must demonstrate reliable respiratory drive, adequate pulmonary gas exchange, and minimal distress.[32]

It is probably best to start weaning by decreasing the parameter that is potentially the most injurious to the patient. For a premature infant receiving a high concentration of inspired oxygen, decreasing the oxygen may be the primary objective. For a term infant with meconium aspiration syndrome requiring high oxygen concentrations and high pressures,

decreasing the pressure first may be important to prevent gas trapping, decrease intrathoracic pressure and pulmonary vascular resistance, and avoid chronic lung injury.

Weaning tends to be a style more than a science. Infants receiving IMV or SIMV are traditionally weaned by reduction in the ventilator rate, while keeping PIP constant or lowering it slowly. Some clinicians prefer to add PSV to the spontaneous breaths to overcome the imposed work of breathing, followed by a further reduction in the mandatory rate. In assist-control ventilation, the PIP is weaned first; weaning the control rate will have no effect as long as the baby is breathing above the control rate. In volume-targeted ventilation, weaning is more straightforward, depending upon the mode, as the ventilator will automatically reduce the pressure.

Babies should be considered ready for extubation when they have been weaned to low ventilator support, exhibit good respiratory drive, and can maintain oxygenation and minute ventilation. The latter may be utilized as an objective measure for readiness for extubation.[33,34]

Postextubation management is still controversial. Some centers use methylxanthine therapy in the periextubation period to stimulate breathing, improve diaphragmatic contractility, and perhaps maintain airway patency. Others prefer to use some form of distending pressure after extubation, such as nasal CPAP or high-flow nasal cannulas to maintain upper airway patency and overcome airway resistance.

Conclusion

Respiratory failure in the newborn may result from numerous causes. Present-day mechanical ventilation offers the clinician a variety of options to approach this problem. Decisions as to which type, mode, and modality of ventilation to choose should be based on an understanding of not only how the ventilator functions, but also on the underlying lung disease and how the individual baby responds to the settings chosen. Careful assessment of the baby through physical examination, laboratory results, and real-time monitoring will dictate the adjustments necessary to achieve adequate gas exchange and to minimize lung injury.

References

1. Greenough A, Milner AD: Mechanisms of respiratory failure. In Sinha SK, Donn SM (eds): Manual of Neonatal Respiratory Care. Armonk, NY, Future Publishing, 2000, pp 94–96.
2. Donn SM, Sinha SK: Advances in neonatal ventilation. In Kurjak A, Chervenak F (eds): Textbook of Perinatal Medicine, 2nd ed. London, Parthenon Publishing Group (in press).
3. Hagus CK, Donn SM: Pulmonary graphics: Basics of clinical application. In Donn SM (ed): Neonatal and Pediatric Pulmonary Graphics: Principles and Clinical Applications. Armonk, NY, Future Publishing, 1998, pp 81–28.
4. Sinha SK, Donn, SM, Gavey J, McCarty M: Randomised trial of volume controlled versus time cycled, pressure limited ventilation in preterm infants with respiratory distress syndrome. Arch Dis Child 1997; 77:F202–F205.
5. Donn SM, Becker MA: Understanding pressure control ventilation. Neonatal Intensive Care 2003; 16:39–43.
6. Carlo WA, Ambalavanan N, Chatburn RL: Basic principles of mechanical ventilation. In Sinha SK, Donn SM (eds): Manual of Neonatal Respiratory Care. Armonk, NY, Future Publishing, 2000, pp 108–121.
7. Donn SM, Sinha SK: Newer techniques of mechanical ventilation: An overview. Semin Neonatol 2002; 7:401–407.
8. Donn SM, Nicks JJ, Becker MA: Flow-synchronized ventilation of preterm infants with respiratory distress syndrome. J Perinatol 1994;14:90–94.
9. Perlman JM, McMenamin JP, Volpe JJ: Fluctuating cerebral blood flow velocity in respiratory distress syndrome: Relationship to subsequent development of intraventricular hemorrhage. N Engl J Med 1983;309:204–209.
10. Donn SM, Sinha SK: Controversies in patient-triggered ventilation. Clin Perinatol 1998;25:49–61.
11. Donn SM, Sinha SK: Newer modes of mechanical ventilation for the neonate. Curr Opin Pediatr 2001;13:99–103.
12. Donn SM, Sinha SK: Invasive and noninvasive neonatal mechanical ventilation. Respir Care 2003;48:1–16.
13. Cannon ML, Cornell J, Tripp-Hamel DS, et al: Tidal volumes for ventilated infants should be determined with a pneumotachometer placed at the endotracheal tube. Am J Respir Care 2000;162:2109–2112.
14. Bunnell JB: General concepts of high-frequency ventilation. In Sinha SK, Donn SM (eds): Manual of Neonatal Respiratory Care. Armonk, NY, Futura Publishing, 2000, pp 226–234.
15. Keszler M: High-frequency jet ventilation and the Bunnell Life Pulse High-Frequency Jet Ventilator. In Sinha SK, Donn SM (eds): Manual of Neonatal Respiratory Care. Armonk, NY, Futura Publishing, 2000, pp 235–241.
16. Clark RH, Gerstmann DR: High-frequency oscillatory ventilation. In Sinha SK, Donn SM (eds): Manual of Neonatal Respiratory Care. Armonk, NY, Futura Publishing, 2000, pp 242–252.
17. Keszler M, Donn SM, Bucciarelli RL, et al: Multicenter controlled trial comparing high-frequency jet ventilation and conventional mechanical ventilation in newborn infants with pulmonary interstitial emphysema. J Pediatr 1991;119:85–93.
18. Courtney SC, Durand DJ, Asselin JM, et al: High-frequency oscillatory ventilation versus conventional mechanical ventilation for very-low-birthweight infants. N Engl J Med 2002;347:643–652.
19. Donn SM, Sinha SK: Respiratory distress syndrome. In Sinha SK, Donn SM (eds): Manual of Neonatal Respiratory Care. Armonk, NY, Futura Publishing, 2000, pp 260–265.
20. Lacaze-Masmonteil T: Exogenous surfactant therapy: Newer developments. Semin Neonatol 2003;8: 433–440.
21. Wiswell TE: Meconium aspiration syndrome. In Sinha SK, Donn SM (eds): Manual of Neonatal Respiratory Care. Armonk, NY, Futura Publishing, 2000, pp 266–272.
22. Walsh MC, Stork EK: Persistent pulmonary hypertension of the newborn: Rational therapy based on pathophysiology. Clin Perinatol 2001;28:609–627.
23. Peckham GS, Fox WW: Physiological factors affecting pulmonary artery pressures in infants with persistent pulmonary hypertension. J Pediatr 1978;93: 1005–1110.
24. Wung JT, James LS, Kilchevsky E, et al: Management of infants with severe respiratory failure and persistence of the fetal circulation without hyperventilation. Pediatrics 1985;76:488–493.
25. Roberts JD, Fineman JR, Morin FC 3, et al: Inhaled nitric oxide and persistent pulmonary hypertension of the newborn. N Engl J Med 1997;336:605–610.
26. Kinsella JP, Neish SR, Abman SH: Low-dose inhalational nitric oxide in persistent pulmonary hypertension of the newborn. Lancet 1992;340: 819–820.
27. Philip AGS: Oxygen plus pressure plus time: The etiology of bronchopulmonary dysplasia. Pediatrics 1975;55:44–48.
28. Northway WH Jr, Rosan RC, Porter DY: Pulmonary disease following respiratory therapy for hyaline membrane disease—Bronchopulmonary dysplasia. N Engl J Med 1967;276:357–368.
29. Coalson JJ: Pathology of the new bronchopulmonary dysplasia. Semin Neonatol 2003;8:73–82.
30. Attar MA, Donn SM: Mechanisms of ventilator-induced lung injury in premature infants. Semin Neonatol 2002;7:353–360.
31. Nicks JJ, Becker MA, Donn SM: Bronchopulmonary dysplasia: Response to pressure support ventilation. J Perinatol 1994;14:495–497.
32. Sinha SK, Donn SM: Weaning newborns from mechanical ventilation. Semin Neonatol 2002;7: 421–28.
33. Wilson BJJr, Becker MA, Linton ME, Donn SM: Spontaneous minute ventilation predicts readiness for extubation in mechanically ventilated preterm infants. J Perinatol 1998;18:436–439.
34. Gillespie LM, White SD, Sinha SK, Donn SM: Usefulness of the minute ventilation test in predicting successful extubation in newborn infants: A randomized controlled trial. J Perinatol 2003;23: 205–207.

Bronchopulmonary Dysplasia

Jeffrey S. Gerdes, MD

Bronchopulmonary dysplasia (BPD) is a chronic lung disorder that follows acute pulmonary diseases such as respiratory distress syndrome (RDS) and primarily affects preterm infants. BPD was originally defined by Northway and associates as the presence of respiratory symptoms, an abnormal chest radiograph, and the need for supplemental oxygen at 28 days of age.[1,2] Because most extremely low birth weight (ELBW) infants (<1000 g) have very immature lungs and have a residual oxygen requirement at 28 days of age, significant BPD has been redefined as chronic lung disease requiring supplemental oxygen at 36 weeks' postmenstrual age. The pathologic findings in this disorder are a chronic inflammatory and reparative cellular and fibrotic response to unresolved acute lung injury. The classical clinical and pathologic findings have evolved over time to a form of "new BPD" occurring in ELBW infants in whom acute lung injury is minimized by antenatal steroids and surfactant treatment. New BPD is characterized histopathologically by disrupted alveolar and vascular development, and less inflammation and fibrosis than seen in classical BPD.[3]

BPD can be identified clinically by chronic respiratory distress, retention of carbon dioxide (hypercapnia), a diminished blood oxygen concentration (hypoxemia), and an abnormal chest radiograph.[4] BPD is a unique phenomenon in pulmonary medicine in that it is a disease in which lung injury and repair are superimposed on a system of ongoing organ growth and development.

BPD is recognized in approximately 30% of preterm babies with birth weights less than 1000 g. Although many cases are relatively mild and have minimal sequelae, some babies exhibit severe chronic lung disease requiring oxygen or respiratory support for months or years. The cause of BPD is multifactorial and includes inherent factors such as lung underdevelopment secondary to prematurity as well as factors ensuing from therapies provided to preterm neonates, such as oxygen administration and mechanical ventilation. The methods of prevention and treatment are as varied as the many possible causes, providing one of the greatest challenges in modern neonatal-perinatal medicine.

Predisposing Factors and Etiologic Mechanisms

Prematurity is one of the major factors predisposing to the development of BPD. Smaller, more premature infants are more likely to develop the disease than are infants born at or near term gestation. However, as noted earlier, BPD is a multifactorial disease (Table 11-1). This chapter presents the case study of baby boy Sam from birth through 6 months of age. You will be asked to analyze a variety of problems related to this infant's condition.

Case Study

Baby boy Sam was born after 25 weeks of gestation, weighing 730 g. His mother had

TABLE 11-1

FACTORS PREDISPOSING TO THE DEVELOPMENT OF BRONCHOPULMONARY DYSPLASIA

Anatomic lung immaturity
Biochemical lung immaturity
Genetic predisposition
Fluid overload
Patent ductus arteriosus
Pneumothorax
Pulmonary interstitial emphysema
Barotrauma from mechanical ventilation
Oxygen toxicity and antioxidant insufficiency
Early development of increased airway resistance
Malnutrition
Lung inflammation and disordered fibrosis
Prenatal exposure to chorioamnionitis or cytokines
Relative adrenal insufficiency

premature cervical dilatation, premature labor, and asthma; she was treated with magnesium sulfate for preterm labor and was given two doses of betamethasone 3 days before delivery to promote lung maturation. Twenty hours before the birth, the membranes ruptured and signs of chorioamnionitis developed. Labor was augmented with oxytocin and progressed to a spontaneous vaginal delivery. Sam had Apgar scores of 5 at 1 minute and 8 at 5 minutes. He was intubated immediately after birth and placed on a pressure-limited ventilator with an inspiratory pressure (IP) of 18 cm H_2O, a positive end-expiratory pressure (PEEP) of 5 cm H_2O, a synchronized intermittent mandatory ventilation (SIMV) rate of 40, and an inspired oxygen concentration (F_{IO_2}) of 0.50. He was treated prophylactically with surfactant and transported on the ventilator to the intensive care nursery (ICN).

Exercise 1

QUESTION

1. What four features of this case history indicate that baby Sam is predisposed to developing BPD?

ANSWER

1. Anatomic immaturity of the lungs, surfactant deficiency, family history of reactive airway disease, and chorioamnionitis.

Anatomic immaturity of the lung structures is a major risk factor for the development of BPD. At 25 weeks' gestation, the lungs are still in the canalicular phase of development and are just beginning the saccular phase, when respiratory saccules appear from the transitional ducts. Interruption of lung development may occur secondary to preterm birth and air breathing when the lung is meant to be fluid filled, and it is certainly disrupted by mechanical ventilation and oxygen therapy. In addition, the immature lung is characterized by an altered collagen composition and decreased elastin concentration compared with the mature lung, resulting in diminished elasticity, which reduces pulmonary compliance on an anatomic basis. Fortunately, the preterm lung has a remarkable potential for remodeling and growth and undergoes an increase in surface area from 0.5 m^2 at 24 weeks' gestation to 4.5 m^2 at term (Fig. 11-1). This growth potential makes recovery from BPD possible.

Surfactant deficiency is an important cause of RDS and contributes to lung injury on a primary basis. Neonates who have RDS are more likely to develop BPD than are those who do not, although it is important to recognize that BPD can develop in preterm neonates who never received oxygen or ventilator treatment. Although surfactant replacement therapy reduces the severity of RDS, the incidence of air leak, and the risk of death, it has not been shown to substantially decrease the incidence of BPD in very tiny premature infants. Further, exposure to antenatal corticosteroids, while reducing the incidence of RDS and intraventricular hemorrhage (IVH), has not been shown to alter the incidence of BPD.

The history of asthma in Sam's mother is also a consideration in this case. *BPD is more likely to develop in babies with a family history of reactive airway disease.* The pathophysiologic basis for this observation remains uncertain, although it is likely due to a predisposition to early reactive airway disease in the neonate, which results in gas trapping and overdistention of the distal air spaces.

The presence of chorioamnionitis is also a major risk factor for the development of BPD. Preterm babies born of mothers with chorioamnionitis have a lower rate of RDS (presumably due to stress) but a higher incidence of BPD than those not exposed to an infected intrauterine environment. It has been hypothesized that chorioam-

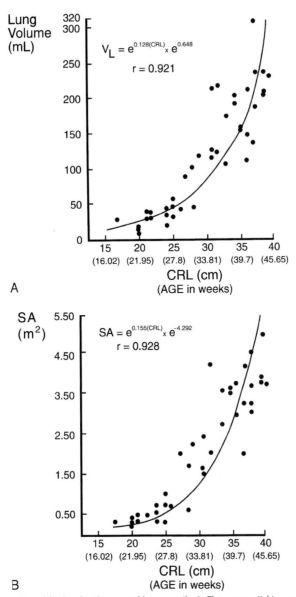

Figure 11-1 Graphic representation of fetal and early neonatal lung growth. **A,** The exponential increase in lung volume between 16 and 45 weeks of gestation, with the corresponding crown-rump length (CRL) at each gestation. **B,** A similar growth pattern for internal surface area of the lung (SA) as a function of gestational age and crown-rump length. (From Langston C, Kida K, Reed M, et al: Human lung growth in late gestation and in the neonate. Am Rev Respir Dis 1984;129:610–611. Reprinted with permission of the American Lung Association.)

nionitis activates an inflammation–lung injury sequence. Inflammatory cytokines interleukin 6 (IL-6), IL-1, IL-8, and tumor necrosis factor (TNF) are present in high levels in the amniotic fluid of babies who go on to develop BPD, and leukocyte elastase concentrations are elevated at birth in the tracheal effluent of these infants. These findings imply that lung inflammation and injury start before birth in the clinical setting of chorioamnionitis.

Case Study *Continued*

Baby Sam responded well to initial stabilization. His ventilator support was reduced rapidly, and he was extubated at 2 hours of age and placed on nasal CPAP (continuous positive airway pressure) at 5 cm H₂O with an F_{IO₂} of 0.23. The initial chest radiograph showed adequate lung volumes with bilateral haziness and some perihilar streaky changes, consistent with *immature lungs or surfactant-treated RDS. Intravenous fluid therapy was given at a rate of 100 to 130 mL/kg/day to maintain serum sodium in the range of 138 to 148 mEq/L and to allow a 10% to 15% weight loss from birth weight. Sam was also started on vitamin A, 5000 units IM three times per week for 28 days. At 72 hours of age, Sam developed carbon dioxide (P_{CO_2}) retention of 50 mm Hg and blood pressure of 43/18 mm Hg, with no change in the physical examination or chest radiograph. No heart murmur was heard, but a patent ductus arteriosus (PDA) with left-to-right shunting was suspected and confirmed by color Doppler echocardiography. A course of indomethacin was administered, with resolution of the PDA. After PDA closure, Sam's CO_2 retention improved, but he developed apnea, which improved on caffeine therapy. Pulmonary function testing on day 5 showed modestly reduced compliance and elevated pulmonary airway resistance.*

Exercise 2

QUESTION

1. What additional elements of this case increase the probability that Sam will develop BPD?

ANSWER

1. PDA and elevated airway resistance.

The presence of a PDA with left-to-right shunting increases interstitial lung water, decreases lung compliance, and elevates lung airway resistance, which ultimately results in an increase in the degree of ventilatory support. Even though the PDA was treated aggressively in this case, the presence of a PDA increases the likelihood of BPD.

Babies with RDS who exhibit high airway resistance during the first week of life are predisposed to the development of BPD. Whether the elevated resistance is causative or symptomatic is unclear. Pulmonary function testing (measurements of lung resistance and compliance) during the first week of life may predict which infants are likely to develop BPD.

QUESTION

2. What factors in this case reduce the probability of developing BPD?

ANSWER

2. Relative fluid restriction, absence of air leak, and minimization of oxygen and ventilator therapies.

This patient was given appropriate intravenous fluid therapy for his weight and gestational age. A larger preterm infant should be restricted to fluids totaling about 80 mL/kg/day, but ELBW infants often require more than 100 mL/kg/day to compensate for insensible water loss. *Retrospective studies have demonstrated an increased incidence of BPD in neonates who received higher fluid volumes than were necessary to maintain euhydration.* Excess fluid administration increases interstitial lung water in patients with RDS because of the capillary leak that accompanies the disease. Further evidence that excess lung fluid is deleterious is the finding of an increased rate of BPD in infants with RDS who do not exhibit the expected diuresis on days 2 to 3.[5] This concept of overhydration predisposing to BPD is tempered, however, by prospective trials in which fluid restriction in neonates with RDS did not prevent the development of BPD.[6]

Fortunately, Sam showed no sign of air leak such as pulmonary interstitial emphysema (PIE) or pneumothorax. These complications can be difficult to manage acutely, and their management often dictates an increase in oxygen and ventilator support. Furthermore, air leak syndromes increase the risk of developing BPD.

Even without air leak, barotrauma (or volutrauma) from mechanical ventilation can cause direct mechanical injury to the developing lung, and *the incidence of BPD is higher in babies who are ventilated with high inspiratory pressures (IP > 30 mm Hg) or who are exposed to high inspiratory oxygen concentrations ($F_{IO_2} > 0.80$) for an extended period.* In this case, Sam was extubated promptly to CPAP and low F_{IO_2}, which minimizes toxicity; however, as noted earlier, even low levels of artificial positive pressure support are foreign to the immature lung and may lead to lung injury. Similarly, even low levels of inspired oxygen and arterial P_{O_2} levels of 50 to 80 mm Hg are higher than levels the fetus is exposed to in utero and may be toxic to the pulmonary epithelial cells. For example, in the STOP-ROP trial of higher versus lower early oxygen treatment, the study group with target Sa_{O_2} of 86% to 92% had a lower rate of BPD than the group with target Sa_{O_2} of 92% to 96%. There are a variety of reasons why the lungs of premature newborn infants may be particularly susceptible to oxidant injury. First, pulmonary host defense mechanisms in preterm infants against oxygen toxicity are diminished relative to the defense mechanisms in the lung of term babies or adults. Not only are there reduced levels of intracellular antioxidant enzymes (superoxide dismutase [SOD], catalase, and glutathione peroxidase), but the usual developmental increase in these enzymes before term birth may not occur in the preterm lung.[7] Extracellular substances that protect against injury, such as vitamin E, ceruloplasmin, and selenium, are also deficient in the preterm lung. Second, the metabolism of alveolar macrophages and surfactant secretion by type II pneumocytes is adversely affected by hyperoxia. In addition to inducing lung cell cytotoxicity, hyperoxic exposure of newborn animals during the early critical periods of lung development has been shown to disrupt normal alveolar development.

The effects of barotrauma or volutrauma are evident in the pathogenesis of BPD; however, the specifics of how different ventilator strategies either contribute to or ameliorate BPD are unclear. Certainly, surfactant treatment reduces the degree of ventilation needed to treat RDS, yet surfactant treatment has not been shown to reduce the incidence of BPD. Early application of CPAP without intubation and ventilation appears to have succeeded in reducing the rate of BPD in some centers, but those results have yet to be replicated or generalized. Early application of HFOV reduces the incidence of BPD in baboons, and in one multicenter study reduced the incidence of BPD in human infants; however, these results have not been replicated, and the data in the study have been insufficient to result in a change in clinical practice.

Pulmonary inflammation contributes to the pathophysiology of pulmonary microvascular injury and altered membrane permeability associated with oxygen toxicity. Although polymorphonuclear neutrophil recruitment is a normal phase of lung healing, persistence of neutrophils, neutrophil secretory products, and cytokines (elastase, arachidonic acid metabolites, interleukins, leukotrienes) may further injure the immature lung. These inflammatory mediators cause connective tissue damage, pulmonary vasoconstriction, pulmonary capillary leak, bronchonconstriction, and further amplification of the inflammatory response.[8,9]

Case Study *Continued*

In the third week of life, Sam continued on nasal CPAP of 5 cm H_2O and an F_{IO_2} of 0.30. He had modest CO_2 retention and mild increased work of breathing on clinical examination. He had episodes of feeding intolerance, and so remained on a slow feeding advance and supplemental hyperalimentation; his maximum caloric intake was 90 kcal/kg/day. One evening his oxygen requirement increased to 0.50 and he developed significant apnea and bradycardia episodes. A chest radiograph showed lower lobe infiltrates, and there was a "left shift" on the white blood cell count. Cultures were obtained and antibiotic therapy initiated. A blood culture subsequently grew Staphylococcus aureus. The respiratory and gastrointestinal symptoms resolved on treatment, but Sam's F_{IO_2} remained elevated at 0.40.

Exercise 3

QUESTION

1. What additional medical conditions increase the probability that Sam will develop BPD?

ANSWER

1. Poor nutrition and pneumonia.

Rapid weight gain and organ growth take place in the fetus between 26 weeks' gestation (when baby Sam was born) and term gestation. Unfortunately, once an infant is born prematurely, our ability to provide adequate nutrition is limited and usually cannot match the effectiveness of the in utero environment. If the poor postnatal nutrition is not corrected, it ultimately leads to nutritional deficiencies that interfere with lung repair and lung growth. In a general sense, malnutrition leads to a catabolic state, which inhibits cell and organ growth. More specifically, however, malnutrition is believed to lead to impaired surfactant production, decreased lung cell replication, and decreased structural alveolar development and septation.

Vitamin A is necessary for epithelial integrity and healing of the airways. Preterm neonates who develop BPD are often deficient in vitamin A, and early vitamin A supplementation reduces the incidence of the disorder.[10] Very low birth weight infants are also prone to develop zinc deficiency; zinc is an important cofactor for many enzymes, including the antioxidant enzyme superoxide dismutase. Inositol positively influences lung development and maturation of surfactant metabolism, and inositol supplementation may reduce the incidence of BPD in preterm infants.[11] Malnutrition can further compromise the already deficient immune system in neonates. Deleterious effects of malnutrition have been demonstrated on both cellular and humoral immunity. These immune deficiencies predispose to the development of intercurrent infections and pneumonia.

Nosocomial pneumonia often causes a clinical deterioration from which neonates with evolving BPD may have difficulty recovering. The infection may result in increased lung injury because the polymorphonuclear leukocytes that enter the lung release elastase and other proteolytic enzymes that cause further lung injury.[12] Viral infections such as adenovirus may cause an obliterative bronchiolitis even in healthy infants, which may exacerbate the small airway disease that is part of BPD. *Ureaplasma urealyticum* colonization or infection has been correlated with the development of BPD, but the extent of this potential problem is not yet understood, and it is not known if treatment affects the course of BPD.

Lung injury and repair in neonates tax an immature respiratory system undergoing a rapid process of growth and development. These developmental changes, along with an immature and diminished response to lung injury, lead to structural and biochemical changes favoring lung repair with fibrosis, a response not commonly observed in the lung healing of adult patients. In uncomplicated RDS that resolves without lung scarring, normal lung reparative phases include transient inflammation, proliferation of type II pneumocytes, and restoration of lung growth and differentiation. When "classical" BPD develops, however, the acute inflammatory phase of RDS evolves into a persistent inflammatory exudative phase. During this time, a period of extensive fibroblast proliferation occurs, with deposition of collagen and lung scarring. When a patient is on mechanical ventilation, the lung is continually exposed to injurious agents such as oxygen and barotrauma, which inhibit the proliferation and biosynthetic functioning of many cells in the lung. Interestingly, however, fibroblast proliferation is not suppressed by hyperoxia; in fact, hyperoxia stimulates alveolar macrophage release of fibronectin and insulin growth factor-1, which stimulate fibroblast migration into the lung. The acute lung injury also damages the pulmonary epithelial, capillary basement membrane, and intercellular matrix architecture, as indicated by the release of elastin degradation products and fibronectin.[13] Finally, the collagen composition of the lungs of infants with BPD is abnormal. Whereas the type I–type III collagen ratio is 2:1 in the lungs of normal adults and 1:6 in the immature lungs of preterm infants without BPD, the ratio in the lungs of infants who died from BPD is greater than 3:1. Because type I collagen is less elastic than type III collagen, the lungs of infants with BPD are inappropriately stiff.

In contrast to "classical" BPD, the lungs of babies with "new BPD" do not develop the same degree of fibrosis, but instead have variable degrees of alveolar underdevelopment.

The Clinical Picture: An Evolving Process

As is evident from the previous discussion, the development of BPD is an evolving process. As such, it is difficult to determine exactly when BPD starts. From a pathophysiologic point of view, BPD starts as soon as the acute lung injury of RDS fails to resolve and the abnormal exudative, reparative, and alveolar developmental processes begin. Biochemical studies of lung inflammation and physiologic studies of pulmonary function suggest that the process begins as soon as 5 to 7 days of age. However, from a practical point of view, in many neonates who show these early signs of chronic lung disease, symptoms resolve within several weeks; thus, they would not be considered to have chronic lung disease.

The traditional operational or epidemiologic definition of BPD was (1) the need for supplemental oxygen, (2) the presence of an abnormal chest radiograph, and (3) clinical symptoms of respiratory distress at 28 days of age. Most older studies of BPD used this definition. However, because very few extremely low birth weight infants would escape the diagnosis using this definition (simply on the basis of anatomic lung immaturity), the modern definition of BPD is the need for supplemental oxygen

TABLE 11-2

DEFINITION OF BRONCHOPULMONARY DYSPLASIA (BPD): DIAGNOSTIC CRITERIA FOR BABIES LESS THAN 32 WEEKS' GESTATIONAL AGE

Time point of assessment: 36 weeks'
   postmenstrual age or discharge to home,
   whichever comes first
Criteria: Treatment with oxygen > 21% for at least
   28 days
Mild BPD: Breathing room air
Moderate BPD: Need for <30% oxygen
Severe BPD: Need for ≥30% oxygen or positive
   pressure (positive-pressure ventilation or
   noncontinuous positive airway pressure)

and an abnormal chest radiograph at 36 weeks' postmenstrual age. In 2000, the NICHD conducted a consensus conference that resulted in a new definition of BPD that allowed for classification of infants with chronic lung disease into mild, moderate, and severe categories (Table 11-2). Most recently, Walsh and associates proposed a new physiologic definition: the inability to maintain an oxygen saturation of 90% or more in room air.[14] This new definition is appealing because it provides a more objective way to determine if an infant needs supplemental oxygen and has BPD.

BPD was first described in 1967 by Northway, a radiologist.[2] Then, as now, the chest radiograph is an important factor in the diagnosis and staging of BPD. The radiographic appearance of "classical" BPD evolves slowly during the first week of life, analogous to the pathophysiologic and clinical evolution noted earlier. In Northway's description, stage I BPD is indistinguishable from RDS, with hazy lung fields, a ground-glass appearance, and air bronchograms (Fig. 11-2A). Stage II BPD (Fig. 11-2B) shows continued or advancing homogeneous opacity of the lung fields at 4 to 10 days of age, when acute RDS should be resolving. The histopathologic correlate of stage II BPD is the development of alveolar and airway epithelial necrosis, with early repair, and exudation into the airways. Cystic change begins in stage III BPD (Fig. 11-2C), in association with early changes of interstitial fibrosis. These changes tend to be diffuse and homogeneous, without gross distortion of lung architecture. The histopathologic findings of stage III BPD are mucosal metaplasia, obliterative

bronchiolitis, and microscopic atelectasis and emphysema (Fig. 11-3A). Stage IV disease (Fig. 11-2D) occurs beyond 1 month of age and is characterized radiographically by gross distortion of the lung architecture, interstitial fibrosis, large cystic areas, hyperinflation, shifting atelectasis, and emphysema (Fig. 11-4). Edward devised a radiographic scoring system for BPD that has been helpful in standardizing diagnosis and data validity for research.[15] Points are assigned for varying degrees of cardiomegaly, hyperinflation, cystic change interstitial fibrosis, and a subjective severity assessment, with a final score ranging from 1 to 10.

In contrast, the radiographic and pathologic changes in the "new BPD" tend to be less severe. The radiographic appearance includes hazy lung fields and mild fibrotic changes; large emphysematous cysts and nonhomogeneous atelectasis (as seen in "classical" BPD) are rarely observed. The hallmark pathologic lesions are large and simplified alveolar ducts and alveoli with simplified acinar development, milder and variable smooth muscle hyperplasia and interstitial fibrosis, and some degree of decreased microvascular development (Fig. 11-3B).

The symptoms and signs of BPD also undergo a developmental process. The classic early signs of RDS (grunting and retractions), which are secondary to diminished lung compliance and functional residual capacity, are gradually replaced with a more chronic respiratory distress characterized by tachypnea, hypoxemia, hypercarbia, wheezing, and retractions secondary to increased airway resistance. These infants have increased work of breathing related to both continued poor compliance and increased airway resistance. Most of them appear chronically ill and fatigued and may require prolonged ventilatory support to lessen the work of breathing.

Case Study *Continued*

By the fourth week of life, Sam was weaned off CPAP and placed on nasal cannula oxygen at 1.5 L/minute flow and F_{IO_2} of 0.40. Sam's P_{CO_2} was 52 mm Hg. His pulmonary function tests demonstrated a modestly low specific compliance of 0.8 mL/cm H_2O/kg and a high airway resistance of 85 cm H_2O/L/second. His flow-volume loops exhibited early signs of expiratory flow limitation

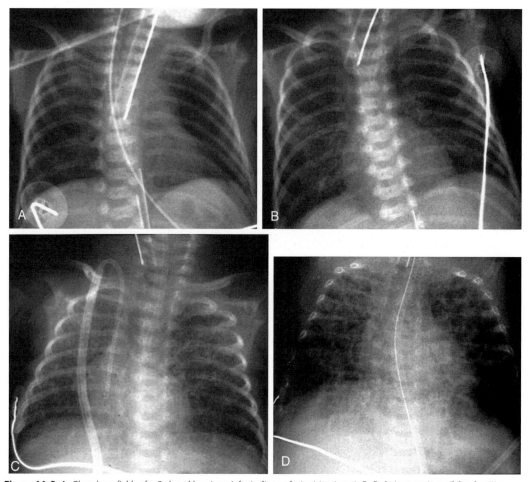

Figure 11-2 A, Clean lung fields of a 3-day-old preterm infant after surfactant treatment. **B,** Early increase in perihilar densities representing pulmonary edema and exudative changes. **C,** Stage III bronchopulmonary dysplasia (BPD) exhibits diffuse cystic changes, with early interstitial fibrosis. **D,** The findings of stage IV BPD include gross distortion of lung architecture, with interstitial fibrosis, large cystic change, shifting atelectasis, and emphysema.

(Fig. 11-5B). He had occasional episodes of wheezing, with a concomitant increase in retractions. He did not exhibit excess weight gain, edema, or other obvious signs of fluid overload. His nutritional status improved, with gradual tolerance of enteral feedings and weaning of his intravenous hyperalimentation. A vitamin A level was 15 µg/mL.

Exercise 4

QUESTION

1. If you were managing baby Sam's oxygenation now at over 4 weeks of age, what range of arterial oxygen saturation values would you try to maintain?

    a. Sao_2 of 82% to 90% to minimize further oxygen toxicity

    b. Sao_2 of 96% to 100% to provide plenty of oxygen to the healing tissues of this chronically ill baby

    c. Sao_2 of 88% to 95% to provide adequate tissue oxygenation and help avoid future complications of BPD

ANSWER

1. c

There are several cogent reasons for maintaining relative normoxemia in a patient with established BPD. During the first month of life, there is some evidence that maintaining lower saturations (82% to 90%) may reduce the incidence of BPD and ROP, but once BPD is established, saturations of 88% to 95% are reasonable. This level of oxygen supplementation should be continued for as long as needed.

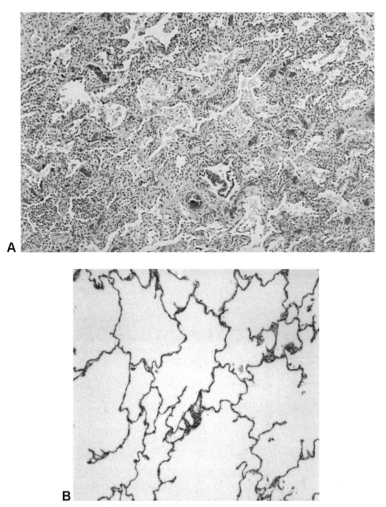

Figure 11-3 **A,** The histopathologic findings of stage III bronchopulmonary dysplasia (BPD) include mucosal metaplasia, obliterative bronchiolitis, and microscopic atelectasis and emphysema. **B,** New BPD in a surfactant-treated infant. Photomicrograph (original magnification, ×50; H&E stain) shows expanded, simplified alveolar ducts, saccules, and alveoli with little or no alveolar septal fibrosis.

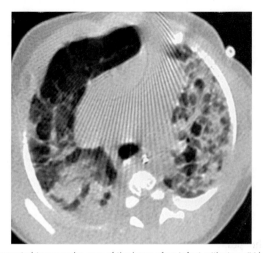

Figure 11-4 A cross-sectional computed tomography scan of the lungs of an infant with stage IV bronchopulmonary dysplasia, demonstrating gross distortion of lung architecture, with cystic emphysema and areas of atelectasis.

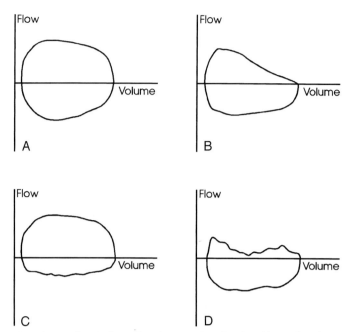

Figure 11-5 Representative pulmonary function flow-volume loops. **A,** Normal tracing with even flow characteristics on inspiration and expiration. **B,** Infants with bronchopulmonary dysplasia often demonstrate limitation of expiratory flow because of small airway damage and bronchospasm. **C,** Subglottic stenosis produces an inspiratory, extrathoracic obstruction on the flow-volume loop. **D,** Tracheo-bronchomalacia exhibits an intrathoracic obstructive pattern, with intermittent airway closure during the expiratory phase.

Oxygen can be used at home if the infant is otherwise ready for discharge but cannot maintain normoxemia in room air.

One of the fundamental tenets of neonatal intensive care is to make sure that every infant is adequately oxygenated. There is, however, a wide range of arterial Po_2 and O_2 saturation values that can achieve this goal and satisfy tissue oxygen needs. In this case, answer a (Sao_2 of 82% to 90%) is incorrect. Although oxygen toxicity may be operative in the pathogenesis of BPD, it is unlikely that continued provision of 40% oxygen by nasal cannula would cause significant further damage. On the contrary, there is evidence suggesting that any degree of chronic hypoxemia may be deleterious to the recovery of BPD patients. Weight gain is better for infants with BPD who are maintained normoxemic than for those with lower levels of oxygenation. Adequate oxygenation may help forestall the development of pulmonary hypertension and right-sided heart strain (cor pulmonale), one of the most serious complications of BPD. The propensity to develop high pulmonary vascular resistance in these patients is due to a combination of factors, including anatomic distortion, with an associated decreased cross-sectional area of the pulmonary vasculature; hypoxic pulmonary vasoconstriction; and pulmonary artery vasoconstriction from elaboration of inflammatory mediators such as leukotrienes.[16] Many infants with BPD are sensitive to oxygen administration and exhibit an acute decrease in pulmonary vascular resistance when the arterial Po_2 value is increased.[17] Recurrent hypoxemia is also likely to be harmful to the developing brain. Babies with chronic BPD and recurrent hypoxic spells are at significant risk for developmental delay.

Answer b (Sao_2 of 96% to 100%) is also incorrect. There is no evidence that hyperoxia is beneficial to an infant with BPD. Furthermore, hyperoxia is one of many factors implicated in the pathogenesis of retinopathy of prematurity.

An equally important and controversial issue is where to maintain this infant's blood carbon dioxide concentration. The current school of thought is to allow "permissive hypercapnia" both in the acute and chronic phases of neonatal lung disease. Allowing Pco_2 levels up to 70 mm Hg. with a pH of 7.20 or higher reduces the duration and intensity of mechanical ventilation, which may decrease the incidence and severity of evolving BPD.

QUESTION

2. Listed here are the medications that have been used for treatment of BPD. Match each

drug with one of its potential mechanisms of action.

Drugs

a. Bronchodilators

b. Diuretics

c. Dexamethasone

Mechanisms of Action

d. Decrease of interstitial edema

e. Airway smooth muscle relaxation

f. Acute improvement of lung function and decreased inflammation

ANSWER

2. a = e, b = d, c = f.

Of the wide variety of drugs used in infants with chronic lung disease, bronchodilators are selected most frequently (Table 11-3). As many as 60% of infants with BPD have reactive airway disease, as defined by the presence of wheezing, an increase in airway resistance after bronchoprovocation, or the response to bronchodilating agents. Bronchiolar smooth muscle hyperplasia and bronchospasm may begin at a very young postnatal age and have been observed in infants with BPD whose postconceptional age is only 26 weeks. Theophylline, caffeine, and albuterol have all been shown to provide acute therapeutic relief for bronchospasm in these babies. Inhalation is the preferred route of administration of albuterol or other β-agonists, because the acute response is better and the side effects are fewer than with oral dosing. Most bronchospasm in babies with BPD can be managed with a β-agonist and without methylxanthines.

Some babies with BPD will benefit from the use of diuretics, even if there are no obvious signs of systemic fluid overload (see Table 11-3). Interstitial water accumulation occurs in the lungs of BPD infants for a variety of reasons, including capillary leak from the damaged epithelium, increased pulmonary capillary pressure, impaired lymphatic drainage due to the distorted architecture, and decreased plasma oncotic pressure from malnutrition or fluid overload. Furosemide is the most frequently studied diuretic in BPD. The administration of furosemide results in a diuresis that minimizes total lung water and raises plasma oncotic pressure. However, furosemide also has important nonrenal effects on pulmonary function, which are evident soon after the dose and well before the effect of diuresis could have taken place. Furosemide causes venodilation, which increases venous capacitance and therefore decreases right ventricular end-diastolic volume and pulmonary capillary pressure. There are also direct effects of furosemide on airway epithelium, which results in decreased chloride and water transport across the epithelium, as well as diminished airway reactivity. Studies of pulmonary mechanics have demonstrated improvement in both lung compliance and lung resistance.

TABLE 11-3

DRUG THERAPY AND DOSAGES FOR NEONATES WITH BRONCHOPULMONARY DYSPLASIA

Drug	Dosage	Comments
Bronchodilators		
Albuterol inhalation	Nebulize 0.1–0.15 mL/kg every 6 hr or metered dose inhaler 1 puff every 6 hr	
Caffeine citrate	Load 20 mg/kg Maintenance 5–10 mg/kg/day	Maintain serum level of 10–25 µg/mL for bronchodilation
Theophylline	Load 6 mg/kg Maintenance 1.1 mg/kg/day every 8 hr	Maintain serum level of 10–15 µg/mL for bronchodilation
Diuretics		
Furosemide (IV or IM)	1 mg/kg once daily or every other day (oral dose, 1 to 3 mg/kg)	Monitor electrolytes, give potassium chloride supplement
Chlorothiazide	20–40 mg/kg/day, divided bid	Monitor electrolytes, give potassium chloride supplement
Spironolactone	1–3 mg/kg/day, divided bid	Monitor electrolytes
Nutritional Supplements		
Vitamin A	5000 U IM 3×/week for 28 days	Normal serum level is 20–50 µg/mL
Vitamin E	25 U/day PO	Normal serum level 1–3 µg/mL
Zinc sulfate	1 mg/kg/day PO	Normal serum level is 70–100 µg/mL

Most studies have used a dose of 1 mg/kg/day, but 1 mg/kg every other day also causes a sustained improvement with fewer side effects. The side effects of furosemide include fluid and electrolyte imbalance (chloride depletion and metabolic alkalosis, hyponatremia), hypercalciuria and nephrolithiasis, osteopenia, and ototoxicity.

The combination of chlorothiazide and spironolactone results in a diuresis similar to that of furosemide, but the effects on pulmonary mechanics are less clear-cut. Whereas earlier studies showed improvement in lung compliance and airway resistance with this therapy, others have demonstrated an adequate diuresis but no improvement in pulmonary function or oxygenation.[18] The safety profile of these drugs is an advantage, however, because fewer side effects (e.g., nephrolithiasis, ototoxicity) have been noted. Spironolactone adds little to the diuretic effect of chlorothiazide and does not prevent the hypokalemia that occurs with the chronic use of diuretics.[19] Infants receiving furosemide or chlorothiazide on a chronic basis often require supplementation with KCl to prevent hypokalemia, hyponatremia, and hypochloremia.

Even though the studies summarized here demonstrated an acute improvement in lung function after diuretic administration, very little long-term data support the efficacy and safety of diuretic therapy for treatment of BPD. Because data are lacking for diuretic use beyond 2 to 14 days' duration, the chronic use of diuretics for BPD should be individualized and not initiated as a routine treatment. Once initiated, however, diuretics are generally continued until the infant no longer requires oxygen therapy.

Once a mainstay of BPD therapy, the use of corticosteroids is now limited to only the most severe, life-threatening cases. Although administration of high-dose dexamethasone to ventilator-dependent infants beyond 2 weeks of age facilitates weaning from respiratory support with improvement in pulmonary function and attenuation of lung inflammation, side effects of decreased somatic growth and impaired neurodevelopmental outcome preclude its use. Since many preterm infants have relative adrenal insufficiency, prevention of BPD has been attempted with early, low-dose physiologic hydrocortisone prophylaxis. Those studies, however, were not completed because of an increased incidence of spontaneous bowel perforation in the treatment group; excess bowel perforation has also been reported in studies of early dexamethasone therapy.[20] Another approach to modulating lung inflammation has been the administration of low-dose inhaled nitric oxide (iNO). The use of iNO in preterm infants is considered off label and controversial. Several recently published randomized clinical trials, including three in the past year, have shown considerable variance in outcomes. These outcomes range from no reduction in the incidence of BPD in ELBW infants to lower incidence of IVH and a significant reduction in the incidence of BPD. Routine use of iNO in preterm infants is not recommended given the variability of outcomes in the current data.

Two other approaches to prevention of BPD include use of inhaled beclomethasone and superoxide dismutase. In clinical trials neither drug reduced the incidence of chronic lung disease, but both showed improvement in long-term pulmonary outcomes without side effects. Early application of inhaled beclomethasone in preterm infants at risk for BPD reduced the need for systemic dexamethasone and ventilatory support[21]; early treatment of similar infants with recombinant superoxide dismutase reduced wheezing and need for bronchodilators at 18 months of age.[22]

As discussed previously, there is enough evidence to suggest that vitamin A reduces the incidence of BPD. Therefore, it makes good clinical sense to administer vitamin A to the highest risk infants (<1250 g birth weight) during the first month of life.[10] Even with this supplementation, many infants with BPD will continue to have insufficient vitamin A levels. It is unknown if supplementation beyond 1 month of age is beneficial.

QUESTION

3. How many calories are needed to allow Sam to grow at an in utero rate?

ANSWER

3. With the increased work of breathing and increased metabolic rate, many infants with BPD require 120 to 150 kcal/kg/day to maintain an adequate weight gain of 15 to 30 g/day.

Enteral feedings should consist of 24 kcal/oz fortified breast milk, if available, or preterm infant formulas, which have added nutrients such as calcium, phosphorus, zinc, and vitamin E. Adequate mineral intake is necessary to prevent osteopenia, or rickets of prematurity, which may occur in chronically ill infants with BPD who do not have an adequate intake of calcium and phosphorus. Older infants with BPD should receive a transitional formula or a formula designed for term infants that is concentrated up to 30 kcal/oz. Additional calories can be supplied by additives such as medium-chain triglyceride (MCT) oil, microlipids, vegetable oil, or baby cereal.

Mechanical problems may also interfere with adequate intake. Some infants with BPD use too much energy trying to suck, swallow, and breathe; other infants are unable to suck because of neurologic deficits. These babies should be given tube feedings as needed to minimize the work of breathing and maximize weight gain. Gastroesophageal reflux is also a common problem in older infants with BPD, which may require treatment with antireflux positioning, cereal-thickened feedings, ranitidine, metoclopramide, or fundoplication in the most recalcitrant cases.

QUESTION

4. Why should carbohydrate additives be used cautiously in infants with BPD?

ANSWER

4. Carbohydrate additives such as Polycose should be used with caution because the high respiratory quotient of carbohydrates generates more carbon dioxide per unit of oxygen consumption, which can lead to hypercarbia or increase work of breathing.

Case Study *Continued*

Baby Sam continued on nasal cannula oxygen and nutrition was optimized. His neonatologist did not treat him with diuretics, believing that low flow oxygen was no more or less toxic than diuretic use. In the sixth week of life, Sam developed intermittent episodes of desaturation associated with increased work of breathing, retractions, and faint wheezing. These episodes decreased in frequency and severity after treatment with albuterol via metered dose inhaler.

Exercise 5

QUESTION

1. What diagnostic workup should be performed at this time?

ANSWER

1. First, rule out pneumonia with chest x-ray, white blood cell count, and blood cultures. Second, consider electrocardiogram (ECG) and echocardiogram. Third, consider pulmonary function testing, airway fluoroscopy, or bronchoscopy.

BPD spells are sudden episodes of hypoxemia and agitation that may occur in older infants with BPD, especially those who are ventilator dependent. The cause of these spells is often unclear, and their diagnosis and management can be frustrating for the clinician. However, an attempt should be made to find a treatable cause and thereby minimize the undesired exposure to hypoxemia.

Sepsis or pneumonia should always be considered in infants with BPD who exhibit instability or deterioration in baseline need for support. A chest x-ray, white blood cell count, and blood and tracheal aspirate cultures (if intubated) should be obtained.

The clinical description of these spells (retractions and cyanosis) appears to indicate an airway problem. However, episodes of hypoxemia could also be due to right-to-left shunting at the atrial level related to right-sided heart strain and pulmonary hypertension, which are symptoms of cor pulmonale. In infants with BPD, normal pulmonary vascular development is disrupted. Chronic hypoxia may lead to hypertrophy of the pulmonary artery smooth muscle, and the anatomic distortion of lung architecture may lead to a decreased total cross-sectional area of the pulmonary vasculature. The resulting pulmonary hypertension causes right-sided heart strain, as well as secondary strain on the left ventricle. Infants with cor pulmonale may have an increase in oxygen and ventilator requirements, a single second heart sound, and hepatomegaly. The ECG usually shows right atrial enlargement and right ventricular hypertrophy. The echocardiogram may document chamber enlargement or hypertrophy and can provide more direct evidence of pulmonary hypertension. A cardiac evaluation should be obtained at 2 months of age in an infant with chronic BPD and then every 1 to 2 months until supplemental oxygen has been discontinued and there are no signs of respiratory distress. Infants with cor pulmonale are administered oxygen to achieve pulmonary vasodilation and diuretics to reduce filling pressure in the right heart. Inotropic agents have not been useful in treating this complication of BPD, but nitric oxide is sometimes used to decrease pulmonary vascular resistance.

As many as 25% of infants with BPD may have systemic hypertension, the exact cause of which is unclear.[2] Antihypertensive medications may be indicated if the systolic blood pressure is consistently greater than 100 mm Hg and the diastolic exceeds 80 mm Hg.

In Sam's case, the presence of retractions during the hypoxic spells suggest either bronchospasm or airway collapse during the spells. As noted earlier, infants with BPD frequently have reactive airway disease responsive to bronchodilators. In addition, tracheobronchomalacia may occur in infants with BPD due to the inherent weakness of the cartilaginous airways of the preterm infant, along with damage to the supporting parenchymal structure of the lung. The diagnosis can be made by demonstrating a characteristic flow-volume loop on pulmonary function tests (Fig. 11-5D) or by performing fluoroscopy or bronchoscopy, during which the airways can be observed to collapse on inspiration as the distending pressure is lowered. There is no specific treatment for this condition. Most infants improve with time as the major airways increase in diameter, although occasionally, an infant requires tracheostomy. With tracheobronchomalacia, there is a theoretical concern with the use of β-agonist bronchodilators, which relax smooth muscle and may reduce the stability of the weakened airways. If albuterol is found to worsen the clinical status, ipraprotrium (an anticholinergic bronchodilator) can be tried, which may minimize proximal airway smooth muscle relaxation.

Another potential airway problem for a chronically ventilated infant with BPD is subglottic stenosis, secondary to prolonged endotracheal intubation. This complication can be detected by demonstrating an extrathoracic obstruction on flow-volume loops during pulmonary function testing (Fig. 11-5C). Subglottic stenosis is confirmed by bronchoscopy; severe cases may require tracheostomy for stabilization of the airway.

Infants with BPD are prone to the development of shifting atelectasis because of anatomic distortion of the airways, mucosal inflammation and edema, and exudative plugging. Treatments include chest physical therapy and positioning of the infant with the atelectatic side elevated. Fiberoptic bronchoscopy may demonstrate airway obstruction by inflammatory granulomas, which may improve with short-term corticosteroid treatment.

Long-Term Follow-up

Case Study *Continued*

By 60 days of age, Sam demonstrated regular weight gain and an increase in respiratory muscle strength. Oxygen therapy was discontinued at 70 days of age, and he was discharged home on PRN albuterol. He received routine immunizations and Synagis to help prevent RSV infection. Following an upper respiratory infection at age 5 months, wheezing developed, requiring a brief hospitalization and treatment with nebulized albuterol. When Sam was 6 months of age, pulmonary function testing showed minor residual abnormalities of compliance, resistance, and expiratory flow limitation (see Fig. 11-5B), but he appeared to be clinically well and thriving, without dyspnea or noticeable respiratory symptoms.

Exercise 6

QUESTION

1. What long-term pulmonary and neurodevelopmental problems might Sam face?

ANSWER

1. Abnormal pulmonary function, recurrent episodes of wheezing, developmental delay and cerebral palsy.

Structural remodeling and physiologic improvements in pulmonary function can occur in infants with chronic lung disease for as long as 10 years. The decreased compliance observed in acute RDS persists in those infants who develop

BPD. However, airway abnormalities are a more significant long-term problem in these infants, with persistence of increased total pulmonary resistance and expiratory flow limitation for up to 3 years. Fifty to 75% of infants with BPD exhibit increased bronchial reactivity demonstrated by methacholine, exercise, or cold-air challenge, and many of these infants have wheezing requiring acute or chronic bronchodilator therapy. At 10 years of age, children with BPD tend to have evidence of hyperinflation. Pulmonary function tests in these children demonstrate an increased residual volume, an improving but still slightly low FEV_1 (forced expiratory volume at 1 second), and abnormal forced expiratory flows. It should be emphasized that most of these children have normal exercise tolerance, although aerobic exercise in BPD children occurs at the expense of a drop in oxygen saturation and a rise in carbon dioxide. In summary, most infants with BPD can be expected to "outgrow"' the disease from the point of view of symptoms, except for wheezing in some cases. The residual pulmonary function abnormalities, although not often noticed by the child or the parents, may persist into adolescence or young adulthood.[24] In extremely severe cases (less than 1% of ventilated preterm neonates) infants with BPD may remain ventilator dependent for months or years.

Infants with BPD are at risk for poor neurodevelopmental outcome because of (1) recurrent episodes of hypoxia in those infants with chronic disease and lability with BPD spells, (2) the association of BPD with intraventricular hemorrhage and periventricular leukomalacia, (3) poor nutrition during periods of critical brain growth, and (4) prolonged hospitalization and prolonged mechanical ventilation, which may preclude normal stimulation and parent-infant interaction. The incidence of developmental delay as measured by low Bayley mental developmental scores ranges from 10% to 45%. Cerebral palsy may occur in 7% to 28% of infants with BPD and these infants may also exhibit a high incidence of early, transient neuromotor problems.

Summary: A Multifactorial Approach to a Multifactorial Disease

BPD is a disease with many underlying causes and predispositions, including immature lung anatomy, physiology, and cell biology; toxicities related to the use of oxygen and ventilators; nutritional deprivation; and infection. Prevention of the disease is not yet within our grasp. However, it is the hope of all clinicians who care for these infants that a multifactorial approach using less invasive respiratory support strategies, surfactant replacement, and antioxidant and anti-inflammatory regimens will lead to a reduction in the incidence of chronic lung disease in preterm neonates (Table 11-4).

Once BPD develops, the primary goal of therapy is to provide an environment that permits lung growth and repair and eventual resolution of the major abnormalities in lung function. The therapies for these babies must include an integrated approach that provides sufficient oxygen, adequate calories for growth, vitamins and minerals for antioxidant defense and repair processes, diuretics and bronchodilators to improve lung function, aggressive therapy of intercurrent infection, and constant attention to appropriate levels of infant stimulation and neurodevelopmental support.

TABLE 11-4

COMPLICATIONS OF BRONCHOPULMONARY DYSPLASIA AND RECOMMENDED THERAPIES

Complication	Therapy
Fluid retention	Diuretics
Bronchospasm	Bronchodilators; diuretics
Intercurrent infection	Antibiotics
Acute respiratory failure	Ensure patent airway Increase ventilatory support Increase bronchodilation and diuresis
Tracheobronchomalacia	Maintain end-distending pressure
Cor pulmonale	Oxygen and diuretic therapy
Neurodevelopmental delay	Ongoing neurodevelopmental assessment, with physical and occupational therapy
Malnutrition	Maximize balanced caloric intake at a minimum of 120 kcal/kg/day Optimize trace element and vitamin intake

References

1. Northway WH, Moss RB, Carlisle KB, et al: Late pulmonary sequelae of bronchopulmonary dysplasia. N Engl J Med 1990;323:1793–1799.
2. Northway WH Jr, Rosan RC, Porter DY: Pulmonary disease following respiratory therapy of hyaline membrane disease: Bronchopulmonary dysplasia. N Engl J Med 1967;276:357–368.
3. Jobe AH, Bancalari E: Bronchoplumonary dysplasia. Am J Respir Crit Care Med 2001;163:1723–1729.
4. Bancalari E, Abdenour GE, Feller R: Bronchopulmonary dysplasia: Clinical presentation. J Pediatr 1979;95:819–822.
5. Spitzer AR, Fox WW, Delivoria-Papadopoulos M: Maximum diuresis—A factor in predicting recovery from respiratory distress syndrome and the development of bronchopulmonary dysplasia. J Pediatr 1981;98:476–479.
6. Van Marter LJ, Leviton A, Allred EN, et al: Hydration during the first days of life and the risk of bronchopulmonary dysplasia in low birth weight infants. J Pediatr 1990;116:942–949.
7. Frank L, Sosenko IRS: Development of the lung antioxidant enzyme system in late gestation: Possible implications for the prematurely born infant. J Pediatr 1987;110:9–14.
8. Stenmark KR, Eyzaguine M, Westcott JY, et al: Potential role of lipid mediators of inflammation in bronchopulmonary dysplasia. Am Rev Respir Dis 1987;136:770–772.
9. Viscardi RM, Muhumuza CK, Rodriguez A, et al: Inflammatory markers in intrauterine and fetal blood and cerebrospinal fluid compartments are associated with adverse pulmonary and neurologic outcomes in preterm infants. Pediatr Res 2004; 55:1009–1017.
10. Tyson JE, Wright LL, Oh W, et al, for the National Institute of Child Health and Human Development Neonatal Research Network: Vitamin A supplementation for extremely-low-birth-weight infants. N Engl J Med 1999;340(25):1962–1968.
11. Hallman M, Pohjavuori M, Bry K: Inositol supplementation in respiratory distress syndrome. Lung 1990;168 (Suppl):877–882.
12. Gerdes JS, Harris MC, Dworanczyk R, et al: Effect of dexamethasone and intercurrent infection on tracheal lavage elastase and proteinase inhibitor in bronchopulmonary dysplasia. Pediatr Res 1986;20: 429A.
13. Gerdes JS, Yoder MC, Douglas SD, et al: Tracheal lavage and plasma fibronectin: Relationship to respiratory distress syndrome and development of bronchopulmonary dysplasia. J Pediatr 1986;108: 601–606.
14. Walsh MC, Wilson-Costello D, Zadell A, et al: Safety, reliability and validity of a physiologic definition of bronchopulmonary dysplasia. J Perinatol 2003;23: 451–456.
15. Edwards DK: Radiology of hyaline membrane disease, transient tachypnea of the newborn and bronchopulmonary dysplasia. In Farrell PM (ed): Lung Development: Biological and Clinical Perspectives, Vol 2. New York, Academic Press, 1982, pp 47–89.
16. Abman SH: Bronchopulmonary dysplasia: "A vascular hypothesis." Am J Respir Crit Care Med 2001;164:1755–1756.
17. Abman SH, Wolfe RR, Accurso FJ, et al: Pulmonary vascular response to oxygen in infants with severe bronchopulmonary dysplasia. J Pediatr 1985;75: 80–84.
18. Kao LC, Warburton D, Cheng MH, et al: Effect of oral diuretics on pulmonary mechanics in infants with chronic bronchopulmonary dysplasia: Results of a double-blind crossover sequential trial. J Pediatr 1984;73:509–514.
19. Hoffman DJ, Gerdes JS, Abbasi S: Pulmonary function and electrolyte balance following spironolactone treatment in preterm infants with chronic lung disease: A double-blind, placebo-controlled, randomized trial. J Perinatol 2000;1:41–45.
20. Watterberg KL, Gerdes JS, Cole CH, et al: Prophylaxis of early adrenal insufficiency to prevent bronchopulmonary dysplasia: A multicenter trial. Pediatrics 2004;114:1649–1657.
21. Cole CH, Colton T, Shah BL, et al: Early inhaled glucocorticosteroid therapy to prevent bronchopulmonary dysplasia. N Engl J Med 1999;340: 1005–1010.
22. Davis JM, Parad RB, Michele T, et al: North American Recombinant Human CuZnSOD Study Group: Pulmonary outcome at 1 year corrected age in premature infants treated at birth with recombinant human CuZn superoxide dismutase. Pediatrics 2003;111:46–476.
23. Abman SH, Warady BA, Lum GM, et al: Systemic hypertension in infants with bronchopulmonary dysplasia. J Pediatr 1984;104:928–931.
24. Blayney M, Kerem E, Whyte LL, et al: Bronchopulmonary dysplasia: Improvement on lung function between 7 and 10 years of age. J Pediatr 1991; 118:201–206.

Suggested Readings

Ambalavanan N, Carlo WA: Bronchopulmonary dysplasia: New insights. Clin Perinatol 2004;31: 613–628.

Autor AP, Frank L, Roberts RJ: Developmental characteristics of pulmonary superoxide dismutase: Relationships to idiopathic respiratory distress syndrome. Pediatr Res 1976;10:154–158.

Bader D, Ramos AD, Lew CD, et al: Childhood sequelae of infant lung disease: Exercise and pulmonary function abnormalities after bronchopulmonary dysplasia. J Pediatr 1987;110:693–699.

Baier RJ, Loggins J, Kruger TE: Failure of erythromycin to eliminate airway colonization with Ureaplasma urealyticum in very low birth weight infants. BMC Pediatr 2003;3:10.

Banks BA, Seri I, Ischiropoulos H, et al: Changes in oxygenation with inhaled nitric oxide in severe bronchopulmonary dysplasia. Pediatrics 1999;103: 610–618.

Barrington KJ: The adverse neuro-developmental effects of postnatal steroids in the preterm infant: A systematic review of RCTs. BMC Pediatr 2001;1:1.

Berman W, Katz R, Yabek SM, et al: Long-term follow-up of bronchopulmonary dysplasia. J Pediatr 1986; 109:45–50.

Bernbaum JC, Williamson-Hoffman M: Chronic lung disease of infancy, bronchopulmonary dysplasia. Prim Care Preterm Infant 1991;5:87–119.

Bhutani VK, Abbasi S: Relative likelihood of bronchopulmonary dysplasia based on pulmonary mechanics in preterm neonates during the first week of life. J Pediatr 1992;120:605–613.

Bonikos DS, Bensch KC, Northway WH: Bronchopulmonary dysplasia: The pulmonary pathologic sequel of necrotizing broncholitis and pulmonary fibrosis. Hum Pathol 1976;7:643.

Bowman CM, Lloyd CL, Scanlon KL, et al: Mechanisms of pulmonary vascular injury and repair: Hyperoxia decreases endothelial cell synthesis of DNA and protein. Am Rev Respir Dis 1986;133:A298.

Brown ER: Increased risk of bronchopulmonary dysplasia in infants with patent ductus arteriosus. J Pediatr 1979;95:865–866.

Brown ER, Stark A, Sosenkin I, et al: Bronchopulmonary dysplasia: Possible relationship to pulmonary edema. J Pediatr 1978;92:982–984.

Bruce MC, Wedig KE, Jentoft N, et al: Altered urinary excretion of elastin cross-links in premature infants who develop bronchopulmonary dysplasia. Am Rev Respir Dis 1985;131:568–572.

Byrne PJ, Piper MC, Darrah J: Motor development at term of very low birth weight infants with BPD. J Perinatol 1989;9:301–306.

Cassell GH, Waites KB, Crouse DT, et al: Association of *Ureaplasma urealyticum* infection of the lower respiratory tract with chronic lung disease and death in very-low-birth-weight infants. Lancet 1988;2: 240–245.

Chandra RK Influence of nutrition-immunity axis on perinatal infection. In Ogra PL (ed): Neonatal Infection, Vol 14. Orlando, FL, Grune & Stratton, 1984, pp 229–245.

Coalson JJ: Pathology of new bronchopulmonary dysplasia. Semin Neonatal 2003;8:73–81.

Committee on Fetus and Newborn: Postnatal costicosteroids to treat or prevent chronic lung disease in preterm infants. Pediatrics 2002;109: 330–338.

Crapo JD, Barry BE, Fascise HA, et al: Structural and biochemical changes in rat lungs occurring during oxygen exposures to lethal and adaptive doses of oxygen. Am Rev Respir Dis 1978;122:123–143.

Davis WB, Rennard SI, Bitterman PB, et al: Pulmonary oxygen toxicity: Early reversible changes in human alveolar structures induced by hyperoxia. N Engl J Med 1983;309:878–883.

Englehardt B, Gerhardt T: Short and long-term effects of furosemide on lung function in infants with bronchopulmonary dysplasia. J Pediatr 1986;109: 1034–1039.

Frank L, Groseclose EE: Oxygen toxicity in newborn rats: The adverse effect of undernutrition. J Appl Physiol 1982;53:1248–1256.

Fujimura M, Kitajima H, Nakayama M: Increased leukocyte elastase of the tracheal aspirate at birth and neonatal pulmonary emphysema. Pediatrics 1993; 92:564–569.

Goldman SL, Gerhardt T, Sonni R, et al: Early prediction of chronic lung disease by pulmonary function testing. J Pediatr 1983;102:613–617.

Greenspan JS, Abbasi S, Bhutani VK: Sequential changes in pulmonary mechanics in the very low birthweight (1000 gm) infants. J Pediatr 1988; 113:732–737.

Greenspan JS, DeGiulio PA, Bhutani VK: Airway reactivity as determined by a cold air challenge in infants with bronchopulmonary dysplasia. J Pediatr 1988; 114:452–454.

Groneck P, Speer CP: Inflammatory mediators and bronchopulmonary dysplasia. Arch Dis Child 1995; 73:F1–F3.

Heldt GP Pulmonary status of infants and children with bronchopulmonary dysplasia. In Merritt TA, Northway WH Jr, Boynton BR (eds): Contemporary Issues in Fetal and Neonatal Medicine, Vol 25. Boston, Blackwell Scientific Publications, 1985, pp 421–438.

Howlett A, Ohlsson A: Inositol for respiratory distress syndrome in preterm infants. Cochrane Database Syst Rev 2003;(4):CD000366.

Husain AN, Siddiqui NH, Stocker JT: Pathology of arrested acinar development in postsurfactant bronchopulmony dysplasia. Hum Pathol 1998;29: 710–717.

Kao LC, Durand DJ, Nickerson BG: Improving pulmonary function does not decrease oxygen consumption in infants with bronchopulmonary dysplasia. J Pediatr 1988;112:616–621.

Kirpalani H, Jordana M, Irving L, et al: Effects of oxygen exposure on human neonatal pulmonary fibroblast proliferation. Pediatr Res 1988;23:512A.

Langston C, Kida K, Reed M, et al: Human lung growth in late gestation and in the neonate. Am Rev Respir Dis 1984;129:607–613.

Lorenz J, Kleinman L, Kotagal U, et al: Water balance in very low birth weight infants, relationship to water and sodium intake and effect on outcome. J Pediatr 1982;101:423–432.

Mallory GB, Chaney LL, Munch RI, et al: Longitudinal changes in lung function during the first three years of life in premature infants with moderate to severe bronchopulmonary dysplasia. Pediatr Pulmonol 1991;11:8–14.

Mariani G, Cifuentes J, Carlo WA: Randomized trial of permissive hypercapnia in preterm infants. Pediatrics 1999;104:1082–1088.

Merritt TA, Cochrane CG, Holcomb K, et al: Elastase and alpha-1-proteinase inhibitor activity in tracheal aspirates during respiratory distress syndrome: Role of inflammation in the pathogenesis of bronchopulmonary dysplasia. J Clin Invest 1983;72: 656–666.

Mirmanesh SJ, Abbasi S, Bhutani VK: Alpha-adrenergic bronchoprovocation in neonates with bronchopulmonary dysplasia. J Pediatr 1992;121: 622–625.

Motoyama EK, Fort MD, Klesh KW, et al: Early onset of airway reactivity in premature infants with bronchopulmonary dysplasia. Am Rev Respir Dis 1987; 136:50–57.

Moylan FMB, Walker AM, Krammer SS, et al: Alveolar rupture as an independent predictor of bronchopulmonary dysplasia. Crit Care Med 1978;6:10–13.

Nickerson BG, Taussig LM: Family history of asthma in infants with bronchopulmonary dysplasia. Pediatrics 1980;65:1140–1144.

NICU Quality Management Report. Burlington, VT, Vermont Oxford Neonatal Network, 2004.

O'Brodovich H, Coates G: Pulmonary clearance of TcDTPA in infants who subsequently develop bronchopulmonary dysplasia. Am Rev Respir Dis 1988;137:210–212.

O'Brodovich HM, Mellins RB: Bronchopulmonary dysplasia: Unresolved neonatal acute lung injury. Am Rev Respir Dis 1985;132:694–709.

Ogden BE, Murphy SA, Saunders GC, et al: Neonatal lung neutrophils and elatase/proteinase inhibitor imbalance. Am Rev Respir Dis 1984;130: 817–821.

Oh W, Poindexter BB, Perritt R, et al: for the Neonatal Research Network: Association between fluid intake and weight loss during the first ten days of life and risk of bronchopulmonary dysplasia in extremely low birth weight infants. J Pediatr 2005;147: 786–790.

Ohki Y, Kato M, Kimura H, et al: Elevated type IV collagen in bronchoaveolar lavage fluid from infants with bronchopulmonary dysplasia. Biol Neonate 2001;79:34–38.

Peltoniemi O, Karli A, Heinonen K, et al: Pretreatment cortisol values may predict responses to hydrocortisone administration for the prevention of bronchopulmonary dysplasia in high-risk infants. J Pediatr 2005;146:632–637.

Rajagopalan L, Abbasi S, Gerdes JS, et al: Tracheobronchomalacia evaluated by airflow mechanics and direct bronchoscopy. Pediatr Res 1988;23:321A.

Roberts RJ, Weisner KM, Bucker JR: Oxygen-induced alterations in lung vascular development in the newborn rat. Pediatr Res 1983;17:368–375.

Rosenfeld W, Concepcion L, Evans H, et al: Serial trypsin inhibitory capacity and ceruloplasmin levels in prematures at risk for bronchopulmonary dysplasia. Am Rev Respir Dis 1986;134:1229–1232.

Rotschild A, Solimano A, Puterman M, et al: Increased compliance in response to salbutamol in premature infants with developing bronchopulmonary dysplasia. J Pediatr 1989;115:984–991.

Rush MG, Engelhardt B, Parker RA, et al: Double-blind, placebo-controlled trial of alternate-day furosemide therapy in infants with chronic bronchopulmonary dysplasia. J Pediatr 1990;117:112–118.

Shennan AT, Dunn MS, Ohlsson A, et al: Abnormal pulmonary outcomes in premature infants: Prediction from oxygen requirement in the neonatal period. Pediatrics 1988;82:527.

Sherman FS: Cor pulmonale. In Merritt TA, Northway WH Jr, Boynton BR (eds): Contemporary Issues in Fetal and Neonatal Medicine, Vol 14, Boston, Blackwell Scientific Publications, 1985, pp 251–262.

Sherman MP, Evans MJ, Campbell LA: Prevention of pulmonary alveolar macrophage proliferation in newborn rabbits by hyperoxia. J Pediatr 1988;112: 782–786.

Shoemaker CT, Reiser KM, Goetzman BE, et al: Elevated ratios of type I/III collagen in the lung of chronically ventilated neonates with respiratory distress. Pediatr Res 1984;18:1176–1180.

Singel BD, Maisels MJ, Ballantine VN: Gastroesophageal reflux to the proximal esophagus in infants with bronchopulmonary dysplasia. Am J Dis Child 1989; 143:1103–1106.

Soll RF: Synthetic surfactant treatment of RDS. In Chalmers I (ed): Oxford Database of Perinatal Trials, version 1.2, disk issue 6, record 5252 (Autumn 1991).

Sotomayor JL, Godinez RI, Borden S, et al: Large airway collapse due to acquired tracheobronchomalacia in infancy. Am J Dis Child 1986;140:367–371.

Stark AR, Waldemar CA, Jon TE, et al, for the National Institute of Child Health and Human Development Neonatal Research Network: Adverse effects of early dexamethasone treatment in extremely-low-birth-weight infants. N Engl J Med 2001;344:95–101.

Sunday ME, Yoder BA, Cuttitta F, et al: Bombesin-like peptide mediates lung injury in a baboon model of bronchopulmonary dysplasia. J Clin Invest 1998; 102:584–594.

Tay-Uyboco JS, Kwiatkowski K, Cates DB, et al: Hypoxic airway constriction in infants of very low birth weight recovering from moderate to severe bronchopulmonary dysplasia. J Pediatr 1989;115: 456–459.

Tepper RS, Morgan WA, Cata K, et al: Expiratory flow limitation in infants with bronchopulmonary dysplasia. J Pediatr 1986;109:1040–1046.

Thibeault DW, Mabry SM, Ekekezie II, et al: Collagen scaffolding during development and its deformation with chronic lung disease. Pediatrics 2003;111: 766–776.

Thibeault DW, Mabry SM, Ekekezie II, Truog WE: Lung elastic tissue maturation and perturbations during the evolution of chronic lung disease. Pediatrics 2000;106:1452–1459.

Tomashefski JF Jr, Oppermann HC, Vawter GE, et al: Bronchopulmonary dysplasia: A morphometric study with emphasis on the pulmonary vasculature. Pediatr Pathol 1984;2:469–487.

Van Marter LJ, Allred EN, Pagano M, et al: Do clinical markers of barotrauma and oxygen toxicity explain interhopsital variation in rates of chronic lung diease? Pediatrics 2000;405:1194–1201.

Van Marter LJ, Leviton A, Kuban KCK, et al: Maternal glucocorticoid therapy and reduced risk of bronchopulmonary dysplasia. Pediatrics 1990;86: 331–336.

Ward JA, Roberts RJ: Effects of hyperoxia on phosphatidylcholine synthesis, secretion, uptake and stability in the newborn rabbit lung. Biochim Biophys Acta 1984;796:42–50.

Watterberg KL, Demers LM, Scott SM, et al: Chorioamnionitis and early lung inflammation in infants in whom bronchopulmonary dysplasia develops. Pediatrics 1996;97:210–215.

Watts JL, Milner R, Zipursky A, et al: Failure of supplementation with vitamin E to prevent bronchopulmonary dysplasia in infants less than 1500 g birth weight. Eur Respir J 1991;4:188–190.

Welty SE: Antioxidants and oxidations in bronchopulmonary dysplasia: There are no easy answers. J Pediatr 2003;143:697–698.

Yeh TF, Lin YJ, Huang CC, et al: Early dexamethasone therapy in preterm infants: A follow-up study. Pediatrics 1998;105:e7.

Yoon BH, Romero R, Jun JK, et al: Amniotic fluid cytokines (interleukin-6, tumor necrosis factor-alpha, interleukin-1B, and interleukin-8) and the risk for the development of bronchopulmonary dysplasia. Am J Obstet Gynecol 1997;177:825–830.

Breathing Disorders

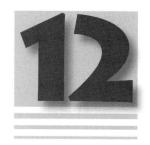

Robert A. Darnall, MD

This chapter reviews conditions that cause alterations in breathing patterns in newborn infants. Some of the clinical problems associated with alterations in respiratory control are shown in Table 12-1. Breathing, or ventilation, is the process of exchange of air between the lungs and the environment, and clearly is essential for life. The physiology involved in the control of respiration is intriguing, and is an example of one of the many cyclic phenomena that take place in nature. Respiration is a short-term cyclic phenomenon that involves the brain, lungs, airways, heart, circulation, peripheral and central sensors, and interconnections among these organ systems. Table 12-2 illustrates examples of respiratory control abnormalities originating in some of these areas. Respiratory instability, periodic breathing, and apnea are the most commonly encountered signs of respiratory control abnormalities in the newborn period. This chapter focuses largely on the diagnosis and management of apnea but also considers the respiratory control abnormalities present in infants with bronchopulmonary dysplasia (BPD). A thorough understanding of how the normal system

functions and the changes that occur during development is essential to the diagnosis and management of abnormal and sometimes life-threatening breathing patterns.

Physiology of the Respiratory Control System

The respiratory control system has both involuntary and voluntary components. The major function of the involuntary control component is the exchange of oxygen and carbon dioxide in the lungs. The relative contributions of the voluntary and involuntary components to the total control of breathing depend on the demands placed on the overall system. For example, during sleep, the involuntary component largely determines the level of ventilation. During other activities, such as exercise, speech, or eating, the voluntary or behavioral control component has more influence. Although the identification of voluntary activities that affect breathing are relatively straightforward in the adult, the study of respiratory control during development from the fetus to the adult has been difficult because of variables that are age related. For example, the time spent sleeping varies significantly in the fetus (who, data suggest, sleeps all the time), the newly born infant (who sleeps most of the time), and the adult (who usually sleeps one third of the time). The fetus and newborn do not respond to voluntary commands in the same way as the adult. Furthermore, measurements in the newborn are most often made in the supine position, compared with the sitting position in the adult. In the newborn

---

TABLE 12-1

COMMON PROBLEMS IN THE NEWBORN RELATED TO RESPIRATORY CONTROL

Apnea of prematurity
Periodic breathing
Upper airway obstruction
Central hypoventilation syndrome
Abnormalities of the central nervous system
Bronchopulmonary dysplasia

TABLE 12-2

STRUCTURES INVOLVED IN RESPIRATORY CONTROL: EXAMPLES OF DISORDERS AND BREATHING PATTERNS

Structure	Disorder	Breathing Pattern
Forebrain	Seizure	Apnea, irregular breathing
Medulla	Arnold-Chiari malformation	Low respiratory rates, hypoventilation
Cervical spinal cord	High cord transection	Respiratory muscle paralysis
Phrenic nerve	Brachial plexus injury, phrenic nerve agenesis	Diaphragmatic paralysis
Diaphragm	Eventration	Increased work by accessory muscles
Lung	Bronchopulmonary dysplasia	Tachypnea, increased work of breathing, apnea
Upper airways	Tracheomalacia, laryngomalacia	Stridor, obstructive apnea

infant, therefore, the voluntary component does not appear to be as active as in the adult. Nevertheless, behaviors such as stretching, crying, and sucking can greatly alter the baseline metabolic respiratory drive. For example, during feeding in the newborn and young infant, breathing can be interrupted to the point that bradycardia, decreases in oxyhemoglobin saturation, and even apnea can occur. Figure 12-1 illustrates the effects of sucking on minute ventilation in two groups of premature infants. Note the almost 50% reduction in minute ventilation during continuous sucking in the younger group.

Organization of the Respiratory Control System

Neuronal elements of respiratory rhythmogenesis that drive the respiratory muscles involved in both the involuntary and the voluntary components of the respiratory control system are shown in Figure 12-2. Normal respiration results from the alternating discharge of several groups of neurons that drive the respiratory muscles. During inspiration, the diaphragm and external intercostal muscles contract, expanding the chest cavity, creating a negative pressure that draws air into the lungs. An important component of inspiration, especially in the newborn, is the pattern of contraction of upper airway muscles that maintains the patency of the pharynx and larynx (see later discussion). Cervical (phrenic nerve) and thoracic lower motor neurons innervate the diaphragm and intercostal muscles. The upper airway muscles are innervated by brain stem neurons with efferents in the glossopharyngeal, vagus, and hypoglossal nerves. In contrast, the elastic recoil forces accumulated during inspiration largely accomplish expiration. As a result, expiratory muscles such as the internal intercostals and abdominals are less active during quiet breathing.

Some behavior affecting breathing is voluntary, in that it involves the cerebral cortex stimulating respiratory lower motor neurons. In the newborn, however, activities that may affect breathing, such as arm and leg movement, crying, and sucking frequently originate in the

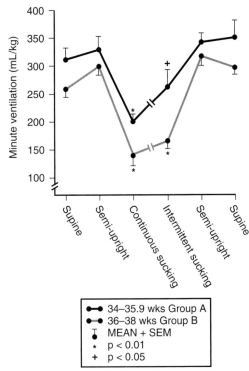

Figure 12-1 Minute ventilation during feeding in two groups of premature infants. Ventilation during the continuous sucking phase is significantly lower than control infants in both groups. Note that greater reduction in ventilation occurs in the more immature group of infants. (Adapted from Mathew OP: Respiratory control during oral feeding. In Mathew OP [ed]: Respiratory Control and Disorders in the Newborn. New York, Marcel Dekker, 2003, p 380; vol 173 in the series by Claude Lenfant [ed]: Lung Biology in Health and Disease.)

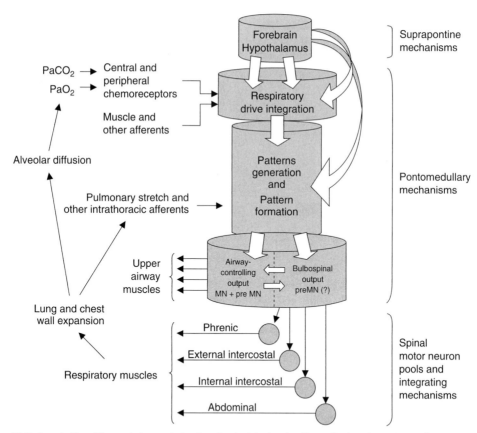

Figure 12-2 Organization of the respiratory control system. Emphasis is placed on the mechanisms for respiratory drive integration and respiratory pattern generation and formation, and their influences on the two main output systems that control the upper airway and respiratory muscles. The behavioral component of the control system with direct connections between the cerebral cortex and the lower motor neurons is not shown. pre-MN. (Adapted from Euler CV: Breathing and behaviour. In Euler CV, Lagercrantz H [eds]: Neurobiology of the Control of Breathing. New York, Raven Press, 1987, p 4.)

brain stem or spinal column and may or may not involve neurons in the cerebral cortex. In contrast, the involuntary component of the control system originates entirely in the medulla and pons. Most of our information about neurons involved in respiration has been derived from the study of small mammals such as the cat and rat. In these species, networks of neurons responsible for rhythm generation are located in the medulla. A group of cells in the rostral ventral medulla in an area termed "the pre-Bötzinger complex" is essential to the network. These neurons exhibit bursting pacemaker properties and are believed to be the "kernel" responsible for respiratory rhythm. The mechanisms responsible for the alternating pattern of inspiration and expiration are not fully understood, but most likely include the characteristics of the individual respiratory neurons, the connections between them, and the resulting network characteristics. Recordings of the activity of neurons that discharge in synchrony with respiration show that

there are several distinct patterns coinciding with different phases of respiration, such as inspiration and expiration. For example, neurons that discharge during inspiration are commonly called inspiratory neurons, and those that fire primarily during expiration are referred to as expiratory neurons. Other groups of neurons discharge only during early expiration or "post-inspiration," whereas some neurons are active during both inspiration and expiration. The activity of these medullary neuronal networks is influenced by many excitatory and inhibitory inputs from chemoreceptors, mechanoreceptors, and other areas of the brain, including the forebrain and the hypothalamus (see Fig. 12-2).

Neurons in the pre-Bötzinger complex synapse with neurons located predominantly in two areas. Mostly inspiratory neurons are located in the dorsal respiratory group (DRG) in the dorsal medulla. A second group of both inspiratory and expiratory neurons is located in the ventral respiratory group (VRG), which lies ventral and lateral to the DRG. Most DRG neurons have direct connections to phrenic or inspiratory intercostal neurons. During quiet breathing, expiration is mostly passive and, therefore, most expiratory neurons are active only when ventilation is increased. The pneumotaxic center, or pontine respiratory group (PRG), consists of groups of neurons in the rostral pons. These cells are thought to be important in terminating inspiration.

Airway Control during Breathing

Maintaining the patency of the upper airway during inspiration is particularly important for the newborn infant because of the airway's propensity to collapse. The airway of the newborn is more compliant than in the adult, and the anatomic arrangement of the upper airway favors obstruction, particularly when the neck is flexed. Figure 12-3 illustrates the various collapsing and dilating forces operating on the newborn airway. During extreme flexion, it appears that the airway can collapse even under conditions of positive pressure. Under normal physiologic conditions, the contractions of the muscles controlling the patency of the upper airway are timed to occur just before

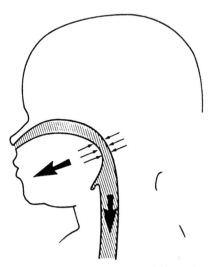

Figure 12-3 Collapsing (*small arrows*) and dilating (*large arrows*) forces acting on the upper airway. This sagittal section of the upper airway demonstrates various forces operating either to collapse the pharynx or to maintain its patency during normal respiration. (Adapted from Miller MJ, Martin RJ: Pathophysiology of apnea of prematurity. In Polin RA, Fox WW [eds]: Fetal and Neonatal Physiology. Philadelphia, WB Saunders, 1992.)

contraction of the diaphragm. Alterations in this timing can promote upper airway obstruction. At the level of the pharynx, the genioglossus muscle plays a major role in maintaining patency by pulling the tongue and hyoid bone toward the mandible. At the level of the larynx, the posterior cricoarytenoid (PCA) muscle opens the vocal cords during inspiration. It has been observed in normal full-term infants that, unlike the coordinated activity observed in adults, the PCA often contracts simultaneously with or even after the diaphragm in a high percentage of breaths.

During expiration, there is also a need to modify airflow through the airways, largely because of the tendency for the lung to collapse secondary to the compliant chest wall of the newborn. This is particularly evident during rapid eye movement (REM) sleep (see later discussion). During early expiration (often termed postinspiration), there is often a residual contraction (mostly of the lateral portions of the diaphragm) and increased activity in the major laryngeal constrictors. This phenomenon has been termed *expiratory braking* and serves to prolong expiratory time and preserve lung volume.

Effects of Arousal and Sleep State on Respiratory Control

The resting breathing pattern of the newborn, particularly the premature newborn, is generally irregular. There is a large degree of breath-to-breath variability accompanied by long stretches of "periodic breathing" in which regular breathing alternates with apnea. The resting breathing pattern of the neonate does not appear to be totally sleep-state dependent, although sleep greatly modulates it. The newborn infant sleeps the majority of the time, and 50% and 90% of that time is REM sleep. Sleep is usually classified by a combination of electroencephalogram (EEG) and behavioral criteria. Quiet or non-REM sleep is difficult to define before 32 weeks' gestation. In general, sleep depresses ventilatory and arousal responses and many respiratory reflexes.

In the adult, as the state changes from wakefulness to sleep, breathing tends to become more regular; metabolic rate and inputs from central and peripheral chemoreceptors largely determine minute ventilation. During sleep, minute ventilation decreases, on average, and is accompanied by a slight increase is Pa_{CO_2}. In the newborn during sleep, brief periods of regular breathing alternate with longer periods of irregular breathing. In both the newborn and the adult, it is likely that sleep removes excitatory inputs from the reticular activating (arousal) system that are normally present during wakefulness. During REM sleep, breathing is irregular, with marked variability in the rate and depth of breathing. In addition, there is loss of muscle activity in intercostal and airway-maintaining musculature. In the newborn, the loss of phasic inspiratory activity in upper airway muscles contributes to a greater risk of upper airway obstruction. The inhibition of respiratory muscle activity, especially those muscles contributing to expiratory braking mechanisms, in combination with the generally compliant chest wall, puts the infant at a mechanical disadvantage, increasing the potential for reduced end-expiratory lung volume. Table 12-3 summarizes the physiologic changes in REM sleep and the effects on respiration.

Periodic breathing, or alternating periods of hyperpnea and apnea, is a common breathing pattern in premature infants and occurs throughout the sleep cycles. As the infant matures, and non-REM (quiet) sleep can be better defined, periodic breathing can be identified in both sleep states. The difference is that during REM sleep, the periodicity is accompanied by irregular breathing, whereas during quiet sleep, the periodic breathing is regular, with breathing and apneic intervals of similar duration. Figure 12-4 shows examples of periodic breathing during REM and non-REM sleep. Although the mechanisms have not been fully elucidated, it is likely that the periods of hyperpnea or hyperventilation may decrease Pa_{CO_2} and reduce the stimulus to breathe, resulting in apnea. The transition from regular to periodic breathing, however, does not usually occur

abruptly. In premature infants, the depth of breathing tends to oscillate in relatively slow cycles. True periodic breathing or apnea emerges when the lowest depth segments of the breathing cycle actually pause.

Thermoregulation, Metabolism, and the Control of Breathing

Metabolic rate increases after birth to meet the demands for growth and heat production. The increased oxygen demand and carbon dioxide production in turn increase respiratory drive. Temperature-related stimulation may be particularly important for sustained breathing after birth. The relatively narrow thermoneutral range of the neonate may also affect respiratory control. Under steady-state conditions, ventilation is closely matched to metabolic rate. Figure 12-5 illustrates the general relationships between ambient and body temperature, metabolism, and ventilation. In the newborn infant, heat production is largely accomplished by the oxidative metabolism of brown fat, producing what is known as nonshivering thermogenesis. Nonshivering thermogenesis is an oxidative process. Infants who are hypoxic, therefore, cannot respond normally to cold stress. In addition, in many species, the metabolic response to cooling is blunted during REM sleep. In the newborn human, however, this does not appear to be the case. As the metabolic rate of brown fat declines, the ability to produce heat by shivering and by regulation of cutaneous blood flow takes precedence. A diurnal rhythm in body temperature develops over the first 2 months of life. In animals, and possibly in human neonates, increasing environmental temperature reduces the gain of respiratory responses. This, combined with the reduced metabolic respiratory drive at

---

TABLE 12-3

PHYSIOLOGIC CHANGES IN RAPID EYE MOVEMENT SLEEP AND EFFECTS ON RESPIRATION

Physiologic Change	Potential Consequences
Decreased intercostals and upper airway muscle tone and phasic respiratory activity	Increased inspiratory chest wall paradoxical movement Susceptibility to upper airway collapse Increased diaphragmatic work of breathing
Decreased response to pulmonary afferent mechanoreceptor feedback	Decreased recruitment of abdominal muscles
Decreased response to peripheral and central chemoreceptor stimulation	Decreased ventilatory and arousal responses to hypercapnia and hypoxia

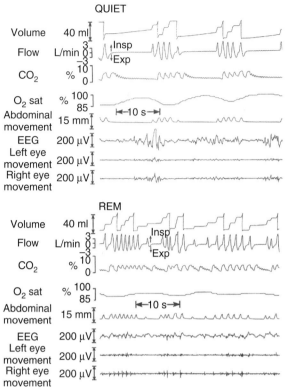

Figure 12-4 Periodic breathing in one preterm infant during quiet and REM sleep. Note that periodic breathing is more regular in quiet sleep; that is, the apneas and breathing intervals are nearly constant, as opposed to the irregular periodicity observed in REM sleep. (Copyright © 2003 from Mathew OP [ed]: Respiratory Control and Disorders in the Newborn. New York, Marcel Dekker, 2003; reproduced by permission of Routledge/Taylor and Francis Group, LLC.)

warmer temperatures, may predispose an infant to develop apnea. In a clinical setting, for example, clusters of apnea can often be observed after a rapid rise in incubator air temperature. Infants who are weaned from their incubators too quickly can also be at increased risk for apnea. In this case, a large energy expenditure is necessary to maintain body temperature, and in extreme cases, this can lead to decreased ability to defend against hypoxia with increasing ventilation, resulting in more apnea and periodic breathing.

Mechanoreflexes

During lung inflation, slowly adapting pulmonary stretch receptors, innervated by the vagus nerve, are stimulated and help to terminate inspiration. This phenomenon is known as the Hering-Breuer inflation inhibition reflex. The reflex appears to be much more active in newborn infants than in adults. There are also rapidly adapting pulmonary receptors, such as

irritant receptors, that can be stimulated both chemically (smoke, noxious gases) and mechanically (particulate matter or changes in airflow). These receptors are located mostly in the larger airways and appear to be poorly developed in premature infants. Their stimulation may augment inspiratory activity, but in older infants, it can also constrict the airway and cause coughing or rapid shallow breathing. The very rapid breathing that occurs after aspiration of meconium or amniotic fluid may be an example of irritant receptor stimulation. In addition, afferents from chest wall proprioceptors convey information about chest wall movement and the forces exerted by respiratory muscles.

The paradoxic reflex of Head was first described in 1889. When the lungs are rapidly inflated, there is a further inspiration, rather than inhibition. This reflex is commonly observed in neonates in the form of a sigh. Sighs are common in premature infants, are more frequent during REM sleep than during quiet sleep, and are also more common during periodic

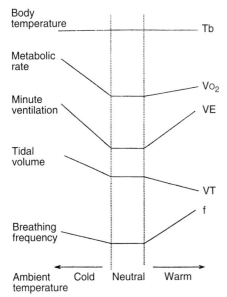

Figure 12-5 Thermoregulation and breathing. Relationship between ambient temperature and body temperature (Tb), metabolic rate ($\dot{V}o_2$), minute ventilation ($\dot{V}e$), tidal volume (V_T), and breathing frequency (f). For modest drops or increases in ambient temperature (as assumed here), Tb does not change. $\dot{V}o_2$ and $\dot{V}e$ have minimal values at thermoneutrality, and V_T increases and decreases, respectively, below and above thermoneutrality; f increases slightly with low ambient temperature and markedly above thermoneutrality. (Adapted from Mortola JP, Gautier H: Interaction between metabolism and ventilation: Effects of respiratory gases and temperature. In Dempsey JA, Pack AI [eds]: Regulation of Breathing. New York, Marcel Dekker, 1995, p 1034.)

breathing. It is thought that the high incidence of sighs in premature infants reflects a greater need for lung recruitment at this age.

Laryngeal Reflexes

The larynx contains mechanoreceptors and chemoreceptors that respond to various stimuli, including pressure and airflow, hyperosmolar solutions, milk, water, and carbon dioxide. Information from these receptors is carried in the superior laryngeal nerve. In older infants and adults, a typical response to the introduction of certain liquids into the larynx includes cough, expiratory efforts, and swallowing. In newborns, however, the response can include apnea and bradycardia, followed by swallowing. This response pattern is most marked in premature infants. In newborn infants, gastroesophageal reflux may stimulate laryngeal receptors, inducing apnea. In animal experiments, apnea caused by electrical stimulation of the superior laryngeal nerve, or by the introduction of water

into the larynx, persists long after the end of the stimulus. In older infants, respiratory syncytial virus (RSV) infection has been associated with laryngeal apnea.

Chemical Regulation of Breathing

Respiratory rate and tidal volume are regulated by feedback mechanisms involving chemoreceptors that sense Pao_2 and $Paco_2$, which in turn trigger changes in minute ventilation to maintain blood gases and pH within some normal range. An increase in $Paco_2$ or a decrease in Pao_2 increases excitatory input to central respiratory neural networks, increasing respiratory muscle activity, augmenting the exchange of carbon dioxide and oxygen. Although blood gas changes in the opposite direction can result in a decrease in minute ventilation, the response is weak compared with the excitatory response. Under normoxic conditions, $Paco_2$ largely determines minute ventilation. In infants with chronic lung disease, however, who often have chronic elevations in $Paco_2$, these responses may be blunted and "hypoxic drive" may become an important determinant of minute ventilation, particularly during sleep.

Response to Hypercapnia. Central chemoreceptors are largely responsible for sensing changes in carbon dioxide and are located in the brain stem, predominantly on the ventral surface of the medulla, but in several other locations as well. Stimulation of these receptors results in an increase in minute ventilation. When exposed to an elevated level of carbon dioxide, several minutes are required to reach a full excitatory response. This relatively slow time course, together with the large body stores of carbon dioxide, helps eliminate rapid changes in ventilation and stabilize breathing.

In the newborn infant, the response to carbon dioxide is usually assessed by measuring respiratory variables after increasing the inspired carbon dioxide concentration (3% to 5%). This response is diminished in immature infants younger than 33 weeks postconceptual age. It has also been reported that the slope of the ventilatory response to hypercapnia is decreased in premature infants with apnea of prematurity compared with those without apnea. A cause-and-effect relationship, however, has not been clearly established. There is also some evidence that the response to carbon dioxide is blunted

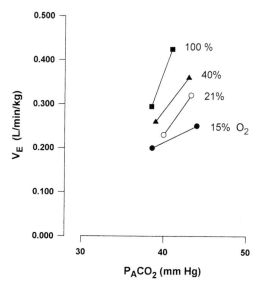

Figure 12-6 Ventilatory response to hypercapnia. Carbon dioxide sensitivity measured in premature infants after achieving steady state at different concentrations of oxygen. The lower the oxygen percentage, the less the response to increased inhaled carbon dioxide. This response is opposite to that seen in adults. (Adapted from Rigatto H: Apnea. Pediatr Clin North Am 1982;29:1105–1116.)

Response to Hypoxia. In the newborn infant, a decrease in Pao_2 causes an initial increase in minute ventilation, followed by a more sustained decrease, often to baseline levels, or even apnea. As shown in Figure 12-7, this "biphasic" ventilatory response to hypoxia is different from that in the older child or adult, in whom the increase in minute ventilation is more sustained. In the fetus, fetal breathing movements are decreased or abolished during hypoxic episodes. Thus, the differences in the responses of the fetus, the newborn, and the adult may represent a developmental continuum. Similar mechanisms may be involved, but the balance and timing of the excitatory and depressive components of the response may change with development. In the biphasic ventilatory response to hypoxia, an initial increase in minute ventilation results from stimulation of peripheral chemoreceptors located primarily in carotid bodies at the junction of the internal and common carotid arteries. The excitatory input from the carotid bodies to the brain stem respiratory centers travels in the carotid sinus branch of the glossopharyngeal nerve and appears to be sustained. It is likely that the late decrease in minute ventilation originates centrally and ultimately overrides the excitatory inputs, resulting in a net decrease in ventilation. The mechanisms responsible for the central "depression"

during periods of REM sleep. Unlike the augmenting effects of hypoxia in the adult, coexisting hypoxia in the newborn diminishes the ventilatory response to carbon dioxide (Fig. 12–6).

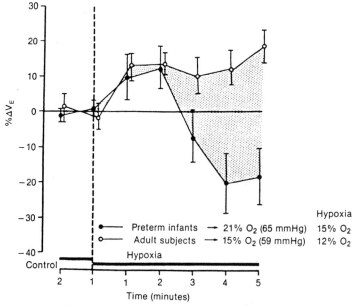

Figure 12-7 Ventilatory response to hypoxia in premature infants and adults. Percent change in ventilation when 15% oxygen was substituted for 21% oxygen in preterm infants (*closed circles*) and when 12% oxygen was substituted for 15% oxygen in adult subjects (*open circles*). The initial increase in ventilation is sustained in adults but not in preterm infants. (Adapted from Rigatto H: Maturation of breathing. In Hunt CE [ed]: Apnea and SIDS. Clin Perinatol 1992;4:739–756.)

of ventilation have not been completely elucidated but probably include changes in metabolism and local perfusion and the production of inhibitory neuromodulators such as adenosine and γ-aminobutyric acid (GABA).

Recent evidence suggests that certain areas in the midbrain or rostral pons may also contribute to the decrease in ventilation produced by hypoxia in the fetus and neonate. It has been postulated that these regions may contain neurons that function as "oxygen sensors" that, when activated, inhibit brain stem respiratory neurons. In addition, in the conscious animal or human, arousal is an important component of the total behavioral response to hypoxia. During REM sleep, this component appears to be blunted.

Maturation of Respiratory Control

The control of lung volume, laryngeal reflexes, patency of the upper airway, and the incidence of apnea all change over the course of maturation. An important characteristic of the respiratory system in the newborn is the highly compliant chest wall. To maintain an adequate end-expiratory lung volume, there must be mechanisms activated to interrupt expiration and initiate inspiration before deflation is complete. This is accomplished by decreasing expiratory time and retarding expiratory airflow by sustained activity of the diaphragm and laryngeal narrowing. Mechanical stability of the respiratory system is a greater challenge in preterm infants, owing in part to their more compliant chest wall. Although many of the breathing strategies used by term infants to defend lung volume are in place, the vulnerability of preterm infants is increased by the longer time spent in REM sleep, a more irregular respiratory rhythm, and frequent breathing pauses. With maturation, chest wall compliance decreases and the mechanical advantage of the chest wall muscles improves, enhancing the mechanical stability of the respiratory system.

The ventilatory response to hypoxia, which is "biphasic" in the early newborn period, also matures with age, becoming more like the adult response within a few weeks of life. Because the pattern of this response is due to the net sum of the excitatory effects of carotid body stimulation and the slightly delayed inhibitory effects of brain stem hypoxia, a change to a more sustained excitatory response could be secondary to a combination of a strengthening of the carotid body response and an attenuation of central inhibition.

Respiratory Control in Infants with Bronchopulmonary Dysplasia

The improved survival of extremely immature neonates over the course of the last 20 years has not been without significant cost. Approximately 30% of infants who weigh less than 1000 g at birth develop chronic lung disease. Our knowledge about the specific abnormalities of respiratory control in infants with bronchopulmonary dysplasia (BPD) is limited. However, there is some information about other groups of infants with chronic lung disease, and it is likely that infants with BPD have similar alterations in respiratory control. More important, infants recovering from severe BPD may be at increased risk for sudden death. It is possible that impaired responses to hypoxia and hypercapnia, together with changes in respiratory control that occur during sleep, may contribute to this increased risk.

Peripheral Chemoreceptors, the Ventilatory Response to Hypoxia, and Chronic Hypoxemia.

Peripheral chemoreceptors play a critical role in the defense against hypoxia and in the control of breathing, and when their function is altered, the clinical consequences can be serious. In animal models, dysfunction of the peripheral chemoreceptors has been linked to severe disturbances in respiratory control mechanisms, an absence of arousal from hypoxia, and, in infants, apparent life-threatening events. Absent or attenuated peripheral chemoreceptor function may, at least in part, explain the significantly increased incidence of SIDS (sudden infant death syndrome) in infants with BPD. Despite oxygen supplementation, infants with BPD usually have varying degrees of hypoxemia (and hypercapnia). Information on the effects of chronic hypoxemia on ventilatory control comes mostly from studies in two groups of subjects: those with cyanotic congenital heart disease, and those who live at high altitudes. Infants with cyanotic congenital heart disease have a blunted response to hypoxemia, and there seems to be a direct relationship between the degree of chronic hypoxemia and the degree of blunting of the ventilatory response to further decreases in Pa_{O_2}. Infants born and raised at a high altitude have a normal ventilatory response to hypoxia at birth but develop a blunted hypoxic response over time. Infants born at sea level, who then move to a high-altitude location, have hypoxic ventilatory responses similar to subjects born at high altitude. It is, therefore, likely that infants with BPD who are chronically hypoxemic also have impaired ventilatory responses to intermittent periods of worsening hypoxemia. In addition, hypoxemia increases both the prevalence of central apneas and the amount of periodic breathing, whereas elevation of oxyhemoglobin saturation to above 93% stabilizes breathing patterns. Thus, chronic hypoxemia from parenchymal damage together with blunted chemosensitivity can result in an impaired ability to respond to further hypoxic insults. This might partially explain the frequent oxyhemoglobin desaturations that are associated with alveolar hypoxia and increased pulmonary resistance in ventilated infants with BPD. In spontaneously breathing infants with BPD, marginal levels of oxygenation are associated with airway constriction and wheezing and changes in lung mechanics, including increases in functional residual capacity (FRC) and decreases in lung compliance. Figure 12-8 illustrates the consequences of chronic hypoxemia in infants with BPD. There is current controversy about oxygen management of preterm infants and a

movement to maintain oxyhemoglobin saturations at lower levels than previously used, to reduce the incidence of retinopathy of prematurity, and to decrease the damaging effects of oxygen on the lung. On the other hand, keeping saturations above 93% in infants with BPD has been associated with decreases in the incidence of sudden unexpected death.

Central Chemoreceptors, the Ventilatory Response to CO$_2$, and Chronic Hypercapnia. Increases in P_{CO_2} and H^+ stimulate central chemoreceptors, which are located near the ventral surface of the medulla and other widespread locations and result in an increase in ventilation in an attempt to normalize pH and P_{CO_2}. The action of CO_2 on medullary chemosensitive neurons is essential for the maintenance of normal breathing, particularly during sleep. There is less information regarding the effects of chronic hypercapnia than regarding the effects of chronic hypoxia. This is largely because hypercapnia rarely occurs alone in a clinical setting, and is almost always accompanied by some degree of hypoxemia. In subjects living at high altitude, the resting Pa_{CO_2} is normal and the ventilatory responses to carbon dioxide are normal, even though the response to hypoxia is blunted. During chronic hypercapnia, as occurs frequently in infants with BPD, renal compensation results in an increase

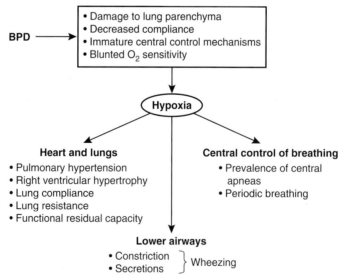

Figure 12-8 Etiology and clinical consequences of hypoxia in bronchopulmonary dysplasia (BPD). (Copyright © 2003 from Mathew OP [ed]: Respiratory Control and Disorders in the Newborn. New York, Marcel Dekker, 2003; reproduced by permission of Routledge/Taylor and Francis Group, LLC.)

in bicarbonate ion concentration, partially restoring the pH toward normal. Thus, for any given increment in $Paco_2$, there is a smaller change in $[H^+]$ at the level of the central chemoreceptors, resulting in a smaller increase in ventilation. In addition, the increase in airway resistance in infants with BPD can result in a decrease in the response to worsening hypercapnia, which may be related to the increased work of breathing associated with the increase in airway resistance.

Chronic Compensatory Metabolic Alkalosis. An elevation in plasma bicarbonate occurs frequently in infants with BPD due to renal compensation for chronic respiratory acidosis. The associated alkalosis in the brain results in a smaller change in $[H^+]$ at the level of the central chemoreceptors for a given increase in $Paco_2$. Overcorrection of pH rarely develops but can be observed with loss of gastric acid with vomiting, unreplaced nasogastric drainage, or diuretic therapy. In these instances, there are further increases in bicarbonate, often associated with an alkalotic pH, hypochloremia, and hypokalemia. The resulting alkalosis at the level of the central chemoreceptors may further reduce ventilatory drive and blunt the ventilatory responses to $Paco_2$.

Breathing during Sleep. As discussed earlier, infants and children are at risk for gas exchange abnormalities during sleep, partly because of the anatomic features of the chest wall and diaphragm. The efficiency of diaphragmatic contraction is relatively poor in newborns and improves with growth. Chest wall compliance, which is high in newborns, also decreases with growth. During REM sleep in infants, the absence of tonic activity of the diaphragm, and both tonic and phasic activity of the intercostal muscles, can lead to decreases in end-expiratory volume and decreased stability of the chest wall (as discussed earlier in this chapter). These changes are exaggerated in infants with chronic lung disease leading to an increase in upper airway resistance, and a further decrease in respiratory drive. Obstructive apneas with associated oxyhemoglobin desaturation, common in infants with BPD, cause frequent arousals that lead to sleep fragmentation and further impairment of respiratory mechanics and drive. Gas trapping in infants with BPD may also put the diaphragm at a further mechanical disadvantage. This is particularly important during REM sleep. The changes that occur during REM sleep cannot be overemphasized. By the age of 6 months, normal infants spend 30% to 50% of their sleep time in REM sleep. The interactive effects of sleep and respiratory control are illustrated in Figure 12-9. The combination of marginal oxygenation, blunted ventilatory responses to hypoxia and hypercapnia, and the normal decreases in ventilatory responses during sleep may result in pathologic hypoventilation and increase the risk for sudden death, particularly during sleep.

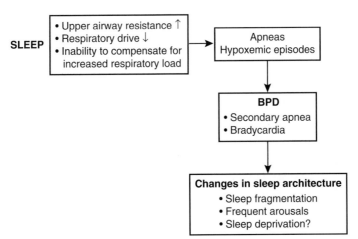

Figure 12-9 Interactive effects of sleep and respiratory control in lung disease. BPD, bronchopulmonary dysplasia. (Copyright © 2003 from Mathew OP [ed]: Respiratory Control and Disorders in the Newborn. New York, Marcel Dekker, 2003; reproduced by permission of Routledge/Taylor and Francis Group, LLC.)

Case Study 1

A full-term infant was observed to have intermittent "spells" of cyanosis during sleep associated with inspiratory "choking" sounds. The nurses also observed apnea associated with some of the spells. Upon physical examination, both nares are patent (evidenced by condensation on a small mirror held under the nostrils). However, you are unable to pass a nasogastric tube through either nostril, and there appears to be more than a normal amount of secretions. When the infant is quiet and awake, breathing appears normal and there are no choking or other abnormal sounds such as stridor. However, when activity increases or the infant cries, choking sounds return, but there is no cyanosis or apnea. There are no associated body movements that might indicate seizure activity.

Exercise 1

QUESTIONS

1. What is the most likely origin of the choking sounds?

2. What might be the contribution of the partially obstructed nasal passages?

3. Why are the choking sounds heard only during sleep or when activity increases?

4. Why do cyanosis and apnea occur only during sleep?

5. What changes in breathing would you expect under the following conditions?

   a. Sudden increase in the environmental temperature

   b. Deep suction of the pharynx

   c. Reflux of gastric contents after or during a feeding

ANSWERS

1. The choking sounds are probably caused by the tongue being drawn backward against the back of the pharynx by the negative pressure in the oral cavity.

2. The partial obstruction of the nares requires that a greater negative pressure be generated to draw air through the nose into the lungs.

3. During REM sleep, the activity of the muscles of the upper airway is decreased or inhibited, thus allowing the tongue to more easily be drawn back against the back of the pharynx. When the infant is crying or active, a greater inspiratory force is generated, drawing the tongue against the back of the pharynx.

4. During sleep, respiratory reflexes are generally depressed, resulting in hypoxia and apnea.

5. a. Apnea can be associated with changes in environmental temperature. In particular, rapid increases in temperature can be associated with apnea clusters.

   b. Deep suction of the pharynx can be associated with apnea and prolonged bradycardia.

   c. Laryngeal receptors are particularly sensitive to acid-containing fluids. Reflux of gastric contents into the larynx can initiate a reflex that includes apnea, bradycardia, swallowing, and (in older infants) coughing.

Case Study 2

An experiment was performed in which the minute ventilation was measured for 5 minutes in a full-term, healthy infant at 2 days of age, breathing room air (21% oxygen) and then measured for an additional 5 minutes while the infant was breathing 15% oxygen.

Exercise 2

QUESTIONS

1. After 1 minute of breathing 15% oxygen, would you expect the minute ventilation to be increased, decreased, or unchanged from that observed while breathing room air?

2. What would you expect the change in minute ventilation to be after 5 minutes of 15% oxygen breathing?

3. How would the adult ventilatory response to 15% oxygen breathing differ from that in this full-term 2-day-old newborn?

4. What would you expect to observe if the experiment were repeated at 3 to 4 weeks of age in this same infant?

5. What would you expect to observe if this experiment were performed on a 26-week gestation infant at 2 days of age? At 3 to 4 weeks to age? At 6 to 8 weeks of age?

ANSWERS

1. The typical ventilatory response of a 2-day-old full-term infant to 1 minute of 15% oxygen breathing would consist of a transient *increase* in minute ventilation, peaking at about 1 to 2 minutes.

2. After 5 minutes of 15% oxygen breathing, minute ventilation would be expected to *decrease* from the peak levels, approximating prehypoxia levels. In some infants, minute ventilation might even decrease to levels below baseline, or they might experience apnea.

3. The adult ventilatory response to hypoxia would be more sustained. However, there might be a slightly delayed decrease in minute ventilation. This has been called a "roll-off" phenomenon and may or may not be caused by mechanisms similar to those causing the more pronounced decrease in the newborn.

4. In a full-term infant at 3 to 4 weeks of age, the ventilatory response to hypoxia would be more like that of the adult, with a sustained excitatory response.

5. In very immature premature infants, the initial increase in minute ventilation in response to hypoxia may be limited or absent. However, as these infants mature, they can exhibit a typical "biphasic" ventilatory response to hypoxia that can persist into the second month of life.

Case Study 3

A male infant was born at 26 weeks' gestation. His hospital course was marked by the development of severe chronic lung disease requiring prolonged mechanical ventilation. An episode of Staphylococcus aureus *pneumonia complicated the course. At 6 months of age, he remained on mechanical ventilation and required an inspired oxygen concentration of 30% to 40%. He was on a number of medications, including oral diuretics and intermittent albuterol. In addition, he received a course of dornase for increased secretions. Sequential chest x-rays demonstrated "migratory atelectasis" and a localized pneumatocele in the right upper lobe. The shifting atelectasis was accompanied by frequent episodes of deterioration requiring transient increases in respiratory support and oxygen needs. On average, his Pa_{O_2} and pH (determined mostly by capillary blood gas*

measurements) were 60 to 65 mm Hg and 7.35 to 7.45, respectively. His oxyhemoglobin saturation ranged from 88% to 92%, and his serum sodium was kept in a normal range by oral supplements. Potassium chloride supplements were also given to control the hypokalemia and hypochloremia. There were frequent episodes of oxyhemoglobin desaturation, especially during sleep.

Exercise 3

QUESTIONS

1. What would this infant's ventilatory response to hypoxia be compared with that of a normal infant of the same age?

2. How would the ventilatory response to hypercapnia be affected by the intermittent hypoxemia and chronic hypercarbia?

ANSWERS

1. Chronic hypoxemia beginning during the postnatal period may impair responses to subsequent episodes of hypoxia. Furthermore, there seems to be a direct relationship between the degree of chronic hypoxemia and the degree of blunting of the ventilatory response to further worsening of hypoxemia.

2. In general, chronic hypoxemia does not limit the ventilatory response to hypercapnia. However, because of renal compensation (which occurs in response to chronic retention of carbon dioxide), the change in $[H^+]$ at the level of the central chemoreceptors would be blunted, thereby limiting the ventilatory response. The increase in airway resistance in these infants may further limit the response to hypercapnia. Inadequate responses to intermittent hypoxia and hypercapnia may contribute to the high risk of sudden death in these patients.

Case Study 4

An otherwise healthy full-term infant was observed to become pale (even cyanotic) during sleep. The infant did not become apneic, although breathing was very shallow, but regular. There were no signs of upper airway obstruction. When the infant was awake, color, activity, and breathing appeared to be *normal. The infant needed to be bundled quite heavily to maintain his temperature in the normal range and there were episodes of diffuse sweating. During an overnight sleep study, in which his response to carbon dioxide was evaluated, the infant had a decreased ventilatory response to breathing 3% CO_2.*

Exercise 4

QUESTIONS

1. What do you think happened to Pa_{O_2} (or oxyhemoglobin saturation) and Pa_{CO_2} during sleep in this infant?

2. Which of the following statements on the relationship between sleep state and breathing patterns are true?

   a. Airway obstruction is less likely to occur during sleep.

   b. Periodic breathing occurs during both REM and non-REM sleep states.

   c. Ventilatory responses are decreased during sleep.

   d. Breathing becomes more regular during REM sleep.

   e. There is a loss of muscle activity in intercostal and airway-maintaining musculature during REM sleep.

3. Assuming there are no other common treatable conditions, what are your thoughts about possible diagnoses?

ANSWERS

1. When this infant hypoventilates during sleep, it would be expected that Pa_{CO_2} would increase and Pa_{O_2} would decrease.

2. b, c, and e are true.

3. Cyanosis during sleep is always abnormal. Hypoventilation occurred only during sleep. There was no apnea but only shallow breathing. One possibility is that the infant has a form of congenital central hypoventilation syndrome (CCHS).

Alveolar hypoventilation in the absence of neuromuscular disease was first described by chance in 1951. The literary reference "Ondine's curse" was applied by Severinghaus and Mitchel in 1962, but after a careful review of the legend of Ondine, Comroe and Sugar concluded that it was not accurately applied.

The use of this term should be discouraged, not only because of the inaccuracy but also because it is physiologically imprecise and may have negative connotations for parents. Mellins described the first pediatric case of congenital idiopathic congenital central hypoventilation syndrome (CCHS) in 1970, and over the ensuing years there have been a number of case reports but probably fewer than 200 living children worldwide. Alveolar hypoventilation occurs when the output from the brain stem centers is deficient. Infants with CCHS typically have normal respiratory rates associated with shallow breathing only during sleep. Apnea is uncommon, but the extent of hypopnea can be quite severe, with tidal volumes lower than physiologic dead space. They have absent or deficient ventilatory and arousal responses to hypercapnia during sleep and variable deficiencies in the ventilatory response to hypoxia. During sleep, there is an absent or negligible arousal response to hypoxia. Table 12-4 lists some of the characteristics of CCHS. CCHS has been associated with lower penetrance anomalies of the autonomic nervous system, including Hirshsprung disease and tumors of neural crest derivatives such as ganglioneuromas and neuroblastomas. Feeding difficulty with esophageal dysmotility in infancy, breath-holding spells, poor temperature regulation with basal body temperature typically below 98°F, and sporadic profuse sweating episodes with cool extremities have been described. Children with CCHS lack a perception of dyspnea but maintain conscious control of breathing. During exercise these children may be at risk for hypercapnia and hypoxia. The perception of anxiety is also decreased among children with

---

TABLE 12-4

CHARACTERISTICS OF CONGENITAL CENTRAL HYPOVENTILATION SYNDROME

Hypoventilation (hypopnea) during quiet sleep, leading to progressive hypercarbia and hypoxemia

Absent or negligible ventilatory and arousal sensitivity to hypercarbia during sleep

Variable deficiency in hypoxic ventilatory responsiveness, with absent or negligible hypoxic arousal responsiveness during sleep

General unresponsiveness to respiratory stimulants

Absence of autoresuscitation (gasping) and perception of asphyxia

Normal ventilation during wakefulness and rapid eye movement sleep except in severely affected patient

Absent or negligible ventilatory sensitivity to hypoxia and hypercarbia when awake

CCHS. A genetic origin of CCHS has long been suspected. Until recently, only low-penetrant predisposing mutations of the RET-glial cell line derived neurotrophic factor (GDNF), endothelin 3, and brain-derived neurotrophic factor (BDNF) pathways had been reported in a few cases of CCHS. In a recent report, 18 of 29 patients with CCHS had heterozygous de novo mutations in *PHOX2B*, a paired-like homeobox gene that is important in the development of autonomic nervous system reflex circuits. Little is known about the origin of ventilatory control anomalies in CCHS. It is speculated that it involves a defect in the integration by the nucleus of the solitary tract and interneurons of the inputs from central CO_2/pH-sensitive chemoreceptors in the carotid body. Several of these structures express *PHOX2B* in mice and humans and fail to form or degenerate in $PHOX2B^{-/-}$ mutants. For a review of this interesting disorder see Weese-Mayer and Silvestri.

Clinical Problems

Among the clinical problems of respiratory control shown in Table 12-1, apnea of prematurity and periodic breathing are encountered most often by neonatologists. Clinically significant apnea (as defined later in the chapter) occurs in more than 50% of infants born at 32 weeks' gestation or less. In contrast, only 7% of infants born at 34 to 35 weeks' gestation are diagnosed with recurrent apnea. It has been assumed that apnea of prematurity represents a developmental phenomenon, because most premature infants cease to have apnea by around 37 weeks postmenstrual age (PMA). Furthermore, it is well accepted that infants with apnea have prolonged latency responses of brain stem auditory evoked responses (suggesting an overall immaturity of the brain stem) and that periodic breathing is more common in premature infants and decreases with advancing postnatal age.

It is best not to think of apnea and periodic breathing as two separate disorders. Indeed they are both components of the same process and most apnea occurs in association with periodic breathing. The common occurrence of periodic breathing and the associated apnea is most likely related to the relative proximity of actual Pa_{CO_2} levels and the CO_2 apneic threshold in the newborn. The CO_2 apneic threshold is that level of Pa_{CO_2}, below which there is no hypercapnic

drive resulting in a cessation of breathing. Figure 12-10 illustrates the relationship between the CO_2 apneic threshold and the baseline or actual Pa_{CO_2} in neonates and adults. In the neonate, the Pa_{CO_2} is much more likely to decrease below the apneic threshold compared to the adult. One can remove the proximity of the actual Pa_{CO_2} and the CO_2 apneic threshold by breathing low concentrations of CO_2; this results in a more regular respiratory pattern. Figure 12-11 illustrates the effect of breathing CO_2 on periodic breathing in comparison to treatment with theophylline. Note that breathing CO_2 eliminates periodic breathing as effectively as theophylline. As shown in Figure 12-12, similar results can be achieved with increasing F_{IO_2} suggesting that carotid body activity contributes to periodic breathing and apnea. Indeed, the strength of the carotid body influence on respiration increases with development paralleling the decrease in the incidence of periodic breathing and apnea.

Although periodic breathing and apnea are clearly "normal" development phenomena, the consequences, including bradycardia and hypoxemia, can be serious and even life-threatening. In most instances, more severe decreases in heart rate and oxyhemoglobin saturation occur with prolonged apnea. However, periodic breathing can also be associated with significant decreases in oxyhemoglobin saturation, especially when there is a progression to apnea. Figure 12-13 shows the progression of periodic breathing to a prolonged central and obstructive apneic episode resulting in significant hypoxemia.

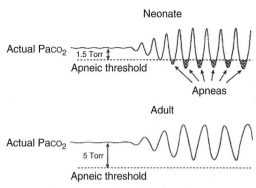

Figure 12-10 Illustration of the relationship between CO_2 apneic threshold and the baseline or actual Pa_{CO_2} levels in neonates and adults. Because of the proximity of these two levels in neonates, Pa_{CO_2} is much more likely to dive below the apneic threshold than in the adult. (Copyright © 2003 from Mathew OP [ed]: Respiratory Control and Disorders in the Newborn. New York, Marcel Dekker, 2003; reproduced by permission of Routledge/Taylor and Francis Group, LLC.)

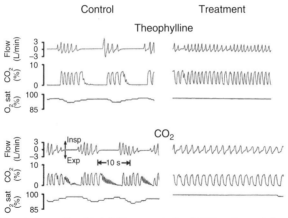

Figure 12-11 The effects of theophylline and low inhaled CO_2 concentration (0.5%) on the respiratory pattern in two preterm infants. Note that CO_2 seems as effective as theophylline to regularize breathing. (Copyright © 2003 from Mathew OP [ed]: Respiratory Control and Disorders in the Newborn. New York, Marcel Dekker, 2003; reproduced by permission of Routledge/Taylor and Francis Group, LLC.)

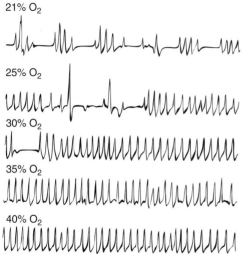

Figure 12-12 An example of the effects of a gradual increase in inspired oxygen on respiratory pattern. Respiratory flow is recorded in one preterm infant, age 16 days, 1600 g. Note the regularization of breathing pattern with increased inspired oxygen. (Copyright © 2003 from Mathew OP [ed]: Respiratory Control and Disorders in the Newborn. New York, Marcel Dekker, 2003; reproduced by permission of Routledge/Taylor and Francis Group, LLC.)

Important recent advances in our understanding of the neurobiology of respiratory control during development include information about groups of neurons responsible for rhythmogenesis, identification of sites of chemoreception in the brain stem, the phenotypes of the neurons involved in chemoreception, and the interaction of upper airway and chest wall muscles in coordinating resultant respiratory muscle and ventilatory responses. Although these advances have increased our understanding of the mechanisms responsible for apnea and periodic breathing, they have not led to substantial clinical advances in either the diagnosis or the management of apnea of prematurity. Apart from the addition of noninvasive measurement of oxygen saturation, monitoring techniques have not substantially changed in the last 25 years.

Recognizing Apnea

The term *apnea*, in its broadest sense, means the cessation of breathing. It should be recognized that some periodic breathing and short respiratory pauses, less than 15 to 20 seconds in duration and unaccompanied by bradycardia or cyanosis, can be normal in both premature and term neonates. In addition, shorter respiratory pauses associated with startles, movement, or defecation are also common. In premature infants the frequency of these short apneic episodes (3 to 15 seconds) is highest during the first weeks of life and decreases over the course of development. The definition of clinically significant apnea varies widely. The definition provided by the National Institutes of Health (NIH) consensus development conference on infantile apnea and home monitoring that took place about 20 years ago continues to provide a working basis for discussion. Most neonatologists continue to consider apnea longer than 20 seconds in duration, or apnea of shorter duration accompanied by bradycardia, and decreases in oxyhemoglobin saturation, "significant apnea"

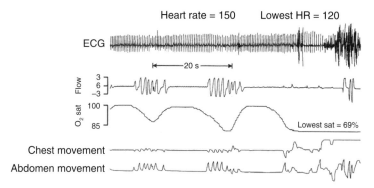

Figure 12-13 An example of a periodic breathing pattern followed by a prolonged mixed apnea, with severe desaturation and a less severe decrease in heart rate. Note the progressive decrease in the levels of oxyhemoglobin saturation during the periodic breathing preceding apnea. The prolonged apnea is mixed with a central component followed by airway collapse and obstruction. (Copyright © 2003 from Mathew OP [ed]: Respiratory Control and Disorders in the Newborn. New York, Marcel Dekker, 2003; reproduced by permission of Routledge/Taylor and Francis Group, LLC.)

or *pathologic apnea* as defined by the NIH consensus conference. Although the phenomenon of apnea is normal in the preterm infant, *pathologic* apnea in the term infant is almost always abnormal and is usually a symptom of another problem such as sepsis, seizure activity, central nervous system abnormality, or a metabolic derangement.

Other terms commonly used to describe apnea include *central, obstructive,* and *mixed apnea.* Central apnea is the absence of breathing efforts. In most cases, this results from a failure of the central nervous system to initiate a breath. However, failure of the neuromuscular junction or muscle paralysis might also cause central apnea, using this definition. Obstructive apnea is the absence of airflow to the lungs, despite appropriate signals from brain stem respiratory centers and an otherwise intact neuromuscular system. This usually results from an upper airway obstruction at the level of the pharynx or larynx. Mixed apnea refers to an episode that has both central and obstructive components. Recently, it has been determined that some degree of narrowing of the airways can occur in up to 45% of episodes of central apnea and in all central apneas lasting more than 20 seconds. This potential obstruction may develop a few seconds after the onset of the apnea and may not persist for the duration of the episode. The association of airway obstruction with apnea is of considerable clinical importance, because bradycardia is more likely to occur when there is an obstruction, regardless of the length of the episode. Significant bradycardia can occur within 1 to 2 seconds of the onset of respiratory efforts against a closed airway. Although these heart rate responses are potentiated by hypoxia, they appear to be reflex in nature, because the bradycardia is relieved within 2 to 3 seconds of the onset of normal breathing.

Other terms defined by the NIH conference include *periodic breathing, apnea of prematurity,* and *symptomatic premature infant.* Periodic breathing is "a breathing pattern in which there are three or more respiratory pauses of greater than 3 seconds duration with less than 20 seconds of respiration between pauses." Apnea of prematurity is "periodic breathing with pathologic apnea in a premature infant." Symptomatic premature infants are "preterm infants who continue to have apnea of prematurity at the time when they would otherwise be ready for discharge." Although no longer referred to by this term, this last group of infants has been the subject of much controversy about the timing of discharge and the issues relating to home monitoring.

Case Study 5

A 7-day-old infant born at 30 weeks' gestation was initially treated with surfactant and mechanical ventilation. He has now recovered sufficiently to require only 28% oxygen by hood. You respond to a monitor alarm, and when you arrive at the bedside, the infant appears to be making respiratory movements and the heart rate is normal. You call up the recorded event, which is shown in Figure 12-14.

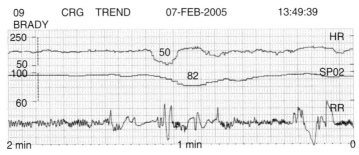

Figure 12-14 An example of a mixed apnea breathing pattern.

Exercise 5

QUESTION

1. Describe what you see in the recording.
2. Would you classify this event as a "brady" as the monitor suggests?

ANSWERS

1. The rapid decrease in heart rate accompanied by what appear to be respiratory movements strongly suggests there are obstructive components to this event. The decrease in heart rate during obstructive apnea is often more rapid than with a central apnea episode. The mechanism is unclear because there is often little or no decrease in oxyhemoglobin saturation, unless the obstruction is prolonged. In some episodes, the obstruction may originate from stimulation of the larynx with secretions or gastric contents, precipitating reflex bradycardia. However, the apparent period of obstruction is preceded by a period in which there are no chest movements. Because this event has both central and obstructive components, the correct designation would be a *mixed* apnea.

2. This is clearly not an isolated bradycardia. It should be classified as an apnea and bradycardia.

Evaluating and Responding to Apnea

The evaluation of apnea depends on the ability to measure respiratory effort and airflow and assess the adequacy of ventilation. Information about chest wall movement, nasal airflow, heart rate, and oxygen saturation are relatively easy to obtain in a research setting. In most clinical situations, however, accurate measurements of chest wall movements and nasal airflow are cumbersome and are not practical for routine use. Infants in the NICU are usually monitored with an impedance monitor that detects heart rate and chest wall movement. Although heart rate can usually be measured with some accuracy, impedance monitors are notorious for giving false indications of chest movement and are sensitive to almost any movement. The use of pulse oximetry has added an important modality, providing information about the degree of oxyhemoglobin desaturation associated with episodic events. Hence, in clinical settings, evidence about the severity of an event can be inferred from observations of changes in heart rate and saturation, but the distinction between an obstructive and a central event can be difficult to determine; it is often deduced from breathing and heart rate patterns.

In the NICU those caring for newborns with apnea respond to any of three alarms: (1) a heart rate alarm (when the heart rate falls below some predetermined level), (2) a respiratory alarm (when there is absence of chest movement in excess of some predetermined time interval), or (3) an oxygen saturation alarm (when the oxygen saturation falls below a predetermined level). Although there is no clear consensus about alarm settings, it is common practice to set the heart rate alarm at 80 to 100 beats per minute, the respiratory alarm at 20 seconds, and the oxygen saturation monitor at 80% to 85%. After arriving at the bedside, the caregiver must first discern which alarm sounded and then determine the presence or absence of apnea and bradycardia and the degree of desaturation or color change in the infant. The degree of severity must be determined, and the decision to intervene must be made. Finally, the details of each event should be recorded including presence of apnea, bradycardia, desaturation, or color change and whether stimulation or bag and mask ventilation were required. Clearly, the initial settings greatly influence any estimation of the frequency of events.

In the majority of events it is the heart rate alarm that sounds. This is largely because it is rare to have a central apnea episode of 20 seconds' duration without an accompanying decrease in heart rate. In the case of mixed events, the apnea duration may be brief, and a rapid drop in heart rate can occur while the infant is making chest movements. In a purely obstructive event, there is no absence of chest wall movement; thus, no apnea is recorded. When responding to a heart rate alarm, it may be difficult to determine whether apnea has actually occurred, because the infant is often found to be breathing when the caregiver arrives. When the infant is nearing discharge, this information is particularly important, because brief episodes of bradycardia, without apnea, may not be considered significant. The use of a monitor with some type of trend display with recording capability is essential for an accurate assessment of episodic events. The most useful display is one in which a 1.5- to 3-minute tracing of respiration is displayed along with heart rate and oxyhemoglobin saturation as a graph (see Fig. 12-13). With this type of display, the caregiver responding to an alarm can make a quick assessment of whether there has been an apneic event (even if the infant has resumed breathing) or whether other types of respiratory disturbances such as periodic breathing or extremely irregular breathing were associated with the bradycardia. We have found that the ability to "call up" a stored event is also of great help, especially near the time of discharge, particularly if there are questions about the significance of the event. Unfortunately, many of the newer monitors also make an attempt to "diagnose" the event as an apnea, bradycardia, or desaturation. The algorithms vary, but are often dependent on the first alarm to be triggered and the alarm criteria. For example, there may be a 15-second apnea with significant bradycardia and desaturation that will be labeled a "bradycardia and desaturation" because the apnea duration did not exceed 20 seconds. In these cases examination of the recorded event can easily identify the correct diagnosis.

To further complicate matters, most heart rate monitors determine heart rate on a "beat-to-beat" basis and set off the alarm regardless of the duration of the bradycardia. Even a few aberrant beats can cause a momentary drop in calculated heart rate, resulting in an alarm. It is unusual to find significant sustained bradycardia unaccompanied by some form of respiratory disturbance in otherwise healthy premature infants with apnea.

Case Study 6

A 28-week gestation male infant was extubated at 5 days of age after a course of respiratory distress syndrome (RDS) treated with surfactant and mechanical ventilation. Aminophylline was started before extubation. At 8 days of age, the theophylline level was 6 μg/mL. At that time, the infant was on nasal continuous positive airway pressure (CPAP) and 26% oxygen. The nurses' apnea log described several episodes of bradycardia with oxyhemoglobin desaturations, but no apnea. Your unit has just started using a new "smart" monitor that has recording capability and makes an attempt to "diagnose" the event. You call up one of the episodes listed as a "bradycardia." The recording is shown in Figure 12-15.

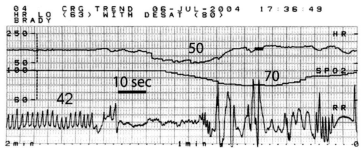

Figure 12-15 An example of a central apnea breathing pattern.

Exercise 6

QUESTIONS

1. Describe what you see in the recording with respect to the compressed impedance respiratory tracing, heart rate, and oxyhemoglobin saturation.

2. Would you call this event an isolated bradycardia?

ANSWERS

1. The respiratory tracing shows a significant pause in breathing (>20 seconds' duration), following what is probably a brief body movement. The apnea is accompanied by a gradual fall in heart rate and, after a slight delay, a fall in oxyhemoglobin saturation to approximately 50%. The relatively slow decrease in heart rate after the onset of apnea and the absence of chest movements suggest that this is an episode of central apnea and is consistent with a diagnosis of an apnea associated with bradycardia and desaturation. Because the infant was extubated recently and is still on CPAP, there may be a contribution from residual lung disease. However, after removal of the CPAP, the apnea did not worsen, suggesting that apnea of prematurity was the dominant factor. The mechanism responsible for the bradycardia in central apnea is not clear. A significant correlation between the degree of desaturation and the degree of bradycardia has been demonstrated. Based on these data, some have postulated that the decrease in heart rate may be due to hypoxic stimulation of the carotid body chemoreceptors in the absence of chest movement. However, these relationships are complex. As can be seen in the tracing, the fall in heart rate appears to precede the fall in oxhyhemoglobin saturation.

2. Although the recording shows that this clearly was a central apnea, the nurses were recording the event as a bradycardia with desaturation according to the monitor's "diagnosis." This should have been classified as an apnea, bradycardia, and desaturation.

Assessing the Significance of Apnea

The definition of pathologic apnea suggested by the NIH consensus conference includes criteria that identify an event as outside the range of normal for a newborn infant and thus is assumed to be clinically significant. It should be recognized, however, that no clear consensus exists as to the optimal alarm settings that should be used in either the hospital or at home for respiration, heart rate, and oxygen saturation. Furthermore, the clinical significance and long-term consequences of persistent apnea, bradycardia, and desaturation continue to be debated.

The degree of hypoxia and the level and duration of bradycardia that are dangerous to the infant are also unclear. Marked sustained bradycardia has been shown to cause changes in cerebral blood flow. However, as determined by a cardiac monitor, transient self-resolving bradycardia is quite common. Some have suggested that self-resolving apnea between 15 and 20 seconds in duration, accompanied by transient bradycardia, may be normal. However, impedance monitors alone fail to diagnose obstructive events associated with brief periods of bradycardia. It may be that most short episodes of bradycardia are associated with brief obstructive events. Nevertheless, there is continuing debate whether these kinds of events should be considered potentially dangerous, warranting continued monitoring either in the hospital or at home. In addition, the approach to heart rate monitoring is highly inconsistent. The heart rate alarm is most often set between 80 and 100 bpm, although both of these values are necessarily arbitrary. For example, if the resting heart rate is 105 bpm, a decrease to 80 bpm may not be either statistically or clinically significant. Perhaps setting the alarm limit at some proportion of the resting heart rate may be a more physiologic approach. However, there is currently no consensus. It seems prudent, therefore, for each nursery to at least develop a consistent approach that can be strictly adhered to by the staff.

The apnea record is often relied on to assess the frequency and severity of events in the nursery. However, based on studies in which nursing assessment of apnea was compared with electronic monitoring techniques with event recording, there is ample evidence that all apneas are not always recorded by clinical observers. Nevertheless, we believe that a combination of trend monitoring (see earlier discussion) with recording capability and good nursing judgment will detect most if not all clinically significant apneas. Those apneas requiring no stimulation because they resolve quickly, and those that are severe enough to require bag and mask ventilation, are usually easy to distinguish. However, in other situations, differences in the "response thresholds" of caregivers make it difficult to distinguish, in retrospect, between a self-resolving event and one that "requires" stimulation. Each nursery must develop a consistent approach to the evaluation of apnea to increase the probability of an accurate assessment of apnea severity.

Diagnosing Apnea of Prematurity

Although apnea of prematurity is a normal developmental condition in premature infants, many other conditions may precipitate or worsen apnea. Therefore, the diagnosis of apnea of prematurity often becomes one of exclusion. Apnea can be a nonspecific or specific sign of other conditions (Table 12-5). Apnea may be a sign of infection, including sepsis, pneumonia, or meningitis. Apnea associated with bacterial infections is usually severe and may be associated with respiratory failure requiring mechanical ventilation. Infants infected with RSV often present with apnea and hypoxemia. Because prolonged hypoxia can be associated with a depression of ventilation, any condition that results in hypoxia can cause apnea. Apnea occurs frequently in infants with chronic lung disease. Infants with congenital heart disease often present with apnea. In most cases, this is secondary to hypoxemia, but it can also occur in infants with acyanotic congenital heart disease. For example, in premature infants, pulmonary congestion from a patent ductus arteriosus can present as an increase in the severity of apnea. Structural abnormalities of the central nervous system can also present as apnea. This should always be suspected in a full-term infant who presents with apnea in the first few days of life. Although apnea can be the sole manifestation of seizure activity, there are usually other associated signs.

Common metabolic disturbances such as hypoglycemia, hyponatremia, acidemia, or hypocalcemia can be associated with apnea. Genetically inherited metabolic disorders can present with apnea. For example, urea cycle disorders, organic acidurias, and medium chain acyl-CoA dehydrogenase deficiency commonly present with apnea. Medications such as narcotics that depress respiration should be considered in the differential diagnosis of apnea. Apnea may be an early sign of magnesium toxicity. Prostaglandin E_1, used to maintain ductal patency in certain ductal-dependent congenital cardiac defects, can produce apnea, particularly if the infant is hypoxemic.

The effect of anemia on the incidence and severity of apnea of prematurity is controversial. Reports in the literature are inconsistent, and there seems to be a lack of consensus in this area. Most would agree that severe anemia should be avoided. Others have suggested that a hematocrit less than 25% associated with

---

TABLE 12-5

CAUSES OF APNEA IN THE NEONATAL PERIOD

Central nervous system
  Apnea of prematurity
  Depression
    Sedatives, narcotics
    Post-anesthesia
    Hypoxia
  Intracranial hemorrhage
  Seizures
  Tumors
  Hyperekplexia
  Hydrocephalus
  Malformation
  Infection
    Meningitis
    Meningoencephalitis
Circulatory system
  Patent ductus arteriosus
  Heart failure
  Shock
Gastrointestinal tract
  Nasopharyngeal reflux
  Gastroesophageal reflux
  Necrotizing enterocolitis
  Nipple feeding
Hematologic
  Severe anemia
Sepsis
  Bacteria
  Viral
  Fungal
Temperature regulation
  Hypothermia
  Hyperthermia
Airway obstruction
  Choanal atresia
  Pierre Robin sequence
  Neck flexion
  Secretions
Reflex
  Passage of nasogastric tube
  Vigorous suction
  Cold stimulus to the face
Metabolic disorders
  Hypoglycemia
  Nonketotic hyperglycinemia
  Urea cycle disorders
Miscellaneous
  Immunization
  Prostaglandin E_1

severe apnea should be treated. Gastroesophageal reflex can cause apnea and can be an important factor in some infants who continue to have apnea beyond term PMA. Almost all premature infants, however, have some degree of reflux for which routine studies and treatment are probably not indicated. Infants with tracheomalacia can have severe apnea that often requires prolonged treatment with CPAP. Partial nasal obstruction can present as "choking" spells and apnea. The obstruction is usually at the level of the pharynx, caused by increased negative pressure in the oral cavity drawing the tongue backward against the back of the pharynx.

Apnea during recovery from anesthesia is well recognized in premature infants. It can be observed even after minor surgical procedures such as herniorrhaphy. Infants with BPD are particularly susceptible. The incidence of apnea in premature infants may increase after administration of immunizations.

Case Study 7

You are called urgently to the normal newborn nursery to assess a 12-hour-old full-term infant who has had a "spell." When you arrive, you discover that the infant had been breastfed and put in the crib next to the mother's bed. Shortly thereafter, the mother found her infant "not breathing" and blue. After vigorous stimulation, the infant resumed spontaneous respiration but was tachypneic. On examination, the infant is pale and has poor peripheral perfusion. The color improves with oxygen administration.

Exercise 7

QUESTION

1. What are the possible causes of this infant's apnea?

ANSWER

1. A sudden, severe episode in an otherwise low-risk full-term infant is rare and should be considered abnormal until determined otherwise. On physical examination, the infant was pale and had poor peripheral perfusion. Although pallor and poor

perfusion might be the result of a recent episode of apnea that might resolve, these findings could also be secondary to a more serious underlying problem such as infection, metabolic disturbance, or congenital heart disease. Sepsis or an acute metabolic disturbance such as hypoglycemia is a primary concern since each can and should be treated, and if left untreated can have serious consequences. Depending on the urgency of the situation and the physical examination findings, the diagnostic workup might include a bedside test-strip for glucose, serum electrolytes, hematocrit or hemoglobin level, arterial blood gas determination, complete blood count, and chest x-ray. Blood cultures should be done and, depending on clinical judgment, antibiotics should be given.

Case Study 8

A male infant born at 28 weeks' gestation received aminophylline prior to extubation. He is now 3 weeks of age and his aminophylline has been switched to caffeine. He is receiving full feedings by gavage and has been gaining weight. He is having five to eight episodes of apnea and bradycardia each day, with occasional events requiring stimulation. You are called to the bedside at 4 AM because shortly after the infant was weighed, several apnea and bradycardia episodes occurred over a period of 2 hours, some of which required stimulation.

Exercise 8

QUESTION

1. What is the most likely cause of this infant's apnea?

ANSWER

1. Although a sudden increase in the frequency and severity of apnea might suggest a serious problem, the sequence of events in this scenario suggests another common cause for apnea clustering. It is common for infants to be removed from the incubator for weighing and other procedures. If, in the process of weighing, the incubator temperature is allowed to fall substantially, the infant may be exposed to a rapidly increasing air

temperature as the incubator attempts to reestablish the original air temperature. This rapid rewarming can precipitate clusters of apnea that are often difficult to distinguish from other causes of increased apnea frequency. Of course, large fluctuations in environmental temperature should be avoided.

Case Study 9

A full-term infant was delivered vaginally after a normal pregnancy, labor, and delivery. The infant was moderately depressed at birth, with Apgar scores of 4 and 7 at 1 and 5 minutes, respectively. The infant's color improved, but he continued to demonstrate shallow breathing and decreased tone. He was evaluated for sepsis, started on antibiotics, and closely observed. Electrolyte, calcium, and glucose levels were normal. You are called to the the infant's bedside 6 hours after his birth because he had a prolonged apneic episode associated with cyanosis, bradycardia, and a marked decrease in oxygen saturation. The nurses report that the infant's eyes were deviated to the right when they first arrived at the bedside. The infant had been successfully resuscitated with a bag and mask, but because of continued apnea, you place an endotracheal tube and begin mechanical ventilation. You observe that the infant is quite hypotonic and makes only intermittent attempts to breathe spontaneously.

Exercise 9

QUESTION

1. What is the most likely cause of this infant's apnea?

ANSWER

1. A prolonged apneic episode in an otherwise healthy full-term infant should be considered abnormal. In this case, the accompanying hypotonia, shallow breathing, and eye devia-tion suggest that the origin may be the central nervous system. Apnea can be the sole sign of seizure activity, but other manifestations, such as eye deviations, are often present. If seizures are suspected, the infant should be treated. The workup may include serum electrolytes and glucose to rule out common metabolic disturbances and an EEG to confirm seizure activity. Imaging of the brain is usually obtained as part of the evaluation.

Case Study 10

A 9-month-old male infant born at 25 weeks' gestation has moderate to severe BPD. He remains oxygen dependent and has developed bilateral hernias. He has had mild apnea, but no episodes have been recorded for 2 weeks. He is taken to the operating room for a hernia repair. After extubation, you are called to the bedside because there have been several episodes of apnea, one of which required bag and mask ventilation.

Exercise 10

QUESTION

1. What is the most likely cause of this infant's apnea?

ANSWER

1. This scenario describes the common problem of apnea during recovery from surgery in premature infants. The cause is unclear, but it appears to be more common when inha-lational anesthetics have been administered. Upper airway muscles are particularly sus-ceptible to the effects of anesthesia, and air-way obstruction may contribute to these events. Infants with chronic lung disease may be more susceptible. In addition, the ventilatory response to intermittent hypoxia may be accompanied by ventilatory depres-sion when the infant is lightly anesthetized. Some clinicians have suggested that all infants be monitored for 24 to 48 hours after a procedure involving a general anesthetic.

Case Study 11

An infant born at 27 weeks' gestation was initially treated with mechanical ventilation and surfactant. A patent ductus arteriosus, suspected clinically at 5 days of age and confirmed by echocardiography, was treated successfully with a course of indomethacin. At 32 weeks PMA, he was receiving aminophylline for apnea of prematurity and had a serum theophylline level of 10 μg/mL. Forty-eight hours before your involvement in this case, there was an increase in the frequency of apnea episodes that required stimulation. Three of the episodes required oxygen administration and use of a mask and bag. The infant appears somewhat pale on examination, and the nurses report that the infant has been more lethargic over the course of the previous 6 to 8 hours. There are no signs of respiratory distress. A hematocrit obtained 2 days previously was 35%.

Exercise 11

QUESTION

1. What is the most likely cause of this infant's apnea?

ANSWER

1. This scenario is common in the NICU and often leads to a workup for sepsis and institution of antibiotic therapy. Early symptoms of infection can be subtle and can be mimicked by repeated episodes of apnea and bradycardia. One needs to use good judgment in these cases. If, based on laboratory testing, sepsis seems unlikely, this may represent a case of worsening apnea of prematurity. A repeat theophylline level may reveal a need for redosing. A repeat loading dose of 1 mg/kg will raise the theophylline level by about 2 μg/mL. After reloading, an increase in the maintenance dose by 10% or 20% may be needed to maintain an adequate level. A hematocrit of 35% is unlikely to be associated with worsening apnea.

Treating Apnea of Prematurity

Otherwise healthy premature infants with mild apnea (frequency < 10/day) who require no intervention or who respond quickly to tactile stimulation probably do not need any additional treatment. When apnea occurs more frequently, the infant is slow to respond to tactile stimulation, or bag and mask ventilation is required, further treatment is indicated. In most cases, this is a matter of medical judgment; there are no standard criteria for starting therapy.

In the past, regular stimulation has been advocated as a form of treatment of apnea of prematu-

rity. These interventions have included tactile stimulation and vestibular-proprioceptive stimulation with a waterbed. Although there are undoubtedly important vestibular-proprioceptive inputs to respiratory control areas of the brain stem, these methods have limited application to the treatment of apnea in today's NICU. Indeed several Cochrane reviews have failed to show significant long-term benefit from kinesthetic stimulation for apnea. Regular tactile stimulation (such as frequent stroking) should not be confused with the tactile stimulation (such as gentle jostling) that continues to be the most time-honored and universally applied first intervention for infants who are experiencing apnea. Other stimulatory treatments, including face air jets, audible alarms, and entrainment devices have also not been shown to be beneficial.

General Principles

A number of general principles are important in the treatment of apnea of prematurity. Specific therapy should be directed at any underlying cause, if one is identified. For example, if intermittent hypoxemia is found by oxygen saturation monitoring, supplemental oxygen should be provided. One should be cautious, however, not to give too much oxygen because of the risk of retinopathy of prematurity. The oxygen saturation should be measured continuously in infants given oxygen for apnea. Oxyhemoglobin saturation levels should generally be kept between 88% and 92%, although older infants with BPD may benefit from higher oxyhemoglobin saturations.

One should be cautious to avoid reflexes that may trigger apnea. Suctioning of the pharynx, for example, should be done carefully. Positions of extreme neck flexion or extension should be avoided, and oral feedings should be initiated cautiously. Avoiding swings in environment temperature may eliminate some clusters of apnea. Cooling infants to the lower end of the thermoneutral environment may reduce the incidence of apnea. However, without measuring oxygen consumption, it is difficult to determine the lower threshold of the thermoneutral range, and there is a risk of needlessly increasing oxygen consumption. Extreme anemia may exacerbate apnea of prematurity. Although controversial, transfusing infants who have a hematocrit of 25% or less is reasonable, if the apnea is severe and aminophylline levels are adequate.

Drug Therapy

The methylxanthines—theophylline, usually in the form of aminophylline, or caffeine—have become the mainstays of treatment for infants with apnea of prematurity. Theophylline and caffeine differ in chemical structure by only one methyl group and share many pharmacologic properties. Their effects on breathing most likely include competitive inhibition of adenosine receptors in the central nervous system. Adenosine is a ubiquitous inhibitory neuromodulator present in all areas of the brain. Xanthines may also improve diaphragmatic contractility and reduce fatigue. Methylxanthines have a number of unwanted side effects, including irritability, tremors, seizures, tachycardia, gastric irritation, water and sodium diuresis, and glucose intolerance. Side effects are more common with aminophylline because of its lower therapeutic index. Both aminophylline and caffeine are metabolized in the liver, and their excretion improves with age. Therefore, the half-life of the methylxanthines is prolonged in preterm infants and exhibits considerable individual variation among infants. Clinically, theophylline rather than aminophylline levels are measured. In premature infants treated with aminophylline, there may be an additional effect of caffeine secondary to conversion of some of the theophylline to caffeine. Therapeutic serum levels of theophylline (5 to 10 µg/mL) or caffeine (8 to 20 µg/mL) are usually free of toxicity. Table 12-6 describes one commonly used treatment regimen for xanthine treatment of apnea.

Nasal Continuous Positive Airway Pressure

CPAP delivered by nasal prongs, nasal mask, or face mask at 2 to 5 cm H_2O pressure has proved effective in the treatment of apnea in some premature infants. Initial studies suggested that the beneficial effects of CPAP are mediated by means of an alteration of the Hering-Breuer reflex, stabilization of the chest

TABLE 12-6

TREATMENT OF APNEA WITH XANTHINES

Feature	Aminophylline	Caffeine
Route of administration	Intravenous initially	Oral, intravenous
Loading dose	4–6 mg/kg (infuse over 30 min)	10 mg/kg caffeine base (20 mg/kg caffeine citrate) × 1
Maintenance dose	1–3 mg/kg q 8–12 hr; start maintenance dose 8–12 hr after loading	2.5–5 mg/kg/dose of caffeine base every 24 hr (starting 24 hr after loading dose) (*Note:* 2 mg caffeine citrate = 1 mg caffeine base)
Clinical considerations	—	Initial half-life is 90–100 hr, decreasing to 6 hr after 60 weeks postmenstrual age
Therapeutic levels	5–10 µg/mL	8–20 µg/mL
Monitoring	Monitor heart rate and check blood glucose periodically during loading-dose therapy; assess for agitation and feeding intolerance; withhold next dose if heart rate exceeds 180 bpm; after maintenance therapy is established, monitor serum trough levels on day 4 of therapy and then 1–2 times/wk; check serum trough level when toxicity is suspected or when apnea spells increase in frequency; if apnea is severe before the fourth day of therapy, obtain serum trough level; if low, give a partial bolus: 1 mg/kg for each 2 µg/mL in serum theophylline concentration	Obtain therapeutic trough levels before fifth dose; cardiovascular, neurologic, or gastrointestinal toxicity reported with levels >40–50 µg/mL; monitor heart rate and hold then reduce dose if >180 bpm; assess for agitation and response to therapy
Precautions	Intramuscular administration causes intense local pain and sloughing	Increased risk of kernicterus with caffeine sodium benzoate due to uncoupling of albumin-bilirubin binding
Adverse reactions	Gastrointestinal upset, arrhythmias, seizures, tachycardia (heart rate >180 bpm warrants determination of serum levels	Restlessness, agitation, vomiting, tachycardia, overdose symptoms include arrhythmias and tonic-clonic seizures

wall with reduction of the intercostal-phrenic inhibitory reflex, or an increase in oxygenation. Although all of these mechanisms may contribute to stabilization of respiration, CPAP has been found to reduce only mixed and obstructive apnea, with little or no effect on central apnea.[76] In addition, it has been demonstrated that CPAP in the range used clinically decreases upper airway resistance in sleeping premature infants. Therefore, it appears likely that CPAP exerts its beneficial effect in infants by splinting the upper airway with positive pressure throughout the respiratory cycle. There is no firm consensus on when to start CPAP clinically. Small premature infants with acute lung disease such as RDS are often extubated to nasal CPAP to facilitate the transition and to stabilize lung volumes and oxygenation. Most are weaned off CPAP within a few days. Others, however, require prolonged periods of treatment with nasal CPAP for apnea. Recently a new device has been introduced that provides high flow (1 to 8 L/minute) heated and humidified gas through loosely fitting nasal prongs (Vapotherm). Some have advocated using this device as a replacement for CPAP for the treatment of apnea in selected infants. Using heated and humidified breathing gas is clearly an advantage over the commonly used nasal cannula that provides cold and only partially humidified gas. However, there is no evidence that Vapotherm can achieve a clinically significant level of CPAP nor that it can adequately treat apnea in infants that require CPAP for treatment. Our own preliminary investigations have shown that the level of CPAP that is achieved with Vapotherm is determined by the flow rate and the nasal and mouth leaks. Because these leaks are rather large, very little continuous positive pressure is achieved. However, when the prongs fit snugly in the nose (and the mouth is closed) a pressure of 4 to 5 cm H_2O can be achieved at a flow rate of 4 L/minute.

Case Study 12

A male infant was delivered at a gestational age of 31 weeks because of maternal preeclampsia. The Apgar scores were 4 and 7, and only blow-by oxygen was required. On day 2 there were two episodes of apnea and bradycardia during sleep, unaccompanied by any metabolic disturbances or signs of infection. The diagnosis of apnea of prematurity is made, and the infant is observed. Over the next several days, the frequency and severity of the apnea increase. He is now 5 days of age and there have been 14 events over the last 24 hours, two requiring stimulation and one of those needing bag and mask ventilation.

Exercise 12

QUESTION

1. When is it appropriate to start treatment?

ANSWER

1. This case study most likely represents worsening apnea of prematurity. It is not always obvious when to start aminophylline or caffeine. In this case, the frequency and severity of these episodes are clearly increasing. We recommend starting methylxanthines if there has been more than one apnea episode (on average) every 2 hours, accompanied by the need to stimulate, especially if bag and mask ventilation was required. A loading dose of 4 to 6 mg/kg of aminophylline would be appropriate, followed by a maintenance dose of 1 to 3 mg/kg every 6 to 12 hours.

Case Study 13

A male infant was born at 27 weeks' gestation, intubated, and given surfactant in the delivery room. Mechanical ventilation was discontinued on day 5 after starting aminophylline. Over the next 4 weeks, there were increasing episodes of apnea and bradycardia (5 to 10/day), and one to two episodes a day required some sort of intervention. He was switched to oral caffeine when enteral feedings were established. Apnea frequency gradually decreased over the next 2 weeks. He is now 33 weeks PMA, and there continues to be approximately one episode every 3 days.

Exercise 13

QUESTION

1. What would you do about the caffeine at this time?

ANSWER

1. This case most likely represents resolution of apnea of prematurity with advancing age.

At some point, a decision must be made about stopping caffeine. As a general guideline, we recommend stopping methylxanthines if the infant has been apnea free for a week at any PMA, or at 34 weeks PMA for aminophylline and at 33 weeks PMA for caffeine (because of the longer half-life). We then wait about 2 days (for aminophylline) or about 7 days (for caffeine) before starting an apnea "countdown." Clearly, there may be exceptions to this guideline, and good clinical judgment must be relied upon in each case.

Case Study 14

A female infant was born at 26 weeks' gestation. She was intubated and given surfactant in the delivery room, and over the next several days, she received a total of three doses of surfactant. On day 3 of life, indomethacin was started for a patent ductus arteriosus. Following the last dose of indomethacin, the ductus was shown to be closed by echocardiography. At 12 days of age, the infant deteriorated, and Staphylococcus epidermidis *was cultured from a blood sample. After a 10-day course of antibiotics, the infant stabilized but remained on a ventilator at moderate settings. The infant was weaned to CPAP from the ventilator at 32 weeks PMA. At 34 weeks PMA she was weaned to high flow nasal cannula (Vapotherm) treatment at 4 L/minute. The flow rate was gradually decreased and at 38 weeks PMA she was switched to standard nasal cannula oxygen. She is now at 40 weeks PMA, and continues to require nasal cannula oxygen at an inspired concentration of 30% to 40%. She had been treated with aminophylline early in her course and continues on caffeine. Other medications include oral diuretics. All feedings are being given enterally. There are occasional episodes of apnea and bradycardia, and some require stimulation. On many occasions, the apnea is associated with a fall in the oxyhemoglobin saturation, requiring a transient increase in the inspired oxygen concentration.*

Exercise 14

QUESTION

1. What will be your discharge criteria for this patient?

ANSWER

1. This infant has reached term and yet continues to have apnea. Keeping in mind that some infants born at this gestation will continue to have apnea of prematurity beyond term, it is often difficult, if not impossible, to distinguish apnea of prematurity from apnea from other confounding conditions. There are several ongoing issues with this patient that might contribute to the persistence of the apnea, including chronic lung disease with continued oxygen requirement, which may be associated with a blunted ventilatory response to intermittent hypoxia and hypercapnia. There is no simple formula for when to discharge these complex patients. In many instances, feedings may also be associated with continued episodes of apnea and bradycardia. In general, we continue to recommend that these infants should be apnea free for 1 week before discharge. If supplemental oxygen continues to be required, it may be appropriate to discharge the infant with oxygen. In this case, monitoring, usually pulse oximetry, should be continued at home.

Case Study 15

A mother carrying a 25-week fetus was transported for possible delivery. A male infant was born at 25 weeks' gestation. The infant's early hospital course included RDS treated with surfactant and oscillatory ventilation. There was no history of amnionitis. Mechanical ventilation was weaned to CPAP at 27 weeks PMA and subsequently to nasal cannula O_2 at 30 weeks PMA. Oxygen therapy was discontinued at 36 weeks PMA. Apnea of prematurity was treated with aminophylline and then caffeine. An attempt to discontinue caffeine was made at 33 weeks PMA, but it was restarted because of recurrent apnea. Caffeine was finally discontinued at 36 weeks PMA. He continued to have apnea that was characterized by one to two episodes per day with 10 to 15 seconds, accompanied by bradycardia (<80 bpm for at least 5 seconds) and oxyhemoglobin desaturation to below 75%. Some of these required stimulation. He is now 39 weeks PMA, and weighs 2200 g. He is taking all feedings by mouth, and is maintaining his temperature in an open crib. However, he continues to have apnea and bradycardia during sleep. These occur at a *frequency of one to two episodes per day and are accompanied by decreases in heart rate to 70 bpm and decreases in oxyhemoglobin saturation to 75% to 80%. Episodes of oxyhemoglobin desaturation also occur during feedings, but these are not thought to be significant.*

Exercise 15

QUESTION

1. What is the next step in management?

ANSWER

1. This infant has reached 39 weeks PMA, recovered from his lung disease, and met all other criteria for discharge, yet he continues to have significant apnea of prematurity. Because the infant was born at 25 weeks' gestation, immature breathing patterns can be expected to continue beyond term. A general recommendation would be to continue to monitor this infant in the hospital until he is apnea free for 7 days and then discharge him without a home monitor.

Case Study 16

A female infant was born at 32 weeks' gestation. She required no resuscitation in the delivery room but developed respiratory distress requiring CPAP for 3 days. She was quickly weaned off oxygen and then developed apnea of prematurity that required treatment with aminophylline and subsequently with caffeine. The caffeine was discontinued at 34 weeks PMA. At 37 weeks PMA, she is maintaining her temperature in a crib and taking all of her feedings by mouth. She had been apnea free for 7 days.

Exercise 16

QUESTION

1. Is this infant ready for discharge?

ANSWER

1. This infant born at 32 weeks' gestation has now reached 37 weeks PMA and has met

all the standard criteria for discharge (including being apnea free for 1 week). She should be discharged home without monitoring. Note that caffeine has a half-life that is considerably longer than aminophylline and should be discontinued so that the infant can be observed for 7 days after levels become negligible. This is usually about 1 week after discontinuing the drug. In this case, the infant was observed for 7 days starting at 36 weeks PMA, 2 weeks after stopping caffeine.

Case Study 17

A female infant was born at 30 weeks' gestation but weighed only 900 g. She required a brief period of mechanical ventilation followed by CPAP therapy. She quickly weaned off oxygen but required aminophylline for apnea of prematurity that was subsequently switched to caffeine. The caffeine was discontinued at 33 weeks PMA. At 35 weeks PMA she continued to have brief apnea that was self-resolving, but she weighed only 1600 g.

At the request of the parents, she was weaned out of her isolette. The parents spent considerable amounts of time at the bedside providing "skin-to-skin kangaroo care"; however, the infant required heavy "bundling" to maintain her temperature when not kangarooing. She was taking all of her feedings by mouth but gained only minimal weight over the week before discharge. She was discharged at 36 weeks PMA on a home monitor.

During the week after discharge you receive reports from the visiting nurses that despite keeping the house at close to 80°F and heavy bundling, her temperature was only 36.5°C. A week after discharge you receive a call from a nearby hospital that the infant had been feeding and became apneic while in the mother's arms. The infant recovered after vigorous stimulation and mouth-to-mouth resuscitation and was brought by the rescue squad to the local hospital. The infant was readmitted to your NICU for further evaluation. It was noted that he hadn't gained any weight since discharge.

Exercise 17

QUESTION

1. What do you think happened to this infant?

ANSWER

1. The infant suffered a cardiorespiratory event at home that was "frightening" to the parents. This event could be correctly diagnosed as an "acute life-threatening event" (ALTE), a term that has replaced the old term "near miss SIDS." This event, however, may have been precipitated by other, perhaps predictable, factors. The frequent "skin-to-skin" care given by the parents in the NICU just prior to discharge may have masked the infant's inability to maintain temperature without exogenous heat. It is possible that the thermal stress experienced by the infant at home precipitated the event that resulted in readmission. Large energy expenditures to maintain body temperature in extreme cases can lead to a decreased ability to defend against hypoxia with increasing ventilation, resulting in more apnea and periodic breathing. After admission, she required care in an isolette for 10 days and that was discontinued when her weight approached 1800 g. Otherwise, she appeared healthy. She had a number of studies to investigate other causes for the event which were all negative. She continued to gain weight over the next week and was discharged home weighing about 2 kg.

Natural History of Apnea of Prematurity and Discharging Infants Home

The decision to discharge an infant who has been hospitalized for several weeks requires good clinical judgment accompanied by a healthy dose of common sense. Traditionally, the criteria for discharge have included evidence of cardiopulmonary and neurologic stability. In practical terms, this means being able to maintain a normal temperature outside the incubator, taking all feedings by mouth, and no longer having significant apnea or bradycardia. Recently, there has been increasing pressure to discharge infants earlier and to reduce the length of hospital stay. Some have advocated a particular weight or PMA as a marker for discharge. For those infants who continue to have apnea but from all other standpoints are ready for discharge, several avenues of management have evolved. Infants at highest risk for continued apnea are those born at 32 weeks' gestation or earlier, especially when prolonged oxygen therapy is needed for residual lung disease. In this group of infants, especially those born at less than 28 weeks' gestation, significant apnea of prematurity often continues beyond 40 weeks PMA. In addition, the corrected age when apnea ceases is inversely correlated with gestational age at birth. Figure 12-16 shows the relationship of the last day of apnea

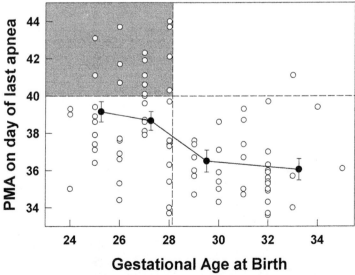

Figure 12-16 Relationship between the gestational age at birth (in weeks) and the postmenstrual age (PMA) on the day of the last episode of apnea. Each open circle represents one infant. The closed circles are the least-square means of the same data compressed into quartiles (means ± SEM). Reference lines have been included at 40 weeks PMA and at 28 weeks' gestational age to illustrate the distribution of infants who experience their last clinically significant apnea at 40 weeks or greater PMA. Nearlhy all such infants were born at 28 weeks of gestation or earlier. (Adapted from Darnall RA, Kattwinkel J, Nattie C, Robinson M: Margin of safety for discharge after apnea in preterm infants. Pediatrics 1997;100:795–801.)

and the gestation at birth in a group of infants born at 32 weeks' gestation or earlier from two tertiary intensive care nurseries. As shown, all but one infant who exhibited apnea beyond 40 weeks corrected age were 28 weeks' gestation or less at birth.

Furthermore, the incidence of apnea persisting beyond 38 weeks postconceptional age is significantly higher in infants born at 24 to 27 weeks, compared with infants born at 28 weeks' gestation. These data are consistent with the idea that the nervous systems of premature infants when they reach 40 weeks PMA are not as mature as the nervous systems of those born at 40 weeks' gestation. Supporting this hypothesis is the observation of more immature patterns of gray-white matter distribution, myelination, and neurobehavior in premature infants who have reached a term PMA compared with infants born at term. Apnea therefore may be an important marker of neurocardiorespiratory immaturity. These observations strongly argue against the advisability of using a fixed weight or PMA for discharge. An infant born at 25 weeks' gestation, for example, may well be less mature and at higher risk for significant apnea when he or she reaches a weight of 1800 g, than an 1800-g baby born at 32 weeks' gestation.

It is the practice of many neonatologists to observe infants with a history of apnea until they have been apnea free for some reasonable period of time off methylxanthines. Most of these infants are discharged without home monitoring. According to one survey of neonatologists, 84% observed infants for at least 5 days and 55% for at least 7 days before discharge without a monitor. Seventy-two percent of neonatologists responded that they usually do not send these infants home on monitors, and only 7% responded that they frequently discharge infants on xanthines. A recent study has confirmed the safety of a period of observation off methylxanthines before discharging an infant home without a monitor. In a population of infants born at 32 weeks' gestation or less from two major academic centers, it was concluded that otherwise healthy premature infants can occasionally have clinically significant apnea events separated by as many as 8 days before the last apnea preceding discharge occurs. Conversely, infants with longer between-apnea intervals often have identifiable risk factors other than apnea of prematurity. In another study,

24-hour recordings were made of nasal airflow, chest wall impedance, and oxyhemoglobin saturation in 187 infants thought to be ready for discharge. The discharge criteria included a 3-day apnea-free period off methylxanthines. In 12 infants, the discharge was delayed because of episodes that were too frequent, too prolonged, or too severe.

Some neonatologists continue to recommend the use of routine cardiorespiratory recordings in premature infants before discharge. This practice continues despite the fact that no relationship has ever been demonstrated between recorded events and apnea of prematurity, between recorded events and apparent life-threatening events, and between recorded events and sudden infant death syndrome (SIDS). In some NICUs, infants are commonly discharged with continuing episodes of apnea on methylxanthines, a home monitor, or both. There appears to be little consistency in the criteria for discharge in these infants, although frequently discharge is considered when the infant reaches an arbitrary PMA or weight (see the earlier discussion). The option of routine home monitoring, as opposed to observing infants in the hospital until they are apnea free for some period of time, remains controversial. It is important to understand that the home monitoring in this instance is for apnea of prematurity and not for prevention of SIDS. Unfortunately, this is an area of clinical practice in which widely differing opinions are often strongly held, but based on little data. There is no current consensus.

Only limited information is available about cardiorespiratory behavior in preterm infants after discharge from the nursery. There are a few reports in the literature, but they are difficult to interpret because of inconsistent discharge criteria, the limited value of impedance monitoring, short recording times, varying criteria for abnormal heart rate and oxyhemoglobin saturation, and the continued use of methylxanthines at home. In one recent report of long-term home monitoring, the most prevalent occurrence was a bradycardic event not associated with detectable apnea. These recordings, however, were based on impedance monitoring and, therefore, could not distinguish obstructive events. The Collaborative Home Infant Monitoring Evaluation (CHIME) study, a multicenter study supported by the National Institute of Child Health and Human Development, and the largest home monitoring study to date, demonstrated that otherwise healthy premature infants can have prolonged episodes of apnea associated with a fall in the oxyhemoglobin saturation and these events continue until 43 weeks PMA. Figure 12-17 illustrates the incidence of significant events in several groups of infants including (1) preterm infants that were at least apnea free for 5 days before discharge, (2) preterm infants that were having apnea at the time of discharge, (3) preterm and term infants who had experienced an ALTE, (4) preterm and term siblings of SIDS infants, and (5) healthy term infants. Note that significant events did not occur beyond 43 weeks PMA in any of the groups. In addition, those preterm infants who were still having apnea at discharge had a higher incidence of events at home compared to preterm infants who were apnea free for at least 5 days prior to discharge. These data are consistent with the understanding that apnea of prematurity is an important marker for neurodevelopment. Recently, the CHIME investigators, in a follow-up study of 443 preterm and 541 full-term infants, reported decreases in mean Mental Developmental Index in infants who had more than five recorded conventional apneic events at home after discharge underscoring the importance of not simply dismissing these events as normal phenomena.

From this apparent confusion, a number of facts are starting to emerge: (1) Some premature infants, especially those born at 28 weeks' gestation or less, continue to have clinically significant apnea beyond term; (2) cardiorespiratory recordings or pneumograms before discharge are not predictive of continuing clinically significant apnea of prematurity; and (3) routine home monitoring of premature infants who have been free of apnea for some period is not warranted. The controversy is largely centered on those infants who have met all other criteria for discharge except for apnea. These infants are generally born at less than 32 weeks' gestation and have a postconceptional age of at least 37 weeks. Even the fundamental issue of which events are clinically significant (i.e., dangerous) is open to question. If there continues to be clinically significant apnea (regardless of the criteria) the question then becomes whether to monitor the infant in the hospital or at home. There are no published data to help answer these questions. In consideration of the timing of discharge, there are other relevant issues (other than apnea), including the capabilities and desires of the parents and regional issues such as access to care. At present, there is no way to predict the safety of the home monitoring for an individual infant, so good clinical judgment and common sense are the guide.

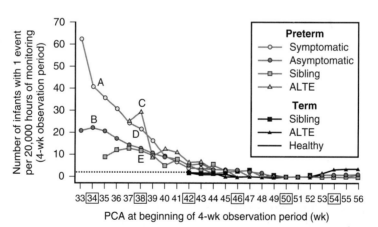

Figure 12-17 Each point represents the number of infants in a given study group who experienced at least one event exceeding the extreme threshold per 20,000 hours of monitor use during a 4-week observation period beginning at the specified PCA week. Poisson analyses were used to calculate relative rates for nonoverlapping 4-week periods (beginning at the PCA weeks enclosed in a box) compared with the reference group of healthy term infants observed from 42 to 45 weeks PCA. Significantly higher relative rates were observed in five groups, labeled A through E on the figure. A, preterm symptomatic group at 34 to 37 weeks (relative rate, 19.7; 95% confidence interval [CI], 4.1–94.0; $P < 0.001$. B, preterm asymptomatic group at 34 to 37 weeks (relative rate, 10.5; 95% CI, 2.4–47.0; $P = 0.002$. C, apparent life-threatening event (ALTE) preterm group at 38 to 41 weeks (relative rate, 14.3; 95% CI, 2.6–80.1; $P = 0.002$). D, preterm symptomatic group at 38 to 41 weeks (relative rate, 10.2; 95% CI, 2.2–47.8; $P = 0.003$). E, preterm asymptomatic group at 38 to 41 weeks (relative rate, 6.0; 95% CI, 1.4–26.5; $P = 0.02$). A sixth group consisted of the siblings of infants who died of sudden infant death syndrome, preterm group at 38 to 41 weeks (relative rate, 5.7; 95% CI, 1.0–31.1; $P = 0.05$). (Adapted from Ramanathan R, Corwin MJ, Hunt CE, et al and The Collaborative Home Infant Monitoring Evaluation Study Group: Cardiorespiratory events recorded on home monitors: Comparison of healthy infants with those at increased risk for SIDS. JAMA 2001;285[17]:2199–207.)

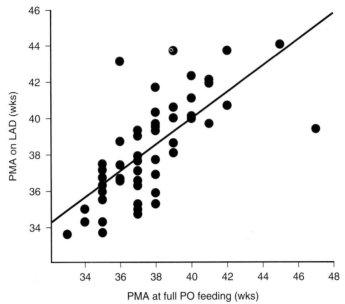

Figure 12-18 Relationship between the postmenstrual age (PMA) on the day of the last apnea and the postmenstrual age when full oral (PO) feedings were achieved. Each point represents a single infant.

Issues related to hospital stay continue to be controversial. A recent study showed that there are significant variations in the length of hospital stay of a large cohort of otherwise healthy preterm infants. The differences derived primarily from the variation in documented duration of time to mature feeding behavior and recurrent apnea. As pointed out by the authors, PMA at the time full oral feedings are achieved and the PMA on the last apnea day are closely linked and are both reasonable indicators of neurodevelopment. Figure 12-18 shows the relationship between the time full oral feedings are achieved and apnea resolution from our NICU. Variations in practice with respect to the management of apnea have important implications in the development of national guidelines for discharging preterm infants. Before meaningful guidelines can be developed, a consensus needs to be reached on what constitutes a "significant apnea or bradycardia" and the monitoring techniques that should be used to detect these events.

Suggested Readings

Alvaro R, Alvarez J, Kwiatkowski K, et al: Small preterm infants (1500 g) have only a sustained decrease in ventilation in response to hypoxia. Pediatr Res 1992;32:403–406.

Amiel J, Laudier B, Attie-Bitach T, et al: Polyalanine expansion and frameshift mutations of the paired-like homeobox gene PHOX2B in congenital central hypoventilation syndrome. Nat Genet 2003;33:1–3.

Anderson JW, Sant'Ambrogio FB, Mathew OP, Sant'Ambrogio G: Water-responsive laryngeal receptors in the dog are not specialized endings. Respir Physiol 1990;79:33–44.

Aubier M, Murciano D, Viires N, et al: Diaphragmatic contractility enhanced by aminophylline: Role of extracellular calcium. J Appl Physiol 1983;54:460–464.

Baird TM: Clinical correlates, natural history and outcome of neonatal apnoea. Semin Neonatol 2003;9: 205–211.

Barrington KJ, Finer N, Li D: Predischarge respiratory recordings in very low birth weight newborn infants. J Pediatr 1996;129(6):934–940.

Boggs DF, Bartlett D: Chemical specificity of a laryngeal apneic reflex in puppies. J Appl Physiol 1982; 53:455–462.

Botham SJ, Isaacs D, Henderson-Smart DJ: Incidence of apnoea and bradycardia in preterm infants following DTPw and Hib immunization: A prospective study. J Paediatr Child Health 1997;33(5):418–421.

Boutroy MJ, Vert P, Royer RJ, et al: Caffeine, a metabolite of theophylline during the treatment of apnea in the premature infant. J Pediatr 1979;94:996–998.

Brouillette RT, Côté A, Hanson MA: Control of breathing. In Gluckman PD, Heymann MA (eds): Pediatrics and Perinatology: The Scientific Basis. London, Arnold, 1996, pp 832–844.

Calder NA, Williams BA, Smyth J, et al: Absence of ventilatory responses to alternating breaths of mild hypoxia and air in infants who have had bronchopulmonary dysplasia: implications for the risk of sudden infant death. Pediatr Res 1994;35(6):677–681.

Coates EL, Li A, Nattie EE: Widespread sites of brain stem ventilatory chemoreceptors. J Appl Physiol 1993;75 (1):5–14.

Committee on Fetus and Newborn, American Academy of Pediatrics: Apnea, sudden infant death syndrome, and home monitoring. Pediatrics 2003;111:914–917.

Committee on Fetus and Newborn, American Academy of Pediatrics: Hospital discharge of the high-risk neonate: proposed guidelines. Pediatrics 1998;102:411–417.

Cordero L, Hon E: Neonatal bradycardia following naso-pharyngeal stimulation. J Pediatr 1971;78:441.

Côté A, Hum C, Brouillette RT, Themens M: Frequency and timing of recurrent events in infants using home cardiorespiratory monitors [see comments]. J Pediatr 1998;132(5):783–789.

Cote CJ, Zaslavsky A, Downes JJ, et al: Postoperative apnea in former preterm infants after inguinal her-niorrhaphy. A combined analysis [see comments]. Anesthesiology 1995;82(4):809–822.

Daily WJ, Klaus M, Meyer HB: Apnea in premature infants: Monitoring, incidence, heart rate changes, and an effect of environmental temperature. Pediat-rics 1969;43:510–518.

Darnall RA: Mild cooling to treat apnea increases oxygen consumption. Pediatr Res 1982;16:284.

Darnall RA, Ariagno RL: The effect of sleep state on active thermoregulation in the premature infant. Pediatr Res 1982;16:512–514.

Darnall RA, Kattwinkel J, Nattie C, Robinson M: Margin of safety for discharge after apnea in preterm infants. Pediatrics 1997;100(5):795–801.

Davies AM, Koenig JS, Thach BT: Upper airway chemor-eflex responses to saline and water in preterm infants. J Appl Physiol 1988;64(4):1412–1420.

Durand M, McEvoy C, MacDonald K: Spontaneous desa-turations in intubated very low birth weight infants with acute and chronic lung disease. Pediatr Pulmo-nol 1992;13:136–142.

Eichenwald EC, Aina A, Stark AR: Apnea frequently per-sists beyond term gestation in infants delivered at 24 to 28 weeks. Pediatrics 1997;100(3 Pt 1):354–359.

Eichenwald EC, Blackwell M, Lloyd JS, et al: Inter-neona-tal intensive care unit variation in discharge timing: Influence of apnea and feeding management. Pedi-atrics 2001;108(4):928–933.

Eichenwald EC, Howell RG, Kosch PC, et al: Develop-mental changes in sequential activation of laryngeal abductor muscle and diaphragm in infants. J Appl Physiol 1992;73(4):1425–1431.

Fewell JE, Kondo CS, Dascalu V, Filyk S: Influence of carotid denervation on the arousal and cardiopul-monary response to rapidly developing hypoxemia in lambs. Pediatr Res 1989;25:473–477.

Garg M, Kurzner SI, Bautista DB, Keens TG: Clinically unsuspected hypoxia during sleep and feeding in infants with bronchopulmonary dysplasia. Pediat-rics 1988;81:635–642.

Garg M, Kurzner SI, Bautista DB, Keens TG: Hypoxic arousal responses in infants with bronchopulmo-nary dysplasia. Pediatrics 1988;82(1):59–63.

Gauda EB, McLemore GL, Tolosa J, et al: Maturation of peripheral arterial chemoreceptors in relation to neo-natal apnoea. Semin Neonatol 2004;9(3):181–194.

Gaultier C, Amiel J, Dauger S, et al: Genetics and early disturbances of breathing control. Pediatr Res 2004;55:729–733.

Gerhardt T, Bancalari E: Apnea of prematurity. I. Lung function and regulation of breathing. Pediatrics 1984;74:58.

Gerhardt T, Bancalari E: Apnea of prematurity. II. Respiratory reflexes. Pediatrics 1984;74:63–66.

Glotzbach SF, Baldwin RB, Lederer NE, et al: Periodic breathing in preterm infants: Incidence and charac-teristics. Pediatrics 1989;84(5):785–792.

Gray PH, Rogers Y: Are infants with bronchopulmonary dysplasia at risk for sudden infant death syndrome? Pediatrics 1994;93(5):774–777.

Guyenet PG, Stornetta RL, Bayliss DA, Mulkey DK: Retro-trapezoid nucleus: A litmus test for the identification of central chemoreceptors. Exp Physiol 2005;90(3):247–257.

Haddad GG, Farber JP: Developmental neurobiology of breathing. Lenfant C (ed): Lung Biology in Health and Disease. New York, Marcel Dekker, 1991.

Henderson-Smart D: Apnea of prematurity. In Beckerman RC, Brouillette RT, Hunt CE (eds): Respiratory Control Disorders in Infants and Children. Baltimore, Williams & Wilkins, 1992, pp 161–177.

Henderson-Smart D: The effect of gestational age on the incidence and duration of recurrent apnoea in new-born babies. Aust Paediatr J 1981;17:273–276.

Henderson-Smart DJ, Butcher-Puech MC, Edwards DA: Incidence and mechanism of bradycardia dur-ing apnoea in preterm infants. Arch Dis Child 1986;61(3):227–232.

Henderson-Smart DJ, Osborn DA: Kinesthetic stimulation for preventing apnea in preterm infants [update of Cochrane Database Syst Rev 2000;(2):CD000373]. Cochrane Database Syst Rev 2002(2):CD000373.

Henderson-Smart DJ, Pettigrew AG, Campbell DJ: Clinical apnea and brainstem neural function in preterm infants. N Engl J Med 1983;308:353–357.

Hodgman JE, Hoppenbrouwers T, Cabal LA: Episodes of bradycardia during early infancy in the term-born and preterm infant [see comments]. Am J Dis Child 1993;147(9):960–964.

Hofer MA: Role of carotid sinus and aortic nerves in respiratory control of infant rats. Am J Physiol 1986;251:811–817.

Hunt CE, Corwin MJ, Baird T, et alThe CHIME Study Group: Cardiorespiratory events detected by home memory monitoring and one-year neurodevelop-mental outcome. J Pediatr 2004;145:465–471.

Hunt CE, McCulloch K, Brouillette RT: Diminished hyp-oxic ventilatory responses in near-miss sudden infant death syndrome. J Appl Physiol 1981;50:1315–1317.

Hüppi PS, Schuknecht B, Boesch C: Structural and neu-robehavioral delay in postnatal brain development of preterm infants. Pediatr Res 1996;39:895–901.

Kattwinkel J, Nearman HS, Fanaroff AA, et al: Apnea of prematurity: Comparative therapeutic effects of cuta-neous stimulation and nasal continuous positive air-way pressure. J Pediatr 1975;86(4):588–592.

Katz-Salamon M: Respiratory control in bronchopul-monary dysplasia. In Mathew OP (ed): Respiratory Control and Disorders in the Newborn. New York, Marcel Dekker, 2003, pp 451–472.

Korner AF, Draemer HC, Haffner ME: Effects of waterbed flotation on premature infants: A pilot study. Pediat-rics 1975;56:361.

Kosch PC, Hutchinson AA, Wozniak JA, et al: Posterior cricoarytenoid and diaphragm activities during tidal breathing in neonates. J Appl Physiol 1988;64:1968–1978.

Kotagal UR, Perlstein PH, Gamblian V, et al: Description and evaluation of a program for the early discharge of infants from a neonatal intensive care unit. J Pediatr 1995;127:285–290.

Kurth CD, LeBard SE: Association of postoperative apnea, airway obstruction, and hypoxemia in former premature infants. Anesthesiology 1991;75(1): 22–26.

Lawson EE: Nonpharmacological management of idiopathic apnea of the premature infant. In Mathew OP (ed): Respiratory Control and Disorders in the Newborn. New York, Marcel Dekker, 2003, pp 335–354.

Lawson EE: Recovery from central apnea: effect of stimulus duration and end-tidal CO2 partial pressure. J Appl Physiol 1982;53:105–109.

Lehtonen L, Martin RJ: Ontogeny of sleep and awake states in relation to breathing in preterm infants. Semin Neonatol 2003;9:229–238.

Lindgren C, Jing L, Graham B, et al: Respiratory syncytial virus infection reinforces reflex apnea in young lambs. Pediatr Res 1992;31:381–385.

Lindgren C, Lin J, Graham BS, et al: Respiratory syncytial virus infection enhances the response to laryngeal chemostimulation and inhibits arousal from sleep in young lambs. Acta Paediatr 1996;85 (7):789–797.

Martin RJ, Difiore JM, Jana L, et al: Persistence of the biphasic ventilatory response to hypoxia in preterm infants. J Pediatr 1998;132(6):960–964.

Martin RJ, Fanaroff AA: Neonatal apnea, bradycardia, or desaturation: Does it matter? [editorial; comment]. J Pediatr 1998;132(5):758–759.

Mathew OP: Maintenance of upper airway patency. J Pediatr 1985;106:863–869.

Mathew OP: Respiratory Control and Disorders in the Newborn. New York, Marcel Dekker, 2003, Vol 173 in the series of Lenfant C (ed): Lung Biology in Health and Disease.

Mathew OP, Roberts JL, Thach BT: Pharyngeal airway obstruction in preterm infants during mixed and obstructive apnea. J Pediatr 1982;100:964–968.

Mellins RB, Balfour HH Jr, Turino GM, Winters RW: Failure of automatic control of ventilation (Ondine's curse): Report of an infant born with this syndrome and review of the literature. Medicine (Baltimore) 1970;49(6):487–504.

Merritt TA, Pillers D, Prows SL: Early NICU discharge of very low birth weight infants: A critical review and analysis. Semin Neonatol 2003;8:95–115.

Milner AD, Greenough A: The role of the upper airway in neonatal apnoea. Semin Neonatol 2003;9:213–219.

Miller D, Schmidt B: Controversies surrounding xanthine therapy. Semin Neonatol 2003;9: 239–244.

Miller MJ, Carlo WA, Martin RJ: Continuous positive airway pressure selectively reduces obstructive apnea in preterm infants. J Pediatr 1985;106(1):91–94.

Miller MJ, Kiatchoosakun P: Relationship between respiratory control and feeding in the developing infant. Semin Neonatol 2003;9:221–227.

Miller MJ, Martin RJ: Pathophysiology of apnea of prematurity. In Polin RA, Fox WW (eds): Fetal and Neonatal Physiology. Philadelphia, WB Saunders, 1991, pp 872–884.

Muttitt SC, Finer NN, Tierney AJ, Rossmann J: Neonatal apnea: diagnosis by nurse versus computer. Pediatrics 1988;82(5):713–720.

National Institutes of Health Consensus Development Conference Statement: Infantile apnea and home monitoring. Pediatrics 1987;79:292–299.

Nattie EE: Central chemoreception. In Dempsey JA, Pack AI (eds): Regulation of Breathing. New York, Marcel Dekker, 1995, pp 473–510.

Newman W, Feltman JA, Devlin B: Pulmonary function studies in polycythemia vera. Am J Med 1951;11: 706–714.

Parmeggiani PL, Rabini D: Shivering and panting during sleep. Brain Res 1967;6:789.

Perlman JM, Volpe JJ: Episodes of apnea and bradycardia in the preterm newborn: impact on cerebral circulation. Pediatrics 1985;76(3):333–338.

Perlstein PH, Edwards NK, Sutherland JM: Apnea in premature infants and incubator-air-temperature changes. N Engl J Med 1970;282(9):461–466.

Pickens DL, Schefft G, Thach BT: Prolonged apnea associated with upper airway protective reflexes in apnea of prematurity. Am Rev Respir Dis 1988;137(1): 113–118.

Poets CF: Gastroesophageal reflux: A critical review of its role in preterm infants. Pediatrics 2004;113(2): e128–e132.

Poets CF: When do infants need additional inspired oxygen—A review of current literature. Pediatr Pulmonol 1998;26:424–428.

Ramanathan R, Corwin MJ, Hunt CE, et al: The Collaborative Home Infant Monitoring Evaluation Study Group: Cardiorespiratory events recorded on home monitors: Comparison of healthy infants with those at increased risk for SIDS. JAMA 2001;285(17): 2199–2207.

Rigatto H, Brady JF, Verduzco RT: Chemoreceptor reflexes in preterm infants: II. The effect of gestational and postnatal age on the ventilatory response to inhaled carbon dioxide. Pediatrics 1975;55:614.

Rigatto H: Periodic breathing. In Mathew OP (ed): Respiratory Control and Disorders in the Newborn. Marcel Dekker, New York, 2003, pp 237–272.

Rigatto H: Ventilatory response to hypoxia. In Oliver TK (ed): Seminars in Perinatology. New York, Grune & Stratton, 1977, pp 363–367.

Sammon MP, Darnall RA: Entrainment of respiration to rocking in premature infants: Coherence analysis. J Appl Physiol 1994;77(3):1548–1554.

Sankaran K, Wiebe H, Seshia MMK, Rigatto H: Immediate and late ventilatory response to high and low O_2 in preterm infants and adult subjects. Pediatr Res 1979;13:875–878.

Sekar KC, Duke JC: Sleep apnea and hypoxemia in recently weaned premature infants with and without bronchopulmonary dysplasia. Pediatr Pulmonol 1991;10(2):112–116.

Severinghaus JW, Mitchell RA: Ondine's curse—Failure of respiratory center automaticity while awake. Clin Res 1962;10:122.

Smith JC, Ellenberger HH, Ballanyi K, et al: Pre-Bötzinger complex: A brainstem region that may generate respiratory rhythm in mammals. Science 1991; 254:726–729.

Spitzer AR, Gibson E: Home monitoring. Clin Perinatol 1992;19:907–926.

Stark AR: Apnea. In Cloherty JP, Stark AR (eds): Manual of Neonatal Care. Philadelphia, Lippincott-Raven, 1998, pp 374–378.

St.-John WM, St.-Jacques R, Li A, Darnall RA: Modulation of hypoxic depressions of ventilatory activity in the newborn piglet by mesencephalic mechanisms. Brain Res 1999;819:147–149.

Tay-Uyboco JS, Kwiatkowska K, Cates DB, et al: Hypoxic airway constriction in infants of very low birth weight recovering from moderate to severe bronchopulmonary dysplasia. J Pediatr 1989;115: 456–459.

Teague WG, Pian MS, Heldt GP, Tooley WH: An acute reduction in the fraction of inspired oxygen increases airway constriction in infants with chronic lung disease. Am Rev Respir Dis 1988;137: 861–865.

Thach BT, Stark AR: Spontaneous neck flexion and airway obstruction during apneic spells in preterm infants. J Pediatr 1979;94(2):275–281.

Thach BT, Tauesch HW: Sighing in human newborn infants: Role of inflation-augmenting reflex. J Appl Physiol 1976;41:502–507.

Waggener TB, Stark AR, Cohlan BA, Frantz ID: Apnea duration is related to ventilatory oscillation characteristics in newborn infants. J Appl Physiol Resp Environ Exer Physiol 1984;57(2):536–544.

Weese-Mayer DE, Hunt CE, Brouillette RT: Alveolar hypoventilation syndromes. In Beckerman RC, Brouillette RT, Hunt CE (eds): Respiratory Control Disorders in Infants and Children. Baltimore, Williams & Wilkins, 1992, pp 231–241.

Weese-Mayer DE, Silvestri JM: Idiopathic congenital central hypoventilation syndrome. Mathew OP (ed): Respiratory Control and Disorders in the Newborn. New York, Marcel Dekker, 2003.

Weiskopf RR, Gabel RA: Depression of ventilation during hypoxia in man. J Appl Physiol 1975;39(6):911–915.

Werthammer J, Brown ER, Neff RK, Taeusch HW: Sudden infant death syndrome in infants with bronchopulmonary dysplasia. Pediatrics 1982;69:301–304.

Upton CJ, Milner AD, Stokes GM: Episodic bradycardia in preterm infants. Arch Dis Child 1992;67(7 Spec No):831–834.

Neonatal Sepsis

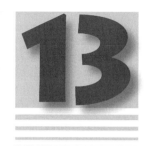

William E. Benitz, MD

The physician who knows syphilis, knows medicine.
Sir William Osler (1849–1919)

What Osler asserted at the beginning of the twentieth century could well be applied to neonatal medicine at the opening of the twenty-first. Like syphilis in decades past, neonatal sepsis is a great masquerader, and neonates with serious bacterial infection can present with almost any sign of illness. There is no doubt that antibiotic therapy is effective, and it is an article of faith that delays in treatment may have disastrous consequences. On the other hand, unnecessary treatment can disrupt mother-infant bonding, interfere with breastfeeding, and invite iatrogenic complications, such as infection with resistant organisms. The approach to neonatal sepsis rests upon three cornerstones: prevention of infection whenever possible; early recognition, evaluation, and treatment of infants who may have serious bacterial infections; and prompt discontinuation of treatment as soon as it is evident that it is no longer necessary.

Neonatal sepsis can be defined as a systemic pathophysiologic response to the presence of microorganisms (or their toxins) in the first 28 days of life. Bacteremia may accompany focal infections of soft tissues, bones, joints, or urinary, gastrointestinal, or respiratory tracts. Most cases of meningitis are complications of bacteremia. These infections are all subsumed within this general discussion of sepsis, but the specifics of each focal infection will not be addressed here. Similarly, viral infections and unusual bacterial infections such as congenital tuberculosis or neonatal Lyme disease, which may present with signs indistinguishable from those of bacterial sepsis, will not be covered in this chapter.

In this chapter, we will track the courses of four neonates with different clinical circumstances. In each case, the opportunities for prevention, appropriate interventions, and critical decision points will be addressed. These case discussions will provide a framework for a discussion of common neonatal bacterial and fungal infections. But first, we will briefly review some aspects of the epidemiology of neonatal sepsis.

Exercise 1

QUESTIONS

1. Which of the following statements about neonatal sepsis are true?

   a. Suspected neonatal sepsis is the most common indication for admission to a neonatal intensive care unit in the United States.

   b. Neonatal sepsis is among the top three causes of neonatal death in the United States.

   c. Efforts to prevent and treat neonatal sepsis have had a substantial impact on neonatal mortality rates attributable to neonatal infections.

   d. Efforts to prevent and treat neonatal sepsis have not had a substantial impact on the rates of neonatal infection.

2. Which of the following statistics most closely approximate the incidence of neonatal sepsis

and meningitis and the mortality rate attributable to neonatal sepsis in the United States and other developed nations?

	Sepsis	Meningitis	Mortality Rate
a. 1 to 5 per 1 million live births	☐	☐	☐
b. 1 to 5 per 100,000 live births	☐	☐	☐
c. 1 to 5 per 10,000 live births	☐	☐	☐
d. 1 to 5 per 1000 live births	☐	☐	☐
e. 1 to 5 per 100 live births	☐	☐	☐

3. Which of the following classifications is most useful in guiding initial management of suspected neonatal sepsis?

    a. Gram-positive/gram-negative/anaerobic/fungal infections

    b. Extremely low birth weight/low birth weight/normal birth weight infants

    c. Male/female gender

    d. Early onset/late onset/nosocomial infections

    e. Focal infection/bloodstream infection/meningitis

ANSWERS

1. a and c are true.

2. Sepsis, d; meningitis, c; mortality rate, c.

3. d.

Epidemiology

Suspected sepsis is the most common working diagnosis for infants admitted to neonatal intensive care units.[1] Of the approximately 4 million infants born each year in the United States, up to 600,000 (15%) are evaluated for possible serious bacterial infections, and as many as 400,000 (10%) may be given empiric antibiotic therapy pending the results of diagnostic tests.[2] However, only a few of these newborn infants are found to have sepsis. Despite recent declines in the incidence of neonatal sepsis, it remains a major cause of neonatal morbidity and death. Worldwide, infections are the most common causes of death in the neonatal period,[3,4] accounting for about 1.6 million neonatal deaths annually in developing countries. Excluding tetanus and diarrhea, sepsis and pneumonia alone account for 28% of neonatal deaths, trailing only prematurity (28% of deaths) in prevalence. In contrast, bacterial sepsis is the sixth most common cause of death in the neonatal period in the United States (after prematurity; birth defects; complications of pregnancy; disorders of the placenta, cord, or membranes; and respiratory distress syndrome),[5] but it remains one of the causes of death most amenable to prevention or effective treatment. The contribution of bacterial infection to the neonatal mortality rate may be significantly underestimated, as postmortem cultures of blood and cerebrospinal fluid demonstrate unsuspected bacterial infections in 10% to 25% of neonatal autopsies.[6,7]

The incidence of neonatal sepsis has been estimated to range between 6 and 9 per 1000 live births,[3] representing fewer than 10% of the infants who undergo diagnostic evaluation and empiric treatment for suspected sepsis. Meningitis is diagnosed in 4 to 11 infants per 10,000 live births.[8,9] National mortality statistics have shown a steady reduction in neonatal deaths attributable to sepsis in the United States since the 1970s[5,10-12] (Table 13-1) to a current rate of approximately 2 per 10,000 live births. These data suggest that prevention efforts, primarily directed toward reduction of the rate of sepsis due to group B streptococcus, have been effective in reducing the overall incidence of this disease. Not all types of sepsis

TABLE 13-1

NEONATAL MORTALITY RATES FROM SEPSIS— UNITED STATES 1979–2002

Epoch	Deaths/ Year	Mortality Rate*	Reference
1979–1981	1808	50.5	10
1986–1988	1643	43.0	10
1992–1994	1521	38.0	10
1995–1998	1185	31.8	11
2002	705	17.5	5,12

*Deaths due to sepsis per 100,000 live births.

have been equally affected, however. CDC surveillance data[13,14] have demonstrated a substantial (approximately 70%) and sustained reduction in attack rates for early onset sepsis caused by group B streptococcus (GBS) (Fig. 13-1). Rates of late onset group B streptococcal sepsis have not changed. The impact of prevention efforts on rates of infection due to other organisms is controversial. Experience at some hospitals suggested that increased use of intrapartum antibiotic prophylaxis has been associated with an increase in the incidence of infection with other organisms, particularly *Escherichia coli*. However, population studies indicate that the rates of gram-negative and *E. coli* infections have been reduced, at least in some settings, but to a lesser extent than early onset GBS infections.[15,16]

The risk of infection increases steeply with decreasing gestational age (Table 13-2)[17] and therefore correlates with low birth weight (Table 13-3).[18] Neonatal sepsis is more common in males than in females.[19] Microorganisms in any of the categories named in Question 3a, as well as viruses, may be responsible for causing sepsis syndrome in neonates, but these infectious agents cannot be distinguished from one another early in the course of the illness. Despite these associations, none of these classifications are of much use in guiding initial management. The location of the infection has important implications for management, but classification by site is not practical early in the

course of the illness. Some focal infections, such as osteomyelitis or septic arthritis, are the result of an antecedent bacteremia, making the focal versus systemic distinction specious. The clinical findings in infants with meningitis are difficult to distinguish from those of infants who have sepsis alone. There are a few focal infections (e.g., perianal abscess) that are rarely associated with systemic dissemination, but these are exceptions, and classification on this basis is not generally a useful guide for initial management.

Neonatal infections are usually classified (according to the age of the infant and clinical setting at the time of onset of the illness) as early onset, late onset, and nosocomial infections. Each of these categories has a characteristic timing of onset, predisposing factors, mode of presentation, and bacteriology. Although different thresholds (ranging from 2 to 10 days of age) have been used to distinguish early from late onset disease, a consensus seems to be developing that early onset sepsis should be defined as those cases that develop in the first 72 hours after birth. Most cases of early onset neonatal sepsis are recognized in the first 48 hours,[20] and nearly all cases of early onset group B streptococcus infection are evident within 24 hours of birth.[21] Late onset neonatal sepsis consists of those cases that present between 3 and 28 days of age. It is useful to distinguish episodes that develop in previously well infants outside the hospital (late onset, or community-acquired infections) from those in

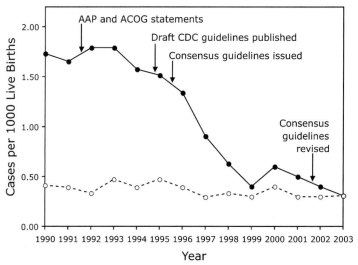

Figure 13-1 Attack rates for neonatal group B streptococcus sepsis in CDC surveillance areas, 1990–2003. Early onset: closed circles, solid line; late-onset: open circles, broken line. (Data from Schrag SJ, Zywicki S, Farley MM, et al: Group B streptococcal disease in the era of intrapartum antibiotic prophylaxis. N Engl J Med 2000;342:15–20 and Centers for Disease Control and Prevention: Active Bacterial Core Surveillance Report. 2005. Available at www.cdc.gov/ncidod/dbmd/abcs/survreports.htm.)

TABLE 13-2

REPRESENTATIVE ODDS RATIOS FOR MATERNAL RISK FACTORS ASSOCIATED WITH EARLY ONSET
NEONATAL SEPSIS

Clinical Finding	Univariate Odds Ratio (95% CI)	Reference
Meconium-stained fluid	1.8 (1.2–2.6)	24
Spontaneous onset of labor before term	1.9 (1.1–3.2)	24
Screening for group B streptococcus (GBS) colonization before delivery	0.48 (0.38–0.61)	88
Medicaid insurance coverage*	1.49 (1.17–1.91)	88
Preterm delivery (< 37 weeks)	1.76 (1.28–2.42)	88
Prolonged rupture of membranes (> 18 hr)	1.80 (1.28–2.53)	88
Inadequate prenatal care*	1.80 (1.37–2.36)	88
Black race	2.20 (1.73–2.80)	88
Maternal age < 20 years	2.64 (1.93–3.60)	88
Previous infant with GBS disease	3.79 (1.30–11.1)	88
Intrapartum fever > 37.5°C†	4.05 (2.17–7.56)	89
Intrapartum fever ≥ 38°C	5.99 (4.28–8.38)	88
Preterm premature rupture of membranes (PPROM)	6.02 (1.95–18.7)	17
Fetal tachycardia > 160 bpm	6.3 (4.0–10)	24
Chorioamnionitis	6.42 (2.32–17.8)	17
Preeclampsia	6.43 (1.73–23.8)	19
Prolonged rupture of membranes > 18 hr (PROM)	5.92 (2.19–16.1)	17
Placental abruption	12.7 (1.88–85.2)	19
Positive rectovaginal GBS culture at 36 weeks†	29.4 (7.44–116)	89
Fetal tachycardia > 160 bpm in last 10 min of labor	55.3 (8.68–345)	25
Positive vaginal GBS culture during labor†	204 (100–419)	26
Gestational age 34–36 weeks‡	3.25 (0.90–11.8)	17
Gestational age 31–33 weeks‡	6.89 (1.56–30.8)	17
Gestational age 28–30 weeks‡	14.8 (3.23–70.3)	17
Gestational age < 28 weeks‡	32.1 (4.19–265)	17

*Not significant in multivariate analysis.
†Odds ratios specific for risk of group B streptococcus sepsis.
‡Reference group: gestational age ≥ 37 weeks.

infants who remain hospitalized (nosocomial, or hospital-acquired infections).[22] The latter may occur in as many as 25% of very low birth weight (VLBW) infants and others who require extended hospitalizations. The characteristics of these conditions will be explored in the following exercises.

Case Study 1

Ms. A was a 24-year-old primigravida who received good prenatal care starting at 12 weeks' gestation. Her estimated date of delivery was established by ultrasonography at 14 weeks. At 29 weeks' gestation, she telephoned her obstetrician's office to report fluid leaking from her vagina for 2 hours. In the obstetrician's office, the fluid was found to be nitrazine positive and positive for

ferning. She denied feeling uterine contractions and none were palpated. She was sent to the hospital for admission to the antepartum unit.

Case Study 2

Ms. B was a 32-year-old gravida 3 para 2 woman whose prior medical history and pregnancies had been uncomplicated. She had good prenatal care and her prenatal laboratory results were unremarkable, except for recovery of group B streptococci from a rectovaginal swab obtained at 35 weeks' gestation. She presented to the Labor and Delivery Unit at 41 weeks' gestation with regular contractions, intact membranes, and cervical dilation to 3 cm. Her membranes ruptured spontaneously an hour after admission. Over the next 4 hours, cervical dilation progressed to only 4 cm. An epidural catheter was

TABLE 13-3

TABLE 13-3

REPRESENTATIVE ODDS RATIOS FOR INFANT CLINICAL SIGNS ASSOCIATED WITH EARLY ONSET
NEONATAL SEPSIS

Clinical Finding	Univariate Odds Ratio (95% CI)	Reference
Male sex	1.75 (1.13–2.70)	19
Retractions	2.41 (1.03–5.63)	90
Lethargy	2.78 (1.14–6.78)	90
Poor feeding	2.85 (1.13–7.19)	90
Apnea	3.75 (1.47–9.56)	90
Abdominal distention	4.10 (1.53–11.0)	90
Hypotension or hypertension	4.42 (1.41–14.0)	90
Irritability	4.84 (1.79–13.2)	90
Pustules	6.4 (1.7–25)	90
Bleeding	6.6 (1.4–32)	90
Decreased peripheral perfusion	7.87 (3.15–19.7)	90
Jaundice (nonphysiologic, no isoimmunization)	8.1 (2.9–23)	19
Tachycardia or arrhythmia	8.20 (3.28–20.6)	90
Vasomotor instability	9.5 (3.1–30)	90
Pallor	20.6 (7.13–60.2)	90
Omphalitis	37 (7.3–180)	90
Purpura	53 (7.1–380)	90
Hyaline membrane disease	71 (9.1–550)	19
Neonatal tachycardia > 160 bpm, persistent	126 (17–940)	91
Birth weight 1500–2499 g*	14.4 (9.2–22.4)	18
Birth weight 1000–1499 g*	47.7 (30.0–76.0)	18
Birth weight 600–999 g*	94.5 (61.0–147)	18
Cord blood metabolic acidosis (pH ≤ 7.18)[†]	56.4 (17.0–188)	92
Twin with group B streptococcus sepsis	≈130	26

*Reference group: birth weight ≥ 2500 g.
[†]Odds ratio specific for risk of group B streptococcus sepsis.

placed, epidural analgesia was initiated, and labor was augmented with Pitocin. Labor continued to progress slowly, and after 12 hours of labor augmentation her cervix had dilated to only 8 cm. At that time, she was found to have an elevated temperature to 38.4°C.

Case Study 3

Ms. C was a healthy 28-year-old woman who presented for delivery of her second child in active labor with intact membranes at 35½ weeks' gestation. Antepartum screening cultures for group B streptococcus colonization had not been performed.

Case Study 4

Ms. D was a 15-year-old high school student who presented to the emergency room with cramping abdominal pain. She denied having been sexually active, but her physical examination showed a fundal height of 25 cm and auscultation confirmed the presence of fetal heart sounds. She was afebrile and her examination was otherwise not remarkable. Obstetric ultrasonography demonstrated an intrauterine pregnancy with fetal measurements consistent with a gestational age of 26 weeks. She was sent to the labor floor for admission. Her initial evaluation showed moderate uterine contractions at intervals of 5 to 7 minutes and cervical dilation to 3 cm with 80% effacement.

Exercise 2

QUESTION

1. Which of the following risk factors for neonatal sepsis are present in each of these pregnant women?

	Case 1	Case 2	Case 3	Case 4
a. Threatened preterm delivery	☐	☐	☐	☐
b. Premature preterm rupture of membranes	☐	☐	☐	☐
c. Prolonged rupture of membranes	☐	☐	☐	☐
d. Intrapartum fever	☐	☐	☐	☐
e. Group B streptococcal colonization	☐	☐	☐	☐
f. Chorioamnionitis	☐	☐	☐	☐
g. Lack of prenatal care	☐	☐	☐	☐

ANSWER

1. Case 1: a, b. Case 2: e. Case 3: a. Case 4: a.

Ms. A has premature (before onset of labor) preterm (before term gestation) rupture of membranes (PPROM), which is a major independent risk factor for neonatal sepsis and also predisposes to preterm delivery. Ms. B is colonized with group B streptococci. Her elevated temperature is attributable to epidural analgesia, which is associated with a gradual increase in maternal temperature up to a maximum of 38.5°C.[23] Ruptured membranes for 16 hours does not meet the criterion for prolonged rupture of membranes (>18 hours). Ms. C is likely to deliver before term. Her GBS colonization status is unknown. Ms. D has preterm labor. Although that may be a consequence of chorioamnionitis, that diagnosis cannot be made from the information available. Lack of prenatal care has not been established as an independent indicator of risk.

Early Onset Sepsis

Maternal Indicators of Risk

Numerous studies have evaluated the relationship between maternal conditions and the risk of neonatal bacterial infection, both in general[17,19,24,25] and for group B streptococcus infections in particular.[26] Representative estimates of the odds ratios for early onset neonatal

sepsis associated with several of these conditions are shown in Table 13-2. Some of these conditions may afford opportunities for intervention to prevent the development of infection, but others occur so late in labor (fetal tachycardia in the last 10 minutes prior to delivery) or typically only become known after delivery (vaginal GBS colonization during labor) that they are not useful as indications for prophylaxis. Others are associated with only small increases in the risk of infection (e.g., meconium staining of the amniotic fluid) or have not been validated as independent risks in multiple studies (fetal tachycardia).

For early onset neonatal infections, the major maternal indicators of neonatal infection risk are PPROM, clinical chorioamnionitis, impending preterm delivery, and risk factors specific for group B streptococcal infections.[26] PPROM (which must be distinguished from PROM) appears to be a particularly powerful predictor of neonatal infection risk, with sepsis developing in up to 15% of these infants overall, and GBS sepsis developing in as many as one third to one half of those whose mothers are GBS-colonized. Chorioamnionitis, at least when diagnosed using stringent clinical criteria (fever > 38.0°C and at least two additional characteristic clinical findings such as fetal tachycardia, maternal tachycardia, maternal leukocytosis, foul-smelling vaginal discharge, or uterine tenderness) also correlates with a neonatal infection rate of up to 20%. Significantly, such findings are present in nearly 90% of women whose infants become infected despite appropriate intrapartum antibiotic prophylaxis. Preterm birth dramatically increases the risk of early onset neonatal infection, both because preterm labor may be caused by subclinical intrauterine infection and because the immune defenses of the preterm infant may be particularly compromised by incomplete transplacental transfer of protective maternal antibodies and immature leukocyte function. The incremental risk is much greater in infants who deliver before 31 weeks' gestation (see Table 13-2). The strong association of early onset sepsis with these perinatal risk factors is a reflection of vertical acquisition of the infecting organisms from the maternal genitourinary tract prior to or during the course of delivery.

Many variables are associated with substantially increased risk of group B streptococcus infection. Many of these, such as race, socioeconomic status, and inner city residence may be surrogate markers for proximal risk indicators, such as maternal colonization, and therefore have limited clinical utility. Others, such as absence of maternal specific opsonizing antibodies, are neither readily recognizable nor currently modifiable by treatment. The CDC consensus guidelines[27] identify five major indicators of risk for early onset GBS sepsis: (1) a prior infant born to the same mother who had invasive GBS disease, (2) GBS bacteriuria during gestation, (3) maternal GBS colonization, (4) preterm delivery before screening for GBS colonization, and (5) intrapartum fever (>38 °C) or prolonged rupture of membranes (>18 hours) in women with unknown GBS colonization. Each of these findings is considered a sufficient indication for intrapartum antibiotic prophylaxis.

Exercise 3

QUESTION

1. Which of the following interventions, if any, would be appropriate in each of these circumstances?

	Case 1	Case 2	Case 3	Case 4
a. Vaginal culture for group B streptococci	☐	☐	☐	☐
b. Ampicillin 2 g IV, then 1 g IV every 6 hours	☐	☐	☐	☐
c. Erythromycin 250 mg IV every 6 hours	☐	☐	☐	☐
d. Gentamicin 80 mg IV every 24 hours	☐	☐	☐	☐
e. Magnesium sulfate IV 4 g × 1, then 2 g/hour	☐	☐	☐	☐
f. Betamethasone 12 mg IM every 24 hours × 2	☐	☐	☐	☐

ANSWER

1. Case 1: a, b, c, f. Case 2: b. Case 3: b. Case 4: a, e, f.

As a patient with PPROM, Ms. A should be given ampicillin and erythromycin prophylaxis.

Because she is at risk of preterm delivery, induction of lung maturity with antenatal steroids (betamethasone) is also appropriate. Ms. B is colonized with GBS, so intrapartum antibiotic prophylaxis with penicillin or ampicillin is indicated. Ms. C has impending preterm delivery with unknown GBS colonization status, so she should also receive intrapartum antibiotic prophylaxis. The objective of treatment for Ms. D is delaying delivery as much as possible with the suppression of labor (e.g., with magnesium sulfate [antibiotics have not been shown to have efficacy in this respect]). Because her delivery is not imminent, antibiotic prophylaxis is not indicated. She should be screened for GBS colonization to determine whether intrapartum prophylaxis should be given in the likely event that delivery before term becomes imminent. Antepartum betamethasone treatment would also be appropriate, although some would not consider it until 28 weeks' gestation.

Maternal Interventions for Risk Reduction

A randomized controlled trial has demonstrated that the risk of infection in infants born to women with PPROM can be reduced by nearly 50% by treatment with intravenous ampicillin (2 g IV every 6 hours) and erythromycin (250 mg IV every 6 hours) for 48 hours, followed by oral amoxicillin (250 mg every 8 hours) and erythromycin (333 mg every 8 hours) for 5 days.[28] The risk of infection associated with clinical chorioamnionitis is reduced by more than 80% with intrapartum antibiotic treatment, which typically consists of broad-spectrum antibiotics, such as ampicillin and gentamicin. The ORACLE II trial, which enrolled more than 600 patients, demonstrated that oral administration of amoxicillin-clavulanic acid, erythromycin, or both had no impact on the risk of subsequent neonatal infection for infants born to women in preterm labor and intact membranes without other signs of infection.[29] Intrapartum intravenous administration of penicillin for prophylaxis against group B streptococcus sepsis is recommended for women with threatened preterm delivery, unless they have had a negative antepartum screening culture within the previous 5 weeks.[27]

There is good evidence that regimens recommended for prevention of early onset group B streptococcal infections are effective.[30] Clinical trials have shown that both penicillin (5 million units IV once, followed by 2.5 million units IV every 4 hours until delivery) and ampicillin (2 g IV once, followed by 1 g IV every 4 hours until delivery), coupled with neonatal prophylaxis with the same agents, reduce the attack rate by approximately 95%. Use of intrapartum prophylaxis alone has been estimated to prevent 80% of the expected cases. The CDC guidelines recommend penicillin, because of its narrower spectrum of activity. Empirical evidence does not show that ampicillin is more likely than penicillin to select for resistant gram-negative organisms.[31] However, it is important to note that adoption of these strategies for prevention of early onset GBS infections has had a dramatic impact on the incidence of this disease (see Fig. 13-1).[13,14] For women who may be allergic to penicillin but who have no history of anaphylaxis, angioedema, or urticaria, cephazolin (2 g IV once, followed by 1 g IV every 8 hours) is the recommended agent. Although there have been no clinical trials of this drug for GBS infections, it is very likely effective because therapeutic levels in the fetus and amniotic fluid are achieved quickly and the organism remains uniformly sensitive. Alternatives recommended for women at high risk for anaphylactic reactions include clindamycin, erythromycin, and vancomycin. GBS is consistently sensitive to vancomycin, but the prevalence of resistance to erythromycin and clindamycin is rapidly increasing (up to 30% and 20% for these drugs, respectively).[32] Therefore, sensitivity testing of GBS strains isolated from prenatal cultures is essential to exclude resistance to these agents prior to their use in intrapartum prophylaxis. In addition, there have been no clinical trials of clindamycin, erythromycin, or vancomycin for prevention of neonatal GBS infection or colonization, and little is known about placental transfer of these agents, so a high level of suspicion for GBS infection in at-risk infants whose mothers were treated with these antibiotics should be maintained.

Case Study 1 *Continued*

Upon admission of Ms. A to the labor suite, swabs of the rectum and lower third of the vagina were obtained and sent for cultures. Treatment with intravenous ampicillin and erythromycin was initiated. After 2 days of intravenous therapy, oral

therapy with amoxicillin and erythromycin was substituted and continued for 5 days. Her rectovaginal cultures were reported negative for GBS. She was discharged home on oral medications, but returned in active labor at 32 weeks' gestation. Because the cervix was already dilated to 5 cm, no tocolytic therapy was attempted.

Case Study 4 *Continued*

Because of her preterm labor, Ms. D was treated with intravenous magnesium sulfate. Despite initial suppression of uterine activity, contractions resumed within a few hours, and cervical dilation had progressed to 5 cm with 90% effacement.

Exercise 4

QUESTIONS

1. With this additional information, how would you characterize the risk of infection in these two cases?

	Case 1	Case 4
a. Very low (1%)	☐	☐
b. Low (1–2%)	☐	☐
c. Moderate (2–5%)	☐	☐
d. High (5–10%)	☐	☐
e. Very high (10%)	☐	☐

2. What interventions would be appropriate now?

	Case 1	Case 4
a. Ampicillin and gentamicin IV	☐	☐
b. Ampicillin, gentamicin, and clindamycin IV	☐	☐
c. Ampicillin, cefotaxime, and metronidazole IV	☐	☐
d. Penicillin IV	☐	☐
e. None of the above	☐	☐

ANSWERS

1. Case 1: d. Case 4: e.

2. Case 1: a, b, c, or e. Case 4: a, b, c, or e.

Even after prophylactic antibiotic treatment of women with PPROM and no GBS colonization (like Ms. A), the residual risk of neonatal sepsis remains substantial at about 8%.[28] Ms D. has an impending delivery of a preterm infant at less than 28 weeks, and her labor is refractory to tocolytic therapy, suggesting that she has chorioamnionitis that is otherwise subclinical. These findings indicate a very high risk for bacterial infection.

Because Ms. A has no evidence of GBS colonization, the CDC guidelines do not recommend intrapartum antibiotic prophylaxis for GBS sepsis. Preterm labor with progression refractory to tocolytic therapy may be an indication for broad-spectrum treatment of suspected chorioamnionitis, using any of the combinations listed in choices a to c. The high risk of infection in their babies—even despite the earlier treatment for Ms. A—would prompt some to recommend treatment anyway. There is no clear consensus on the most appropriate management of either of these women.

Peripartum Risk Evaluation

Assessment of risk, and reassessments as additional information becomes available, may be quite difficult. The impact of individual findings on the risk of infection may be estimated using the odds ratios shown in Tables 13-2 and 13-3, along with knowledge of the overall attack rate for neonatal sepsis. Unless all of the odds ratios included are obtained from the same multivariate regression, however, it is not appropriate to simply apply multiple odds ratios in sequence to estimate the risk in infants with multiple findings. For example, the odds ratio for neonatal infection in a preterm infant born at 27 weeks' gestation and 900 g birth weight would *not* be approximately 3200, as might be suggested by multiplication of the univariate odds ratio for gestation less than 28 weeks (32) by that for birth weight less than 1000 g (approximately 100), because these findings are not independent variables. Nonetheless, infants with multiple findings (maternal, neonatal, or laboratory) are at greater risk than infants with only a single risk factor. Conversely, appropriate interventions may significantly reduce the risk of neonatal infection,[30] and should not be treated as indicators of incremental risk. Synthesis of multiple observations into a single estimate of risk to guide management decisions—either to perform additional diagnostic tests or to initiate or terminate treatments—is the central challenge of these endeavors.

Case Study 1 *Continued*

Ms. A progressed to spontaneous vaginal delivery of a baby boy weighing 1720 g. The labor was unremarkable, without intrapartum fever, fetal tachycardia, uterine tenderness, or abnormal contraction patterns. No intrapartum antibiotics were administered. Arterial cord blood gases included a pH of 7.22, Pco$_2$ of 52 mm Hg, and Po$_2$ of 21 mm Hg. Boy A was vigorous, required no resuscitation, had Apgar scores of 7 and 9, and was admitted to the NICU. There were no signs of respiratory distress and he had satisfactory pulse oximeter readings in room air.

Case Study 2 *Continued*

Because of her known colonization with GBS and a history of penicillin allergy, Ms. B was treated with intravenous clindamycin, beginning soon after admission. After 16 hours of Pitocin augmentation, she delivered a vigorous 3250-g girl with Apgar scores of 6 and 8 at 1 and 5 minutes of age. There was a mild fetal tachycardia to 170 to 180 beats per minute, along with several variable decelerations to fetal heart rates in the 80s over the last 20 minutes of labor. Cord blood gases showed an arterial pH of 7.12, Pco$_2$ of 55 mm Hg, and Po$_2$ of 19 mm Hg. Resuscitation consisted of stimulation and brief administration of blow-by oxygen. On arrival in the NICU, baby girl B was slightly dusky and mildly tachypneic.

Case Study 3 *Continued*

Ms. C had rapid progression of labor and precipitous delivery of a 2830-g boy. Baby boy C had Apgar scores of 8 and 9. He began breast-feeding in the delivery room and his physical examination on admission to the well-baby nursery was entirely benign.

Case Study 4 *Continued*

Uterine contractions and cervical dilation continued to progress, despite tocolytic therapy. Fetal heart rate monitoring showed fetal tachycardia to 180 to 200 beats per minute with reduced variability, and Ms. D complained of uterine tenderness and developed a fever to 38.8°C shortly before delivery. Baby D was a 765-g baby girl who had Apgar scores of 3, 5, and 7 at 1, 5, and 10 minutes, respectively. She required intubation and received her first dose of surfactant in the delivery room. She was then admitted to the NICU for continuing intensive care.

Exercise 5

QUESTION

1. What additional indicators of infection are exhibited by each of these newborn infants?

	Case 1	Case 2	Case 3	Case 4
a. Abnormal fetal heart rate tracing	☐	☐	☐	☐
b. Clinical chorioamnionitis	☐	☐	☐	☐
c. Precipitous delivery	☐	☐	☐	☐
d. Low Apgar score	☐	☐	☐	☐
e. Tachypnea	☐	☐	☐	☐
f. Cyanosis	☐	☐	☐	☐
g. Acidosis	☐	☐	☐	☐
h. Respiratory distress	☐	☐	☐	☐
i. Apnea	☐	☐	☐	☐
j. Intrapartum exposure to antibiotics	☐	☐	☐	☐
k. None	☐	☐	☐	☐

ANSWER

1. Case 1: k. Case 2: a, e, f, g. Case 3: k. Case 4: a, b, d, g.

Neonatal Signs of Early Onset Sepsis

Early onset infections are often characterized by fulminant onset, multisystem involvement, and prominent signs of respiratory failure and circulatory collapse. The early manifestations are frequently less dramatic, and can be subtle. At birth, infected fetuses may be depressed, have persistently low Apgar scores, and require resuscitation and continuing support. Signs of infection include respiratory distress (grunting, retractions, tachypnea, cyanosis), circulatory disturbances (pallor, mottling, cool extremities, hypotension), thermal instability (usually hypothermia), behavioral changes (poor feeding, lethargy, hypotonia), gastrointestinal dysfunction (abdominal distention, vomiting—especially if bilious), and hypoglycemia. Infants with meningitis may have a bulging fontanel, seizures, nuchal rigidity, and opisthotonus, but these specific signs are late and unreliable findings. Representative odds ratios associated with various potential signs of neonatal sepsis are shown in Table 13-3. Notably, many signs commonly believed to be strongly associated with sepsis—including tachypnea, grunting, cyanosis, abnormal muscle tone, and seizures—are quite nonspecific and have odds ratios that are not statistically significant. These findings should suggest, but cannot confirm, the diagnosis of neonatal sepsis. In addition, more than half of infants with early onset sepsis are asymptomatic at birth[33]; therefore, relying on signs of illness as indicators of the diagnosis is inappropriate. Yet, any sign of illness in a neonate can be a sign of bacterial infection; therefore, this diagnosis is included in the differential diagnosis for the majority of infants admitted to neonatal intensive care.

Exercise 6

QUESTION

1. Which of the following diagnostic tests are appropriate for each of these newborn infants?

	Case 1	Case 2	Case 3	Case 4
a. White blood cell count with differential	☐	☐	☐	☐
b. C-reactive protein level	☐	☐	☐	☐
c. Lumbar puncture for CSF analysis	☐	☐	☐	☐
d. Blood culture	☐	☐	☐	☐
e. Urine culture	☐	☐	☐	☐
f. Endotracheal aspirate for Gram stain and culture	☐	☐	☐	☐
g. Cultures of umbilical stump and ear canal	☐	☐	☐	☐
h. Chest radiographs	☐	☐	☐	☐
i. None of the above	☐	☐	☐	☐

ANSWER

1. Case 1: a, d. Case 2: a, c, d, h. Case 3: i. Case 4: a, c, d, f, h.

Despite several reassuring findings and his mother's prior treatment, baby boy A remains at significant risk. He should at least have a minimal evaluation for possible sepsis. Despite appropriate intrapartum prophylaxis, baby girl B has several indicators of increased risk, including the history of maternal GBS colonization, fetal tachycardia, metabolic acidosis, and signs of respiratory distress; she should have a complete diagnostic evaluation for bacterial sepsis. She is not intubated, so endotracheal fluid is not available. Baby boy C has only minimal risk factors for sepsis (slight prematurity and possibly precipitous delivery), with no signs of illness; no diagnostic studies are indicated. Ms. D has developed clear signs of clinical chorioamnionitis (fetal tachycardia, uterine tenderness, and fever) and baby girl D is obviously ill; a complete diagnostic evaluation (including culture of a tracheal aspirate) is indicated.

Diagnostic Evaluation

Definitive laboratory confirmation or exclusion of the presence of serious bacterial infection relies upon the results of cultures of body fluids. Because culture results are likely to become available only after a day or more, numerous hematologic and immunologic markers of the inflammatory response to infection have been evaluated as potential diagnostic tools for neonatal infection. Unfortunately, the available data indicate that the accuracy of these tests is poor, particularly at the time of initial evaluation.[34] The ideal tests would allow immediate identification of infants with bacterial infection, as well as rapid determination of at-risk infants who are not infected. This would allow for timely treatment for those infected and eliminate unnecessary treatment. No tests that approximate this ideal exist as yet.

The complete blood count with differential and platelet count is the most widely relied upon initial diagnostic test for neonatal sepsis. Findings suggestive of infection include abnormal total white blood cell count ($<5000/mm^3$ or $>25,000/mm^3$, $30,000/mm^3$, or $21,000/mm^3$ at birth, 12 to 24 hours of age, and after the first day, respectively), increased absolute or relative numbers of immature granulocytes (>1500 per mm^3, immature:mature ratio ≥ 0.3, or immature:total ratio > 0.15), low platelet counts ($\leq 150,000/mm^3$), or the presence of toxic granulations, Döhle bodies, or vacuoles in the granulocytes. Each of these findings has limited sensitivity, specificity, or both. The test performance can be improved to some extent by combining observations into a summative score, but even this fails to produce a cutoff value for which the sensitivity and specificity both exceed 90%.[35] Among infants admitted to the NICU at birth for immediate evaluation, the hematologic score had a sensitivity of only 63% and specificity of only 55%, improving to 100% and 73%, respectively, after 12 to 24 hours,[36] so this test is inadequate for screening for sepsis immediately after birth. Furthermore, the criteria for and reproducibility of counting immature neutrophil forms or for recognition of degenerative morphologic changes are neither clearly defined nor easily implemented. Finally, the diagnostic accuracy of hematologic tests for neonatal sepsis has been evaluated only in relatively small sample populations, consisting of a few hundred infants, including only a few dozen with sepsis. Most likely, these tests enjoy their current widespread acceptance for lack of alternatives.

The unsatisfactory performance of the complete blood count has prompted investigations of other markers of the inflammatory process. One of the most extensively studied is the serum concentration of C-reactive protein.[37] As for the hematologic changes associated with sepsis, there is a delay in the C-reactive protein response, with elevated levels becoming apparent 12 to 24 hours after the onset of infection. This test, therefore, lacks sensitivity at the time of evaluation of most infants with suspected sepsis, particularly those without clinical signs of illness who are being evaluated because of maternal factors. Inclusion of C-reactive protein as a component of a "sepsis screen" is therefore not supported by empirical evidence. In that setting, an elevated level might provide an additional indication for initiation of empiric antibiotic therapy, but a normal level should not be sufficiently reassuring to preclude treatment of an infant otherwise deemed to be at risk. A major limitation of C-reactive protein measurements is the lack of specificity, because serum levels of this protein can be elevated in response to a variety of noninfectious conditions, including traumatic and ischemic injuries.

Many other markers of acute inflammation have been evaluated as potential diagnostic tools. Several, including serum levels of procalcitonin, interleukins (IL-6, IL-8), and tumor necrosis factor (TNF-α), and cell-surface concentrations of markers such as CD11b and CD64, are elevated early in the course of an infection and have been characterized as "early sensitive" markers of sepsis, in contrast to the "late" response of C-reactive protein.[38] Although these measurements show promise, none has demonstrated sensitivity sufficient to support a decision to withhold treatment at the onset of suspected neonatal infection. The best results have been found when these tests are used as components of a panel of tests, often including hematologic values and other markers of inflammation (C-reactive protein, haptoglobin, erythrocyte sedimentation rate), particularly when early and late markers are combined. Adoption of these newer tests into routine clinical practice awaits results of larger studies demonstrating their utility.

Blood culture remains the definitive diagnostic tool for identification of neonatal sepsis, and is the gold standard against which all other diagnostic tests are measured. Positive results, augmented by sensitivity testing on the isolated organisms, are extremely useful in guiding antimicrobial treatment. Blood for culture prior to initiation of antibiotic therapy should be obtained whenever possible. The optimal technique, including the ideal volume of blood and number of cultures necessary remains to be established. In most instances, a single specimen of 1 mL inoculated into an aerobic culture bottle is sufficient. Cultures from multiple sites may be useful to distinguish contamination with relatively nonpathogenic organisms (e.g., coagulase-negative *Staphylococcus*) from invasive disease. Organisms recovered in cultures obtained from a newly inserted umbilical catheter are likely to represent true pathogens. Otherwise, cultures from indwelling vascular catheters may be difficult to interpret, as the organisms isolated may represent only colonization of the catheter. There is good reason to believe that culture results are not always definitive, because nearly 20% of infants whose autopsies identify bacterial infection as the cause of death have had negative blood cultures.[39] The false negative rate is unknown, but may be as high as 40%.[40]

Some sources advocate inclusion of a blood culture as a component of a "sepsis screen" for infants for whom initiation of antibiotic therapy is not immediately intended. The usefulness of this common practice is uncertain. For infants whose likelihood of infection is low enough to permit withholding antibiotic therapy, the diagnostic yield will be small. Conversely, delaying initiation of treatment in patients with a substantial probability of bacteremia risks an adverse outcome. Finally, if a change in an infant's condition is sufficient to prompt administration of antibiotics, it may be an indication of the onset of bacteremia subsequent to culture. Therefore, it is important to obtain a new set of cultures (including a blood culture) prior to initiating treatment.

Cultures of endotracheal aspirates may have utility in newly intubated infants who have respiratory distress and radiographic evidence of pulmonary infiltrates.[41,42] In 320 such infants, 25 (8%) had positive cultures of fluid obtained from the trachea, including 11 (3%) whose blood cultures were sterile.[41] Positive cultures of tracheal fluid from infants who have been intubated for several hours or more are likely to represent only colonization of the instrumented airway and have no utility.[43,44] Urine cultures are rarely positive in the first 3 days after birth,[45,46] so this test need not be included in the evaluation of suspected early onset sepsis. Superficial cultures, including surface cultures of the placenta, gastric aspirates, rectum, skin, umbilical stump, nasopharynx, and external ear canal, may be useful to determine neonatal colonization but have no utility in diagnosing neonatal infection. Positive cultures from these sites do not provide evidence for, and negative results do not exclude, invasive disease. Routine use of surface cultures is not recommended.[47]

The question of whether lumbar punctures should be included in the initial diagnostic evaluation of infants with possible sepsis may be one of the most controversial in neonatal medicine, with recommendations ranging from *always* to *virtually never*. There is agreement that infants with signs clearly referable to the central nervous system, such as seizures or a bulging fontanel, merit investigation of the cerebrospinal fluid. Infants with bacterial meningitis are likely to be clinically ill,[48] and the yield of lumbar punctures is low in the first week after birth.[49] It may be reasonable to omit this evaluation in asymptomatic neonates undergoing evaluation because of maternal risk factors, such as intrapartum fever. In addition, few premature infants with uncomplicated respiratory distress syndrome are found to have meningitis,[50] so these infants may not require lumbar punctures. There is little consensus about other circumstances. The prevalence of bacterial meningitis among infants with bacterial sepsis has decreased substantially in recent decades, from historical values of 25% or more in those with early onset disease and greater than 90% for those with late onset group B streptococcus or *Listeria* sepsis in the 1970s to about 5% in the 1990s.[20] These data support the argument that lumbar punctures may be superfluous. However, blood cultures are sterile in a substantial proportion (15% to more than 50%) of infants with bacterial meningitis.[51–53] Culture of the CSF prior to initiation of treatment may therefore represent the only opportunity to make a specific bacteriologic diagnosis. Appropriate selection of patients for lumbar puncture during evaluation for early onset sepsis remains a major challenge. A middle ground may be performance of lumbar punctures in sick infants (excluding premature infants with uncomplicated respiratory distress syndrome) and omitting it in those who appear clinically well.

Radiographic imaging has a limited and ancillary role in diagnosis of neonatal sepsis. The lungs are often the portal of entry for infections acquired from infected amniotic fluid, and sepsis is very often associated with pneumonia or respiratory distress. Findings on chest radiographs are not diagnostic for infection, however, as they may be indistinguishable from those associated with aspiration of meconium or other fluids, retained fetal lung fluid, respiratory distress syndrome, or congestive heart failure. Chest radiographs are, therefore, not likely to be informative in neonates without signs of respiratory compromise, and abnormal findings should be considered suggestive but not diagnostic for bacterial infection. The presence of a pleural effusion should prompt consideration of sepsis, however, as effusions are common with bacterial infections but unusual with other common respiratory disorders.

The infant whose mother has been treated with intrapartum antibiotics (such as baby girl B) presents a particular management challenge. Although use of intrapartum antibiotics reflects recognition of a finding associated with an elevated risk of sepsis, it should not be viewed as an automatic indication for diagnostic assessment or treatment of the newborn infant. For example, maternal GBS colonization at delivery increases the risk of early onset GBS disease to approximately 20 per 1000 live births[26]; intrapartum prophylaxis alone is expected to reduce that risk by 80%,[30] to the overall population attack rate of approximately 4 per 1000, which is not sufficient to merit diagnostic investigation or treatment. In contrast, the residual attack rates may be as high as 5% following intrapartum treatment of clinical chorioamnionitis[54] and 8% following antepartum treatment for PPROM,[28] so those infants deserve a careful diagnostic evaluation and empiric treatment until sepsis can be excluded. Evaluation and treatment are clearly indicated for infants who are clinically ill. The sample algorithm provided by the CDC to guide care of asymptomatic infants in this circumstance suggests selection of infants less than 35 weeks' gestation or whose mothers received antibiotic prophylaxis for less than 4 hours prior to delivery for a "limited evaluation."[27] Because evidence to support these recommendations is not definitive, however, this algorithm is given as an example and is not intended to exclude other approaches. The minimum requirement for all such babies is careful observation in the hospital for at least 48 hours, or a minimum of 24 hours for infants who meet stringent criteria (term gestation, no clinical signs of illness, adequate prophylaxis at least 4 hours prior to delivery, experienced caregiver at home, and access to telephone and transportation).[27]

Case Study 1 *Continued*

Boy A's initial blood counts included a white blood cell count of 22.7×10^9/L with 37% segmented neutrophils and 26% band forms and a platelet count of 180×10^9/L. Because of the left-shifted differential, he then had a comprehensive evaluation for possible sepsis. His cerebrospinal fluid studies included a white blood cell count of $22/mm^3$, red blood cell count of 5200 per mm^3, protein of 90 mg/dL, and glucose of 43 mg/dL, and a negative Gram stain.

Case Study 2 *Continued*

A sepsis screen, consisting of a complete blood count, C-reactive protein level, and blood culture, was obtained. The blood count was 9.7×10^9/L with 48% segmented neutrophils and 14% bands. The C-reactive protein level was 0.8 mg/dL.

Exercise 7

QUESTIONS

1. What organisms might you expect to recover from blood cultures in each of the forementioned cases?

	Case 1	Case 2	Case 3	Case 4
a. Anaerobes	☐	☐	☐	☐
b. Group B streptococcus	☐	☐	☐	☐
c. *Candida* species	☐	☐	☐	☐
d. *Escherichia coli*	☐	☐	☐	☐
e. *Listeria monocytogenes*	☐	☐	☐	☐
f. *Staphylococcus aureus*	☐	☐	☐	☐
g. *Pseudomonas aeruginosa*	☐	☐	☐	☐
h. *Klebsiella pneumoniae*	☐	☐	☐	☐
i. Coagulase-negative *staphylococcus*	☐	☐	☐	☐
j. *Serratia marcescens*	☐	☐	☐	☐
k. *Haemophilus influenzae*	☐	☐	☐	☐
l. *Streptococcus viridans*	☐	☐	☐	☐
m. *Enterobacter cloacae*	☐	☐	☐	☐
n. None	☐	☐	☐	☐

2. What treatment, if any, should be provided?

	Case 1	Case 2	Case 3	Case 4
a. Ampicillin and gentamicin IV	☐	☐	☐	☐
b. Cefazolin PO	☐	☐	☐	☐
c. Ampicillin and cefotaxime IV	☐	☐	☐	☐
d. Vancomycin and cefotaxime IV	☐	☐	☐	☐
e. Oxacillin and gentamicin IV	☐	☐	☐	☐
f. No antibiotic therapy	☐	☐	☐	☐

TABLE 13-4

ORGANISMS ASSOCIATED WITH EARLY ONSET NEONATAL SEPSIS

Group B streptococcus
Escherichia coli
Haemophilus influenzae
Enterococcus species
Streptococcus viridans
Listeria monocytogenes
Staphylococcus, coagulase-negative
Staphylococcus aureus
Pseudomonas aeruginosa
Enterobacter species
Klebsiella species
Other gram-negative enteric organisms

Data from Edwards RK, Clark P, Sistrom CL, et al: Intrapartum antibiotic prophylaxis 1: Relative effects of recommended antibiotics on gram-negative pathogens. Obstet Gynecol 2002;100:534–539; Isaacs D, Fraser S, Hogg G, et al: *Staphylococcus aureus* infections in Australasian neonatal nurseries. Arch Dis Child Fetal Neonatal Ed 2004;89:F331– F335; Stoll BJ, Gordon T, Korones SB, et al: Early onset sepsis in very low birth weight neonates: A report from the National Institute of Child Health and Human Development Neonatal Research Network. J Pediatr 1996;129:72–80; and Daley AJ, Isaacs D: Ten-year study on the effect of intrapartum antibiotic prophylaxis on early onset group B streptococcal and *Escherichia coli* neonatal sepsis in Australasia. Pediatr Infect Dis J 2004;23:630–634.

ANSWERS

1. Cases 1, 2, 4: b, d, e, f, g, h, i, k, l, m. Case 3: n.

2. Case 1: a or c. Case 2: a or c. Case 3: f. Case 4: a or c.

The bacteriology of early onset neonatal sepsis is summarized in Table 13-4. Despite appropriate antepartum treatment for PPROM, baby boy A remains at significant risk for serious infection. His hematologic findings are not reassuring, so empiric treatment is necessary. Some providers would argue that this screening step was not necessary, and that empiric treatment was indicated because of the risk associated with PPROM alone. Baby girl B has clinical signs of illness. The reassuring hematologic findings, in which the slightly elevated ratio of immature to mature (I:M) granulocytes is the only abnormal result, should not dissuade her doctors from treating her. Baby boy C does not need treatment, but (like all neonates) should be observed for signs of developing infection. Baby girl D is quite ill and needs immediate treatment.

Treatment of Early Onset Neonatal Sepsis

Selection of appropriate antibiotic therapy requires familiarity with the bacteriology of neonatal infections. Early onset infections are most frequently caused by *Escherichia coli*, group B streptococcus, *Haemophilus influenzae*, *Enterococcus* species, and other enteric gram-negative bacilli (see Table 13-4). *Listeria monocytogenes*, once a common cause of neonatal sepsis, is now relatively uncommon.[55] Coagulase-negative *Staphylococcus* and *Staphylococcus aureus* are re-emerging as important causes of early onset disease.[31,56,57] Anaerobes, yeast, and *Serratia* have all been reported as causes for early onset infection, but are rare.

Empiric treatment of early onset infection should include antibiotics effective for both gram-positive and gram-negative organisms. This is usually achieved using a combination of a broad-spectrum penicillin (usually ampicillin) and either an aminoglycoside (gentamicin, except when resistance to older aminoglycosides is common) or a third-generation cephalosporin (such as cefotaxime). Ampicillin is effective against group B streptococcus, *Enterocous*, *Listeria*, and many strains of *E. coli*. Gentamicin is effective for *E. coli*, *Klebsiella*, and other gram-negative enteric organisms. The third-generation cephalosporins are similarly effective for these gram-negative organisms, but are less effective than penicillin for group B streptococcus and are inactive against *Enterococcus* and *Listeria*. Isolation, identification, and sensitivity testing of a specific organism should prompt adjustment of the antibiotic regimen to permit treatment with the least toxic and most narrow-spectrum effective agents. Isolation of group B streptococcus, for example, might lead to substitution of penicillin alone for the initial empiric regimen (although some sources recommend dual therapy with gentamicin as well for the first few days because of enhanced killing kinetics). Conversely, isolation of a resistant gram-negative organism might mandate changing to meropenem and amikacin.

Case Study 4 *Continued*

Following admission to the NICU, baby girl D continued to require assisted ventilation and support with dopamine and hydrocortisone for hypotension. She was empirically treated with ampicillin and cefotaxime. On the second day, her blood culture was reported positive for E. coli, which was resistant to both ampicillin and third-generation cephalosporins. She was treated with meropenem and gentamicin for 14 days. By 3 weeks of age, she had been extubated for 5 days, was having rare episodes of apnea and bradycardia on nasal CPAP at 7 cm H$_2$O and 24% oxygen, and was tolerating feedings of maternal breast milk that provided approximately half of her fluid intake. The remainder of her nutrition was provided as parenteral nutrition administered via her umbilical venous catheter.

Exercise 8

QUESTION

1. Identify at least five risk factors for late onset or nosocomial infection in baby girl D.

ANSWER

1. Extreme prematurity, extremely low birth weight, postnatal steroid exposure, broad-spectrum antibiotic therapy, prolonged assisted ventilation, prolonged parenteral nutrition, prolonged use of an indwelling central venous catheter, nasal administration of incompletely humidified gas.

Late Onset and Nosocomial Infection

Risk Factors

The risk of late onset GBS infections is increased by prematurity, by maternal GBS colonization, in infants of mothers who are black or under 20 years of age, in hospitalized infants,[58] and by lack of specific opsonizing maternal antibody levels. These risk factors are not readily amenable to modification, and intrapartum interventions have had no impact on the incidence of late onset disease[13,14] (see Fig. 13-1). With these exceptions, community-acquired late onset infections (Table 13-5) are generally not closely associated with risk factors identifiable in the perinatal period because of the different mode of transmission of these infections, which can be acquired from other caregivers, the environment, or the infant's mother.

TABLE 13-5

ORGANISMS ASSOCIATED WITH COMMUNITY-ACQUIRED LATE ONSET NEONATAL SEPSIS

Group B streptococcus
Listeria monocytogenes
Klebsiella species
Enterococcus species
Enterobacter species
Escherichia coli
Streptococcus pneumoniae
Neisseria meningitidis
Haemophilus influenzae

Data from Greenberg D, Shinwell ES, Yagupsky P, et al: A prospective study of neonatal sepsis and meningitis in southern Israel. Pediatr Infect Dis J 1997;16:768–773; Brown JC, Burns JL, Cummings P: Ampicillin use in infant fever: A systematic review. Arch Pediatr Adolesc Med 2002;156:27–32; and Baker MD, Bell LM: Unpredictability of serious bacterial illness in febrile infants from birth to 1 month of age. Arch Pediatr Adolesc Med 1999;153:508–511.

TABLE 13-6

ORGANISMS ASSOCIATED WITH NOSOCOMIAL NEONATAL SEPSIS

Staphylococcus, coagulase-negative
Candida species
Staphylococcus aureus
Enterococcus species
Enterobacter species
Escherichia coli
Streptococcus viridans
Klebsiella species
Acinetobacter species
Pseudomonas aeruginosa
Group B streptococcus
Other gram-negative enteric organisms

Data from Greenberg D, Shinwell ES, Yagupsky P, et al: A prospective study of neonatal sepsis and meningitis in southern Israel. Pediatr Infect Dis J 1997;16:768–773; Gaynes RP, Edwards JR, Jarvis WR, et al: Nosocomial infections among neonates in high-risk nurseries in the United States. National Nosocomial Infections Surveillance System. Pediatrics 1996;98:357–361; Stoll BJ, Gordon T, Korones SB, et al: Late-onset sepsis in very low birth weight neonates: A report from the National Institute of Child Health and Human Development Neonatal Research Network. J Pediatr 1996;129:63–71; and Jiang JH, Chiu NC, Huang FY, et al: Neonatal sepsis in the neonatal intensive care unit: Characteristics of early versus late onset. J Microbiol Immunol Infect 2004;37:301–306.

Nosocomial infections (Table 13-6) are largely independent of maternal conditions, except to the extent that extreme prematurity

or extremely low birth weight are the major predisposing factors for late hospital-acquired infections.[59] Other conditions associated with an increased risk of nosocomial infections (Table 13-7) include prolonged use of: assisted ventilation, parenteral nutrition, indwelling central venous catheters, and exposure to broad-spectrum antibiotics, or trauma to the nasal mucosa by inadequately humidified oxygen administered by nasal CPAP or cannula. In very low birth weight infants, nosocomial coagulase-negative staphylococcal bacteremia has been linked to the use of intravenous lipids (OR 9.4, 95% CI 1.2–74.2), central venous catheters (OR 2.0, 1.1–3.9), mechanical ventilation (OR 3.2, 1.3–7.6), or peripheral vein catheters (OR 2.6, 1.0–6.5) within the previous week.[60] Coagulase-negative staphylococcal infections also tend to occur 3 to 7 days after initiation of cannula oxygen or nasal CPAP,[61] implicating these treatments as contributing factors in this infection. *Candida* infections are specifically associated with postnatal use of corticosteroids,[62] use of H_2-receptor antagonists, extensive prior antibiotic use, vascular catheters, and prolonged parenteral nutrition, lipid administration, and assisted ventilation.[63]

Case Study 3 *Continued*

Baby boy C was discharged home with his mother at 2 days of age. He did well and was gaining weight at his first clinic visit. At 3 weeks of age, Ms. C called his pediatrician because he had been refusing to breastfeed for several hours. She had observed no other changes in behavior. When seen in the pediatrician's office, he was quiet but awake and responsive, with normal vital signs and a benign physical examination. He showed no interest in feeding, refusing to go to breast or suck from a bottle.

Case Study 4 *Continued*

At 3 weeks of age, baby girl D began having frequent episodes of apnea and bradycardia requiring resuscitation with bag-mask assisted ventilation. These episodes were accompanied by recurrent abdominal distention and bilious emesis.

TABLE 13-7

REPRESENTATIVE ODDS RATIOS FOR CLINICAL RISK FACTORS ASSOCIATED WITH
NOSOCOMIAL NEONATAL SEPSIS

Clinical Finding	Multivariate Odds Ratio (95% CI)
All Infants—All Organisms[59]	
Parenteral nutrition	1.54 (1.01–2.34)
Transfer from another hospital	1.57 (1.13–2.19)
Nasogastric tube	1.90 (1.24–2.91)
Tracheal intubation > 5 days	3.84 (1.50–9.83)
Nasal cannula > 5 days	6.47 (2.97–14.1)
Nasopharyngeal cannula > 5 days	15.5 (5.30–45.1)
Necrotizing enterocolitis	15.6 (5.76–42.2)
Umbilical artery catheter > 5 days	16.5 (5.37–50.5)
Umbilical vein catheter > 5 days	21.2 (10.6–42.2)
Birth weight < 1500 g*	8.42 (5.23–13.6)
Birth weight 1500–2500 g*	4.17 (2.90–6.00)
VLBW Infants—All Organisms[93]	
Cesarean delivery	1.17 (1.01–1.36)
Decrease of 1 wk in gestational age	1.21 (1.17–1.25)
Patent ductus arteriosus	1.23 (1.05–1.44)
Mechanical ventilation	1.69 (1.37–2.08)
Bronchopulmonary dysplasia	1.94 (1.62–2.34)
Necrotizing enterocolitis	2.80 (2.15–3.66)
VLBW Infants—*Candida*[63]	
H_2 blockers	2.44 (1.11–5.29)
Lipid use > 7 days	2.91 (1.22–7.19)
Parenteral nutrition > 5 days	2.93 (1.11–8.39)
Apgar < 5 at 5 minutes	3.40 (1.32–8.08)
Shock	3.55 (1.61–7.73)
Exposure to > two antibiotics	3.83 (1.44–11.4)
Central vascular catheter	3.94 (1.48–12.3)
Gestational age < 32 weeks	4.00 (1.20–14.4)
Length of stay > 7 days	5.33 (1.23–48.4)
Tracheal intubation	10.7 (1.66–450)

*Reference group: birth weight > 2500 g.

Exercise 9

QUESTION

1. Which of the following diagnostic tests are appropriate for these infants?

	Case 3	Case 4
a. White blood cell count with differential	☐	☐
b. C-reactive protein level	☐	☐
c. Lumbar puncture for CSF analysis	☐	☐
d. Blood culture	☐	☐
e. Urine culture	☐	☐
f. Endotracheal aspirate for Gram stain and culture	☐	☐
g. Abdominal radiographs	☐	☐
h. Chest radiographs	☐	☐
i. None of the above	☐	☐

ANSWER

1. Case 3: a, c, d, e. Case 4: a, c, d, e, g.

Baby boy C is now exhibiting clinical signs consistent with late onset sepsis, and the changes in baby D's behavior may be indications of nosocomial infection. These clinical syndromes and the rationale for selection of these diagnostic tests are discussed in the following section.

Clinical Manifestations

Late onset community-acquired infections are typically indolent in onset and associated with relatively subtle and nonspecific signs, such as fever, lethargy, and poor feeding. Signs of circulatory or respiratory failure are unusual, as are focal findings on physical examination.

Nosocomial infection in hospitalized neonates may also present in an indolent fashion, with gradual development of increasing respiratory instability (increasing oxygen requirement, more frequent episodes of apnea and bradycardia), hypotension, feeding intolerance (gastric residuals, abdominal distention, vomiting), thermal instability, lethargy, or metabolic disturbances (metabolic acidosis, hyperglycemia or hypoglycemia, elevated triglyceride levels) (Table 13-8).[64] Catastrophic decompensations can occur with rapid development of profound apnea, poor perfusion with skin mottling and cold extremities, and urgent requirement for initiation of intensive care, including assisted ventilation and cardiotonic drugs. The latter pattern of presentation is particularly common in infants with necrotizing enterocolitis (NEC), which may have a fulminant onset and rapid progression.

Diagnostic Evaluation

The mainstays of diagnostic evaluation beyond the first 3 days of life remain the complete blood count and blood culture. The interpretation of these tests is similar in early and late onset settings. In evaluating infants for nosocomial infection, however, thrombocytopenia should prompt consideration of coagulase-negative *Staphylococcus* or *Candida* as potential causative organisms, as that finding is particularly frequent and often disproportionate to other signs of illness in infants with those infections.

Similarly, acute-phase reactants such as C-reactive protein and other markers of inflammation are subject to the same limitations encountered in the early onset setting. One difference that applies to both hematologic and immunologic screening tests is their higher sensitivity for late onset and nosocomial infections. This likely is a result of the fact that infants evaluated beyond the immediate postnatal period are all exhibiting signs of illness and are, therefore, at a more advanced stage of the infection, as opposed to evaluations for early onset disease, which are frequently prompted by maternal conditions, rather than by signs of illness in the baby. The sensitivity and negative predictive value of blood counts and C-reactive protein levels, even when normal, are not sufficient to rule out use of antibiotic therapy in a sick infant.

Few infants with late onset sepsis (developing outside the hospital) present with prominent signs of respiratory compromise requiring endotracheal intubation; so the opportunity for tracheal aspirate cultures rarely presents itself. The utility of such cultures in the occasional infant with late onset disease who does require intubation has not been studied. The airways of infants who have been intubated for days or weeks are typically colonized with many organisms that are ordinarily recognized as pathogens, including *Staphylococcus aureus, Pseudomonas, Acinetobacter, Klebsiella, E. coli, Enterobacter,* and *Citrobacter.*[43,44] Cultures of tracheal aspirates from such infants are, therefore, not useful. One exception may be identification of endotracheal colonization by yeast in intubated very low birth weight infants, which is associated with a very high likelihood of development of systemic candidiasis.[65] In contrast to the first 3 days of life, urine cultures are often useful in the evaluation of infants with suspected late onset or

---

TABLE 13-8

REPRESENTATIVE UNIVARIATE ODDS RATIOS FOR INFANT CLINICAL SIGNS ASSOCIATED WITH NOSOCOMIAL SEPSIS IN VLBW INFANTS

Clinical Finding	Odds Ratio (95% CI)
Temperature instability	0.78 (0.45–1.66)
Leukocytosis (WBC $> 20 \times 10^9$/L)	1.12 (0.76–1.66)
Gastrointestinal problems	1.26 (0.92–1.72)
Immature:mature neutrophil ratio > 0.2	1.39 (0.97–1.97)
Feeding intolerance	1.40 (1.00–1.96)
Increase in apnea/bradycardia	1.58 (1.14–2.18)
Hyperglycemia (> 140 mg/dL)	1.63 (1.00–2.66)
Neutropenia ($< 1.5 \times 10^9$/L)	1.68 (0.99–2.85)
Increase in oxygen requirement	1.78 (1.29–2.45)
Increase in assisted ventilation	1.80 (1.31–2.47)
Lethargy or hypotonia	2.11 (1.52–2.92)
Unexplained metabolic acidosis	2.21 (1.42–3.44)
Hypotension	3.49 (2.09–5.82)

Data from Fanaroff AA, Korones SB, Wright LL, et al: Incidence, presenting features, risk factors and significance of late onset septicemia in very low birth weight infants. The National Institute of Child Health and Human Development Neonatal Research Network. Pediatr Infect Dis J 1998;17:593–598.

nosocomial infections.[45,46] Urinary tract infection resulting from ascending infection (often associated with urinary tract anomalies) may lead to bacteremia, or the kidneys and urine may be infected hematogenously. Urine specimens for culture should be obtained by suprapubic aspiration[66,67] or urethral catheterization. Bag or "clean-catch" urine specimens from neonates are frequently contaminated (often with a single dominant organism) making recognition of such contamination based upon the presence of multiple different organisms unreliable.

As is the case with early onset infections, the role of lumbar puncture in evaluation of late onset disease or nosocomial infection is controversial. The case for obtaining cerebrospinal fluid for analysis and culture in these settings is more compelling because these infants have clinical signs of disease. Second, meningitis is quite common in infants who return to the hospital with signs consistent with late onset community-acquired sepsis. Earlier recognition of this association has reduced the proportion of infants with late onset sepsis who develop meningitis, from more than 90% to about 25%, but this risk remains substantial. Third, meningitis was diagnosed in 5% of VLBW infants who had cerebrospinal cultures performed as part of evaluations for nosocomial infections after 3 days of age.[68] Because many infants with bacterial meningitis do not have positive blood cultures, cultures of CSF may provide the only bacteriologic diagnosis. Most infants who need evaluation for late onset nosocomial sepsis, therefore, should have CSF obtained for culture before (or very soon after) initiation of antibiotics. Some infants, especially the VLBW infants, are truly too unstable and fragile to tolerate the stress of positioning for performance of a lumbar puncture, but these very sick infants are precisely the ones most likely to have meningitis. Radiographic studies also provide ancillary rather than diagnostic information. Infants with late onset, community-acquired sepsis usually do not have focal respiratory or abdominal findings, so radiographic studies are typically not indicated. Nosocomial infection often takes the form of ventilator-associated pneumonia, which may be identified on chest radiographs. Nosocomial infection in low-birth-weight infants frequently is associated with necrotizing enterocolitis or septic ileus, so abdominal radiographs may be quite useful, particularly if they reveal the characteristic signs of NEC (intestinal pneumatosis, portal venous gas, or free intraperitoneal air).

Exercise 10

QUESTIONS

1. What organisms might you expect to recover from blood cultures from each of these infants?

	Case 3	Case 4
a. Anaerobes	☐	☐
b. Group B streptococcus	☐	☐
c. *Candida* species	☐	☐
d. *Escherichia coli*	☐	☐
e. *Listeria monocytogenes*	☐	☐
f. *Staphylococcus aureus*	☐	☐
g. *Pseudomonas aeruginosa*	☐	☐
h. *Klebsiella pneumoniae*	☐	☐
i. Coagulase-negative staphylococcus	☐	☐
j. *Serratia marcescens*	☐	☐
k. *Haemophilus influenzae*	☐	☐
l. *Streptococcus viridans*	☐	☐
m. *Enterobacter cloacae*	☐	☐
n. None	☐	☐

2. What treatment, if any, should be provided for each of the infants in case studies 3 and 4?

	Case 3	Case 4
a. Ampicillin and gentamicin IV	☐	☐
b. Cefazolin PO	☐	☐
c. Ampicillin and cefotaxime IV	☐	☐
d. Vancomycin and cefotaxime IV	☐	☐
e. Oxacillin and gentamicin IV	☐	☐
f. Give IVIG 750 mg/kg IV	☐	☐
g. No antibiotic therapy	☐	☐

ANSWERS

1. Case 3: b, e, h, l, m. Case 4: a, c, d, f, g, h, i, l, m.

2. Case 3: c. Case 4: d or e.

Treatment

Selection of optimal empiric antibiotic therapy requires knowledge of the identity and sensitivity patterns of the organisms responsible for late onset and nosocomial infections, both in general and at each facility. Community-acquired, late onset disease is most commonly caused by group B streptococcus, *E. coli*, and *Listeria monocytogenes*, but may be associated with enterococci, *Streptococcus pneumoniae*, and other gram-negative enteric organisms as well (see Table 13-5).[22,69,70] These infections usually respond well to treatment with ampicillin and a third-generation cephalosporin, such as cefotaxime or ceftriaxone. In locales where infection with *Listeria* and enterococci is rare, inclusion of ampicillin may not be necessary.[69]

The organisms responsible for nosocomial infections (see Table 13-6)[22,71,72] and their susceptibility to antibiotics are heavily influenced by patterns of antibiotic use and other local factors, many of which are not well understood. In most settings, the coagulase-negative staphylococci are the most prevalent cause of nosocomial infections. In facilities where these organisms are predominantly susceptible to penicillinase-resistant penicillins (e.g., methicillin), oxacillin or nafcillin is an appropriate choice for initial treatment of nosocomial infections. In many areas, however, most coagulase-negative staphylococci are resistant to penicillins, so it is more appropriate to include vancomycin in the initial empiric antibiotic regimen. *Staphylococcus aureus* is re-emerging as a cause of nosocomial infections. Although oxacillin or nafcillin would usually be the agent of choice for *S. aureus*, strains resistant to methicillin (MRSA) are now frequently encountered in many locations, providing another reason for selection of vancomycin as an initial agent. Nosocomial infections may also be caused by gram-negative enteric organisms, requiring empiric therapy with an aminoglycoside. Unless resistance to gentamicin is common in your facility, gentamicin is an appropriate choice for initial treatment, with newer aminoglycosides (tobramycin, amikacin, or netilmicin) reserved for organisms found to be resistant. *Candida* species are also common causes of nosocomial infection, especially in debilitated very low birth weight infants who have been treated with prior courses of broad-spectrum antibiotics or with systemic corticosteroids (including hydrocortisone in moderate doses).[62] On rare occasions, it may be appropriate to include amphotericin B in the initial empiric regimen. *Candida* infections are typically indolent rather than rapidly progressive, so it is more often appropriate to defer initiation of specific antifungal therapy until invasive yeast infection is documented by culture. If there is evidence of *Candida* meningitis, flucytosine (which crosses the blood-brain barrier much more readily than amphotericin) should be added to the antifungal regimen.[73] Newer antifungal agents, such as caspofungin,[74] should be reserved for management of resistance or refractory infections. Anaerobic infections are relatively unusual in neonates, but may be seen in association with necrotizing enterocolitis, especially with bowel perforations.

Despite the well-recognized relationship between immunologic immaturities with an increased risk of sepsis, the absence of specific opsonizing antibodies and readily depleted marrow granulocyte reserves, interventions to correct these deficits have not been proved effective.[75] Although several clinical trials have shown encouraging results, there is still insufficient evidence to support routine use of intravenous immunoglobulin (IVIG) for either proven or suspected neonatal sepsis. Trials of granulocyte colony-stimulating factor or granulocyte-monocyte colony-stimulating factor have demonstrated increases in circulating granulocyte counts, but not a reduction in mortality rate. Although data from several small trials suggest a favorable effect of granulocyte transfusion on mortality rates, the criteria for patient selection and dose amount, frequency, and duration are unknown. Granulocyte preparations are not routinely available and the best methods for preparation have not been defined. In addition, transfusions of white blood cells have been associated with sequestration of activated leukocytes in the lung and consequent hypoxemia and respiratory distress, acute fluid overload, graft-versus-host disease, and transmission of viral infections. These innovative therapies deserve further investigation, but are not ready for application outside of properly designed clinical trials.

Case Study 2 *Continued*

Baby girl B had persistent tachypnea and a progressive requirement for supplemental oxygen. Antibiotic therapy with intravenous ampicillin and gentamicin was initiated, but she developed hypotension that was poorly responsive to volume repletion and dopamine infusion. In addition, she was intubated and received assisted ventilation. Arterial blood gases on 75% oxygen, tidal volumes of 7 mL/kg, PEEP 7, mean airway pressure of 18, and rate of 36 breaths per minute included a pH of

7.03, Pco_2 of 48 mm Hg, Po_2 of 58 mm Hg, and a base excess of –17.

Exercise 11

QUESTION

1. What are the next steps in management of this baby?

   a. Increase ventilator rate to 42

   b. Administer sodium bicarbonate 6 mEq IV

   c. Begin inhaled nitric oxide

   d. Place a central venous catheter

   e. Transport to an ECMO (extracorporeal membrane oxygenation) center

ANSWER

1. b, d, e.

   Baby girl B is now developing signs of septic shock, likely due to GBS sepsis. Although her progressive respiratory failure does not yet qualify her for ECMO support (oxygenation index is only 23), she already has significant metabolic acidosis, which should be treated with sodium bicarbonate and more aggressive hemodynamic support. Development of significant metabolic acidosis is an ominous sign, so consideration should be given to initiation of extracorporeal life support (ECMO).

Complications of Neonatal Sepsis

Complications of neonatal sepsis are numerous, diverse, and common. A review of their management is beyond the scope of these exercises. It will have to suffice to note that the early complications include severe infections (meningitis, empyema, abscess), failure of multiple organ systems (respiratory failure, shock, renal failure), and vascular or thrombotic events (purpura, limb ischemia, stroke). Neonates with sepsis should always be cared for in a facility that is prepared to undertake the next level of intervention required to meet their needs, at least until they have reached the convalescent stage of illness. A high degree of vigilance for evolving complications is always warranted. Monitoring the hematologic and immunologic response to

treatment may be helpful. For example, persistently elevated C-reactive protein levels may be a sign of poor response to treatment or development of a complication, such as a subdural empyema during treatment of bacterial meningitis.[76,77]

Case Study 1 *Continued*

Treatment with intravenous ampicillin and gentamicin was initiated. On the second day after birth, cultures of blood and CSF remained sterile, and C-reactive protein levels for the first two mornings after admission remained less than 1 mg/dL.

Case Study 2 *Continued*

Because of rapidly progressive shock and respiratory failure, baby girl B was placed on venoarterial ECMO. With this support, blood gases improved and the metabolic acidosis gradually resolved. The following morning, the blood culture obtained upon admission was reported positive for group B streptococcus.

Case Study 3 *Continued*

Boy C was admitted to the hospital for evaluation for possible late onset sepsis. His white blood cell count was 6.8×10^9/L, with 24% segmented neutrophils and 32% band forms. His cerebrospinal fluid showed 450 white blood cells and 2200 red blood cells per mm^3 with a glucose of 22 mg/dL and protein of 210 mg/dL. The Gram stain showed moderate numbers of granulocytes, but no organisms were identified. The following day, the CSF culture was reported positive for group B streptococcus. Blood and urine cultures remained sterile. The C-reactive protein level was 9.7 mg/dL.

Case Study 4 *Continued*

The complete blood count included a white blood cell count of 18.2×10^9/L, with 34% segmented and 27% band neutrophils, a platelet count of 28×10^9/L, and a C-reactive protein level of 4.2 mg/dL. Twenty-four hours after it was obtained, the blood culture from baby girl D yielded gram-positive cocci in clusters. The following day, the organism was identified as S. aureus, with the following *sensitivity results: resistant to tetracycline and trimethoprim-sulfisoxazole; sensitive to penicillin, methicillin, cephalothin, and vancomycin.*

Exercise 12

QUESTIONS

1. Which antibiotics should be used?

	Case 1	Case 2	Case 3	Case 4
a. Penicillin	☐	☐	☐	☐
b. Ampicillin	☐	☐	☐	☐
c. Oxacillin or nafcillin	☐	☐	☐	☐
d. Vancomycin	☐	☐	☐	☐
e. Gentamicin	☐	☐	☐	☐
f. No antibiotics	☐	☐	☐	☐

2. What should be the duration of treatment for these infants?

	Case 1	Case 2	Case 3	Case 4
a. Stop treatment now	☐	☐	☐	☐
b. Complete 5 days of treatment	☐	☐	☐	☐
c. Complete 10 days of treatment	☐	☐	☐	☐
d. Complete 14 days of treatment	☐	☐	☐	☐
e. Treat until C-reactive protein is normal	☐	☐	☐	☐

ANSWERS

1. Case 1: f. Case 2: a or b, and e. Case 3: a or b, and e. Case 4: a.

2. Case 1: a. Case 2: c or d (see following discussion). Case 3: d. Case 4: d.

Baby boy A has reassuring laboratory studies, including persistently normal C-reactive protein levels and negative cultures, and has no clinical manifestations of a latent infection. His antibiotic therapy can be safely discontinued. Girl B has culture-proven GBS sepsis and will need a full course of treatment with IV antibiotics. Her antibiotic regimen should include gentamicin for 2 to 3 days and either ampicillin or penicillin for at least 10 days. If meningitis cannot be excluded by examination of cerebrospinal fluid obtained after she is no longer anticoagulated for ECMO, a 14-day course of treatment is indicated. The sterile blood culture notwithstanding, boy C has confirmed GBS meningitis and should also be treated with gentamicin for 2 to 3 days and ampicillin or penicillin for 14 days. Girl D has *S. aureus* sepsis, but with an unusual, highly sensitive organism, so completion of treatment with penicillin is appropriate.

Duration of Treatment

The duration of treatment for suspected neonatal sepsis is guided by two considerations. First, for infants who are unlikely to be infected, what findings provide sufficient reassurance (formally, negative predictive value) to ensure that discontinuation of empiric treatment is both safe and timely? Second, for infants in whom the diagnosis of sepsis is confirmed, how long must treatment continue to ensure that there will be a minimal chance for recurrence or relapse of the infection?

Using modern detection systems, nearly all positive blood cultures will yield bacterial growth within 48 hours.[78] In a baby who is otherwise doing well, a negative blood culture at that time provides a high negative predictive value. The greatest utility of C-reactive protein levels is the high sensitivity of sequential levels obtained over the first 48 hours after the onset of illness.[37] In the absence of profound neutropenia, two normal levels separated by 24 hours, with the first delayed at least 8 hours from the decision to begin empiric treatment, have a very high negative predictive value and provide excellent evidence that it is safe to discontinue antibiotics. These findings (particularly in infants who are no longer, or never were, ill) provide ample reassurance that antibiotic therapy can be safely discontinued.

The generally recommended duration of treatment for neonatal infections is based more on tradition and somewhat "magical" numbers rather than strong empirical evidence. For sepsis without meningitis, the usual recommendation is 10 days for gram-positive, 14 days for gram-negative, and 21 days for yeast infections. For meningitis, the recommendations are increased to 14 and 21 days for gram-positive and gram-negative infections. The optimal duration for *Candida* meningitis is unclear. Other infections may require an even longer course of treatment—3 to 4 weeks for osteomyelitis or 6 weeks for endocarditis, for example—but these conditions are, fortunately, unusual in neonates. Some experts advocate continuation of antibiotics for a fixed interval (often 10 or 14 days) after documentation of sterility of the infected body fluid (blood or CSF, for example). Serial C-reactive protein levels have also been suggested as a guide for determining the duration of antibiotic therapy in neonates with probable or confirmed sepsis. Published data indicate that stopping treatment upon normalization of C-reactive protein levels in infants with a clinical diagnosis of sepsis, but without positive cultures, is likely safe.[79,80] These observations should not be extrapolated to infants with culture-proven sepsis, however, as the number of such patients in whom this approach has been evaluated is very small.

Exercise 13

QUESTION

1. How should the parents of these infants be counseled about the prognosis for each baby?

	Case 1	Case 2	Case 3	Case 4
a. Risk of death is less than 1%	☐	☐	☐	☐
b. Risk of death is about 5%	☐	☐	☐	☐
c. Risk of death is about 10%	☐	☐	☐	☐
d. Risk of death is about 20%	☐	☐	☐	☐
e. Neurodevelopmental outcome is normal in less than 10%	☐	☐	☐	☐
f. Neurodevelopmental outcome is normal in over 50%	☐	☐	☐	☐
g. Neurodevelopmental outcome is normal in about 90%	☐	☐	☐	☐
h. Neurodevelopmental outcome is normal in about 98%	☐	☐	☐	☐

ANSWER

1. Case 1: a, h. Case 2: d, f. Case 3: c, f. Case 4: b, f.

Case fatality rates in neonates with sepsis have fallen dramatically, from more than 85% before the advent of antibiotics[81] to 15% to 20% by the 1990s.[9,82] Increased survival of low birth weight infants and changes in perinatal care have substantially altered the patterns of neonatal infection, making data from earlier decades of limited use. Recent data, based on the experience at Ohio State University from 1986 through 2002, show a higher case fatality rate for early onset cases (21%) than for late onset cases (11%).[82] Because there has been a downward trend in case fatality rates for early onset sepsis (due to lower mortality rates for early onset gram-negative infections) and an upward trend for late onset infections (due to increasing mortality rates for gram-negative and fungal infections and increasing numbers of VLBW infants surviving to acquire such infections), the case fatality rate for late onset infections exceeded that for early onset disease in the most recent time period (1998–2002) (Table 13-9). Unlike earlier data, which did not suggest a dependence of case fatality rates for early onset sepsis on the identity of the responsible organism, the case fatality rates in those infected with *E. coli* (33%) or *Pseudomonas* (100%) are higher than in those with early onset group B streptococcus infections (13%) (Table 13-10). Higher case fatality rates for early onset *E. coli* sepsis (19%) as compared to group B streptococcus (7%) have been confirmed in a comparison of outcomes of these conditions.[83] One large series of early onset GBS cases from the early 1990s reported a case fatality rate of only 2.3%.[21] The higher case fatality rates seen with early onset *E. coli* sepsis may reflect differences in the host population rather than pathogenicity of organisms. Infants infected with gram-negative organisms are often smaller and less mature.[72] In addition they are more likely to be infected with a resistant organism following prolonged antepartum antibiotic therapy.[16] Among very low birth weight infants, the case fatality rate with early onset sepsis is approximately 25%.[57] The case fatality rates for late onset infections vary enormously, from 6% for infections due to gram-positive cocci to 28% for those caused by gram-negative bacilli.[82] Mortality rates of nearly 100% have been reported for *Pseudomonas* and other highly resistant enteric organisms. VLBW infants with late onset infection have a higher case fatality rate (17%), with nearly half of all deaths occurring after 2 weeks of age in this group.[72] Case fatality rates for late onset infections among VLBW infants are strongly related to the identity of the infectious organisms: 10%

TABLE 13-9

CASE FATALITY RATES FOR NEONATAL SEPSIS 1986–2002

Bloodstream Infection (BSI)	1986–1991	1992–1997	1998–2002	Total
Early Onset BSI				
Gram-positive cocci	18%	7%	20%	15%
Gram-negative bacilli	33%	28%	15%	26%
Total	25%	20%	16%	21%
Late Onset BSI				
Gram-positive cocci	6%	5%	8%	6%
Gram-negative bacilli	7%	20%	43%	28%
Fungi	8%	6%	27%	13%
Total	6%	8%	18%	11%

Data from Cordero L, Rau R, Taylor D, et al: Enteric gram-negative bacilli bloodstream infections: 17 years' experience in a neonatal intensive care unit. Am J Infect Control 2004;32:189–195.

TABLE 13-10

CASE FATALITY RATES IN NEONATAL SEPSIS

Infectious Agents	Early Onset		Late Onset	
	Cases	Died (%)	Cases	Died (%)
Gram-Positive Cocci				
Group B streptococcus	40	13%	3	0%
Staphylococcus aureus	4	25%	25	4%
Enterococcus faecalis	2	0%	27	7%
Coagulase-positive staphylococcus	0	—	290	6%
Streptococcus pneumoniae	2	50%	0	—
Total	48	15%	345	6%
Gram-Negative Bacilli				
Klebsiella pneumoniae	3	0%	31	16%
Enterobacter cloacae	0	—	15	7%
Escherichia coli	40	33%	32	19%
Pseudomonas aeruginosa	3	100%	16	81%
Serratia marcescens	0	—	6	17%
Acinetobacter baumannii	1	0%	1	100%
Haemophilus influenzae	15	7%	0	—
Other gram-negative bacilli	7	14%	1	100%
Total	69	26%	102	28%
Fungi				
Candida albicans	—	—	51	16%
Candida parapsilosis	—	—	11	9%
Malassezia furfur	—	—	4	0%
Torulopsis glabrata	—	—	4	0%
Total	—	—	70	13%
Total (all)	117	21%	516	11%

Data from Cordero L, Rau R, Taylor D, et al: Enteric gram-negative bacilli bloodstream infections: 17 years' experience in a neonatal intensive care unit. Am J Infect Control 2004;32:189–195.

for those with gram-positive infections, 40% for those with gram-negative infections, and 28% for fungal infections. Mortality rates are lowest for group B streptococcus (3%) and coagulase-negative *Staphylococcus* (10%) and highest for *Pseudomonas* (62%), *E. coli* (41%), and *Enterobacter* (40%).[72] Current case fatality statistics specific for community-acquired late onset infections are not available.

Case fatality rates are substantially greater in infants with meningitis than in those with sepsis not complicated by meningitis. In infants with early onset meningitis, the case fatality rate is 18%, compared to 10% in infants with uncomplicated bacteremia.[83] Case fatality rates for meningitis are higher for infants with low birth weight (34% for those <1500 g versus 6.5% for those >1500 g) and for those with disease caused by gram-negative organisms (29% versus 11% for other organisms).[83] Recent data from the NICHD Neonatal Network for VLBW infants also demonstrated a high case fatality rate (23%) associated with late onset meningitis,[68] with higher risk of death in those infected with gram-negative organisms (41%) or fungi (32%) than for those with gram-positive agents (15%).

Neurodevelopmental impairments, including cerebral palsy and developmental delays, were found in 40% of infants with meningitis but in only 7% of infected infants without meningitis.[84,85] Neurologic sequelae in the latter group may be a consequence of injury associated with activation of the immune and coagulation cascades by a systemic inflammatory response.[86] Sequelae of neonatal meningitis include cerebral palsy (in 9% of survivors), learning problems (8%), seizures (7%), and sensorineural hearing loss (3%).[8] Disability is more likely following meningitis caused by *E. coli* (60%) than in cases of group B streptococcus meningitis (35%).[8] Very low birth weight infants with meningitis are substantially more likely to have neurodevelopmental impairments (50%) than comparable infants without meningitis (20%).[87] Nonetheless, the majority of infants who survive neonatal sepsis have good neurodevelopmental outcomes.

References

1. Spitzer AR, Kirkby S, Kornhauser M: Practice variation in suspected neonatal sepsis: A costly problem in neonatal intensive care. J Perinatol 2005;25:265–269.
2. Escobar GJ: The neonatal "sepsis work-up": Personal reflections on the development of an evidence-based approach toward newborn infections in a managed care organization. Pediatrics 1999;103: 360–373.
3. Vergnano S, Sharland M, Kazembe P, et al: Neonatal sepsis: An international perspective. Arch Dis Child Fetal Neonatal Ed 2005;90:F220–F224.
4. Bryce J, Boschi-Pinto C, Shibuya K, et al: WHO estimates of the causes of death in children. Lancet 2005;365:1147–1152.
5. Anderson RN, Smith BL: Deaths: Leading causes for 2002. Natl Vital Stat Rep 2005;53:1–89.
6. Eisenfeld L, Ermocilla R, Wirtschafter D, et al: Systemic bacterial infections in neonatal deaths. Am J Dis Child 1983;137:645–649.
7. Pierce JR, Merenstein GB, Stocker JT: Immediate postmortem cultures in an intensive care nursery. Pediatr Infect Dis 1984;3:510–513.
8. Harvey D, Holt DE, Bedford H: Bacterial meningitis in the newborn: A prospective study of mortality and morbidity. Semin Perinatol 1999;23:218–225.
9. May ML, Daley AJ, Donath S, et al: Early onset neonatal meningitis in Australia and New Zealand,

10. 1992–2002. Arch Dis Child Fetal Neonatal 2005;90:F324–F327.
10. Stoll BJ, Holman RC, Schuchat A: Decline in sepsis-associated neonatal and infant deaths in the United States, 1979 through 1994. Pediatrics 1998;102: e18.
11. Lukacs SL, Schoendorf KC, Schuchat A: Trends in sepsis-related neonatal mortality in the United States, 1985–1998. Pediatr Infect Dis J 2004;23: 599–603.
12. Martin JA, Hamilton BE, Sutton PD, et al: Births: Final data for 2002. Natl Vital Stat Rep 2003; 52:1–113.
13. Schrag SJ, Zywicki S, Farley MM, et al: Group B streptococcal disease in the era of intrapartum antibiotic prophylaxis. N Engl J Med 2000;342:15–20.
14. Centers for Disease Control and Prevention: Active Bacterial Core Surveillance Report, 2005. Available at www.cdc.gov/ncidod/dbmd/abcs/surv-reports.htm.
15. Isaacs D, Royle JA, Australasian Study Group for Neonatal Infections: Intrapartum antibiotics and early onset neonatal sepsis caused by group B Streptococcus and by other organisms in Australia. Pediatr Infect Dis J 1999;18:524–528.
16. Moore MR, Schrag SJ, Schuchat A: Effects of intrapartum antimicrobial prophylaxis for prevention of group-B-streptococcal disease on the incidence and ecology of early onset neonatal sepsis. Lancet Infect Dis 2003;3:201–213.
17. Yancey MK, Duff P, Kubilis P, et al: Risk factors for neonatal sepsis. Obstet Gynecol 1996;87:188–194.
18. Gladstone IM, Ehrenkranz RA, Edberg SC, et al: A ten-year review of neonatal sepsis and comparison with the previous fifty-year experience. Pediatr Infect Dis J 1990;9:819–825.
19. Soman M, Green B, Daling J: Risk factors for early neonatal sepsis. Am J Epidemiol 1985;121: 712–719.
20. Baltimore RS, Huie SM, Meek JI, et al: Early onset neonatal sepsis in the era of group B streptococcal prevention. Pediatrics 2001;108:1094–1098.
21. Bromberger P, Lawrence JM, Braun D, et al: The influence of intrapartum antibiotics on the clinical spectrum of earlyonset group B streptococcal infection in term infants. Pediatrics 2000;106:244–250.
22. Greenberg D, Shinwell ES, Yagupsky P, et al: A prospective study of neonatal sepsis and meningitis in southern Israel. Pediatr Infect Dis J 1997;16: 768–773.
23. Lieberman E, Lang JM, Frigoletto F, et al: Epidural analgesia, intrapartum fever, and neonatal sepsis evaluation. Pediatrics 1997;99:415–419.
24. Spaans WA, Knox AJ, Koya HB, et al: Risk factors for neonatal infection. Aust NZ J Obstet Gynaecol 1990;30:327–330.
25. Schiano MA, Hauth JC, Gilstrap LC: Second-stage fetal tachycardia and neonatal infection. Am J Obstet Gynecol 1984;148:779–781.
26. Benitz WE, Gould JB, Druzin ML: Risk factors for early onset group B streptococcal sepsis: Estimation of odds ratios by critical literature review. Pediatrics 1999;103:e77.
27. Schrag S, Gorwitz R, Fultz-Butts K, et al: Prevention of perinatal group B streptococcal disease. Revised guidelines from CDC. MMWR Recomm Rep 2002;51:1–22.
28. Mercer BM, Miodovnik M, Thurnau GR, et al: Antibiotic therapy for reduction of infant morbidity after preterm premature rupture of the

membranes. A randomized controlled trial. JAMA 1997;278:989–995.

29. Kenyon SL, Taylor DJ, Tarnow-Mordi W: Broad-spectrum antibiotics for spontaneous preterm labour: The ORACLE II randomised trial. ORACLE Collaborative Group. Lancet 2001;357:989–994.

30. Benitz WE, Gould JB, Druzin ML: Antimicrobial prevention of earlyonset group B streptococcal sepsis: Estimates of risk reduction based on a critical literature review. Pediatrics 1999;103:e78.

31. Edwards RK, Clark P, Sistrom CL, et al: Intrapartum antibiotic prophylaxis 1: Relative effects of recommended antibiotics on gram-negative pathogens. Obstet Gynecol 2002;100:534–539.

32. Manning SD, Foxman B, Pierson CL, et al: Correlates of antibiotic-resistant group B streptococcus isolated from pregnant women. Obstet Gynecol 2003; 101:74–79.

33. Chen KT, Ringer S, Cohen AP, et al: The role of intrapartum fever in identifying asymptomatic term neonates with early onset neonatal sepsis. J Perinatol 2002;22:653–657.

34. Fowlie PW, Schmidt B: Diagnostic tests for bacterial infection from birth to 90 days—A systematic review. Arch Dis Child Fetal Neonatal Ed 1998;78:F92–F98.

35. Rodwell RL, Leslie AL, Tudehope DI: Early diagnosis of neonatal sepsis using a hematologic scoring system. J Pediatr 1988;112:761–767.

36. Greenberg DN, Yoder BA: Changes in the differential white blood cell count in screening for group B streptococcal sepsis. Pediatr Infect Dis J 1990;9:886–889.

37. Benitz WE, Han MY, Madan A, et al: Serial serum C-reactive protein levels in the diagnosis of neonatal infection. Pediatrics 1998;102:E41.

38. Ng PC: Diagnostic markers of infection in neonates. Arch Dis Child Fetal Neonatal Ed 2004;89:F229–F235.

39. Squire E, Favara B, Todd J: Diagnosis of neonatal bacterial infection: Hematologic and pathologic findings in fatal and nonfatal cases. Pediatrics 1979;64:60–64.

40. Kellogg JA, Ferrentino FL, Goodstein MH, et al: Frequency of low level bacteremia in infants from birth to two months of age. Pediatr Infect Dis J 1997;16:381–385.

41. Sherman MP, Goetzman BW, Ahlfors CE, et al: Tracheal aspiration and its clinical correlates in the diagnosis of congenital pneumonia. Pediatrics 1980;65:258–263.

42. Ruderman JW, Srugo I, Morgan MA, et al: Pneumonia in the neonatal intensive care unit. Diagnosis by quantitative bacterial tracheal aspirate cultures. J Perinatol 1994;14:182–186.

43. Thureen PJ, Moreland S, Rodden DJ, et al: Failure of tracheal aspirate cultures to define the cause of respiratory deteriorations in neonates. Pediatr Infect Dis J 1993;12:560–564.

44. Cordero L, Sananes M, Dedhiya P, et al: Purulence and gram-negative bacilli in tracheal aspirates of mechanically ventilated very low birth weight infants. J Perinatol 2001;21:376–381.

45. Tamim MM, Alesseh H, Aziz H: Analysis of the efficacy of urine culture as part of sepsis evaluation in the premature infant. Pediatr Infect Dis J 2003;22:805–808.

46. Visser VE, Hall RT: Urine culture in the evaluation of suspected neonatal sepsis. J Pediatr 1979;94:635–638.

47. Fulginiti VA, Ray CG: Body surface cultures in the newborn infant. An exercise in futility, wastefulness, and inappropriate practice. Am J Dis Child 1988;142:19–20.

48. Fielkow S, Reuter S, Gotoff SP: Cerebrospinal fluid examination in symptom-free infants with risk factors for infection. J Pediatr 1991;119:971–973.

49. Schwersenski J, McIntyre L, Bauer CR: Lumbar puncture frequency and cerebrospinal fluid analysis in the neonate. Am J Dis Child 1991;145:54–58.

50. Weiss MG, Ionides SP, Anderson CL: Meningitis in premature infants with respiratory distress: Role of admission lumbar puncture. J Pediatr 1991;119:973–975.

51. Visser VE, Hall RT: Lumbar puncture in the evaluation of suspected neonatal sepsis. J Pediatr 1980;96:1063–1067.

52. Shattuck KE, Chonmaitree T: The changing spectrum of neonatal meningitis over a fifteen-year period. Clin Pediatr (Phila) 1992;31:130–136.

53. Wiswell TE, Baumgart S, Gannon CM, et al: No lumbar puncture in the evaluation for early neonatal sepsis: Will meningitis be missed? Pediatrics 1995;95:803–806.

54. Mecredy RL, Wiswell TE, Hume RF: Outcome of term gestation neonates whose mothers received intrapartum antibiotics for suspected chorioamnionitis. Am J Perinatol 1993;10:365–368.

55. Sadow KB, Derr R, Teach SJ: Bacterial infections in infants 60 days and younger: Epidemiology, resistance, and implications for treatment. Arch Pediatr Adolesc Med 1999;153:611–614.

56. Isaacs D, Fraser S, Hogg G, et al: Staphylococcus aureus infections in Australasian neonatal nurseries. Arch Dis Child Fetal Neonatal Ed 2004;89:F331–F335.

57. Stoll BJ, Gordon T, Korones SB, et al: Early onset sepsis in very low birth weight neonates: A report from the National Institute of Child Health and Human Development Neonatal Research Network. J Pediatr 1996;129:72–80.

58. Lin FY, Weisman LE, Troendle J, et al: Prematurity is the major risk factor for late-onset group B streptococcus disease. J Infect Dis 2003;188:267–271.

59. Moro ML, De Toni A, Stolfi I, et al: Risk factors for nosocomial sepsis in newborn intensive and intermediate care units. Eur J Pediatr 1996;155:315–322.

60. Avila-Figueroa C, Goldmann DA, Richardson DK, et al: Intravenous lipid emulsions are the major determinant of coagulase-negative staphylococcal bacteremia in very low birth weight newborns. Pediatr Infect Dis J 1998;17:10–17.

61. Kopelman AE, Holbert D: Use of oxygen cannulas in extremely low birthweight infants is associated with mucosal trauma and bleeding, and possibly with coagulase-negative staphylococcal sepsis. J Perinatol 2003;23:94–97.

62. Botas CM, Kurlat I, Young SM, et al: Disseminated candidal infections and intravenous hydrocortisone in preterm infants. Pediatrics 1995;95:883–887.

63. Saiman L, Ludington E, Pfaller M, et al: Risk factors for candidemia in neonatal intensive care unit patients. The National Epidemiology of Mycosis Survey study group. Pediatr Infect Dis J 2000;19:319–324.

64. Fanaroff AA, Korones SB, Wright LL, et al: Incidence, presenting features, risk factors and significance of late onset septicemia in very low birth weight infants. The National Institute of Child Health and Human

Development Neonatal Research Network. Pediatr Infect Dis J 1998;17:593–598.

65. Rowen JL, Rench MA, Kozinetz CA, et al: Endotracheal colonization with Candida enhances risk of systemic candidiasis in very low birth weight neonates. J Pediatr 1994;124:789–794.

66. Nelson JD, Peters PC: Suprapubic aspiration of urine in premature and term infants. Pediatrics 1965;36:132–134.

67. Slosky DA, Todd JK: Diagnosis of urinary tract infection. The interpretation of colony counts. Clin Pediatr (Phila) 1977;16:698–701.

68. Stoll BJ, Hansen N, Fanaroff AA, et al: To tap or not to tap: High likelihood of meningitis without sepsis among very low birth weight infants. Pediatrics 2004;113:1181–1186.

69. Brown JC, Burns JL, Cummings P: Ampicillin use in infant fever: A systematic review. Arch Pediatr Adolesc Med 2002;156:27–32.

70. Baker MD, Bell LM: Unpredictability of serious bacterial illness in febrile infants from birth to 1 month of age. Arch Pediatr Adolesc Med 1999;153: 508–511.

71. Gaynes RP, Edwards JR, Jarvis WR, et al: Nosocomial infections among neonates in high-risk nurseries in the United States. National Nosocomial Infections Surveillance System. Pediatrics 1996;98:357–361.

72. Stoll BJ, Gordon T, Korones SB, et al: Late-onset sepsis in very low birth weight neonates: A report from the National Institute of Child Health and Human Development Neonatal Research Network. J Pediatr 1996;129:63–71.

73. Houmeau L, Monfort-Gouraud M, Boccara JF, et al: [Candida meningitis, in a premature infant, treated with liposomal amphotericin B and flucytosine.] Arch Fr Pediatr 1993;50:227–230.

74. Odio CM, Araya R, Pinto LE, et al: Caspofungin therapy of neonates with invasive candidiasis. Pediatr Infect Dis J 2004;23:1093–1097.

75. Suri M, Harrison L, Van de Ven C, et al: Immunotherapy in the prophylaxis and treatment of neonatal sepsis. Curr Opin Pediatr 2003;15:155–160.

76. Peltola H, Luhtala K, Valmari P: C-reactive protein as a detector of organic complications during recovery from childhood purulent meningitis. J Pediatr 1984;104:869–872.

77. Sabel KG, Hanson LA: The clinical usefulness of C-reactive protein (CRP) determinations in bacterial meningitis and septicemia in infancy. Acta Paediatr Scand 1974;63:381–388.

78. Kaiser JR, Cassat JE, Lewno MJ: Should antibiotics be discontinued at 48 hours for negative late-onset sepsis evaluations in the neonatal intensive care unit? J Perinatol 2002;22:445–447.

79. Ehl S, Gering B, Bartmann P, et al: C-reactive protein is a useful marker for guiding duration of antibiotic therapy in suspected neonatal bacterial infection. Pediatrics 1997;99:216–221.

80. Philip AG, Mills PC: Use of C-reactive protein in minimizing antibiotic exposure: Experience with infants initially admitted to a well-baby nursery. Pediatrics 2000;106:E4.

81. Dunham EC: Septicemia in the newborn. Am J Dis Child 1933;45:229–253.

82. Cordero L, Rau R, Taylor D, et al: Enteric gram-negative bacilli bloodstream infections: 17 years' experience in a neonatal intensive care unit. Am J Infect Control 2004;32:189–195.

83. Mayor-Lynn K, Gonzalez-Quintero VH, O' Sullivan MJ, et al: Comparison of early onset neonatal sepsis caused by Escherichia coli and group B Streptococcus. Am J Obstet Gynecol 2005;192:1437–1439.

84. Horn KA, Meyer WT, Wyrick BC, et al: Group B streptococcal neonatal infection. JAMA 1974;230: 1165–1167.

85. Bennet R, Bergdahl S, Eriksson M, et al: The outcome of neonatal septicemia during fifteen years. Acta Paediatr Scand 1989;78:40–43.

86. Neufeld MD, Frigon C, Graham AS, et al: Maternal infection and risk of cerebral palsy in term and preterm infants. J Perinatol 2005;25:108–113.

87. Doctor BA, Newman N, Minich NM, et al: Clinical outcomes of neonatal meningitis in very-low birth-weight infants. Clin Pediatr (Phila) 2001;40: 473–480.

88. Schrag SJ, Zell ER, Lynfield R, et al: A population-based comparison of strategies to prevent early onset group B streptococcal disease in neonates. N Engl J Med 2002;347:233–239.

89. Boyer KM, Gadzala CA, Burd LI, et al: Selective intrapartum chemoprophylaxis of neonatal group B streptococcal early onset disease. I. Epidemiologic rationale. J Infect Dis 1983;148:795–801.

90. Spector SA, Ticknor W, Grossman M: Study of the usefulness of clinical and hematologic findings in the diagnosis of neonatal bacterial infections. Clin Pediatr (Phila) 1981;20:385–392.

91. Graves GR, Rhodes PG: Tachycardia as a sign of early onset neonatal sepsis. Pediatr Infect Dis 1984;3:404–406.

92. Montgomery DM, Stedman CM, Robichaux AG, et al: Cord blood gas patterns identifying newborns at increased risk of group B streptococcal sepsis. Obstet Gynecol 1991;78:774–777.

93. Makhoul IR, Sujov P, Smolkin T, et al: Pathogen-specific early mortality in very low birth weight infants with late-onset sepsis: A national survey. Clin Infect Dis 2005;40:218–224.

Patent Ductus Arteriosus

Nick Evans, DM, MRCPCH

The ductus arteriosus (DA) creates some of the most difficult diagnostic and therapeutic dilemmas in neonatal medicine. These challenges are most apparent in the care of the very preterm baby, because in about a third of babies born before 30 weeks' gestation, the normal postnatal constriction of the ductus arteriosus will fail. The resultant hemodynamics can have important consequences in both the systemic and pulmonary circulations of these babies. Furthermore, persistent patency of the ductus arteriosus may result in a range of adverse outcomes for preterm babies. On the other hand, as highlighted in Case Study 1, sometimes even normal physiologic closure can create a life-threatening situation for a baby.

Case Study 1

An apparently healthy term baby has a routine examination on day 2 of life. A soft systolic murmur is heard, but the rest of the cardiovascular examination is normal, with normal color, heart sounds, peripheral pulses, and precordial impulses.

Exercise 1

QUESTIONS

1. How likely is it that this murmur represents structural heart disease?

2. How likely is it that this murmur is due to a patent ductus arteriosus (PDA)?

3. What are the common causes of murmurs in this postnatal period?

4. Should this baby have an echocardiogram?

ANSWERS

1. It is unlikely but possible. Most soft murmurs in the early postnatal period reflect transitional circulatory changes or benign structural abnormalities such as small muscular ventricular septal defects.

2. It is not likely. Although often quoted as causing murmurs, PDA is actually an uncommon cause of an innocent transitional murmur in term babies. This reflects the fact that, although functional closure may not occur for up to 3 to 4 days in some term babies, the duct is well constricted and so the volume of the shunt is not sufficient to generate a murmur. Occasionally, these "slow to close" normal ducts will generate a murmur.

3. Flow murmurs from the left pulmonary artery and physiologic tricuspid incompetence would be the most common transitional hemodynamic murmurs. Overall, small benign muscular ventricular septal defects would be the most common reason for murmurs heard on routine newborn examination.

4. This depends on the availability of echocardiography. This baby is still only on day 2 of life, so it would be reasonable to review in 1 to 2 days to see if the murmur persists. It is difficult to accurately exclude significant congenital heart disease on clinical examination, so if the murmur persists, an

echocardiogram would be appropriate. This also serves to alleviate parental anxiety.

Case Study 2

A term baby has been progressing well until day 5 of life, when you are called to the postnatal ward because the baby has suddenly become very pale. On arrival you find the baby pale and shocked with respiratory distress. The peripheral pulses are weak, cardiac impulses are increased, and liver is enlarged to 4 cm below the costal margin.

Exercise 2

QUESTIONS

1. What is the most likely diagnosis?
2. What specific therapy is most likely to improve the baby's condition?

ANSWERS

1. This is likely to be a ductal dependent systemic circulation such as hypoplastic left heart syndrome or critical coarctation. When the ductus closes, the systemic blood flow is cut off and the baby collapses.

2. It is life saving in this situation to open up the ductus with an intravenous infusion of prostaglandin E_1 (0.05 to 0.1 µg/kg/min). Prompt diagnosis is the critical issue. These babies are often treated as septicemic, leading to diagnostic delays.

Normal Physiology of the Ductus Arteriosus

The fetal ductus arteriosus links the main pulmonary artery with the descending aorta. High pulmonary vascular resistance is maintained by constricted pulmonary arterioles and preferentially directs the right ventricular output from right to left through the ductus into the descending aorta and hence back to the placenta. Anatomically, the ductus is a continuation of the main pulmonary artery that is slightly offset to the left so it can describe an arch into the descending aorta (Fig. 14-1). The presence of the

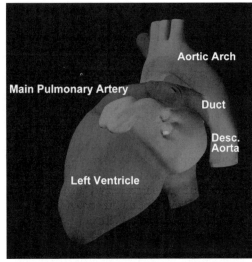

Figure 14-1 Image of a model of the heart viewed from the left side to demonstrate the anatomic relationships of the ductus arteriosus. It can be seen how the ductus is a continuation of the main pulmonary artery that is slightly offset to the left to allow it to describe an arch into the descending aorta. (See also Color Plate.)

ductal arch in fetal echocardiography makes in utero assessment of the aortic arch very difficult. Fetal ductal patency is maintained by high circulating levels of prostaglandins, particularly PGE_2. During the last trimester, the ductus prepares for closure at birth by developing a more muscular wall. In addition, the ductal muscle becomes less sensitive to the dilating effects of PGE_2 and more sensitive to the vasoconstricting effect of oxygen.[1]

After birth, the rising arterial Po_2 causes powerful constriction of the muscle in the wall of the ductus. Complete closure occurs in two phases. The first is functional closure in which the muscle constriction obstructs the flow of blood. The second is structural closure, which results from ischemia and necrosis of the intima.[2] During the phase of functional closure, it is possible for the ductus to reopen, either spontaneously, as can occur in premature babies, or therapeutically in response to prostaglandins as discussed in Case Study 2.

QUESTIONS

3. Which of these two pulmonary artery Doppler traces shows patency of the ductus arteriosus? (See figure at top of page 251.)

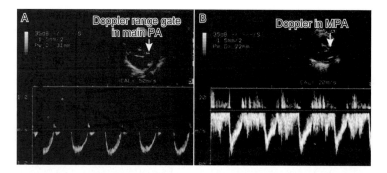

4. Which of the two color Doppler images below shows a patent ductus arteriosus? (See also Color Plate.)

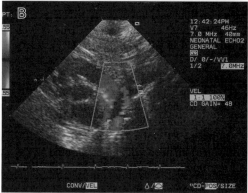

ANSWERS

3. Part B shows the characteristic diastolic turbulence of a left-to-right ductal shunt. Part A shows the normal pattern of systolic forward flow in the main pulmonary artery with minimal diastolic flow.

4. Part A shows a patent ductus marked by the red (flow toward transducer) stream in the middle of the two blue (flow away from the transducer) streams of the left pulmonary artery (left) and descending aorta (right). Part B shows just the two blue streams and the ductus is closed.

Doppler Echocardiography

Much of our current understanding of the ductus comes from study with Doppler echocardiography, so it is important to be familiar with what these ultrasound techniques can assess. The ductus can be directly imaged with two-dimensional (2D) ultrasound. Widely patent ducts with little constriction are readily apparent on 2D imaging, but constricted ducts need color Doppler to assess patency. Color Doppler codes blood according to direction of flow, and as seen in Figure 14-2, this allows accurate assessment of ductal patency by showing movement of blood through the ductus. Color Doppler also allows assessment of the degree of ductal constriction. This can also be seen in Figure 14-2, which contrasts a well-constricted ductus with an unconstricted ductus.

Color Doppler also allows some assessment of the direction of shunting but accurate assessment of direction of shunting requires pulsed Doppler. Pulsed Doppler plots direction and velocity of blood flow against time. Direction of ductal shunting depends on the relative pressure at each end. Figure 14-3 shows the range of patterns of shunting from left to right (when aortic pressures exceed pulmonary) to bidirectional (when the pressures are more similar) to right to left (when pulmonary pressure exceeds aortic).

Normal Closure of the Ductus Arteriosus

In *term babies*, the ductus constricts after birth but does not close immediately. Within the first 12 hours after birth, some shunting of blood

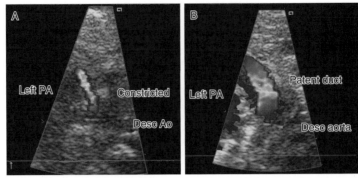

Figure 14-2 This figure shows two preterm PDAs studied within the first 6 hours after birth. Both color Doppler flow studies show predominantly blue stream of blood flow away from transducer in the main and left pulmonary artery with a patent ductus and the red stream of a left-to-right ductal shunt toward the transducer. **A** shows a well-constricted PDA and **B** shows a poorly constricted PDA. (See also Color Plate.) (From Evans N: Current controversies in diagnosis and treatment of patent ductus arteriosus. Adv Neonatal Care 2003;3:168–177, copyright 2003, with permission from The National Association of Neonatal Nurses.)

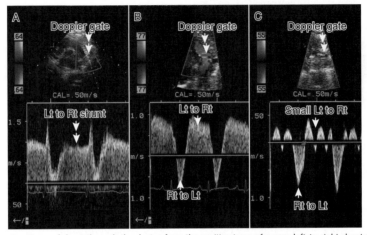

Figure 14-3 Different patterns of shunt through the ductus from the positive trace of a pure left-to-right shunt (**A**) to bidirectional (**B**) to predominantly negative trace of a right-to-left shunt (**C**). (See also Color Plate.) (From Evans N: Current controversies in diagnosis and treatment of patent ductus arteriosus. Adv Neonatal Care 2003;3:168–177, copyright 2003, with permission from The National Association of Neonatal Nurses.)

through the DA will be apparent on color Doppler in most term babies.[5] However, most of these ducts will be well constricted, so the volume of the shunt will be small. After 48 hours, most ducts in term babies will be functionally closed, although a few may be apparent after this time.[4] PDA is not a common cause of benign transitional murmurs in the newborn period, particularly those heard after the first 24 hours.[5] However, at term gestation the ductus arteriosus can be slower to close and cause a murmur that is found on routine examination. Most PDAs found in the first week in term babies will close spontaneously, but they should be followed to ensure that they do close.

In *uncomplicated preterm babies* with minimal respiratory problems, the ductus arteriosus closes in much the same time frame as in term babies.[3,6] Such cohorts of preterm babies tend to be in the gestational age range above 27 weeks, but

this observation does highlight that, in the right environment, the immature ductus will close spontaneously. However, in about a third of babies born before 30 weeks, the DA fails to close. The primary intrinsic problem of the immature duct is lack of muscle; this will compromise chances of functional as well as structural closure as the power of the muscle contraction may not be sufficient to induce the intimal ischemia necessary. There are also extrinsic factors, such as increased circulating prostaglandin levels, that may play a role.[7] This persisting patency has been associated with a range of complications of prematurity, including chronic lung disease, intraventricular hemorrhage, and necrotizing enterocolitis. Thus, the possibility of reducing these complications through prompt diagnosis and appropriate treatment of PDA has been the focus of much research interest in neonatology. The rest of this chapter will deal with the diagnosis, hemodynamic consequences, and treatment of this persisting patency of the preterm ductus.

Case Study 3

A 26-week-gestation boy was delivered precipitously without time for antenatal steroids to be administered to his mother. He is 12 hours old, ventilated with moderate pressures for respiratory distress syndrome (RDS) and has received surfactant. His mean blood pressure is 27 mm Hg and his cardiovascular examination is normal with normal pulses, precordial impulse, and no murmur.

Exercise 3

QUESTIONS

1. What risk factors does this baby have for PDA?
2. Does the normal clinical examination at 12 hours exclude a significant PDA at that time?

ANSWERS

1. Lower gestational age is the main risk factor for most complications of prematurity including PDA. Other risk factors in this baby include the lack of antenatal steroids and the presence of significant hyaline membrane disease (HMD).
2. No. When compared to echocardiographic markers of hemodynamic significance, it is normal for significant PDAs to be clinically silent on day 1 with the majority of significant PDAs being clinically silent up to day 3.

Case Study 4

A 27-week-gestation baby is still on the ventilator on day 6 of life and no weaning in pressures or oxygen has been possible for the last 2 days. The cardiovascular examination is normal.

Exercise 4

QUESTIONS

1. Is a PDA a likely explanation for this baby's failure to wean from the ventilator?
2. What changes in the blood pressure parameters might suggest a PDA in this case?

ANSWERS

1. No. Clinical signs of PDA become progressively more accurate through the first week of life, so a normal clinical examination at this age would make a PDA unlikely. It would not, however, completely exclude a PDA, and for a baby who is failing to wean from ventilation it would be reasonable to request an echocardiogram.
2. Increased pulse pressure is commonly quoted as a sign of PDA. However, when this has been examined systematically, there is no difference in pulse pressure over the first week between babies with or without significant PDAs. PDAs seem to cause a similar reduction in both systolic and diastolic (and therefore mean) pressure without affecting pulse pressure.

Diagnosis of PDA in Preterm Babies

Clinical Signs

The traditional teaching about PDA in preterm babies has been that left-to-right shunting will be minimal immediately following birth because of raised pulmonary artery pressures. It has been generally assumed that as pulmonary pressure falls, the left-to-right shunt increases and the classic physical signs appear. These signs include a long systolic murmur at the upper sternal edge, bounding peripheral pulses, increased pulse pressure, and increased precordial cardiac impulses. Although this may have been true in the era before the use of antenatal steroids, ventilation, and surfactant, the current relevance of this thinking is questionable. Recent echocardiographic studies have demonstrated that markers of hemodynamic significance (discussed later in the chapter) are often present from the first few hours after birth and that when these have been compared systematically with the above-mentioned physical signs, each of the classic signs (murmur, full pulses and active precordium) has a very low sensitivity for detecting a PDA.[8] Clinically silent ductal shunting is the norm on the first two postnatal days.[8,9] The accuracy of physical signs increases after day 4 such that by days 6 and 7, PDA can be diagnosed clinically with reasonable accuracy. However, by echocardiographic criteria, the PDA will have been shunting significantly for an average of 2 days (range 1 to 4 days) before it becomes clinically apparent. Contrary to popular belief, there is no difference in pulse pressure between preterm babies with or without a significant PDA during the first week. In fact, there tends to be a similar negative effect on both systolic and diastolic pressure with a resultant reduction in mean blood pressure.[10] Even toward the end of the first week, not all PDAs will generate physical signs. A high level of suspicion is needed, particularly in babies who are failing to wean from ventilation or who have persistent hypotension.

Echocardiographic Diagnosis

Accurate diagnosis of a PDA requires echocardiography, which allows assessment of patency, degree of constriction, and direction of shunting.[11] There are a variety of indirect methods to diagnose PDA, and of these, the most accurate and easiest to learn is a Doppler study in the main pulmonary artery. The left-to-right shunt through the duct produces the characteristic diastolic turbulence on the Doppler velocity pattern. This method is reasonably accurate but only discloses whether the duct is open or closed, not how significant it is. The best way to determine patency is by direct imaging with color Doppler because of the more complete information obtained about the duct. It does take longer to learn; however, development of these skills should be well within the reach of most neonatologists.[12,13]

Echocardiographic determination of patency is easy; more controversial are the criteria that should be applied to determine hemodynamic significance. In cardiology, the size of a left-to-right shunt is often expressed as the ratio of pulmonary to systemic blood flow (Qp:Qs); this in turn can be derived by measuring both ventricular outputs with Doppler. In studies we have performed, the ductal measure that had the closest correlation with Qp:Qs was the minimum diameter within the course of the duct as measured from the color Doppler as shown in Figures 14-2A and B.[14] In babies less than 1500 g during the first week of life, if the diameter was over 2 mm, the pulmonary blood flow is usually more than twice the systemic. This is consistent with the laws of fluid dynamics, which dictate that the volume of blood passing across a PDA will be determined by the internal diameter and the pressure differential across the duct. The latter is reflected in the velocity of the shunt. Velocity is not an important determinant of shunt size in the first week because it falls into quite a narrow range during this time (usually less than 2 m/second).[14]

More blood flows through a duct in systole than in diastole, but because there is less flow in diastole in the two circulations it connects, the disturbances in flow in the pulmonary and systemic circulations produced by a duct are most apparent in diastole. Therefore, retrograde diastolic flow in the descending aorta and increased velocity in the left pulmonary artery (during diastole) are both useful markers of a significant left-to-right shunt (Fig. 14-4).[14,15]

Preterm Ductal Constriction

The early postnatal constriction of the ductus in babies born before 30 weeks is characterized by great variation.[16–18] This ranges across a spectrum from those in whom the duct constricts in similar fashion to a term baby to those in whom the constriction fails completely. This range of early ductal constriction is shown in Figure 14-5 in which the ductal minimum diameter, as assessed by color Doppler, is plotted against gestation in a cohort of 124 preterm babies at 5 hours of age. This range of constriction determines not only the hemodynamic significance of the ductal shunt at the time but also predicts persisting patency.[16,18] The ductus tends to close in babies with good early ductal constriction (smaller diameters, see Fig. 14-5). The ductus is much more likely to stay open in babies with poor early constriction (larger diameters in Fig. 14-5). The solid triangles in Figure 14-5 highlight the babies in whom the duct later became clinically apparent and required treatment. It can be seen that most of the babies who needed treatment had a DA diameter above the median at 5 hours of age.

Direction of Preterm Ductal Shunting

There are a few preterm babies in whom high pulmonary artery pressure is clinically very important. However, in most preterm babies, the pulmonary artery pressure is below systemic pressures and the dominant direction of shunting is left to right. In the 124 babies studied at 5 hours described in Figure 14-5, 52% had a pure left-to-right shunt, 42% had a bidirectional shunt but a mean of 75% of the cardiac cycle was left to right, and just 2% had a right-to-left shunt.[17]

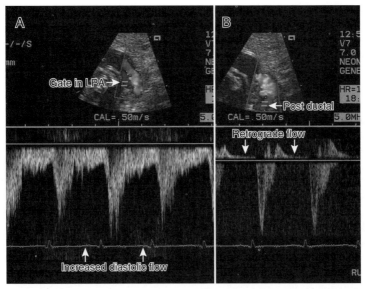

Figure 14-4 The disturbance of diastolic flow is seen in the circulations on either side of a significant duct. A shows the increased velocity diastolic flow in the left pulmonary artery, and B shows the retrograde diastolic flow in the postductal descending aorta. (See also Color Plate.)

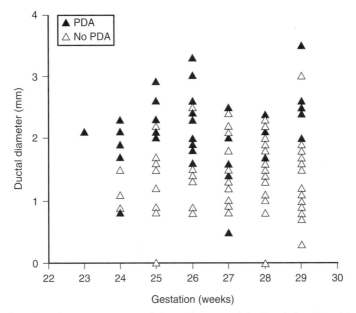

Figure 14-5 Ductal color Doppler diameter at an average of 5 hours of age in 124 babies born before 30 weeks' gestation. Echocardiographic information was not used in clinical care, and the solid triangles represent babies who went on to develop a clinically apparent PDA.

Significance of Early Preterm Ductal Shunting

In babies in whom the DA has failed to constrict, significant volumes of blood can move out of the systemic circulation into the pulmonary circulation, even in the early postnatal hours. Very preterm babies are at high risk of low systemic blood flow in the first 12 hours after birth. This occurs in about a third of babies born before 30 weeks. The negative effect of ductal shunting on the systemic circulation may be most apparent in this early period.[17] By the time the DA is diagnosed clinically, most babies are protecting their systemic circulation well. This effect on early systemic blood flow may be the pathway by which PDA is associated with ischemic complications such as necrotizing enterocolitis (NEC) and intraventricular hemorrhage (IVH). The effect on the pulmonary circulation is more difficult to measure, but based on estimating pulmonary to systemic flow ratios from relative biventricular outputs, pulmonary blood flows that are twice systemic are not uncommon in the early period. Pulmonary blood flow will increase over the first 24 to 48 hours as the flow in both circulations increases. This can reduce pulmonary compliance and may be related to hemorrhagic pulmonary edema or pulmonary hemorrhages. Pulmonary hemorrhages commonly occur within the first 48 hours, suggesting an early clinical impact of high pulmonary blood flow.[18]

Summary

Early preterm ductal constriction is very variable. The predominant direction of shunting is left to right. In babies in whom the duct fails to constrict, very significant shunts can occur even in the early postnatal period, draining blood from the systemic circulation and overloading the pulmonary circulation. Clinical diagnosis is of limited accuracy in the early postnatal period; accurate diagnosis requires echocardiography.

Case Study 5

A 26-week-gestation baby is 4 days old and still ventilated for RDS. He has normal urine output, normal platelets, and no abdominal distention. He has bounding pulses, an active precordium, and an easily heard systolic murmur. An echocardiogram shows a 2.5-mm PDA with left-to-right shunt and retrograde diastolic descending aortic flow.

Exercise 5

QUESTIONS

1. Should this PDA be treated?
2. If you think it should be treated, should it be treated medically or surgically?
3. If you think it should be treated medically, what drug should be used?
4. What outcomes are improved by treating a PDA at this time?

ANSWERS

1. Many neonatologists would treat this duct because it is clinically apparent and fulfills echocardiographic criteria of significance.
2. Medical. Surgery is a significant intervention and there is no evidence that it is superior to medical treatment.

3. Either indomethacin or ibuprofen. The latter is preferred by some because there are fewer renal side effects and the short-term reductions of organ blood flow seen with indomethacin are less apparent with ibuprofen. Neither drug has been shown to be clearly superior in terms of efficacy of ductal closure or important clinical outcomes.
4. We don't know. This approach of waiting for clinical signs before treating is the most commonly used PDA treatment protocol; however, treating versus not treating a PDA like this has never really been compared in a trial. What evidence we have (see later discussion) doesn't show major outcome differences.

Case Study 6

A 25-week-gestation baby, ventilated and given surfactant at birth for RDS, is now 3 hours old with improving ventilation parameters.

Exercise 6

QUESTIONS

1. Should this baby be given prophylactic medical treatment for PDA?
2. If so, what drug should be used?
3. What outcomes are improved by giving prophylactic PDA treatment?

ANSWERS

1. From this information, the evidence for such treatment is not clear.
2. Probably indomethacin. Indomethacin is better studied and has produced improvement in short-term outcomes that has not been apparent (to date) for prophylactic ibuprofen.
3. Prophylactic indomethacin reduces rate of later PDA, need for PDA ligation, and major IVH; however, no improvements in longer term neurodevelopmental outcome have been shown.

Case Study 7

A 28-week-gestation baby was ventilated from soon after birth for HMD and is now on day 3 of life with slow improvement of ventilation parameters. The cardiovascular examination is normal, but an echocardiogram is ordered to screen for a PDA. It shows a 3-mm PDA with left-to-right shunt and retrograde diastolic descending aortic flow.

Exercise 7

QUESTIONS

1. Should this PDA be treated at this time?
2. What outcomes have been shown to be improved by treating a clinically silent PDA at this time?

ANSWERS

1. Probably not, there is no clear evidence that would support treating at this time.
2. In trials, no differences in outcomes have been shown by treating on day 3 compared to waiting for day 7. At a pragmatic level, the more mature a baby is, the more likely the duct will close spontaneously.

Treatment of the Preterm Infant with a PDA

The two dominant questions with respect to treatment of PDA are how to treat and, much more controversially, when to treat.[17]

Treatment Methods

Surgical or Medical Treatment

Surgical ligation of PDA within a neonatal intensive care unit (NICU) is mainly influenced by availability. There is no evidence in the literature that surgery is preferable as a first-line treatment to medical treatment. The Collaborative Trial[18] addressed this issue, and babies randomized to primary treatment with surgery had higher rates of pneumothorax and retinopathy of prematurity. Most clinicians use surgical ligation when a symptomatic PDA has failed to close with medical treatment. Whether ligating the PDA after failed medical treatment protects babies from adverse outcomes has not been tested.

Drug Therapy

Indomethacin or Ibuprofen? Indomethacin has been used for many years in neonatology and it has been shown to successfully close 75% to 90% of PDAs.[20] This benefit comes with the potential harms of a range of well-recognized side effects including oliguria, gastrointestinal bleeding and perforation, hyponatremia, and transient reductions in blood flow to organs such as the brain and intestine. Indomethacin is a nonspecific prostaglandin synthetase inhibitor, and any drug of this class would probably close the ductus. Ibuprofen is the best studied alternative to indomethacin. Ibuprofen has less short-term negative effects on organ blood flow than indomethacin,[21,22] but it is not clear whether this translates to better outcomes. Randomized trials comparing ibuprofen and indomethacin suggest similar efficacy with duct closure and possibly a reduced incidence of transient renal side effects with ibuprofen.[23]

Dosage Regimen. Ibuprofen is usually given at 10 mg/kg daily for 3 days.[23] In early studies, indomethacin was given at 0.2 mg/kg every 12 hours for three doses. This recommended dose was modified to 0.1 mg/kg daily for 6 days, after two randomized trials suggested this regimen achieved similar closure rates with fewer side effects.[24,25] More recently, Tammela and coworkers[26] showed that 0.2 mg/kg followed by two doses of 0.1 mg/kg at 12-hour intervals was as effective as the six daily doses of 0.1 mg/kg with no difference in side effects. Giving each dose as an infusion over 20 to 60 minutes appears to limit some of the negative effects on organ blood flow.[27,28] With wider availability of echocardiographic surveillance, it may be possible to give even shorter courses of indomethacin, depending on the individual response. The immediate constrictive effect of indomethacin is variable, but there is a measurable and significant response by 2 hours after the first dose.[29] Some studies[30,31] have used echocardiographic surveillance to shorten the course of indomethacin, with no obvious adverse effect on closure rates. Most neonatologists would avoid using indomethacin when there is renal dysfunction or evidence of intestinal compromise because of the renal and gastrointestinal side effects. It is advisable to reduce fluid intake when using indomethacin. Some neonatologists withhold feeds; however, there is no evidence that this reduces the risk of gastrointestinal side effects.

Timing of Treatment

Timing remains the main unresolved issue in relation to the management of the preterm

PDA. There are broadly three approaches to the timing of PDA treatment: treating when the duct becomes clinically symptomatic, targeted presymptomatic treatment, and prophylactic treatment. None of these approaches has shown unequivocal benefits in terms of outcome.[17]

Treatment for Symptomatic PDA

Although this is probably the most widely used approach, there is no evidence it makes any difference in outcomes. It has the advantage that fewer babies will be exposed to the potential adverse effects of prostaglandin synthetase inhibitors. The disadvantage is that the ductus will usually have been hemodynamically significant for some time prior to treatment, and it may be too late to make a difference. The six trials of this approach are somewhat dated (1978 and 1983) and limited by the early introduction of open label treatment in the placebo arms. Therefore, conservative versus active medical treatment was not really tested; rather, early versus delayed medical treatment was compared. When these trials are meta-analyzed, babies randomized to indomethacin needed less subsequent treatment for PDA, but there were no differences in other outcomes, including chronic lung disease and mortality rate.[17] These results do suggest that if your protocol is to wait until a PDA becomes clinically apparent, then there is nothing lost by waiting a bit longer to see if it will close spontaneously.

Presymptomatic Treatment

This strategy usually involves echocardiographic screening for the duct at a certain age and treating those ducts that are still patent. Of the seven trials that used this approach, only one was published after 1990.[17] That trial by Van Overmeire and associates,[32] published in 2001, is the largest and the most important. In this trial, babies were randomized on the basis of an echocardiographically patent duct, to treatment on day 3 or waiting and treating if the duct was still patent on day 7. The group treated on day 3 received more indomethacin and had oliguria but there were no differences in respiratory outcomes or mortality rates. Combined adverse outcomes were higher in the early treated group. Therefore, this trial confirmed that there was no improvement in outcomes from treating on day 3. In view of the early hemodynamic effects of ductal shunting, it may be that even day 3 treatment is too late.

Prophylactic Indomethacin

Most of the recent studies of PDA treatment have used this approach; there are 19 randomized trials enrolling 2872 babies in the Cochrane Review.[33] All the studies involved randomized high-risk babies to indomethacin or placebo within the first 24 hours. In most trials, the intervention was initiated within the first 6 hours. The meta-analysis shows that prophylactic indomethacin reduces the incidence of later PDA, PDA ligation, grade 3 or 4 IVH, and ultrasound evidence of periventricular leukomalacia (PVL) or ischemic changes. Unfortunately, this hasn't been demonstrated to improve respiratory outcomes, mortality rates, or neurodevelopmental outcomes at 2 years of age, which was the primary outcome of the large multicenter TIPP trial[34,35] or at school age in the previous large trial of prophylactic indomethacin.[35] There was no evidence of any harm, particularly with respect to necrotizing enterocolitis or gastrointestinal perforation. Therefore, there are some short-term benefits to prophylactic indomethacin but no clear long-term advantage.[34,35] Two trials have examined the effect of prophylactic ibuprofen; both have demonstrated a reduced frequency of PDA but no differences in other outcomes, including IVH.[36,37]

The disadvantage of this approach is that all babies are exposed to the potential adverse effects of therapy. However, the prophylactic approach to PDA treatment is the only one that has been shown to have benefits of any sort. In view of the lack of evidence of any harm, it could be argued that if you're going to treat PDAs at all, then this is the best strategy to use.

Future Directions

Current evidence does not allow unequivocal recommendations about how and when to treat the preterm PDA. Considering the potential early hemodynamic impact of ductal shunting, it may well be that closure after the first 24 hours is too late. On the other hand, the effect of prophylactic indomethacin may be limited by the fact that many babies are receiving a potentially toxic drug that they don't need. The ideal treatment would be to give early indomethacin to those we know will have adverse effects from a patent duct. We don't have a perfect predictive test but the fact that the degree of early ductal constriction predicts persisting patency offers a potential way to target very early treatment more accurately. Considering Figure 14-5, if we had treated the 50% of babies with a ductal diameter above the median, then most of the babies who developed a symptomatic PDA would have been treated within a few hours of birth. The possibility of using early echocardiography to target treatment of PDA in the early postnatal period merits further investigation. It would be limited to NICUs with access to echocardiography, and neonatologists around the world are developing echocardiographic skills in increasing numbers.[38]

How Should the Ductus Arteriosus Be Managed?

The lack of clear evidence about how best to treat the patent ductus arteriosus means that the reader may encounter a whole range of different approaches to this problem in different NICUs. At one end of the spectrum is the view that the lack of evidence of outcome benefit from clinical trials suggests that preterm ductal shunting is "physiologic," and as such, the only indication for treatment of a PDA should be intractable heart failure.[39] At the other end of the spectrum is the view that evidence of short-term benefits and lack of evidence of harm would support the prophylactic use of indomethacin. I am not aware of formal surveys of practice in this area, but my impression is that the commonest approach is still to wait for development of clinical signs or symptoms of a PDA, such as hypotension or failure to wean from ventilation, before treating with indomethacin or ibuprofen. Most NICUs reserve surgery for when medical treatment fails, but the threshold for proceeding to surgery varies.

The approach in my service reflects the philosophy described previously of giving early treatment targeted on the basis of the degree of early ductal constriction defined by color Doppler echocardiography. We perform echocardiography within the first 6 hours of life in all babies born before 28 weeks and in 28- and 29-week gestations, if there are risk factors such as lack of antenatal steroids or significant lung disease requiring ventilation. If the minimum diameter of the color Doppler shunt within the course of the ductus is more than 2 mm, we would treat with indomethacin 0.1 mg/kg with two further doses of 0.1 mg/kg repeated at 24-hour intervals. If the duct is less than 2 mm, we would not treat early, but would observe all infants clinically, and have a low threshold for repeat echocardiography if clinical evidence or possible signs of a PDA developed over subsequent days. We would usually treat with indomethacin if evidence of a PDA emerged, but if a baby was stable on minimal respiratory support (e.g., on CPAP in a low F_{IO_2}), we might observe for a period to see if the duct closes spontaneously. In babies in whom the ductus fails to close after the first course of medical treatment, we often try a second course, but this approach has been rarely efficacious. We try to avoid surgery in these babies, and if a baby with a medically resistant ductus was stable, we would adopt an expectant approach. However, if the baby was unstable or deteriorating from a respiratory point of view and there was clear echocardiographic evidence of hemodynamic significance, we would refer the infant for ligation. Using this approach, PDA ligation is an uncommon event in our service. In babies born before 28 weeks, the rate of surgical ligation of the PDA is about 3% and it is very unusual for us to ligate a PDA in babies born after 27 weeks.

I would emphasize that we have no clear evidence that this approach is the correct one. We see it as a refinement of the prophylactic approach for which there is arguable evidence of benefit, but good evidence of no harm.

Conclusion

In conclusion, the hemodynamic impact of ductal shunting often occurs much earlier than traditionally believed, in the first 24 to 48 hours after birth. Constriction of the duct in the first few hours after birth is very variable and predicts both hemodynamic significance at the time and subsequent persisting patency. This would suggest that treatment to close the duct needs to be given early to make a difference. Currently the only treatment approach that has been shown to make a difference to *any* outcome is prophylactic early indomethacin. Whether this approach is adopted will depend on the relative value placed on the short-term outcomes (that are improved) against the long-term outcomes, about which we have no evidence of change.

References

1. Evans N, Henderson-Smart D: Cardiorespiratory adaptation to extrauterine life. In Rodeck CH, Whittle MJ (eds): Fetal Medicine: Basic Science and Clinical Practice. London, Churchill Livingstone, 1999, pp 1045–1052.

2. Clyman RI, Chan CY, Mauray F, et al: Permanent anatomic closure of the ductus arteriosus in newborn baboons: The roles of postnatal constriction, hypoxia, and gestation. Pediatr Res 1999;45: 19–29.

3. Evans N, Archer LNJ: Postnatal circulatory adaptation in term and healthy preterm neonates. Arch Dis Child 1990;65:24–26.

4. Lim MK, Hanretty K, Houston AB, et al: Intermittent ductal patency in healthy newborn infants: Demonstration by color Doppler flow mapping. Arch Dis Child 1992;67:1217–1218.

5. Arlettaz R, Archer N, Wilkinson AR: Natural history of innocent heart murmurs in newborn babies: Controlled echocardiographic study. Arch Dis Child Fetal Neonatal Ed 1998;78:166–170.

6. Reller MD, Ziegler ML, Rice MJ, et al: Duration of ductal shunting in healthy preterm infants: An echocardiographic color flow Doppler study. J Pediatr 1988;112:441–446.

7. Kluckow M, Evans NJ, Leslie G, Rowe J: Prostacyclin concentrations and transitional circulation in preterm infants requiring mechanical ventilation. Arch Dis Child 1999;80:F34–F37.

8. Skelton R, Evans N, Smythe J: A blinded comparison of clinical and echocardiographic evaluation of the preterm infant for patent ductus arteriosus. J Paediatr Child Health 1994;30:406–411.

9. Davis P, Turner-Gomes S, Cunningham K, et al: Precision and accuracy of clinical and radiological signs in premature infants at risk of patent ductus arteriosus. Arch Pediatr Adolesc Med. 1995;149: 1136–1141.

10. Evans N, Moorcraft J: Effect of patency of the ductus arteriosus on blood pressure in very preterm infants. Arch Dis Child 1992;67:1169–1173.

11. Evans N, Kluckow M, Osborn DA: Diagnosis of patent ductus arteriosus. Neoreviews 2004;5:86–97.

12. Evans N, Malcolm G: Practical echocardiography for the neonatologist. Structural and transitional haemodynamic problems of the newborn. A multimedia CD-ROM. Royal Prince Alfred Hospital. 2002. Accessed at www.cs.nsw.gov.au/rpa/neonatal.

13. Skinner J, Alverson D, Hunter s (eds): Echocardiography for the Neonatologist. London, Churchill Livingston, 2000.

14. Evans N, Iyer P: Assessment of ductus arteriosus shunt in preterm infants supported by mechanical ventilation: Effect of inter-atrial shunting. J Pediatr 1994;125:778–785.

15. Suzumura H, Nitta A, Tanaka G, Arisaka O: Diastolic flow velocity of the left pulmonary artery of patent ductus arteriosus in preterm infants. Pediatr Intl 2001;43(2):146–151.

16. Kluckow M, Evans N: Early echocardiographic prediction of symptomatic patent ductus arteriosus in preterm infants undergoing mechanical ventilation. J Pediatr 1995;127:774–779.

17. Kluckow M, Evans N: Low superior vena cava flow and intraventricular hemorrhage in preterm infants. Arch Dis Child 2000;82:F188–F194.

18. Kluckow M, Evans N: Ductal shunting, high pulmonary blood flow pulmonary hemorrhage. J Pediatr 2000;137:68–72.

19. Knight DB: The treatment of patent ductus arteriosus in preterm infants. A review and overview of randomised trials. Semin Neonatol 2001;6:63–73.

20. Gersony WM, Peckham GJ, Ellison RC, et al: Effects of indomethacin in premature infants with patent ductus arteriosus: The results of a national collaborative trial. J Pediatr 1983;102:895–906.

21. Mosca F, Bray M, Lattanzio M, et al: Comparative evaluation of the effects of indomethacin and ibuprofen on cerebral perfusion and oxygenation in preterm infants with patent ductus arteriosus. J Pediatr 1997;131:549–554.

22. Pezzati M, Vangi V, Biagiotti R, et al: Effects of indomethacin and ibuprofen on mesenteric and renal blood flow in preterm infants with patent ductus arteriosus. J Pediatr 1999;135:733–778.

23. Van Overmeire B, Smets K, Lecoutere D, et al: A comparison of ibuprofen and indomethacin for closure of patent ductus arteriosus. N Engl J Med 2000;43:674–681.

24. Hammerman C, Aramburo MJ: Prolonged indomethacin therapy for the prevention of recurrences of patent ductus arteriosus. J Pediatr 1990;117: 771–776.

25. Rennie JM, Cooke RWI: Prolonged low dose indomethacin for persistent ductus arteriosus of prematurity. Arch Dis Child 1991;66:55–58.

26. Tammela O, Ojala R, Iivainen T, et al: Short versus prolonged indomethacin therapy for patent ductus arteriosus in preterm infants. J Pediatr 1999;134: 552–557.

27. Colditz P, Murphy D, Rolfe P, Wilkinson AR: Effect of infusion rate of indomethacin on cerebrovascular responses in preterm neonates. Arch Dis Child 1989;64:8–12.

28. Edwards AD, Wyatt JS, Richardson C, et al: Effects of indomethacin on cerebral haemodynamics in very preterm infants. Lancet 1990;335: 1491–1495.

29. Osborn DA, Evans N, Kluckow M: Effect of early targeted indomethacin on the ductus arteriosus and blood flow to the upper body and brain in the preterm infant. Arch Dis Child 2003;88:F477–F482.

30. Dumas de la Roque E, Fayon M, Babre F, et al: Minimal effective dose of indomethacin for the treatment of patent ductus arteriosus in preterm infants. Biol Neonate 2002;81:91–94.

31. Su BH, Peng CT, Tsai CH: Echocardiographic flow patterns of patent ductus arteriosus: A guide to indomethacin treatment in premature infants. Arch Dis Child 1999;81:F197–F200.

32. Van Overmeire B, Van de Broek H, Van Laer P, et al: Early versus late indomethacin treatment for patent ductus arteriosus in premature infants with respiratory distress syndrome. J Pediatr 2001; 138:205–211.

33. Fowlie PW, Davis PG: Prophylactic intravenous indomethacin for preventing mortality and morbidity in preterm infants. Cochrane Database of Syst Rev 2002(Issue 4).

34. Schmidt B, Davis P, Moddemann D, et al: Trial of indomethacin prophylaxis in preterms investigators. Long-term effects of indomethacin prophylaxis in extremely-low-birth-weight infants. N Engl J Med 2001;344:1966–1972.

35. Vohr BR, Allan WC, Westerveld M, et al: School-age outcomes of very low birth weight infants in the indomethacin intraventricular hemorrhage prevention trial. Pediatrics 2003;111:e340.

36. Dani C, Bertini G, Reali MF, et al: Prophylaxis of patent ductus arteriosus with ibuprofen in preterm infants. Acta Paediatr 2000;89:1369–1374.

37. Van Overmeire B, Allegaert K, Casaer A, et al: Prophylactic ibuprofen in premature infants: A multicentre, randomised, double-blind, placebo-controlled trial. Lancet 2004;364:1945–1949.

38. Evans N: Echocardiography on neonatal intensive care units in Australia and New Zealand. J Paediatr Child Health 2000;36:169–171.

Color Plate

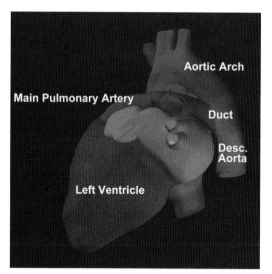

Figure 14-1 Image of a model of the heart viewed from the left side to demonstrate the anatomic relationships of the ductus arteriosus. It can be seen how the ductus is a continuation of the main pulmonary artery that is slightly offset to the left to allow it to describe an arch into the descending aorta.

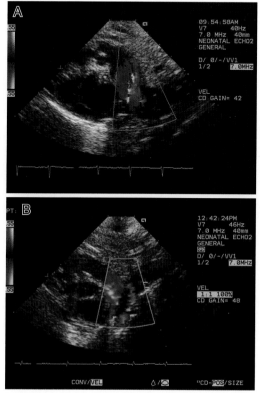

Figure accompanying Chapter 14, Exercise 2, Question 4.

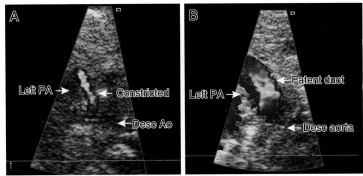

Figure 14-2 This figure shows two preterm PDAs studied within the first 6 hours after birth. Both color Doppler flow studies show predominantly blue stream of blood flow away from transducer in the main and left pulmonary artery with a patent ductus and the red stream of a left-to-right ductal shunt toward the transducer. **A** shows a well-constricted PDA and **B** shows a poorly constricted PDA. (From Evans N: Current controversies in diagnosis and treatment of patent ductus arteriosus. Adv Neonatal Care 2003;3:168–177, copyright 2003, with permission from The National Association of Neonatal Nurses.)

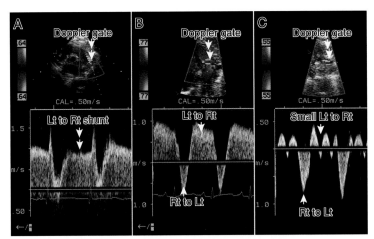

Figure 14-3 Different patterns of shunt through the ductus from the positive trace of a pure left-to-right shunt (**A**) to bidirectional (**B**) to predominantly negative trace of a right-to-left shunt (**C**). (From Evans N: Current controversies in diagnosis and treatment of patent ductus arteriosus. Adv Neonatal Care 2003;3:168–177, copyright 2003, with permission from The National Association of Neonatal Nurses.)

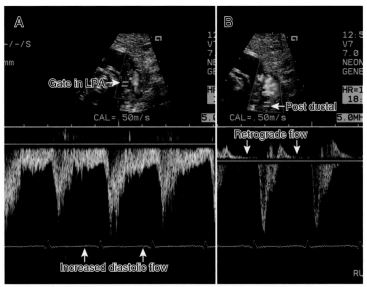

Figure 14-4 The disturbance of diastolic flow is seen in the circulations on either side of a significant duct. **A** shows the increased velocity diastolic flow in the left pulmonary artery, and **B** shows the retrograde diastolic flow in the postductal descending aorta.

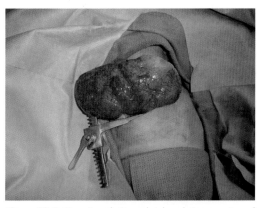

Figure 22-5 Operative photograph taken during resection of an emphysematous lobe.

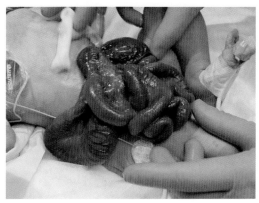

Figure 22-7 Abdominal wall defect with exposed viscera.

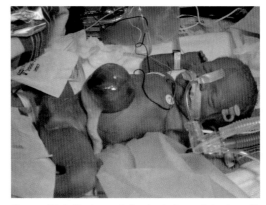

Figure 22-8 Classic centrally located omphalocele with covering membrane.

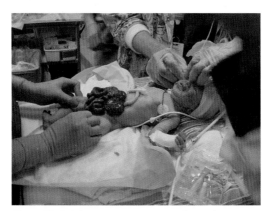

Figure 22-9 Delivery room preparation of a newborn. Intravenous access has been obtained and an orogastric tube is in place.

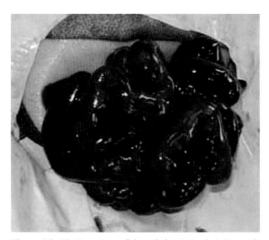

Figure 22-13 Necrotic small bowel due to malrotation with volvulus.

Hypotension in the Newborn Infant

Martin Kluckow, FRACP, PhD

Hypotension is a common finding in the neonatal intensive care unit, where it occurs in up to 30% of very low birth weight (VLBW) infants in the early postnatal period. Furthermore, 16% to 52% are treated with volume expansion and up to 39% need vasopressor treatment.[1] The management of hypotension varies from institution to institution and among clinicians.[1] The variability in management practice ranges from the assessment and measurement of blood pressure to the assessment of the need for treatment and, when necessary, which treatment. Lack of good evidence for both when to treat low blood pressure and whether treatment benefits the long-term outcome of infants underlies this uncertainty. As the blood pressure is the most easily obtained parameter of cardiovascular impairment, clinicians tend to focus on the actual blood pressure and aim to achieve a set number, rather than trying to understand the underlying pathophysiologic mechanisms that have led to a low blood pressure in a particular infant. An understanding of the underlying physiology will allow more specific and targeted management of hypotension.

This chapter addresses the underlying physiologic variables that determine the blood pressure. These need to be understood in the context of the changes occurring in the transitional circulation, particularly in the preterm infant and to a lesser extent in the term infant. The key concept is that blood pressure is just one aspect of the cardiovascular assessment of the neonate. Understanding the reasons for cardiovascular insufficiency allows for a more directed treatment of hypotension.

Case Study 1

Baby boy A was born at 30 weeks of gestation weighing 1650 g. His mother had an antepartum hemorrhage and an emergency cesarean section. There was no time for antenatal betamethasone. Apgar scores were 6 at 1 minute and 7 at 5 minutes. He required resuscitation with bag and mask after birth and required an inspired fraction of oxygen (F_{IO_2}) of 0.30 to maintain oxygen saturation above 88%. He was transferred to the neonatal intensive care unit and nursed in an incubator in F_{IO_2} of 0.3. Intravenous fluids at 80 mL/kg/day were commenced via a peripheral vein. The nursing staff are concerned that he is "poorly perfused."

Exercise 1

QUESTIONS

1. What clinical and physiologic variables relevant to the cardiovascular system might be contributing to the observation of "poor perfusion"?

2. Which of the following factors are responsible for initiating or controlling the circulatory transition?

   a. Oxygen

   b. Cold stress

   c. Epinephrine

   d. Glucocorticoids

   e. Endothelin

   f. Nitric oxide

3. How would you further assess this infant's cardiovascular system?

4. What are the two physiologic determinants of blood pressure?

ANSWERS

1. The infant is premature and undergoing circulatory transition. There may be shunting of blood at both ductal and atrial levels. In addition, the rapid changes in afterload associated with preterm delivery can impair myocardial performance. This infant may have suffered some hypoxic/ischemic insult due to the antepartum hemorrhage, further impairing myocardial function. There is some degree of respiratory distress that may be due either to immaturity of the lungs or to pulmonary congestion. He may also be hypothermic and peripherally vasoconstricted.

2. Oxygen, epinephrine, nitric oxide, endothelin. Shortly after delivery, the severing of the umbilical vessels and inflation of the lungs with air lead to a sudden increase in the resistance in the systemic circulation and a change of blood flow, such that the complete cardiac output now passes through the pulmonary as well as the systemic circulation. The partial pressure of oxygen in the blood is increased, which leads to reduced pulmonary vascular tone and constriction of the ductus arteriosus. At birth there is a surge in the plasma epinephrine and norepinephrine levels, which appears to be a response to decreased oxygenation, decreased environmental temperature, severing of the umbilical cord, and labor and delivery. The surge in catecholamines at birth is responsible for the postnatal increase in cardiac output and myocardial contractility. Glucocorticoids have an effect on vasomotor tone but usually after the transitional period. Nitric oxide and endothelin are responsible for the resting tone of blood vessels and both are higher in the newborn infant, also suggesting a role in the transition.

3. The usual method used to obtain further information regarding an infant's cardiovascular system is to measure the blood pressure—invasively or noninvasively. The measurement obtained is then compared with normative values for infants at 30 weeks' gestation on day 1 of life. Other options include measuring cardiac output and cardiac function using echocardiography and obtaining the arterial acid-base status to look for any evidence of metabolic acidosis.

4. Arterial blood pressure is determined by the product of cardiac output and peripheral vascular resistance. Cardiac output is influenced by preload or blood volume and myocardial contractility. The peripheral vascular resistance will be determined by the vascular tone.

The Transitional Circulation

In utero, the fetal communications of the foramen ovale and ductus arteriosus result in a lack of separation between the left and right ventricular outputs, making it difficult to quantitate their individual contributions. The combined cardiovascular output in human fetuses estimated by the noninvasive Doppler technique steadily rises to about 400 mL/kg/minute at term.[2] The systolic function of the ventricles is determined by the basic physiologic principles of preload (distention of the ventricle with blood prior to contraction), contractility or the intrinsic ability of the myocardial fibres to contract, afterload (the combined resistance of the blood, the ventricular walls, and the vascular beds), and the heart rate. The fetus has a limited ability to respond to changes in these determinants of cardiac output.[3] An infant who is born prematurely still has a developing myocardium, so it is likely that some of these fetal limitations are also experienced by the myocardium of the premature infant. Furthermore, there is a marked difference in the influence of determinants of cardiac output in the newborn premature infant, with a dramatically increased afterload compared to the relatively low resistance placenta and changes in preload from the effects of inflation of the lungs (often by positive pressure ventilation). The newborn ventricle is more sensitive to changes in afterload, such that small changes can have large effects if the preload and contractility are not maximized.[3]

Shortly after delivery, the severing of the umbilical vessels and inflation of the lungs with air leads to a sudden increase in the resistance in the systemic circulation and a change of blood flow, such that the complete cardiac output now passes through the pulmonary as well as the systemic circulation. In normal full-term infants, the ductus arteriosus functionally closes by the second day of life and the right ventricular pressure falls to adult levels by about 2 to 3 days after birth.[4,5] Functional constriction and closure of the ductus is subsequently followed by anatomic closure. In contrast, in the preterm infant, there is frequently a failure of complete closure of both the foramen ovale and the ductus arteriosus in the usual short time frame due to immaturity of the mechanisms involved.[6] As a result, blood may now flow preferentially from aorta to pulmonary artery resulting in a relative loss of blood from the systemic circulation and excessive flow through the pulmonary circulation. This systemic to pulmonary shunting can occur in the first hours of life, with recirculation of 50% or more of the normal cardiac output back into the lungs[7]; the myocardium subsequently attempts to compensate by increasing the total cardiac output. Agata and associates studied the changes occurring in the left ventricular (LV) output from fetal to neonatal life in 34 normal term infants.[8] They found a twofold increase in the LV output at 1 hour of age, resulting primarily from an increased stroke volume, rather than increased heart rate. Furthermore, Drayton and Skidmore demonstrated that the left-to-right shunt through the ductus averaged about 60 mL/kg/minute soon after birth[9] indicating that a significant proportion of this increase is likely to be passing through the ductus arteriosus. This marked increase was reduced by 25% by 24 hours of life and the authors postulate that the decline in cardiac output may be partly due to the concurrent decrease in the amount of ductal shunt by 24 hours of age.[10–12]

Neural and Humoral Determinants of Blood Pressure and Vascular Tone

The regulation of blood pressure is complex and involves both the neural and endocrine systems. The role played by each of these main regulating systems can be either at a central or peripheral level. The autonomic nervous system, particularly the sympathetic outflow, plays an important role in the transition from fetal to neonatal life. Input from arterial baroreceptors located in the great vessels and cardiopulmonary receptors in the heart and great veins provide information regarding changes in pressure and changes in blood volume. In addition, they influence blood pressure via sympathetic nervous system activity.

The fetus and newborn both rely on a number of endocrine mechanisms to enable response to stress and regulate vasomotor tone. The sympathoadrenal system is made up of the sympathetic nervous system, the adrenal medulla, and islets of chromaffin tissue adjacent to the abdominal aorta. Catecholamine receptors (adrenoreceptors) are classified into the α_1-receptors, α_2-receptors and β-receptors.[13] In addition there are two major types of dopaminergic receptors.[14] These receptors may act together or have opposite effects in the same organ (e.g., α_1- and α_2-receptors cause vasoconstriction of peripheral blood vessels, while β-receptors mediate vasodilatation). There is an organ-specific alteration of the number of adrenoreceptors during development in the fetus and neonate. This maturational change in adrenoreceptors may account for the different responses seen in preterm infants to sympathomimetic drugs, such as the increased sensitivity to the pressor effects of dopamine.[15] In premature infants, dopamine-induced activation of the α-adrenergic receptor and the consequent increase in blood pressure occurs at a lower weight adjusted dose than in more mature infants.[15]

In response to stimuli such as hypoxemia, the fetus produces both epinephrine and norepinephrine. This response is proportional to the change in Po_2 and increases with the gestational age.[16] β-Adrenergic stimulation increases the heart rate and the myocardial and pulmonary blood flow. α-Adrenergic stimulation increases the arterial blood pressure and decreases the combined ventricular output as well as blood flow to the renal and peripheral circulations.[17] At birth there is a surge in the plasma epinephrine and norepinephrine levels, which appears to be a response to decreased oxygenation, decreased environmental temperature, labor and delivery, and severing of the umbilical cord.[18] The surge in catecholamines at birth is responsible for the postnatal increase in cardiac output and myocardial contractility.[19]

Glucocorticoids are potentially vasoactive, particularly in the preterm infant. They have a broad spectrum of actions, some of which involve modulation of β-adrenoreceptors in blood vessel walls and the myocardium, enhancing sensitivity to catecholamines.[20] Antenatal corticosteroid treatment appears to improve postnatal blood pressure and protect against both intraventricular hemorrhage and patent ductus arteriosus.[21] Refractory hypotension in newborn infants may be responsive to exogenous steroid treatment.[22,23] There is some controversy as to whether there is evidence of diminished cortisol secretion in infants with hypotension.[24,25] Some of the variation in these studies may be due to the pulsatile secretion of cortisol in the premature infant.[26]

The neurohypophyseal-vasopressin system matures early and arginine vasopressin (AVP) can be detected in the pituitary gland of humans after the 11th week of gestation.[27] In the fetus the role of arginine vasopressin appears to be in response to stress, redirecting blood to the umbilical-placental, cerebral, and coronary circulations with a subsequent increase in oxygen delivery. Plasma AVP levels are increased in the newborn infant and may play a role in lung fluid reabsorption as well as the rise in blood pressure occurring in the early neonatal period. It has an antidiuretic and pressor effect, acting mainly via a strong vasoconstrictor effect. The renin-angiotensin-aldosterone system also develops early in fetal life and plays an important role in the maintenance of blood pressure and response to fetal hemorrhage in experimental animals.[28] Plasma renin, angiotensin II, and aldosterone levels are all increased immediately after birth and progressively decrease after this. The increase at birth appears to be mediated primarily by sympathetic stimulation. The renin-angiotensin-aldosterone system at birth has an important role in maintaining arterial blood pressure and increasing renal tubular sodium reabsorption.

Another potentially important influence on the vasomotor tone at birth is nitric oxide (NO) which is produced within the endothelial cell by the enzyme nitric oxide synthase. NO diffuses from the endothelial cells to adjacent smooth muscle cells and causes an increase in cyclic guanosine monophosphate concentration, eventually resulting in smooth muscle relaxation. The ongoing production of NO is responsible for maintenance of resting vascular tone and this mechanism occurs in the fetus early in gestation.[29] Endogenous nitric oxide has recently been demonstrated to be a crucial element in the maintenance of vasomotor tone and is likely an important mediator of the transitional changes occurring at birth.[30]

Endothelin (ET-1), a potent vasoconstricting peptide, has variable effects in the circulation of the fetus and newborn. Intrapulmonary infusion of ET-1 in the fetus and newborn causes an initial vasodilatation followed by vasoconstriction; however, systemic infusion of ET-1 causes sustained vasoconstriction without initial vasodilatation.[29] Circulating levels of ET-1 are known to be high in the fetal and newborn transitional circulation.[31–35] Endothelin levels on the first day of life progressively decrease[36] and infants with respiratory distress syndrome have higher levels of endothelin than other preterm infants.[31] ET-1 is, therefore, likely to play an important role in the transitional circulation, both in relation to the changes in pulmonary vascular tone and in the closure of the ductus arteriosus.[37]

Physiologic Determinants of Blood Pressure

Arterial blood pressure is determined by the product of cardiac output and peripheral vascular resistance. Cardiac output is influenced by preload or blood volume and myocardial contractility. The peripheral vascular resistance is determined by the vascular tone; in the presence of an unconstricted ductus arteriosus, the peripheral vascular resistance is affected by vascular tone in both the systemic and pulmonary circulations as the open ductus arteriosus exposes the left ventricle to resistance changes within the pulmonary circulation. Myocardial contractility is difficult to assess in the newborn because measurements such as echocardiographic assessment of fractional shortening is influenced by the asymmetry of the ventricles caused by the right ventricular dominance in utero. Some studies have found a relationship between myocardial dysfunction and hypotension,[38] but others have not,[39] even though a similar measurement method was used. Assessment of myocardial contractility may be more reliable if a load independent measure such as the relation between wall stress and corrected velocity of circumferential shortening is used.[118] Similarly, blood volume correlates poorly with blood pressure in hypotensive neonates.[40,41] The unique characteristics of the newborn cardiovascular system indicate that the systemic blood pressure is closely related to changes in the systemic vascular resistance. Systemic vascular resistance cannot be measured directly, so the measurement of cardiac output or systemic blood flow becomes an important element of the understanding of the newborn cardiovascular system.

In the absence of accurate measures of cardiac output and systemic vascular resistance clinicians have tended to rely on the blood pressure as the sole indicator of circulatory compromise. However, there is only a weak relationship between mean blood pressure and cardiac output in infants with a closed ductus arteriosus[39] (Fig. 15-1). Relying on the blood pressure alone can lead the clinician to make incorrect assumptions about the underlying physiology of the cardiovascular system. Many hypotensive preterm infants actually have a normal or high left ventricular output.[42,43] One of the reasons for this probably relates to the effect of a hemodynamically significant ductus arteriosus that causes an increase in left ventricular output and a reduction in the overall systemic vascular resistance. Changes in the peripheral vascular resistance of the infant may cause a difference in the underlying cardiac output that does not affect the blood pressure; thus, two infants with the same blood pressure may have markedly different cardiac outputs and physiologies.

The physiologic determinants of blood pressure may affect blood pressure in multiple ways—via an effect on cardiac performance (and thus cardiac output) or by altering the vascular resistance (or sometimes by altering both). Furthermore, systemic blood pressure increases with advancing gestational age and postnatal age.

Case Study 2

Baby boy B was born at 26 weeks of gestation weighing 890 g. His mother had premature labor and was given two doses of betamethasone 48 hours prior to delivery. The membranes ruptured 2 hours prior to birth. There was no evidence of clinical chorioamnionitis. Apgar scores were 6 at 1 minute and 7 at 5 minutes. At 2 minutes of age, he was intubated due to poor respiratory effort and ventilated using synchronized intermittent mandatory ventilation (SIMV) at an inspiratory pressure of 25 cm H_2O, a positive end-expiratory pressure (PEEP) of 5 cm, a ventilator rate of 40, and an inspired oxygen concentration (F_{IO_2}) of 0.50. He was transferred to the intensive care unit and treated with surfactant at 30 minutes of age. There was a rapid reduction in the F_{IO_2} to 0.28; however, the other ventilator settings remained the same. Intravenous fluids at 80 mL/kg/day were commenced via an umbilical vein catheter (positioned at the junction of inferior vena cava and right atrium and confirmed on x-ray).

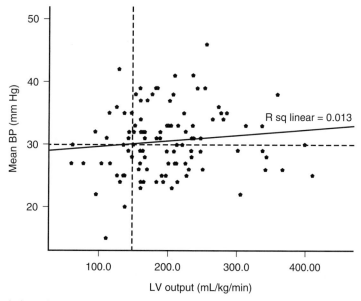

Figure 15-1 This graph shows the weak relationship (R = 0.14) between mean systemic blood pressure (BP) and simultaneously measured left ventricular (LV) output. Some infants with a mean BP greater than 30 mm Hg have critically low cardiac output (<150 mL/kg/minute) and conversely some infants with normal LV output have low mean blood pressure.

QUESTIONS

1. What is the most accurate way to measure baby B's blood pressure?

2. In the neonate, what are the alternatives to direct measurement of blood pressure through a catheter?

ANSWERS

1. Invasively, utilizing either a correctly positioned umbilical artery catheter with pressure transducer or a peripherally inserted arterial catheter placed into an artery such as the radial or posterior tibial artery.

2. Noninvasive measurement utilizing an oscillometric device with an adequate sized cuff; a cuff width-to-arm ratio of 0.45 to 0.55 improves the accuracy of noninvasive measurement.

Measuring the Blood Pressure

Blood pressure measurement is the most readily available gauge of cardiovascular adequacy in the newborn infant. Therefore, many clinicians base cardiovascular management decisions around this single piece of information. Invasive measurement of the arterial blood pressure using a fluid-filled catheter and pressure transducer is usually performed either via an indwelling umbilical artery catheter in the descending aorta or a peripherally placed arterial catheter. There is a strong correlation between blood pressure obtained via a peripheral artery catheter and that obtained from an umbilical artery.[44] Noninvasive measurement of blood pressure by use of validated oscillometric techniques, such as the Dinamap instrument, was first described in 1979.[45] The agreement between direct and indirect measures of BP is generally good.[46–50] The noninvasive technique is more problematic in the VLBW infant, as it is more dependent on choice of the appropriate cuff size.[51] In the newborn a cuff width-to-arm ratio between 0.45 and 0.55 increases the accuracy of indirect BP measurements when compared to direct measures.[52] Accuracy of the invasive BP is dependent on proper use of equipment, including accurate placement of the transducer, proper calibration

of the system, and avoidance of blockages or blood clots in the catheter line, all of which can result in an erroneous measurement of BP.

An umbilical arterial catheter was inserted with the tip positioned at T8 to T10, in the high position. The first arterial blood pressure obtained after calibration of the arterial line and transducer showed a systolic BP of 30 mm Hg, diastolic BP of 18 mm Hg, with a mean BP of 23 mm Hg.

QUESTION

3. Does baby B have hypotension?

ANSWER

3. Yes, according to both of the usual definitions of hypotension (mean BP less than gestational age in weeks or an absolute level of <30 mm Hg). The mean BP is also low according to established norms.

Normal Blood Pressure and Definition of Hypotension

Reference ranges and guidelines regarding what constitutes hypotension in newborn infants are variable. As with many parameters in neonatology, defining a normal BP range in infants who are undergoing intensive care is difficult. The current definitions are not related to physiologic end points such as maintenance of organ blood flow or tissue oxygen delivery. Instead they define hypotension on gestational and postnatal age-dependent norms using population statistics such as the 10th and 90th percentile limits or 95% confidence intervals.

There are now several data sets available to assist in defining the normal range of blood pressure in the newborn infant[52–57] (Fig. 15-2). These data sets are deficient in a number of ways: they often include both invasive and noninvasive measures, data from "sick" and well infants combined, and data collected retrospectively. Furthermore, there were a surprisingly small number of infants below 1000 g.

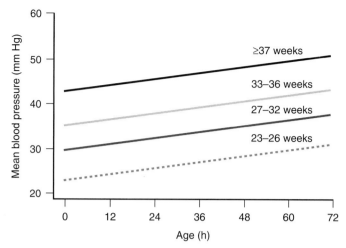

Figure 15-2 Nomogram showing normal ranges for mean blood pressure (BP) in infants of different gestational and postnatal ages. (Reproduced with permission from Nuntnarumit P, Yang W, Bada-Ellzey HS: Blood pressure measurements in the newborn. Clin Perinatol 1999;26:981.)

In practice there are generally two definitions of early hypotension in widespread use:

Early hypotension can be defined as mean blood pressure less than 30 mm Hg in any gestation infant in the first days of life. This definition is based on pathophysiologic associations between cerebral injury (white matter damage or intraventricular hemorrhage) and mean blood pressure less than 30 mm Hg[53,58] and to a lesser degree on more recent data looking at maintenance of cerebral blood flow (CBF) measured by NIRS over a range of blood pressures suggesting a reduction in CBF at a particular mean blood pressure.[59,60] It is worth noting in this regard that according to population-based data the 10th percentile for infants of all gestational ages is at or above 30 mm Hg at day 3 of life. However, in more immature infants the normal mean blood pressure can be *lower* than 30 mm Hg in the first 3 days, emphasizing that it is simplistic to use a single value for blood pressure across a range of gestation and postnatal ages.[52]

Early hypotension has also been defined as mean blood pressure less than the gestational age in weeks, which roughly correlates with the 10th percentile for age in some of the normative data just presented.[53,61] This definition has also been supported by published guidelines, such as the Joint Working Group of the British Association of Perinatal Medicine.[62] Again, this rule of thumb applies mainly in the first few days of life, after which there is a gradual increase in the mean blood pressure such that by day 3

most premature infants have a mean blood pressure above 30 mm Hg.[52]

Exercise 2 *Continued*

QUESTION

4. What are some possible reasons why baby B had a low blood pressure?

ANSWER

4. Excessive ventilation with overdistention of the lungs impeding venous return to the heart, myocardial insufficiency (usually transient) due to prematurity, large patent ductus arteriosus, inappropriate vasodilation of peripheral blood vessels compared to circulating blood volume.

Case Study 2 *Continued*

A chest x-ray showed overdistention of the lungs with 10 ribs visible and a narrow-looking heart. The first arterial blood gas showed a respiratory alkalosis with a P_{CO_2} of 28 mm Hg. After administration of 10 mL/kg of normal saline over half an hour and reduction in the ventilator settings from 25/5 to 20/4 cm H_2O, the blood pressure improved to 40/25 mm Hg with a mean of 33 mm Hg. An echocardiogram at 8 hours of age demonstrated a small patent ductus arteriosus which appeared to be constricting.

Clinical Determinants of Blood Pressure

Gestational Age and Postnatal Age

Both gestational age and postnatal age are major determinants of the systemic blood pressure. Most of the nomograms and tables for normal BP values demonstrate this influence. In many of these studies, BP is higher in more mature infants and progressively increases with postnatal age. The reasons BP increases with postnatal age are unclear, but are probably related to changes in the underlying vascular tone mediated by increased levels of some of the humoral regulators already discussed. At the same time, there are temporal physical changes in the transitional circulation such as closure of the ductus arteriosus.

Use of Antenatal Glucocorticoid Therapy

Some evidence suggests that sick preterm infants may have a relative adrenocorticoid insufficiency and that this may be one of the underlying causes of cardiovascular dysfunction in this group.[63–65] Low cortisol levels have been documented in hypotensive infants requiring inotropic support.[25] The use of antenatal glucocorticoids to assist in fetal lung maturation may also have the positive effect of improving neonatal blood pressure. The likely mechanism for this is via increasing β-adrenergic receptor expression, thereby increasing sensitivity to endogenous catecholamines in the myocardium and peripheral vasculature.[66] Randomized controlled trials of the use of antenatal glucocorticoid have shown variable effects on the neonatal blood pressure. In some trials there was an increase in the mean blood pressure of VLBW infants in the treated group with a decreased need for inotropic support.[67,68] However, other trials have shown little difference between the mean blood pressures of infants whose mothers did or did not receive antenatal steroids.[69,70]

Perinatal Asphyxia

Asphyxiated infants are often thought to be hypotensive or poorly perfused and volume is often routinely administered. There is, however, little evidence that this group of infants is hypovolemic[71] unless there has been specific blood loss or a tight nuchal cord that has resulted in an imbalance of blood volume distribution between the fetus and the placenta. Administration of excessive volume in the setting of asphyxia, with the possibility of an underlying myocardial injury being present, may result in fluid overload and congestive heart failure. In this situation, the judicious use of an inotrope such as dopamine or dobutamine is preferable.[72,73]

Blood Loss

Acute blood loss in the newborn can result from prenatal events (e.g., twin-twin transfusion syndrome or antepartum hemorrhage), intrapartum events (e.g., a tight nuchal cord), or postnatal events (e.g., large subgaleal hematoma or hemorrhage into an organ such as the liver or brain). Acute blood loss may result in significant hypotension, but this effect may be delayed by immediate compensatory mechanisms. Similarly, a drop in the infant's hemoglobin level may not be seen immediately following a significant hemorrhage.

Positive Pressure Ventilation

Many infants in the intensive care unit, particularly those born less than 30 weeks' gestation, will require positive pressure respiratory support in the first days of life. Surfactant deficiency is the main reason for needing positive pressure support, but there may be contributions from sepsis and immaturity of the lungs unrelated to surfactant deficiency. The use of high ventilation pressures in the premature infant who has a relatively small chest can result in unwanted interference with cardiac function. Function may be impaired by a reduction in the preload from reduced systemic or pulmonary venous return. In addition, there may be direct compression of cardiac chambers resulting in a reduced stroke volume or an increase in afterload, particularly of the right ventricle. A reduction in right ventricular output translates to a reduction in the systemic cardiac output, as the right and left sides of the heart are serially connected.

The effect of increasing mean airway pressure on cardiac output has been studied in animal models and adults, where it has been shown that increasing PEEP results in a reduction in the cardiac output. At low PEEP levels, the reduction appears mainly to be due to reduced preload, but at higher PEEP levels the effects of increased afterload and decreased contractility become more important.[74] There have been fewer studies done in premature infants, but the same observations have been made. Trang studied stepwise increases in the PEEP in mechanically ventilated infants and found a fall off in the systemic oxygen delivery if the PEEP was greater than 6 cm H_2O and a reduction in cardiac output at a PEEP of 9 cm H_2O.[75] Another group assessed premature infants (mean gestational age 29 weeks) before and during treatment with mechanical ventilation for severe respiratory distress syndrome and found a reduction in left ventricular dimensions and filling rates resulting in a decrease of cardiac output by about 40% compared to control values.[76] Interestingly, the blood pressure did not change significantly in the group in which cardiac output dropped. In longitudinal clinical studies of blood pressure and blood flow, mean airway pressure has a consistently negative influence on both mean blood pressure[39,77] and on systemic blood flow.[78,79]

Case Study 3

Baby boy C was born at 26 weeks of gestation weighing 1060 g. His mother had premature labor and was given one dose of betamethasone 24 hours prior to delivery. The membranes ruptured 24 hours prior to birth; however, there was no evidence of clinical chorioamnionitis. Apgar scores were 4 at 1 minute and 6 at 5 minutes. He was intubated immediately after birth and ventilated (SIMV) at an inspiratory pressure of 22 cm H_2O, a PEEP of 5 cm H_2O, a rate of 40, and an F_{IO_2} of 0.70. He was transferred to the intensive care unit, where he was nursed on an overhead radiant warmer and treated with surfactant at 20 minutes of age. There was a gradual reduction in the F_{IO_2} to 0.40; however, the ventilator settings remained unchanged. Intravenous fluids at 100 mL/kg/day were commenced via an umbilical vein catheter positioned at the junction of inferior vena cava and right atrium (confirmed on x-ray). An umbilical arterial catheter was also inserted with the tip positioned at T8–T10. The chest x-ray showed hyaline membrane disease with reasonable lung expansion. The infant received two boluses of 10 mL/kg of normal saline due to poor perfusion in

the first 3 hours of life. Ampicillin and gentamicin were begun. The first arterial blood pressure (BP) obtained after calibration of the arterial line and transducer showed a systolic BP of 38 mm Hg, diastolic BP of 25 mm Hg, with a mean BP of 30 mm Hg. At about 8 hours of age the arterial BP had slowly dropped to 34/16 mm Hg with a mean BP of 23 mm Hg. By that time, the ventilator settings had been tapered to 20/5 at a rate of 40 and an F_{IO_2} 0.28. The infant had a capillary refill time of less than 2 seconds and a normal arterial blood gas. An echocardiogram to assess cardiac function was obtained at 10 hours of age, which demonstrated a structurally normal heart with adequate contractility and normal venous filling. There was, however, a large patent ductus arteriosus (PDA) with a predominantly left-to-right shunt. A decision to treat the large PDA with 0.2 mg/kg of indomethacin was made. Within 2 hours the blood pressure had improved to 38/24 with a mean BP of 30 mm Hg.

Exercise 3

QUESTIONS

1. Why did this infant become hypotensive?
2. Was the PDA the cause of this infant's low blood pressure?

ANSWERS

1. Myocardial impairment due to prematurity, patent ductus arteriosus, inappropriate peripheral vasodilation, sepsis fluid loss (e.g., free water loss).
2. Yes, a large PDA might cause these symptoms.

Patent Ductus Arteriosus

A patent ductus arteriosus may not be recognized clinically in the first days of life because the flow through it is generally not turbulent and therefore no murmur is audible.[80] Despite this, the flow is almost always left to right or bidirectional with a predominant left-to-right pattern.[7] A PDA is usually thought to be associated with a low diastolic BP but some data now suggest that it is associated with both low diastolic and systolic BP, making PDA one of the possible causes of systemic hypotension.[81] As clinical detection of a PDA in the first days of life is inaccurate, an echocardiogram is required for early diagnosis. The size of the patent ductus on a color Doppler measurement in the first 24 hours of life has been correlated with the probability of developing a symptomatic PDA.[82] After day 4 of life, the classical clinical signs of a murmur, such as bounding pulses and a hyperdynamic precordium, become evident, making clinical detection much more accurate.[80]

Systemic Vascular Resistance

There is an inverse relationship between the systemic vascular resistance and cardiac output in all newborn infants, including those who are sick or ventilated.[83] This relationship may be particularly important with the use of inotropes, such as dopamine, when increasing the peripheral vascular resistance may increase blood pressure but have no impact on, or even decrease, the cardiac output.[84] The peripheral resistance varies markedly in the preterm infant and can be affected by numerous factors, including the maturity of the sympathoadrenal system[85] environmental temperature, carbon dioxide level,[83] patency of the ductus arteriosus (which exposes the left ventricle to the combined pulmonary and systemic vascular resistance),[86] presence of vasoactive hormones such as prostacyclin, and the presence of sepsis. The resulting effects on blood flow may be significant but the impact can only be recognized by measuring the blood flow.

Case Study 4

An infant born at 26 weeks of gestation and weighing 810 g has a blood pressure at 8 hours of age of 38/24 mm Hg with a mean of 28 mm Hg. The left ventricular output measured by Doppler ultrasound is 140 mL/kg/minute (below the normal range of 200 to 300 mL/kg/minute). In the next bed is an infant born at 25 weeks of gestation and weighing 760 g who is also 8 hours old and has a blood pressure of 28/18 mm Hg with a mean BP of only 23 mm Hg. This infant has a left ventricular output measured by Doppler ultrasound of 350 mL/kg/minute, slightly higher than the normal range.

Exercise 4

QUESTION

1. What factors might explain this apparent paradox of a normal BP (as defined by mean BP > GA criteria) and low cardiac output in the first infant and a low BP and normal to high cardiac output in the second infant?

ANSWER

1. Differences in the peripheral vascular resistance (possibly medication induced) and the presence of a ductus arteriosus.

The infant born at 26 weeks' gestation was commenced on a dopamine infusion (8 μg/kg/minute) at age 5 hours for a low systemic BP and responded with an increase in BP. The increase in peripheral vascular resistance and afterload with dopamine resulted in a reduced cardiac output despite the increase in BP.

The infant born at 25 weeks' gestation had a large unconstricted ductus arteriosus with left-to-right shunt on echocardiography. The resulting decreased total peripheral resistance and increased pulmonary blood flow led to an increase in the left ventricular output to maintain systemic blood flow, but despite this physiologic response, the BP remained low.

QUESTION

2. What other measures can be used in the newborn infant to assess the cardiovascular adequacy and what are the limitations of these measures?

ANSWER

2. Capillary refill time, urinary output, pulse rate, invasive and noninvasive measures of the cardiac output. Limitations are discussed in the following section.

Diagnosis of Cardiovascular Compromise

Because of the wide variation in blood pressure levels at varying gestations and postnatal ages, some authors have cautioned against simply treating low BP only, and suggest that the clinician should look for some other evidence of hypoperfusion such as increased capillary return, oliguria, or a metabolic acidosis.[54] However, assessment of the adequacy of the cardiovascular system of the preterm infant is more problematic than in older children or adults. Measures of cardiovascular function that are used in older children and adults, such as pulmonary wedge pressure, central venous pressure, and thermodilutional cardiac output are impractical because of the size and fragility and frequent presence of cardiac shunting in the preterm infant. Assessment usually consists of a clinical appraisal of the perfusion using capillary filling times and urine output and the documentation of the pulse rate and blood pressure. The acid base balance and evidence of lactic acidosis are a further adjunct to this assessment. All of these parameters have limitations in the newborn.

Exercise 5

QUESTION

1. Capillary refill time is often used as an indicator of inadequate blood pressure or cardiac output in the preterm infant. The specificity of the capillary filling time in predicting low systemic blood flow is above 90% when the refill time is:

    a. ≥ 2 seconds

    b. ≥ 3 seconds

    c. ≥ 4 seconds

    d. Never

ANSWER

1. c. A recent study documenting the relationship between a measure of systemic blood flow and capillary refill time showed a capillary refill time of 3 seconds or more had only 55% sensitivity and 80% specificity for predicting low systemic blood flow, and an extremely increased capillary refill time of 4 seconds or more correlated better with low flow states.[90]

Capillary Filling Time

This is a somewhat arbitrary assessment of the cardiovascular system and is often based on an overall impression of the adequacy of the perfusion of the skin. Despite this limitation, it is widely utilized as a proxy for both cardiac output and peripheral resistance in infants. Several techniques to allow standardization of assessment have been described and normal values have only recently been documented for neonates.[87] A number of confounding factors can make the capillary refill time potentially inaccurate, including different techniques used (site tested, pressing time), interobserver variability, ambient temperature,[88] medications, and immaturity of skin blood flow control mechanisms. Tibby and associates showed only a weak relationship between the capillary refill time and other hemodynamic measures such as the stroke volume index in a group of older children receiving intensive care.[89] A more recent study documenting the relationship between a measure of systemic blood flow and capillary refill time showed a capillary refill time of 3 seconds or more had only 55% sensitivity and 80% specificity for predicting low systemic blood flow. An extremely increased capillary refill time of 4 seconds or more correlated better with low flow states (Table 15-1).[90]

Urine Output

Urine production and output is useful in assessing cardiovascular well-being in the older child. However, the immature renal tubule in infants less than 32 weeks postconceptual age is inefficient at concentrating urine and therefore may be unable to reduce urine flow in the face of a high serum osmolality.[91] As a result, even if the glomerular filtration rate is decreased markedly, there may be little or no change in urine output. In addition, accurate measurement of urinary output is not easy in infants, generally requiring a urinary catheter with size limitations, making free drainage difficult.

Pulse Rate

In adults a rising pulse rate is usually indicative of hypovolemia. The mechanism relies on a mature autonomic nervous system, with detection of reduced blood volume (and blood pressure) via baroreceptors and a subsequent increase in the heart rate. Infants have a faster baseline heart rate, and a modest increase may not be noticed. In addition, there are many

TABLE 15-1

DIAGNOSTIC ACCURACY OF BLOOD PRESSURE, CAPILLARY REFILL TIME, AND CENTRAL-PERIPHERAL TEMPERATURE DIFFERENCES FOR LOW SYSTEMIC BLOOD FLOW IN PRETERM (<30 WEEKS' GESTATION) INFANTS

Measurement	Sensitivity	Specificity	Predictive Values	
			Positive	Negative
Mean blood pressure < 30 mm Hg	59	77	36	90
Mean blood pressure < gestational age in weeks	30	88	34	85
Capillary refill time ≥ 3 seconds	55	80	33	91
Capillary refill time ≥ 4 seconds	29	96	55	88
Central-peripheral temperature difference ≥ 2°C	40	69	23	83

From Osborn DA, Evans N, Kluckow M: Clinical detection of low upper body blood flow in very premature infants using blood pressure, capillary refill time, and central-peripheral temperature difference. Arch Dis Child Fetal Neonatal Ed 2004;89:F168–F173.

influences on the heart rate in the immediate postnatal period, and it should not be relied on as an accurate assessment of cardiovascular well-being.

Exercise 6

QUESTION

1. What are the limitations in measuring cardiac output in the newborn infant?

ANSWER

1. The physical size of both term and preterm infants has precluded the use of such measures, especially in the group of infants less than 30 weeks' gestation. Another issue specific to premature infants is the potential inaccuracy of the dye dilution and thermodilution methods in the presence of intracardiac shunts (the ductus arteriosus and the foramen ovale).

Cardiac Output and Myocardial Contractility

Hemodynamic measures such as pulmonary artery thermodilution and mixed venous oxygen saturation monitoring are commonly used in adult intensive care units to allow accurate assessment of the cardiovascular system. However, both of these methods are invasive and generally require the use of a catheter within the pulmonary blood vessels. The physical size of both term and preterm infants precludes the use of such measures, especially in the group of

infants less than 30 weeks' gestation. Another issue specific to premature infants is the potential inaccuracy of the dye dilution and thermodilution methods in the presence of intracardiac shunts (the ductus arteriosus and the foramen ovale). As a result, noninvasive methods of measuring cardiac output such as echocardiography are being used with greater frequency. Doppler ultrasound was first used to noninvasively measure cardiac output in neonates in 1982[92] and has subsequently been shown to be superior to more invasive techniques in children, neonates, and premature infants.[93] The expected coefficient of variation when using Doppler compares favorably to that of indicator dilution and thermodilution.

As noted earlier, assessment of myocardial contractility in the neonate is difficult because the echocardiographic measures of fractional shortening or ejection fraction are adversely influenced by the asymmetry of the ventricles caused by the right ventricular dominance in utero. There is variability between studies examining the relationship between myocardial dysfunction and hypotension,[38,39] even though a similar measurement method was used. Assessment of myocardial contractility using a load independent measure such as the relation between wall stress and corrected velocity of circumferential shortening may be more reliable, although there is little validation of this technique in the preterm population.[118]

Systemic Blood Flow

Mean blood pressure does not necessarily equate with left ventricular output in preterm infants, even in the subgroup in whom the ductus arteriosus has closed (see Fig. 15-1).[39,42] Similarly, the use of near infrared spectroscopy has shown that cerebral blood flow is independent of the systemic blood pressure—even in the physiologic range.[94,95] Further problems arise in assessing systemic blood flow in the preterm infant due to the persistence of components of the in utero circulation in postnatal life, as a result of failure or delay in the normal circulatory transition. The assumption that the left and right ventricular outputs are identical is not necessarily correct in the preterm infant. Increased blood flowing through the patent ductus arteriosus (ductal shunt) will be reflected in a falsely elevated left ventricular output (increased by up to 100%) and the blood flowing through a patent foramen ovale (atrial shunt) will be reflected in a falsely elevated right ventricular output (Fig. 15-3).[86]

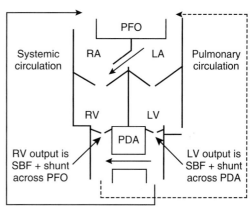

Figure 15-3 Diagram demonstrating the points where right and left ventricular output are measured using Doppler ultrasound. The right ventricular output will consist of the combined systemic venous return (systemic blood flow [SBF]) and any left-to-right shunting across the patent foramen ovale (PFO). The left ventricular output will consist of the total pulmonary venous return (SBF) and the blood destined to cross the patent ductus arteriosus (PDA).

Relationship Between Blood Pressure, Cardiac Output, and Peripheral Resistance

Hypotension may be associated with low cardiac output, more accurately described as low systemic blood flow (SBF). Systemic blood flow falls dramatically in many extremely premature infants in the first hours of life and this reduction in flow is usually associated with high vascular resistance. A substantial proportion of these infants will initially have "normal" blood pressure (i.e., they are in "compensated shock"). About 80% of extremely preterm infants who develop low SBF will also become hypotensive. Using hypotension to direct cardiovascular interventions, however, will result in a considerable delay in treatment of infants with low SBF and some infants with low SBF may not be recognized at all (Fig. 15-4). Hypotension may also be associated with normal or even a high SBF,

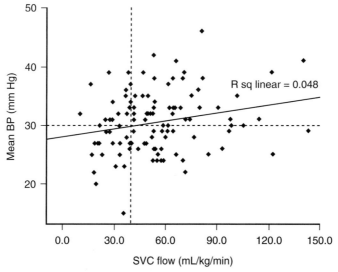

Figure 15-4 Demonstrates the poor relationship between superior vena cava (SVC) flow at age 5 hours, a measure of blood flow, and the simultaneously measured invasive mean blood pressure ($R^2 = 0.05$). Some infants with a mean blood pressure (BP) greater than 30 mm Hg have critically low SVC flow (<40 mL/kg/minute) and conversely some infants with normal SVC flow have low mean blood pressure (as defined by <30 mm Hg). A similarly poor relationship is seen between left ventricular output and mean blood pressure.

as frequently occurs in the preterm infant with persisting hypotension after the first days of life or those with "hyperdynamic" sepsis. These infants generally exhibit a low systemic vascular resistance.

Risks Associated with Cardiovascular Compromise

One of the important aims of provision of intensive care to sick newborn infants is the maintenance of tissue oxygenation, in particular to the cerebral circulation. Avoidance of impaired cerebral perfusion and subsequent ischemic damage is a significant concern and the main reason for treatment of hypotension. Cerebral blood flow, which is important in determining cerebral oxygen delivery, is determined by the relationship between perfusion pressure, systemic blood flow, and the vascular resistance of the cerebral circulation. It is suggested that the process of cerebral autoregulation allows maintenance of a constant cerebral blood flow in the face of variations in the blood pressure, systemic blood flow, and resistance. Lou and associates[96] were the first to suggest that sick preterm infants may have lost the capability to autoregulate, resulting in a pressure-passive cerebral circulation, which is more vulnerable to fluctuations in blood pressure (resulting in low cerebral blood flow if there is systemic hypotension). The relationship between cerebral blood flow and mean arterial blood pressure in preterm neonates is still unclear. Tyszczuk and associates found cerebral blood flow was independent of mean BP in infants between 24 and 34 weeks' gestation, suggesting preservation of autoregulation in some hypotensive infants.[94] In contrast, other groups have found significant relationships between mean arterial blood pressure and cerebral vascular oxygenation, providing evidence of pressure passive cerebral circulation in preterm infants who are hypotensive.[59,60] These authors have suggested a "cut point" of mean BP at 30 mm Hg to be the point where cerebral blood flow begins to decline in very preterm infants.[60] In contrast, there is some evidence to support the concept that cardiac output and the tissue oxygen extraction may be more important factors than blood pressure in maintaining cerebral tissue oxygenation. Several studies have demonstrated that cerebral fractional oxygen

extraction is not related to hypotension, suggesting that sufficient oxygen to meet cerebral demand is delivered even in the presence of hypotension.[95,97,98] An increase in the cardiac output in some infants with hypotension may explain this observation. Recent investigations have suggested that autoregulation is intact in most preterm babies, but is compromised in a subgroup that seem to be at particularly high risk of peri/intraventricular hemorrhage (PIVH).[99,100] It has been suggested that infants suffering severe IVH are more likely to have blood pressure passive changes in cerebral blood flow[53,58-60,100] and oxygenation in the first days of life.

Peri/Intraventricular Hemorrhage

A number of studies have described an association between low mean blood pressure and subsequent PIVH.[53,56,58,101] Those initial observations led to current recommendations for treatment of hypotension. Despite these statistical associations, large population-based studies have not found systemic hypotension to be an independent risk factor for PIVH in VLBW infants.[102]

Periventricular Leukomalacia

The potential relationship between low cerebral blood flow and white matter injury in the preterm infant has led to concerns that hypotension may be an antecedent of periventricular leukomalacia (PVL). Observational data have shown a relationship between hypotension (often mean BP below 30 mm Hg) and adverse cranial ultrasound findings.[58] However, larger studies have failed to identify systemic hypotension as an independent risk factor for white matter injury.[103,104]

Long-Term Neurodevelopmental Outcome

Hypotension in VLBW infants has been correlated with longer term adverse neurodevelopmental outcome.[105,106] A study of systemic blood flow in VLBW infants demonstrated an independent relationship between low systemic blood flow (particularly the duration of the insult) and adverse neurodevelopmental outcome at 3 years of age.[107]

Treatment of Cardiovascular Compromise

The appropriate management of hypotension in the neonate will differ according to the associated features, as demonstrated by the following case histories. The clinician must take into account a number of factors, including the infant's gestational age, postnatal age, and measures of cardiovascular adequacy such as cardiac output/systemic blood flow and associated pathologic processes. In addition, an understanding of the underlying risk factors for hypotension and low systemic blood flow (e.g., immature gestational age or infants with significant ventilatory requirements) is important. An early echocardiogram can assist greatly in the diagnostic process by providing information about the presence, size, and direction of the ductus arteriosus shunt, presence of pulmonary hypertension, assessment of cardiac contractility, adequacy of venous filling, and cardiac output or systemic blood flow.

Before treating hypotension, patent ductus arteriosus, hypovolemia from blood or fluid loss, pneumothorax, use of excessive mean airway pressure, sepsis, and relative adrenocortical insufficiency should first be considered and managed appropriately. A measurement error (transducer height in comparison to patient's right atrium, calibration of the transducer, blood clot in the measurement catheter) should be ruled out. Available therapeutic options that have a physiologic basis for efficacy and have been subjected to clinical trial include volume loading (crystalloid or colloid), pressor/inotropic agents, and hydrocortisone and other steroids. Table 15-2 summarizes the mechanisms of action of the potential therapies and evidence for their use in preterm infants. Table 15-3 suggests an approach to the use of these therapies according to the likely underlying mechanism of cardiovascular compromise.

Case Study 5

Baby girl D was born at 24 weeks of gestation weighing 660 g. Her mother had premature labor and was given two doses of intramuscular betamethasone over the 48 hours prior to delivery. The membranes ruptured at the time of birth. There was no evidence of clinical chorioamnionitis. The mother had a cesarean section due to an unstable lie. Baby D had Apgar scores of 4 at 1 minute and 7 at 5 minutes. She was intubated because of poor respiratory effort at 1 minute of age and ventilated (SIMV) at an inspiratory pressure of 20 cm H_2O, a PEEP of 5 cm H_2O, a ventilator rate of 40, and an F_{IO_2} of 0.35. She was transferred to the neonatal intensive care unit and treated with surfactant replacement therapy at 30 minutes of age. There was a rapid reduction in the F_{IO_2} to 0.21 and the ventilator settings were reduced to 18/4 cm H_2O at a rate of 40. Intravenous fluids at 100 mL/kg/day were commenced via an umbilical vein catheter positioned at the junction of inferior vena cava and right atrium, and an umbilical arterial catheter was inserted and advanced to T8–T10 (confirmed on x-ray). The first arterial BP obtained after calibration of the arterial line and transducer was normal. However, by 6 hours of age, measurements showed a systolic BP of 29 mm Hg, diastolic BP of 16 mm Hg, with a mean BP of 22 mm Hg. She appeared pink with a capillary refill time of less than 2 seconds and a normal acid base balance (although P_{CO_2} was noted to be 37 mm Hg). A single bolus of 10 mL/kg of normal saline made no difference to the BP.

Exercise 7

QUESTIONS

1. Does baby D have low blood pressure?

2. What treatment(s) would you use if you decide to treat the low BP reading?

3. Which kind of volume replacement is most appropriate for hypotensive preterm infants who have no evidence of an absolute volume loss?

   a. 5% albumin

   b. Normal (isotonic) saline

   c. Fresh frozen plasma

   d. Blood

ANSWERS

1. Yes, according to standard nomograms or the two conventional definitions of mean BP less than GA or absolute BP less than 30 mm Hg.

TABLE 15-2

CARDIOVASCULAR INTERVENTIONS USED IN PRETERM INFANTS IN THE FIRST DAY

Intervention	Dose	Receptors/Effects	Indications	Considerations	Evidence
Volume (normal saline or colloid)	10–15 mL/kg	Short-term ↑SBF	Hypovolemia suspected—perinatal blood loss, infant pale with ↑HR	No evidence improved outcome; excess fluid associated with increased mortality rate; PDA and CLD	Cohort[118] SR of RCTs[137]
Dobutamine	10–20 µg/kg/min	β: ↑contractility, ↓PVR/SVR → ↑SBF	First line for low SBF Pulmonary hypertension Asphyxia	Corrects hypotension in 60%; tachycardia if no volume expansion	SR of RCTs[118,127]
Dopamine	2–10 µg/kg/min	Dopamine: ↑renal blood flow. β: ↑contractility, ↓PVR/SVR α: ↑SVR Net effect: ↑BP, ∅SBF	Hypotension. Consider second line for low SBF	In hypotensive infants may increase cerebral blood flow	SR of RCT[118,127]
	>10 µg/kg/min	α >> β → ↑↑SVR ↑↑PVR Net effect: ↑↑ BP, ∅ or ↓ SBF	Refractory hypotension Septic shock	May substantially reduce SBF	SR of RCT[118,127]
Epinephrine	0.05–0.375 µg/kg/min	β > α: ↑BP, ?↑SBF ↑SVR > PVR	Hypotension. Consider second line for low SBF	In hypotensive infants may increase cerebral blood flow	RCT[129]
	>0.375 µg/kg/min	α > β: ↑↑BP, ↑SVR > PVR Net effect: ?↓SBF	Refractory hypotension Septic shock	May substantially reduce SBF	None in preterm
Hydrocortisone	2–10 mg/kg/day in 2–4 divided doses	↑SVR, ↑BP, unknown effect on SBF	Refractory hypotension Adrenal insufficiency	Early steroids associated with intestinal perforation. High-dose steroids ↑BSL	RCT[24]
Dexamethasone	0.25 mg/kg single dose	↑SVR, ↑BP, unknown effect on SBF	Refractory hypotension Adrenal insufficiency	Early steroids associated with intestinal perforation. High-dose steroids ↑BSL	RCT[134]
Milrinone	0.75 µg/kg/min × 3 hours, then 0.2 µg/kg/min	Type III phosphodiesterase inhibitor: ↑contractility, ↓SVR, ↓PVR →↑SBF	Low SBF	May cause hypotension	Pilot study[133]

↑, increase; ↓, decrease; →, leads to; ∅, no change; BP, blood pressure; CLD, chronic lung disease; HR, heart rate; PDA, patent ductus arteriosus; PVR, pulmonary vascular resistance; RCT, randomized controlled trial; SBF, systemic blood flow; SR, systematic review; SVR, systemic vascular resistance.
From Osborn DA: Diagnosis and treatment of preterm transitional circulatory compromise. Early Hum Dev 2005;81:413.

TREATMENT OPTIONS ACCORDING TO UNDERLYING MECHANISM OF CARDIOVASCULAR COMPROMISE

Patient Type	Clinical Issues	Cardiovascular Parameters	Suggested Management
Extreme preterm infant	Early low SBF	Normal or low BP Low SBF/cardiac output Large PDA High systemic vascular resistance Poor myocardial contractility	Saline 10–20 mL/kg Dobutamine 10–20 µg/kg/min—adjust to SBF Second line: Add dopamine 5 µg/kg/min titrate to BP
Preterm infant	Low BP after first 24–48 hours	Normal/high SBF Low systemic vascular resistance	Dopamine 5 µg/kg/min titrated to BP
Preterm infant with PDA	Low BP ± PDA signs	Low BP Large PDA, left to right shunt	Indomethacin first, then address SBF and BP Saline 10–20 mL/kg
Term or preterm infant with asphyxia	Myocardial damage	Normal or low BP Poor myocardial contractility Low SBF	Dobutamine 10–20 µg/kg/min—adjust to SBF Second line: Add dopamine 5 µg/kg/min titrate to BP or epinephrine
Term or preterm infant with suspected sepsis—high output	High output cardiac failure secondary to sepsis	Normal or low BP High SBF Low systemic vascular resistance/capillary leak	Volume replacement—may require more than 20 mL/kg Dopamine 5 µg/kg/min titrated to BP Second line: Epinephrine 0.05 µg/kg/min titrated to BP
Term or preterm infant with suspected sepsis—low output	Sepsis and poor myocardial function	Normal or low BP Normal or low SBF High systemic vascular resistance	Saline 10–20 mL/kg Dobutamine 10–20 µg/kg/min—adjust to SBF Second line: (Low SBF) Epinephrine 0.05 µg/kg/min Second line: (Hypotension) Add dopamine 5 µg/kg/min titrate to BP or epinephrine
Infant with mainly respiratory distress—often term	Pulmonary hypertension	Normal or low BP Normal or low SBF High pulmonary vascular resistance	Dobutamine 10–20 µg/kg/min—adjust to SBF Second line: Epinephrine 0.05 µg/kg/min Pulmonary vasodilators—nitric oxide
Infant with acute fluid loss (intraventricular/pulmonary hemorrhage)	Acute hypovolemia	Normal or low blood pressure Poor venous filling pressures	Volume replacement—may require more than 20 mL/kg, including blood transfusion Dopamine 5 µg/kg/min titrated to BP Second line: Epinephrine 0.05 µg/kg/min titrated to BP
Infant with structural or acquired heart disease (e.g., left-sided obstructive lesions, myocarditis)	Acute cardiac failure and shock, acidosis	Low BP, low SBF Cardiogenic shock	Dobutamine 10–20 µg/kg/min or dopamine 5–10 µg/kg/min Specific treatment such as prostaglandin E_1

BP, blood pressure; PDA, patent ductus arteriosus; SBF, systemic blood flow.
Modified from Kluckow M, Osborn D: Hypotension in the neonate. In Burg FD, Ingelfinger JE, Polin RA, et al (eds): Current Pediatric Therapy, 18th ed. Philadelphia, Elsevier, 2006.

2. Options include: more volume, dopamine, dobutamine, other inotropes, and indomethacin or ibuprofen.

3. b. Normal saline

After two further doses of normal saline (10 mL/kg each) the infant was looking noticeably more edematous and the F_{IO_2} had climbed to 0.45. The BP had increased marginally to 32/22 with a mean BP of 24 mm Hg. An echocardiogram performed at 16 hours showed a large unconstricted patent ductus arteriosus with a left-to-right shunt with some left atrial dilation.

Options for Treating Low Blood Pressure in Neonates

Option 1: Closing the Ductus Arteriosus

A large and unconstricted ductus arteriosus can be associated with hypotension in the first 24 hours of life.[81] Early assessment of the ductus arteriosus in infants who are hypotensive for no apparent reason may allow diagnosis of a large PDA and treatment with a cyclooxygenase inhibitor such as indomethacin or ibuprofen. However, there are no trials using cyclooxygenase inhibitors to treat hypotension, despite some evidence that they assist in maintenance of normal systemic blood flow.[108] The trials of prophylactic indomethacin have shown a reduced incidence of PIVH, and stabilization of the transitional circulation (following closure of the ductus arteriosus) may be one mechanism for this effect. This positive effect, however, must be weighed against the potential risk of reducing cerebral blood flow by using indomethacin.[109] As the hemodynamic effect of a large unconstricted PDA (>1.5 mm on color Doppler measurement)[82] on the transitional circulation of the preterm infant can be significant and sometimes result in other complications, such as pulmonary edema,[110] treatment with an initial dose of 0.2 mg/kg of indomethacin followed by a maintenance dose (0.1 mg/kg per dose daily for up to 5 days) is reasonable.

Option 2: Further Volume Expansion

Hypotension in the preterm infant is rarely associated with hypovolemia unless there has been perinatal blood loss. Hypovolemia should be suspected where there is pallor associated with tachycardia, especially in the setting of peripartum blood loss or a very tight nuchal cord. Infants with sepsis, particularly of later onset, may have significant hypovolemia due to leakage of fluid into tissue spaces and may benefit from volume expansion. In addition, hypovolemia may be observed in infants with necrotizing enterocolitis or other abdominal conditions and some infants with subgaleal hematomas or other intracavity hemorrhage. Studies of the relationship between the blood volume and systolic BP in premature infants have demonstrated a poor correlation, suggesting that *low blood volume is not synonymous with low BP*.[40,41,111] Similarly, other groups have found that infants with hypotension and associated acidosis have reduced left ventricular output and impaired cardiac contractility.[38] The usefulness of volume expansion in this setting is questionable, as it may lead to a worsening of cardiac function. Routine use of volume expansion in preterm infants on the first day of life to improve outcomes is not supported by current evidence.[112]

There appears to be little difference in the efficacy between crystalloid and colloid solutions in the treatment of systemic hypotension.[113,114] There have been recent concerns over the use of 5% albumin in older children and adults in intensive care settings and association with increased morbidity.[115] Colloid solutions are more expensive than normal saline and are derived from donated blood with the risk of infection. In the preterm infant the increased capillary permeability may allow leakage of albumin into the extravascular compartment with subsequent tissue fluid retention, which may impair gas exchange in the lung or may cause injury to the brain. Randomized trials have shown improvement in blood pressure in hypotensive infants given volume, but no change in short- or long-term outcomes. In infants who have had an identified fluid loss such as a hemorrhage at the time of delivery or excessive transepidermal water loss with excessive weight loss from use of radiant heat, the volume should be replaced with the type of fluid lost (e.g., a blood transfusion or increased administration of free water). Volume expansion usually increases the left ventricular output, but it is less effective than inotropes at increasing the blood pressure. One trial showed dopamine to be more effective than plasma in improving the blood pressure in normotensive infants.[116] Observational studies have shown a short-term improvement in blood flow after volume expansion.[90]

Accurate diagnosis of hypovolemia is difficult in the neonate, although measurement of central venous pressure from an umbilical venous catheter placed in the right atrium may provide some useful data. Inotropes are not as effective in the presence of hypovolemia, so it is reasonable to initially treat hypotension with 10 to 20 mL/kg of normal saline administered over 30 to 60 minutes. Trials that have used a volume load prior to administration of a vasodilating inotrope such as dobutamine reported no reflex tachycardia in response to the inotrope, suggesting that volume load may lessen the reduction in preload that potentially occurs with the vasodilation. In an infant requiring positive pressure respiratory support, even if the infant is not hypovolemic, a volume load may increase the central venous pressure sufficiently to improve venous return to the heart. As there is an association between excess fluid administration in premature infants and adverse outcomes, including patency of the ductus arteriosus, necrotizing enterocolitis, chronic lung disease,[117] and even death, excessive or inappropriate administration of volume should be avoided. Early initiation of an inotrope should be considered if normalization of the BP is not achieved with a single dose of volume replacement.

Option 3: Dopamine

Prior to instituting a dopamine infusion an echocardiogram was performed. The heart was structurally normal and there was a constricting ductus arteriosus. There was no shunting at atrial level. Cardiac contractility and filling appeared normal. The left ventricular output was measured at 180 mL/kg/minute (normal range > 150 mL/kg/minute). Dopamine (10 μg/kg/minute) was instituted and the BP slowly increased to 38/25 mm Hg with a mean BP of 30 mm Hg. A repeat echocardiogram 4 hours later (with the BP in an acceptable range) showed that the left ventricular output had dropped to 130 mL/kg/minute and was now outside the normal range.

QUESTION

4. Why has the left ventricular output decreased?

ANSWER

4. Dopamine has a predominantly α-receptor effect on the peripheral vasculature, resulting in peripheral vasoconstriction. This action is effective at increasing the blood pressure, but because of the inability of the fetal/preterm myocardium to respond adequately to sudden changes in the afterload, the increase in blood pressure may come at the expense of a reduction in the cardiac output.

Inotropes and vasopressors have been used in neonates for many years in the treatment of hypotension. They were introduced without proper randomized and blinded trials, and there is still no evidence that use of these agents improves important neonatal outcomes. Studies that have been undertaken have focused on the effect on blood pressure, and it is only recently that the effects of these medications on cardiac output (the main determinant of oxygen delivery to tissues) have been studied.[84,118] Inotropes and pressors that have been used in neonates include dopamine, dobutamine, epinephrine, isoprenaline, and milrinone. The mechanisms of action of these vasoactive agents are complex and affected by the developmental maturation of the cardiovascular and autonomic nervous systems. Consequently, these agents can alter the relationship between the systemic blood pressure and systemic blood flow. If only the blood pressure is monitored, a change in the blood flow may not be appreciated.

Dopamine is the most commonly used pressor agent in the treatment of neonates. Dopamine is a precursor to both epinephrine and norepinephrine, but is also a naturally occurring catecholamine. It is involved in the control of hormone release in the central nervous system and in renal tubular homeostasis. There is a family of specific dopamine receptors that are widely expressed throughout the vascular system, including the kidney. Dopamine administered exogenously acts via these dopaminergic and adrenergic receptors, with varying effects at different doses. At lower doses it acts via increasing myocardial contractility in a dose-dependent fashion, but at higher doses (>10 μg/kg/minute) peripheral vasoconstriction and increased afterload play an increasing role in its effect on blood pressure. It is this increase in the afterload that may also affect cardiac function, particularly in the preterm infant where the immature ventricle may not be as able to maintain cardiac output with increasing peripheral vascular resistance. Therefore, lower doses of dopamine or use of an inotrope with less peripheral vaso-constrictive effect may be prudent in the preterm infant. There is a significant degree of variability in response to dopamine dose between individual infants, with gestational age being an important variable. Most infants have a cardiovascular response to dopamine in a dose range below 20 μg/kg/minute with the majority of low-birth-weight infants responding to a dopamine dose of less than 10 μg/kg/minute.[24,84,119] Improvements in blood pressure and left ventric-ular function have been seen at doses as low as 2 μg/kg/minute.[15,72,120] Accordingly, dopa-mine should be initially started at a low to medi-um dose (2 to 5 μg/kg/minute) and increased according to the response of the BP. Most clini-cians are reluctant to increase the dose of dopa-mine to more than 20 μg/kg/minute due to concerns of excessive peripheral vasoconstric-tion, even though there is little evidence of harm if hypotension is being treated.[14,121] At doses at or above 10 μg/kg/minute, addition of a second pharmacologic agent is preferred. Tachyphylaxis to dopamine is common; low doses may have a significant clinical effect initially, but with time, increasing doses of dopamine or addition of another agent is needed.[122]

Dopamine may also cause some degree of pulmonary vasoconstriction[123]; however, this effect seems to be of only minimal clinical sig-nificance.[14] This is most likely because the dopamine-induced increase in systemic blood pressure with subsequent reduction in the degree of right-to-left shunting through fetal channels is more important than any pulmo-nary vasoconstriction induced by dopamine. Therefore, the clinical effectiveness of dopamine in an infant with pulmonary hypertension will depend upon the hemodynamic findings such as patency and direction of ductal shunting, ventricular function, and peripheral vascular resistance.

Option 4: Dobutamine

Prior to instituting a dobutamine infusion, an echocardiogram was performed. The heart was structurally normal and there was a constricting ductus arteriosus. There was no shunting at atrial level. Cardiac contractility and filling appeared *normal. The left ventricular output was measured at 180 mL/kg/minute (normal range >150 mL/kg/minute). Dobutamine was instituted (7 μg/kg/minute and titrated slowly up to 10 μg/kg/minute) and the BP slowly increased to 35/22 mm Hg with a mean BP of 27 mm Hg. A repeat echocardiogram 4 hours later with the BP now in an acceptable range showed that the left ventricular output had increased to 210 mL/kg/minute, remaining in the normal range.*

QUESTION

5. Why was the cardiac output maintained when dobutamine was used as the initial inotropic agent?

ANSWER

5. Dobutamine not only has an inotropic action, but the peripheral vascular effect results in vasodilation and afterload reduction. This can favorably alter the balance between blood pressure and cardiac output in the preterm infant, particularly in the first 24 hours of life.

Dobutamine is a synthetic catecholamine that increases myocardial contractility via the myo-cardial adrenergic receptors[124] but also has a peripheral vasodilatory effect. In contrast to dopamine, dobutamine does not rely on the release of endogenous catecholamines for its action.[14] These properties make dobutamine particularly suited to treatment of hypotension in neonates where associated myocardial dys-function and low cardiac output is com-mon.[84,125] Use of dobutamine is less likely to be effective when there is significant peripheral vasodilation already established (e.g., neonatal sepsis). Without echocardiography to assess cardiac function and the effect of afterload it is difficult to decide the best first-line inotrope. In some cases (e.g., neonatal sepsis) it will be clear that dopamine is most appropriate, but in other situations in which the BP is not significantly abnormal or the hypotension is due to myocardial damage from asphyxia, dobutamine may be more appropriate. In general, dopamine is more useful as a first-line inotrope than dobutamine after the first few days of life when the specific hemody-namic circumstances related to the circulatory transition are resolved. Cardiovascular response to dobutamine has been demonstrated at doses as low as 5 μg/kg/minute[126] and increases in cardiac output and systemic blood flow occur at doses of 10 to 20 μg/kg/minute.[84,118]

Dobutamine has been compared to dopamine in several randomized trials but, as with dopamine, has never been subjected to trial against placebo or no treatment in newborns. Systematic review of five randomized trials found that dopamine is better than dobutamine at increasing blood pressure in hypotensive preterm infants, but to date has not been better at improving clinical outcomes (including intraventricular hemorrhage and PVL) in hypotensive infants.[127] In contrast, in infants with low systemic blood flow in the first day, dobutamine was better at increasing blood flow than dopamine.[118] Similarly, infants who received dobutamine as treatment for hypotension in a randomized trial were more likely to increase their cardiac output as well as the blood pressure than infants who received dopamine.[84] An understanding of the mechanism of action of both of these drugs and their effect on the various vascular beds in the preterm infant is important to guide their appropriate use.

Case Study 6

Baby boy E was born at 31 weeks of gestation weighing 1420 g. His mother had preterm prolonged rupture of the membranes for 3 weeks and received oral antibiotics. She developed premature labor and was given two doses of intramuscular betamethasone 2 weeks prior to delivery. There was evidence of clinical chorioamnionitis with maternal fever and uterine tenderness. The mother had an emergency cesarean section. Baby E had Apgar scores of 3 at 1 minute and 8 at 5 minutes. He was intubated shortly after birth and ventilated at an inspiratory pressure of 22 cm H_2O, a PEEP of 5 cm H_2O, a rate of 40, and an F_{IO_2} of 0.60. He was transferred to the intensive care unit and treated with surfactant replacement therapy at 20 minutes of age. Antibiotics were administered over the first 60 minutes of life. The initial invasive blood pressure obtained via a peripheral radial arterial catheter at 45 minutes of age showed a systolic BP of 38 mm Hg, a diastolic BP of 22 mm Hg and a mean BP of 28 mm Hg. There was a progressive worsening of his condition, necessitating high frequency

oscillatory ventilation to maintain oxygenation and carbon dioxide removal at age 3 hours. The blood pressure fell progressively over the next few hours to 25/16 mm Hg with a mean BP of only 20 mm Hg. A persistent mixed metabolic and respiratory acidosis developed with a need to increase the F_{IO_2} to 1.0. The capillary refill time was over 4 seconds and pulses were barely palpable in all limbs.

Exercise 8

QUESTIONS

1. What is the likely cause of baby E's low blood pressure?

2. What measures would you implement for management of the low blood pressure?

ANSWERS

1. Sepsis. *Escherichia coli* was isolated from blood cultures at 12 hours of age.

2. Management should include a bolus of volume replacement, use of an inotrope/pressor (dopamine, possibly epinephrine), adjustment of antibiotic regimen, and possibly glucocorticoid therapy. The very low and often very resistant hypotension associated with fulminant sepsis is a very difficult management challenge. The infant is often pathologically vasodilated and may even be in a high output state. As a result, management is best directed toward replacing volume and starting pressors, which result in peripheral vasoconstriction such as dopamine and epinephrine.

Baby E received two boluses of 10 mL/kg of normal saline due to poor perfusion in the first 3 hours of life. Dopamine at a dose of 10 μg/kg/minute was commenced and then increased to 20 μg/kg/minute after no response within the first half hour. An epinephrine infusion was begun at 0.05 μg/kg/minute and increased up to 0.2 μg/kg/minute, with only a slight improvement in the systolic blood pressure. An echocardiogram showed a structurally normal heart that had poor contractility. There was evidence of raised pulmonary arterial pressures with a pure right-to-left shunt at both ductal and atrial levels and very poor right ventricular output. Nitric oxide at 10 to 20 ppm was begun without significant effect and the infant died of presumed fulminant sepsis at 8 hours of life.

Adrenaline (Epinephrine)

Adrenaline (epinephrine) is an endogenous catecholamine released from the adrenal gland medulla in response to stress. At low doses it enhances myocardial contractility and causes some peripheral vasodilation via β-adrenergic effects. At higher doses there is a significant α-adrenergic effect causing peripheral vasoconstriction and increased afterload. Despite limited data for efficacy in neonates, epinephrine is often used in refractory hypotension.[128] In a single trial comparing low-moderate dose dopamine and low-dose epinephrine in hypotensive very preterm infants in the first day of life, similar increases were reported in cerebral blood flow and oxygenation as measured by near infrared spectroscopy. Both inotropes were equally efficacious at increasing blood pressure. No other clinical benefits to either inotrope were reported.[129] Because epinephrine at higher doses has a peripheral vasoconstrictive effect, it may be of particular use in infants with pathologic peripheral vasodilation due to septic shock. The dose range used in neonates ranges from 0.05 μg/kg/minute up to 2.6 μg/kg/minute.[128]

Milrinone

Milrinone is a phosphodiesterase-3 inhibitor that increases intracellular cyclic AMP. It has both a positive inotropic effect (particularly improving myocardial diastolic function) and a peripheral vasodilatory effect. This combination of actions is potentially very efficacious in preterm infants in the first hours of life, when the immature myocardium is struggling against the increased afterload of the postnatal circulation. Milrinone has been shown to be effective in treatment of low cardiac output syndrome (LCOS), seen in up to 25% of infants after cardiac surgery. This syndrome is associated with a rise in systemic and pulmonary vascular resistances.[130] The ability of the myocardium to adapt to an increased afterload is compro-

mised by the effects of cardiac bypass, in much the same way the myocardium of the preterm infant in transition may be compromised. Milrinone significantly increases cardiac output in infants with LCOS.[131] In the multicenter randomized PRIMICORP study, there was a dose-dependent reduction of incidence of LCOS when milrinone was used preventively in infants after cardiac surgery.[132] A single pilot study of the use of milrinone in preterm infants using a modified dosing regimen to prevent low blood flow has been published. When used in an appropriate dose range the potential side effect of significant hypotension was not seen and all infants maintained adequate cardiac output when compared to historical control subjects.[133]

Exercise 9

QUESTIONS

1. In hypotensive newborn infants who require treatment, which of the following statements are true and which are false?

   a. Dopamine consistently increases both blood pressure and cardiac output in VLBW infants.

   b. Dopamine is better at increasing BP than dobutamine.

   c. The maximal safe dose of dopamine is 20 μg/kg/minute.

   d. Dopamine should not be used in infants with evidence of pulmonary hypertension owing to its adverse vasoconstrictive effect on the pulmonary vasculature.

2. Of the inotropes used in the treatment of hypotension, which one of the following acts as an inhibitor of phosphodiesterase?

   a. Dopamine

   b. Epinephrine

   c. Milrinone

   d. Dobutamine

   e. Isoprenaline

ANSWERS

1. True: b. False: a, c, d.

2. c. Milrinone.

Case Study 7

Baby girl F was born at 26 weeks of gestation weighing 1050 g. Her mother had preeclampsia, necessitating emergency delivery by cesarean section. Baby F had Apgar scores of 6 at 1 minute and 8 at 5 minutes. She was maintained on continuous positive airway pressure (CPAP) of 6 cm H_2O in less than 30% oxygen for the first 2 weeks. A percutaneous long line was placed on day 3 and enteral feedings were commenced on day 2. Feedings were increased slowly; however, there were several episodes of intolerance necessitating a temporary cessation. On day 10 she had an increasing number of apneas and became progressively more lethargic and poorly perfused with capillary refill time increasing to over 4 seconds. She was intubated and mechanically ventilated (pressures of 22/5 cm H_2O, rate of 40, and an F_{IO_2} of 0.50) and a peripheral arterial line was inserted in the right radial artery. The first arterial BP obtained after calibration of the arterial line and transducer showed a systolic BP of 32 mm Hg, diastolic BP of 18 mm Hg with a mean BP of 25 mm Hg. There was a mild metabolic acidosis. Antibiotics were administered. A single bolus of 10 mL/kg of normal saline made no difference to the BP. Over the next 4 hours she became progressively worse and developed overt neonatal shock with a BP of 28/18 mm Hg (mean BP of 22 mm Hg), weak peripheral pulses, and worsening respiratory function.

Exercise 10

QUESTION

1. What treatment is indicated at this time?

ANSWER

1. Treatment would involve the following:

   Further volume and fluid resuscitation

   Dopamine 10 µg/kg/minute—escalating rapidly to 20 µg/kg/minute (or possibly introduction of a second pressor such as dobutamine if a rapid improvement is not seen after dopamine at 10 µg/kg/minute)

   Consideration of epinephrine if dopamine dose required is above 20 µg/kg/minute or earlier if a rapid clinical response to dopamine is not seen

   Glucocorticoids if hypotension is pressor resistant

In this case all these treatments were administered in rapid succession but despite these interventions the infant continued to deteriorate with a low BP. A random serum cortisol level was taken (subsequently found to be <5 mg/dL) and treatment with hydrocortisone (1 mg/kg/dose twice daily) was begun. Within 1 hour of the first dose of hydrocortisone the BP rapidly improved to within the normal range and the infant's clinical condition gradually improved. The long line was removed and a Pseudomonas species was grown from both the blood culture and the tip of the long line.

Corticosteroids

Glucocorticoids affect multiple organ systems, including the cardiovascular system. There is some evidence that premature infants have an immature hypothalamic-pituitary-adrenal axis and have an inadequate response to stress, including the adrenal responses to hypotension.[23,25,64] Relative adrenal insufficiency is thought to be an increasingly important variable in the failure of effective circulatory and pulmonary transition in the extremely preterm infant. Recent case reports and clinical trials have highlighted the usefulness of both dexamethasone and hydrocortisone in increasing blood pressure. The effect is marked in the setting of hypotension unresponsive to standard therapy. Two clinical trials have indicated the usefulness of corticosteroids in hypotensive preterm infants.[24,134] Several case series have also reported positive responses to hydrocortisone or dexamethasone in infants with refractory hypotension.[22,23,135,136] No long-term neurodevelopmental outcomes were reported from any of these studies. As significant short-term (especially spontaneous intestinal perforation) and long-term side effects are being identified with the use of glucocorticoids in the preterm infant, caution is advised in their use.

Case Study 8

Baby boy G was born at 41 weeks of gestation weighing 3220 g. His mother had ruptured membranes for over 24 hours and developed a mild

fever toward the end of labor. Baby G was delivered vaginally and had Apgar scores of 7 at 1 minute and 8 at 5 minutes. He was initially well and transferred to the postnatal ward area. He began breastfeeding and remained well until just over 48 hours of life, when he was noted to be more lethargic and not interested in feeding. Physical examination showed a normal axillary temperature, a respiratory rate of 80 bpm, and a pulse rate of 170/minute. He was poorly perfused with capillary refill time increasing to over 4 seconds. Both brachial and femoral pulses were difficult to palpate. There was no heart murmur. A noninvasive blood pressure (right arm) using an oscillometric technique was measured at 35/22 mm Hg with a mean BP of 29 mm Hg. Saturation monitoring revealed an oxygen saturation of 85% in room air. An arterial blood gas showed a metabolic acidosis with a pH of 7.18. A sepsis screen (full blood count and inflammatory markers) was initially negative.

Exercise 11

QUESTIONS

1. What are the most likely diagnoses?
2. What further management should be instituted?

ANSWERS

1. Sepsis or congenital heart disease
2. Management would involve the following:

   Establish intravenous access, take blood cultures and treat with antibiotics

   Establish intra-arterial access for acid-base and BP monitoring

   Perform a chest x-ray to assess cardiac size and lung fields

   If possible, obtain an echocardiogram to exclude structural heart disease and assess cardiac function

   Commence inotropes—dobutamine or dopamine at a dose of 5 to 10 µg/kg/minute

   Provide respiratory support if needed

   He was intubated and mechanically ventilated using SIMV (pressures of 22/5 cm H_2O, rate of 45, and an F_{IO_2} 0.30) and a peripheral arterial line was placed in the right radial artery. The first arterial BP obtained after calibration of the arterial line and transducer showed a systolic BP of

35 mm Hg, diastolic BP of 22 mm Hg, with a mean BP of 28 mm Hg. Antibiotics were administered. The chest x-ray showed an enlarged cardiac shadow with evidence of increased pulmonary blood flow. Owing to persistent hypotension and evidence of congestive cardiac failure, he was started on a dobutamine infusion at a rate of 10 µg/kg/minute. An echocardiogram demonstrated hypoplastic left-sided heart syndrome with a constricting ductus arteriosus.

QUESTION

3. What treatment should now be considered?

ANSWERS

3. Maintain ductal patency with prostaglandin E_1 and avoid hyperventilation and supplemental oxygen if possible to limit pulmonary blood flow; consider surgical relief of left-sided heart obstruction once medically stabilized.

Other Causes of Hypotension in the Newborn

Cardiogenic shock due to congenital heart disease, in particular left-sided obstructive lesions, should also be taken into account in the differential diagnosis of causes of hypotension. Similarly, myocardial dysfunction from either congenital cardiomyopathy or myocarditis may result in congestive cardiac failure and hypotension. Echocardiography is essential to making these diagnoses.

Management Guidelines for Hypotension

As demonstrated by the case histories and exercises within this chapter, the appropriate treatment of hypotension depends upon the underlying physiologic and pathologic circumstances. There is a range of treatments available to treat hypotension in the newborn, but there is a worrisome lack of data or clinical trials linking the available treatments to improved mortality rate and neonatal outcomes. Assumptions are made about the effectiveness of these treatments either based on short-term outcomes, such as improvement in blood pressure, or by epidemiologic associations of both short- and long-term neurologic injury with various levels of systemic hypotension. Despite these limitations, some insight into the appropriate combination of therapies can be obtained by looking beyond the measurement of blood pressure and beginning to assess other parameters that impact cardiovascular adequacy. The underlying cause for cardiovascular compromise should be sought from the history and the physical examination and by utilizing all available diagnostic information.

The variability in systemic vascular resistance in the newborn infant appears to be of much greater importance in determining blood pressure than it is in older children and adults. Accordingly clinicians need to incorporate this factor into therapeutic decisions regarding hypotension. Infants with normal or high left ventricular output and systemic hypotension are likely to have a vasodilated peripheral vasculature. In these cases, treatment of a large ductus arteriosus (if present) and vasopressors that have a vasoconstrictive effect on the peripheral vasculature will have the most significant effect on blood pressure. In the case of a preterm infant in the first day of life with low cardiac output and an immature myocardium sensitive to increased afterload, the use of an agent that causes peripheral vasoconstriction may further reduce systemic blood flow. In this case, dobutamine, which has a vasodilatory effect on the periphery, may be a better choice of inotrope. In infants who remain hypotensive, the addition of dopamine or epinephrine to gently increase vascular resistance, titrated to the minimally acceptable blood pressure, is logical. Infants with refractory hypotension may benefit from low-dose corticosteroid therapy. Preterm or term infants with evidence of perinatal asphyxia and multiorgan dysfunction require careful management of fluid balance to prevent volume overload and subsequent cardiac failure—in this group of infants, inotropic agents with significant afterload reduction effects (dobutamine and milrinone) are probably the most useful. Infants with hypotension presenting outside the immediate postnatal period (or transitional period) commonly have bacterial sepsis. This group of infants generally will have decreased peripheral vascular resistance and hypovolemia from capillary leakage and require urgent fluid resuscitation and inotropes with vasoconstricting properties. Because these infants may also have relative adrenal insuffi-

ciency, they also should be considered candidates for low-dose steroid therapy.

The pulmonary circulation should also be considered when selecting an appropriate treatment for hypotensive infants. Higher pulmonary vascular resistance is often found in the immature preterm infant with low cardiac output and in the ventilated term infant with high oxygen requirements (persistent pulmonary hypertension). Pulmonary hypertension can be treated selectively by the use of inhaled nitric oxide. Cardiac pressors have varying effects on the pulmonary vasculature; dobutamine reduces both systemic and pulmonary vascular resistance, dopamine increases both systemic and pulmonary vascular resistance (especially at higher doses), and epinephrine tends to increase systemic more than pulmonary vascular resistance. Dopamine may decrease the right-to-left shunts associated with pulmonary hypertension but, paradoxically, can result in reduced cardiac output in those infants with existing impaired myocardial function. Table 15-3 outlines the suggested use of available therapies for management of cardiovascular compromise according to the underlying pathophysiologic circumstances.

As the clinician develops a more thorough understanding of the different clinical scenarios that lead to the presentation of hypotension or cardiovascular compromise, treatment algorithms will become increasingly useful. A number of authors have attempted to summarize the different possible therapeutic approaches according to the information available. Figure 15-5 shows an approach to the management of hypotension based purely on clinical information. Without data regarding the actual cardiac output or systemic blood flow, it is still possible to make some assumptions about the underlying physiology. However, an echocardiogram is invaluable in the assessment process of cardiovascular inadequacy/hypotension because it provides additional information regarding the size and shunt direction of the ductus arteriosus, assessment of myocardial contractility, assessment of myocardial filling, and measurement of the cardiac output (which provides indirect information about peripheral vascular resistance). Figure 15-6 summarizes the approach to management of hypotension using the additional information provided by an echocardiogram. This allows more specific customization of treatment options according to the needs of the individual patient.

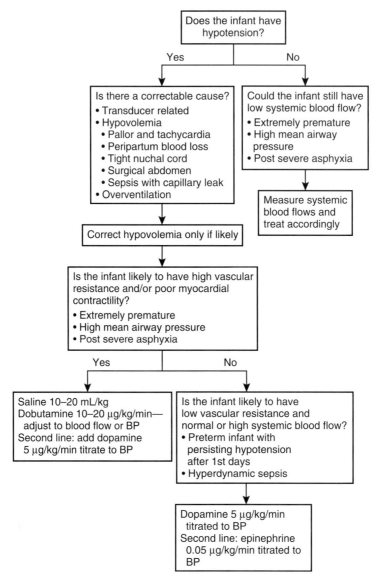

Figure 15-5 Treatment of cardiovascular compromise based on clinical findings. (Adapted from Kluckow M, Osborn D: Hypotension in the neonate. In Burg FD, Ingelfinger JE, Polin RA, et al [eds]: Current Pediatric Therapy, 17th ed. Philadelphia, Elsevier, 2005.)

Conclusion

Systemic blood pressure is dependent on both systemic blood flow (cardiac output) and systemic vascular resistance, and consequently, the relationship between blood pressure and blood flow is not constant. Some infants, in particular premature infants, have a significant reduction in the systemic blood flow in the first day of life, which will not always be recognized by measuring blood pressure alone. Low systemic blood flow, with or without hypotension, is associated with significant morbidity.

Determining whether the infant is likely to have high or low vascular resistance is important in directing treatment of the underlying cause. The underlying pathophysiology of cardiovascular compromise in the neonate is variable, and treatment should be tailored to these differences. Although there is a large body of clinical experience in the use of inotropes, pressors, and corticosteroids in the newborn infant, there is an absence of evidence that these interventions result in the improvement of significant outcomes and prevention of neurodevelopmental disability or death.

SUSPECTED CARDIOVASCULAR
COMPROMISE

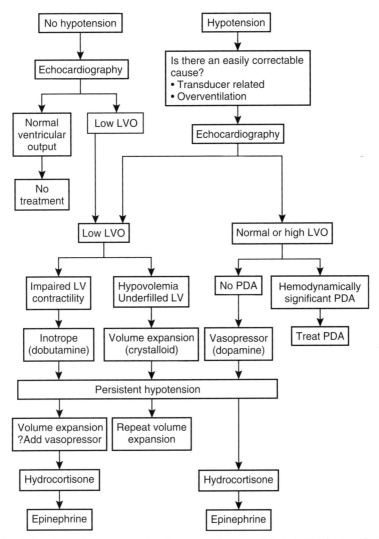

Figure 15-6 Treatment of cardiovascular compromise based on echocardiographic findings. LVO, left ventricular output; LV, left ventricle; PDA, patent ductus arteriosus. (Adapted from Subhedar N: Treatment of hypotension in newborns. Semin Neonatol 2003;8:413.)

References

1. Al Aweel I, Pursley DM, Rubin LP, et al: Variations in prevalence of hypotension, hypertension, and vasopressor use in NICUs. J Perinatol 2001;21:272.
2. Allan LD, Chita SK, Al-Ghazali W, et al: Doppler echocardiographic evaluation of the normal human fetal heart. Br Heart J 1987;57:528.
3. Teitel DF: Physiologic development of the cardiovascular system in the fetus. In Polin RA, Fox WW (eds): Fetal and Neonatal Physiology. Philadelphia, WB Saunders, 1998, pp 827–836.
4. Mahoney LT, Coryell KG, Lauer RM: The newborn transitional circulation: A two-dimensional Doppler echocardiographic study. J Am Coll Cardiol 1985;6:623.
5. Gentile R, Stevenson G, Dooley T, et al: Pulsed Doppler echocardiographic determination of time of ductal closure in normal newborn infants. J Pediatr 1981;98:443.
6. Evans N, Iyer P: Longitudinal changes in the diameter of the ductus arteriosus in ventilated preterm infants: Correlation with respiratory outcomes. Arch Dis Child Fetal Neonatal Ed 1995;72:F156–F161.
7. Evans N, Iyer P: Assessment of ductus arteriosus shunt in preterm infants supported by mechanical ventilation: Effects of interatrial shunting. J Pediatr 1994;125:778.
8. Agata Y, Hiraishi S, Oguchi K, et al: Changes in left ventricular output from fetal to early neonatal life. J Pediatr 1991;119:441.
9. Drayton MR, Skidmore R: Ductus arteriosus blood flow during first 48 hours of life. Arch Dis Child 1987;62:1030.
10. Hiraishi S, Misawa H, Oguchi K, et al: Two-dimensional Doppler echocardiographic assessment

of closure of the ductus arteriosus in normal newborn infants. J Pediatr 1987;111:755.

11. Alverson DC, Eldridge MW, Johnson JD, et al: Effect of patent ductus arteriosus on left ventricular output in premature infants. J Pediatr 1983;102:754.

12. Evans N, Iyer P: Incompetence of the foramen ovale in preterm infants supported by mechanical ventilation. J Pediatr 1994;125:786.

13. Marcus C, Bronnegard M, Carlstedt-Duke J: Fetal and neonatal development of hormone receptors. In Polin RA, Fox WW (eds): Fetal and Neonatal Physiology. Philadelphia, WB Saunders, 1998, pp 176–190.

14. Seri I: Cardiovascular, renal and endocrine actions of dopamine in neonates and children. J Pediatr 1995;126:333.

15. Seri I, Rudas G, Bors Z, et al: Effects of low-dose dopamine infusion on cardiovascular and renal functions, cerebral blood flow, and plasma catecholamine levels in sick preterm neonates. Pediatr Res 1993;34:742.

16. Jones CT, Robinson RO: Plasma catecholamines in foetal and adult sheep. J Physiol 1975;248:15.

17. Barrett CT, Heymann MA, Rudolph AM: Alpha and beta adrenergic receptor activity in fetal sheep. Am J Obstet Gynecol 1972;112:1114.

18. Iwamoto HS: Endocrine regulation of the fetal circulation. In Polin RA, Fox WW (eds): Fetal and Neonatal Physiology. Philadelphia, WB Saunders, 1998, pp 961–970.

19. Padbury J, Agata Y, Ludlow J, et al: Effect of fetal adrenalectomy on catecholamine release and physiologic adaptation at birth in sheep. J Clin Invest 1987;80:1096.

20. Stein HM, Oyama K, Martinez A, et al: Effects of corticosteroids in preterm sheep on adaptation and sympathoadrenal mechanisms at birth. Am J Physiol 1993;264:E763–E769.

21. Crowley P: Prophylactic corticosteroids for preterm birth. Cochrane Database Syst Rev 2000; CD000065.

22. Fauser A, Pohlandt F, Bartmann P, et al: Rapid increase of blood pressure in extremely low birth weight infants after a single dose of dexamethasone. Eur J Pediatr 1993;152:354.

23. Helbock HJ, Insoft RM, Conte FA: Glucocorticoid-responsive hypotension in extremely low birth weight newborns. Pediatrics 1993;92:715.

24. Bourchier D, Weston PJ: Randomised trial of dopamine compared with hydrocortisone for the treatment of hypotensive very low birthweight infants. Arch Dis Child Fetal Neonatal Ed 1997;76:F174–F178.

25. Scott SM, Watterberg KL: Effect of gestational age, postnatal age, and illness on plasma cortisol concentrations in premature infants. Pediatr Res 1995;37:112.

26. Metzger DL, Wright NM, Veldhuis JD, et al: Characterization of pulsatile secretion and clearance of plasma cortisol in premature and term neonates using deconvolution analysis. J Clin Endocrinol Metab 1993;77:458.

27. Levina SE: Endocrine features in development of human hypothalamus, hypophysis, and placenta. Gen Comp Endocrinol 1968;11:151.

28. Iwamoto HS: Neuroendocrine regulation of cardiovascular, fluid and electrolyte homeostasis. In Gluckman PD, Heymann M (eds): Pediatrics and Perinatology: The Scientific Basis. London, Arnold, 1998, pp 520–529.

29. Ziegler JW, Ivy DD, Kinsella JP, et al: The role of nitric oxide, endothelin, and prostaglandins in the transition of the pulmonary circulation. Clin Perinatol 1995;22:387.

30. Endo A, Ayusawa M, Minato M, et al: Endothelium-derived relaxing and contracting factors during the early neonatal period. Acta Paediatr 1997;86:834.

31. Kaapa P, Kero P, Ekblad H, et al: Plasma endothelin-1 in the neonatal respiratory distress syndrome. Ann Chir Gynaecol Suppl 1994;208:110.

32. Kojima T, Isozaki-Fukuda Y, Takedatsu M, et al: Circulating levels of endothelin and atrial natriuretic factor during postnatal life. Acta Paediatr 1992; 81:676.

33. Kojima T, Isozaki-Fukuda Y, Takedatsu M, et al: Plasma endothelin-1 like immunoreactivity levels in neonates. Eur J Pediatr 1992;151:913.

34. Kumar P, Kazzi NJ, Shankaran S: Plasma immunoreactive endothelin-1 concentration in cord blood of normal term neonates. Am J Perinatol 1995;12:113.

35. Yoshibayashi M, Nishioka K, Nakao K, et al: Plasma endothelin levels in healthy children: High values in early infancy. J Cardiovasc Pharmacol 1991;17 (Suppl 7):S404–S405.

36. Malamitsi-Puchner A, Economou E, Efstathopoulos T, et al: Endothelin 1–21 plasma concentrations on days 1 and 4 of life in healthy and ill preterm neonates. Biol Neonate 1995;67:317.

37. Coceani F, Kelsey L, Seidlitz E: Evidence for an effector role of endothelin in closure of the ductus arteriosus at birth. Can J Physiol Pharmacol 1992; 70:1061.

38. Gill AB, Weindling AM: Echocardiographic assessment of cardiac function in shocked very low birth weight infants. Arch Dis Child 1993;68:17.

39. Kluckow M, Evans N: Relationship between blood pressure and cardiac output in preterm infants requiring mechanical ventilation. J Pediatr 1996; 129:506.

40. Bauer K, Linderkamp O, Versmold HT: Systolic blood pressure and blood volume in preterm infants. Arch Dis Child 1993;69:521.

41. Barr PA, Bailey PE, Sumners J, et al: Relation between arterial blood pressure and blood volume and effect of infused albumin in sick preterm infants. Pediatrics 1977;60:282.

42. Pladys P, Wodey E, Beuchee A, et al: Left ventricle output and mean arterial blood pressure in preterm infants during the first day of life. Eur J Pediatr 1999;158:817.

43. Lopez SL, Leighton JO, Walther FJ: Supranormal cardiac output in the dopamine- and dobutamine-dependent preterm infant. Pediatr Cardiol 1997; 18:292.

44. Butt WW, Whyte HW: Blood pressure monitoring in neonates: Comparison of umbilical and peripheral artery measurements. J Pediatr 1984;105:630.

45. Ramsey MI II: Noninvasive automatic determination of mean arterial pressure. Med Biol Eng Comput 1979;17:11.

46. Kimble KJ, Darnall RA Jr, Yelderman M, et al: An automated oscillometric technique for estimating mean arterial pressure in critically ill newborns. Anesthesiology 1981;54:423.

47. Lui K, Doyle PE, Buchanan N: Oscillometric and intra-arterial blood pressure measurements in the

neonate: A comparison of methods. Aust Paediatr J 1982;18:32.

48. Colan SD, Fujii A, Borow KM, et al: Noninvasive determination of systolic, diastolic and end-systolic blood pressure in neonates, infants and young children: Comparison with central aortic pressure measurements. Am J Cardiol 1983;52:867.

49. Park MK, Menard SM: Accuracy of blood pressure measurement by the Dinamap monitor in infants and children. Pediatrics 1987;79:907.

50. Emery EF, Greenough A: Non-invasive blood pressure monitoring in preterm infants receiving intensive care. Eur J Pediatr 1992;151:136.

51. Dannevig I, Dale HC, Liestol K, et al: Blood pressure in the neonate: Three non-invasive oscillometric pressure monitors compared with invasively measured blood pressure. Acta Paediatr 2005;94:191.

52. Nuntnarumit P, Yang W, Bada-Ellzey HS: Blood pressure measurements in the newborn. Clin Perinatol 1999;26:981.

53. Watkins AM, West CR, Cooke RW: Blood pressure and cerebral haemorrhage and ischaemia in very low birthweight infants. Early Hum Dev 1989;19:103.

54. Versmold HT, Kitterman JA, Phibbs RH, et al: Aortic blood pressure during the first 12 hours of life in infants with birth weight 610 to 4,220 grams. Pediatrics 1981;67:607.

55. Emery EF, Greenough A: Neonatal blood pressure levels of preterm infants who did and did not develop chronic lung disease. Early Hum Dev 1992; 31:149.

56. Cunningham S, Symon AG, Elton RA, et al: Intraarterial blood pressure reference ranges, death and morbidity in very low birthweight infants during the first seven days of life. Early Hum Dev 1999; 56:151.

57. Lee J, Rajadurai VS, Tan KW: Blood pressure standards for very low birthweight infants during the first day of life. Arch Dis Child Fetal Neonatal Ed 1999;81:F168–F170.

58. Miall-Allen VM, de Vries LS, Whitelaw AG: Mean arterial blood pressure and neonatal cerebral lesions. Arch Dis Child 1987;62:1068.

59. Tsuji M, Saul JP, du PA, et al: Cerebral intravascular oxygenation correlates with mean arterial pressure in critically ill premature infants. Pediatrics 2000;106:625.

60. Munro MJ, Walker AM, Barfield CP: Hypotensive extremely low birth weight infants have reduced cerebral blood flow. Pediatrics 2004;114:1591.

61. Hegyi T, Carbone MT, Anwar M, et al: Blood pressure ranges in premature infants. I. The first hours of life. J Pediatr 1994;124:627.

62. Development of audit measures and guidelines for good practice in the management of neonatal respiratory distress syndrome: Report of a joint working group of the British Association of Perinatal Medicine and the research unit of the Royal College of Physicians. Arch Dis Child 1992;67:1221.

63. Ng PC, Lam CW, Fok TF, et al: Refractory hypotension in preterm infants with adrenocortical insufficiency. Arch Dis Child Fetal Neonatal Ed 2001;84: F122–F124.

64. Watterberg KL: Adrenal insufficiency and cardiac dysfunction in the preterm infant. Pediatr Res 2002;51:422.

65. Hanna CE, Jett PL, Laird MR, et al: Corticosteroid binding globulin, total serum cortisol, and stress in extremely low-birth-weight infants. Am J Perinatol 1997;14:201.

66. Sasidharan P: Role of corticosteroids in neonatal blood pressure homeostasis. Clin Perinatol 1998; 25:723.

67. Moise AA, Wearden ME, Kozinetz CA, et al: Antenatal steroids are associated with less need for blood pressure support in extremely premature infants. Pediatrics 1995;95:845.

68. Demarini S, Dollberg S, Hoath SB, et al: Effects of antenatal corticosteroids on blood pressure in very low birth weight infants during the first 24 hours of life. J Perinatol 1999;19:419.

69. LeFlore JL, Engle WD, Rosenfeld CR: Determinants of blood pressure in very low birth weight neonates: Lack of effect of antenatal steroids. Early Hum Dev 2000;59:37.

70. Leviton A, Kuban KC, Pagano M, et al: Antenatal corticosteroids appear to reduce the risk of postnatal germinal matrix hemorrhage in intubated low birth weight newborns. Pediatrics 1993;91:1083.

71. Yao AC, Lind J: Blood volume in the asphyxiated term neonate. Biol Neonate 1972;21:199.

72. DiSessa TG, Leitner M, Ti CC, et al: The cardiovascular effects of dopamine in the severely asphyxiated neonate. J Pediatr 1981;99:772.

73. Walther FJ, Siassi B, Ramadan NA, et al: Cardiac output in newborn infants with transient myocardial dysfunction. J Pediatr 1985;107:781.

74. Biondi JW, Schulman DS, Soufer R, et al: The effect of incremental positive end-expiratory pressure on right ventricular hemodynamics and ejection fraction. Anesth Analg 1988;67:144.

75. Trang TT, Tibballs J, Mercier JC, et al: Optimization of oxygen transport in mechanically ventilated newborns using oximetry and pulsed Doppler-derived cardiac output. Crit Care Med 1988; 16:1094.

76. Maayan C, Eyal F, Mandelberg A, et al: Effect of mechanical ventilation and volume loading on left ventricular performance in premature infants with respiratory distress syndrome. Crit Care Med 1986; 14:858.

77. Skinner JR, Boys RJ, Hunter S, et al: Pulmonary and systemic arterial pressure in hyaline membrane disease. Arch Dis Child 1992;67:366.

78. Kluckow M, Evans N: Low superior vena cava flow and intraventricular haemorrhage in preterm infants. Arch Dis Child Fetal Neonatal Ed 2000; 82:188.

79. Evans N, Kluckow M: Early determinants of right and left ventricular output in ventilated preterm infants. Arch Dis Child Fetal Neonatal Ed 1996; 74:F88.

80. Skelton R, Evans N, Smythe J: A blinded comparison of clinical and echocardiographic evaluation of the preterm infant for patent ductus arteriosus. J Paediatr Child Health 1994;30:406.

81. Evans N, Moorcraft J: Effect of patency of the ductus arteriosus on blood pressure in very preterm infants. Arch Dis Child 1992;67:1169.

82. Kluckow M, Evans N: Early echocardiographic prediction of symptomatic patent ductus arteriosus in preterm infants undergoing mechanical ventilation. J Pediatr 1995;127:774.

83. Fenton AC, Woods KL, Leanage R, et al: Cardiovascular effects of carbon dioxide in ventilated preterm infants. Acta Paediatr 1992;81:498.

84. Roze JC, Tohier C, Maingueneau C, et al: Response to dobutamine and dopamine in the hypotensive very preterm infant. Arch Dis Child 1993;69:59.

85. Pourcyrous M, Bada HS, Korones SB, et al: Significance of serial C-reactive protein responses in neonatal infection and other disorders. Pediatrics 1993;92:431.

86. Kluckow M, Evans N: Low systemic blood flow in the preterm infant. Semin Neonatol 2001;6:75.

87. Strozik KS, Pieper CH, Roller J: Capillary refilling time in newborn babies: Normal values. Arch Dis Child Fetal Neonatal Ed 1997;76:F193–F196.

88. Schriger DL, Baraff L: Defining normal capillary refill: Variation with age, sex, and temperature. Ann Emerg Med 1988;17:932.

89. Tibby SM, Hatherill M, Murdoch IA: Capillary refill and core-peripheral temperature gap as indicators of haemodynamic status in paediatric intensive care patients. Arch Dis Child 1999;80:163.

90. Osborn DA, Evans N, Kluckow M: Clinical detection of low upper body blood flow in very premature infants using blood pressure, capillary refill time, and central-peripheral temperature difference. Arch Dis Child Fetal Neonatal Ed 2004;89:F168–F173.

91. Linshaw MA: Concentration of the urine. In Polin RA, Fox WW (eds): Fetal and Neonatal Physiology. Philadelphia, WB Saunders, 1998, pp 1634–1653.

92. Alverson DC, Eldridge M, Dillon T, et al: Noninvasive pulsed Doppler determination of cardiac output in neonates and children. J Pediatr 1982;101:46.

93. Walther FJ, Siassi B, Ramadan NA, et al: Pulsed Doppler determinations of cardiac output in neonates: Normal standards for clinical use. Pediatrics 1985;76:829.

94. Tyszczuk L, Meek J, Elwell C, et al: Cerebral blood flow is independent of mean arterial blood pressure in preterm infants undergoing intensive care. Pediatrics 1998;102:337.

95. Kissack CM, Garr R, Wardle SP, et al: Cerebral fractional oxygen extraction in very low birth weight infants is high when there is low ventricular output and hypocarbia but is unaffected by hypotension. Pediatr Res 2004;55:400.

96. Lou HC, Lassen NA, Friis-Hansen B: Impaired autoregulation of cerebral blood flow in the distressed newborn infant. J Pediatr 1979;94:118.

97. Wardle SP, Yoxall CW, Weindling AM: Peripheral oxygenation in hypotensive preterm babies. Pediatr Res 1999;45:343.

98. Weindling AM, Kissack CM: Blood pressure and tissue oxygenation in the newborn baby at risk of brain damage. Biol Neonate 2001;79:241.

99. Perlman JM, McMenamin JB, Volpe JJ: Fluctuating cerebral blood-flow velocity in respiratory-distress syndrome. Relation to the development of intraventricular hemorrhage. N Engl J Med 1983;309:204.

100. Pryds O, Greisen G, Lou H, et al: Heterogeneity of cerebral vasoreactivity in preterm infants supported by mechanical ventilation. J Pediatr 1989;115:638.

101. Bada HS, Korones SB, Perry EH, et al: Mean arterial blood pressure changes in premature infants and those at risk for intraventricular hemorrhage. J Pediatr 1990;117:607.

102. Heuchan AM, Evans N, Henderson Smart DJ, et al: Perinatal risk factors for major intraventricular haemorrhage in the Australian and New Zealand Neonatal Network, 1995–1997. Arch Dis Child Fetal Neonatal Ed 2002;86:F86–F90.

103. Perlman JM, Risser R, Broyles RS: Bilateral cystic periventricular leukomalacia in the premature infant: Associated risk factors. Pediatrics 1996;97:822.

104. de Vries LS, Regev R, Dubowitz LM, et al: Perinatal risk factors for the development of extensive cystic leukomalacia. Am J Dis Child 1988;142:732.

105. Low JA, Froese AB, Galbraith RS, et al: The association between preterm newborn hypotension and hypoxemia and outcome during the first year. Acta Paediatr 1993;82:433.

106. Goldstein RF, Thompson RJJr, Oehler JM, et al: Influence of acidosis, hypoxemia, and hypotension on neurodevelopmental outcome in very low birth weight infants. Pediatrics 1995;95:238.

107. Hunt RW, Evans N, Rieger I, et al: Low superior vena cava flow and neurodevelopment at 3 years in very preterm infants. J Pediatr 2004;145:588.

108. Osborn DA, Evans N, Kluckow M: Effect of early targeted indomethacin on the ductus arteriosus and blood flow to the upper body and brain in the preterm infant. Arch Dis Child Fetal Neonatal Ed 2003;88:F477–F482.

109. Patel J, Roberts I, Azzopardi D, et al: Randomized double-blind controlled trial comparing the effects of ibuprofen with indomethacin on cerebral hemodynamics in preterm infants with patent ductus arteriosus. Pediatr Res 2000;47:36.

110. Kluckow M, Evans N: Ductal shunting, high pulmonary blood flow, and pulmonary hemorrhage. J Pediatr 2000;137:68.

111. Wright IM, Goodall SR: Blood pressure and blood volume in preterm infants. Arch Dis Child Fetal Neonatal Ed 1994;70:F230–F231.

112. A randomized trial comparing the effect of prophylactic intravenous fresh frozen plasma, gelatin or glucose on early mortality and morbidity in preterm babies: The Northern Neonatal Nursing Initiative [NNNI] Trial Group. Eur J Pediatr 1996;155:580.

113. Emery EF, Greenough A, Gamsu HR: Randomised controlled trial of colloid infusions in hypotensive preterm infants. Arch Dis Child 1992;67:1185.

114. So KW, Fok TF, Ng PC, et al: Randomised controlled trial of colloid or crystalloid in hypotensive preterm infants. Arch Dis Child Fetal Neonatal Ed 1997;76:F43–F46.

115. Nadel S, De Munter C, Britto J, et al: Albumin: Saint or sinner? Arch Dis Child 1998;79:384.

116. Gill AB, Weindling AM: Randomised controlled trial of plasma protein fraction versus dopamine in hypotensive very low birthweight infants. Arch Dis Child 1993;69:284.

117. Van Marter LJ, Leviton A, Allred EN, et al: Hydration during the first days of life and the risk of bronchopulmonary dysplasia in low birth weight infants. J Pediatr 1990;116:942.

118. Osborn D, Evans N, Kluckow M: Randomized trial of dobutamine versus dopamine in preterm infants with low systemic blood flow. J Pediatr 2002;140:183.

119. Klarr JM, Faix RG, Pryce CJ, et al: Randomized, blind trial of dopamine versus dobutamine for treatment of hypotension in preterm infants with respiratory distress syndrome. J Pediatr 1994;125:117.

120. Seri I, Tulassay T, Kiszel J, et al: Cardiovascular response to dopamine in hypotensive preterm neonates with severe hyaline membrane disease. Eur J Pediatr 1984;142:3.

121. Perez CA, Reimer JM, Schreiber MD, et al: Effect of high-dose dopamine on urine output in newborn infants. Crit Care Med 1986;14:1045.

122. Seri I, Evans J: Addition of epinepherine to dopamine increases blood pressure and urine output in critically ill extremely low birth weight infants with uncompensated shock. Pediatr Res 1998;43:194A.

123. Kliegman R, Fanaroff AA: Caution in the use of dopamine in the neonate. J Pediatr 1978;93:540.

124. Ruffolo RR Jr: The pharmacology of dobutamine. Am J Med Sci 1987;294:244.

125. Martinez AM, Padbury JF, Thio S: Dobutamine pharmacokinetics and cardiovascular responses in critically ill neonates. Pediatrics 1992;89:47.

126. Stopfkuchen H, Queisser-Luft A, Vogel K: Cardiovascular responses to dobutamine determined by systolic time intervals in preterm infants. Crit Care Med 1990;18:722.

127. Subhedar NV, Shaw NJ: Dopamine versus dobutamine for hypotensive preterm infants. Cochrane Database Syst Rev 2003; CD001242.

128. Heckmann M, Trotter A, Pohlandt F, et al: Epinephrine treatment of hypotension in very low birthweight infants. Acta Paediatr 2002;91:566.

129. Pellicer A, Valverde E, Elorza MD, et al: Cardiovascular support for low birth weight infants and cerebral hemodynamics: A randomized, blinded, clinical trial. Pediatrics 2005;115:1501.

130. Wernovsky G, Wypij D, Jonas RA, et al: Postoperative course and hemodynamic profile after the arterial switch operation in neonates and infants. A comparison of low-flow cardiopulmonary bypass and circulatory arrest. Circulation 1995;92:2226.

131. Chang AC, Atz AM, Wernovsky G, et al: Milrinone: Systemic and pulmonary hemodynamic effects in neonates after cardiac surgery. Crit Care Med 1995;23:1907.

132. Hoffman TM, Wernovsky G, Atz AM, et al: Efficacy and safety of milrinone in preventing low cardiac output syndrome in infants and children after corrective surgery for congenital heart disease. Circulation 2003;107:996.

133. Paradisis M, Evans N, Osborn D, et al: Pilot study of milrinone for prevention of low systemic bood flow in very preterm infants using an optimised pharmacokinetic profile. Pediatr Res 2004;55:525A.

134. Gaissmaier RE, Pohlandt F: Single-dose dexamethasone treatment of hypotension in preterm infants. J Pediatr 1999;134:701.

135. Seri I, Tan R, Evans J: Cardiovascular effects of hydrocortisone in preterm infants with pressor-resistant hypotension. Pediatrics 2001;107:1070.

136. Kopelman AE, Moise AA, Holbert D, et al: A single very early dexamethasone dose improves respiratory and cardiovascular adaptation in preterm infants. J Pediatr 1999;135:345.

137. Osborn DA, Evans N: Early volume expansion for prevention of morbidity and mortality in very preterm infants. Cochrane Database Syst Rev 2004; CD002055.

Congenital Heart Disease in the Neonate

Gil Wernovsky, MD, and S. David Rubenstein, MD

Congenital heart disease (CHD) is the most common birth defect in the human species, affecting 8 per 1000 live births. Approximately 20% of these children require surgery in the neonatal period (referred to subsequently as "critical" CHD), and an additional 20% to 30% present as newborns and require surgery later in the first year of life. With the exception of infants born prematurely, neonates with CHD represent the largest diagnostic group of children in many neonatal intensive care units. It is beyond the scope of this chapter to review all the different structural defects that may present in the newborn period; rather, a general construct will be presented for the initial diagnosis, stabilization, and management of the newborn with suspected or confirmed CHD. Although there are literally hundreds of different defects, the newborn with critical CHD presents to medical attention in a limited number of (and occasionally overlapping) ways: visible cyanosis, circulatory collapse and shock, arrhythmias, asymptomatic with a heart murmur, and increasingly, with the diagnosis made prenatally.

The Fetal Circulation and Physiologic Changes with Birth

The birth of a neonate represents a time of intense and multifaceted physiologic change and adaptation. Prior to birth the fetus relies on the mother for all aspects of life, including temperature control; accretion of carbohydrates, fats, and protein; waste product elimination; and respiratory gas exchange. After birth,

a neonate must be able to perform those functions and many more independently. Almost immediately after birth, unique postnatal adaptations occur in the cardiorespiratory system to allow independence and extrauterine survival. These changes that allow the successful transition from the fetal cardiopulmonary circulation to the neonatal circulation are complex in nature and are associated with both anatomic and physiologic alterations. During this time of transition from the in utero environment to extrauterine life, a so-called transitional circulation is present, but only until well-described anatomic changes occur, such as obliteration of the ductus arteriosus and closure of the foramen ovale. A brief review of the normal transition from fetal to neonatal circulation follows.

The fetus develops in a relatively hypoxemic environment, normal for the fetus but with levels of Pa_{O_2} that are too low to sustain life for a child or adult. From a physiologic perspective with regard to oxygen delivery, the fetus should be considered as a recipient of venous blood after the highly metabolically active placenta has extracted oxygen from the placental circulation. The highest Pa_{O_2} in the fetus is no greater than 30 to 35 mm Hg and is found within the umbilical vein. This relative fetal hypoxemia is associated with significant pulmonary vasoconstriction, which creates high pulmonary artery pressure and low pulmonary blood flow. In addition, the interrelationships between vasoactive mediators, present locally in the pulmonary vascular endothelium and in the pulmonary circulation, including but not limited to the vasoconstrictors thromboxane and endothelin and the vasodilating prostaglandins and nitric oxide, have a causative and direct role in creating this high pulmonary vascular resistance. No greater than 10% of combined ventricular output (Table 16-1) enters the pulmonary arterial circulation distal to the ductus arteriosus because pulmonary artery pressure is equal to or greater than systemic pressure, and the two circuits, which are independent in postnatal life, are interconnected in fetal life by the ductus arteriosus and foramen ovale (Fig. 16-1). Of note is that the most highly oxygenated blood in the fetus returns to the fetal heart through the ductus venosus and "streams" directly into the left atrium from the right atrium across the foramen ovale, supplying the developing fetal central nervous system with the most highly oxygenated blood in the fetus (see the broader lines and arrows in Fig. 16-1). The blood returning to the right atrium from the head and neck flows into the right ventricle and is ejected into the pulmonary artery from where most of the blood crosses the ductus arteriosus to perfuse the organs supplied by the thoracic and abdominal aorta and their distal branches. The high hemoglobin concentration of the fetus, which is secondary to hypoxia-induced increases in fetal erythropoietin levels, allows adequate fetal tissue oxygen delivery despite the low Pao_2 values encountered in the in utero environment.

Prior to birth, systemic and pulmonary pressures are equal, but a significant decrement in pulmonary pressure (and vascular resistance) can be noted by 3 hours of life. This relaxation in pulmonary vasomotor tone and the subsequent decrease in pulmonary artery pressure are multifactorial in origin, but clearly more nitric oxide and less endothelin are present after birth when compared to fetal life. Successful ventilation of the lungs with gas is also crucial in the

TABLE 16-1

BLOOD FLOW THROUGH THE MAJOR VESSELS OF THE FETAL LAMB AS A PERCENTAGE OF CARDIAC OUTPUT

Area of Blood Flow	Percentage of Combined Output of Both Ventricles ($\pm$ SE)
Right and left ventricles	100
Right ventricle	45 $\pm$ 1.2
Left ventricle	55 $\pm$ 1.2
Thoracic inferior vena cava (IVC)	76 $\pm$ 1.5
IVC flow to right atrium	29 $\pm$ 1.6
IVC flow through foramen ovale	46 $\pm$ 1.6
Superior vena cava + coronary veins	15 $\pm$ 0.9
Lungs	10 $\pm$ 1.6
Ductus arteriosus	35 $\pm$ 2.4
Aortic isthmus	38 $\pm$ 205
Hindpart of body	19 $\pm$ 2.6
Umbilical flow	57 $\pm$ 2.0

Adapted from Dawes GS, Matt JC, Widdicombe JG: The foetal circulation in the lamb. J Physiol 1954;126 (3):563–587.

FETAL CIRCULATION

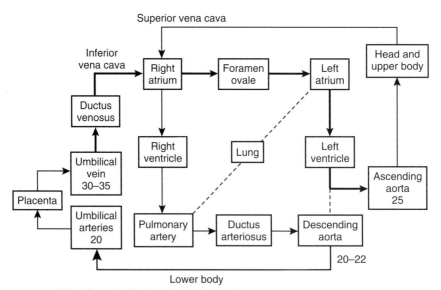

Figure 16-1 Diagram of blood flow in the fetal circulation. The most highly oxygenated blood of the fetus follows the path of the broader arrows. All numerical values represent Po_2.

adaptation process. As shown in Figure 16-2, ventilation of the lungs of fetal lambs with a gas mixture that enhances oxygenation and reduces carbon dioxide levels is associated with increased pulmonary blood flow when compared to unventilated control subjects. Increasing the Pao_2 and decreasing the $Paco_2$ of the alveolar gas and blood by altering the concentrations of oxygen and carbon dioxide of the inhaled gas further

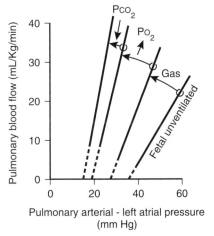

Figure 16-2 This graph demonstrates the right ventricular pressure and pulmonary blood flow as related to pulmonary vascular resistance in an unventilated fetal lung, the fetal lung ventilated with a gas mixture that maintains the Po_2 and Pco_2 of the fetal blood at fetal levels, and a gas mixture that increases Po_2 of fetal level to neonatal levels and decreases Pco_2 of fetal blood to neonatal levels.

augments pulmonary blood flow. The increased flow is directly related to the decrease in pulmonary vascular resistance that occurs after ventilating the lungs with gas and relieving the hypoxia and hypercarbia of the normal in utero environment.

With resection of the umbilical cord and loss of the low resistance placental circulation at birth, systemic resistance increases, producing a higher systemic blood pressure when compared to pulmonary arterial blood pressure. As the hypoxia of fetal life is relieved, both the ductus arteriosus and ductus venosus start to close, resulting in an increase in pulmonary blood flow and left atrial filling (preload). The increased left atrial filling raises left atrial pressure, which closes the foramen ovale. These changes are shown in Figures 16-3 and 16-4, which demonstrate transitional and neonatal circulation, respectively.

Failure of elevated pulmonary vascular resistance to decrease postnatally can result in persistence of both intracardiac (foramen ovale) and extracardiac (ductus arteriosus) right-to-left shunting, producing central cyanosis. Those infants may be misdiagnosed as having cyanotic congenital heart disease. Several factors are known to be associated with pulmonary hypertension and include fetal distress with or without the passage and aspiration of meconium, aspiration of amniotic fluid, chronic intrauterine

TRANSITIONAL CIRCULATION

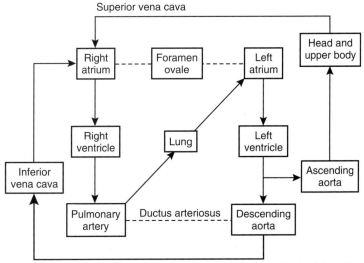

Figure 16-3 Transitional circulation. This figure demonstrates the changes in pulmonary and systemic blood flow during the transition from fetal to neonatal circulation. The dotted lines represent decreasing flow from the right atrium and pulmonary artery to the left atrium and descending aorta, respectively, with resultant increase in blood flow through the lungs.

NEONATAL CIRCULATION

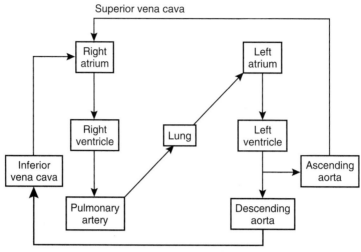

Figure 16-4 Neonatal circulation.

"hypoxia" with medial hypertrophy of medium-sized pulmonary arterioles, parenchymal lung diseases characterized by decreased functional residual capacity, and perhaps chronic maternal ingestion of ibuprofen or prolonged treatment with indomethacin. In infants with persistent pulmonary hypertension, ventilation and adequate oxygenation are important because oxygen is a pulmonary artery vasodilator and carbon dioxide a vasoconstrictor. An echocardiogram is necessary to make certain that suspected pulmonary hypertension is truly present and is unrelated to either left atrial or pulmonary venous obstruction.

Physical Examination of the Neonate with Suspected Congenital Heart Disease

Except for percussion, which has minimal, if any, value in the neonatal physical examination, the other classical components of the physical examination—inspection, palpation, and auscultation—remain important in the evaluation of a critically ill neonate.

Inspection

Always take the time to evaluate every neonate with your eyes before performing palpation or auscultation. First and foremost, evaluate the state of alertness. A term neonate should be in a flexed posture with spontaneous movement

of all extremities and should have a lusty cry. Jaundice should not be visible in the first day of postnatal life and petechiae (other than perhaps over the presenting part) and central cyanosis should never be present. Acrocyanosis, or cyanosis of the hands and feet, is a normal finding in neonates and probably relates to sluggish blood flow with continued oxygen extraction by the tissues in the most distal parts of the upper and lower extremities. The neonate with CHD should not have an altered state of alertness, except in the increasingly rare case of cardiovascular collapse and hypotension as seen in hypoplastic left heart syndrome (HLHS) after ductal closure; the findings of encephalopathy with pallor, petechiae, and jaundice early on should lead toward the diagnosis of infection or a metabolic disorder. The respiratory effort should be unlabored and there should not be audible grunting or retractions of the intercostal or subcostal regions with inspiration. The volume of the chest should increase symmetrically with inspiration; however, the anteroposterior diameter of the chest should not appear "barrel-shaped" or increased. Dyspnea, increased work of breathing, as opposed to tachypnea, increased rate of breathing (respiratory rate > 60 breaths per minute, counted for a full minute), suggests primary lung disease as an etiology for respiratory distress or cyanosis, not CHD, unless pulmonary venous drainage is obstructed at any level from the mitral valve back toward the pulmonary veins. Respiratory distress that begins in the first few hours of postnatal life is usually a manifestation of underlying parenchymal lung disease, not heart disease. Differential cyanosis, or cyanosis of the lower body without cyanosis of the upper body, may be seen in some babies with abnormalities of the aortic arch. Apnea does not usually occur in neonates with CHD. Edema is not a usual sign of congestive heart failure in the neonate, except as may be seen in neonates with hydrops fetalis.

Palpation

Always include palpation in the physical examination and evaluation of every neonate, but especially those with suspected CHD. Increased precordial activity to palpation is not normal, and usually is associated with right ventricular overload or hypertension. You will need to palpate the precordium of many normal neonates before easily deciding if a particular neonate has a hyperdynamic precordium. It is very important to palpate the peripheral pulses. Femoral pulses should always be palpable, and should be equal in volume and pulsation to those of the axillary arteries. Palpating radial arterial pulses for the diagnosis of CHD in neonates should be supplanted by palpation of axillary pulses, which are much easier to feel. If pulses are very easy to feel, consider a diastolic runoff creating a widened pulse pressure as an etiology, such as in a neonate with patent ductus arteriosus (PDA) or arteriovenous (AV) malformation. Thrills are not commonly felt in neonates, and the presence of a thrill would be a significant tip to semilunar valve obstruction, or significant AV valve insufficiency. Do not forget to palpate the abdomen for the size and location of the liver. The normal liver of a neonate may extend 1 to 2 cm below the right costal margin in the midclavicular line, but no further. Hepatomegaly is one of the key physical findings of right ventricular failure or dysfunction. A midline or left-sided liver may be a clue as to the presence of CHD before any other significant signs and symptoms are present. Remember to feel for a temperature differential between the skin of the abdomen and the distal extremities. That disparity may be present in neonates with sepsis or in those with cardiac-related abnormalities of perfusion.

Auscultation

The quality and intensity of the second heart sound is an important clue to identifying an infant with CHD. A loud second heart sound suggests increased pulmonary blood flow or pulmonary hypertension. A single second heart sound (difficult to appreciate at first, but when discovered, a big help in diagnosis) suggests either the absence (atresia) of one of the semilunar valves or malposition of the semilunar valves as in a neonate with transposition of the great vessels (TGV). Make note of where you hear the heart tones the loudest; if the heart is in the right side of the chest, in the absence of a left-sided pneumothorax or left-sided space-occupying lesion, suspect CHD in a dusky or cyanotic neonate.

Murmurs detected in the immediate newborn period are not indicative of CHD in and of themselves; they may represent flow across a transiently insufficient tricuspid valve (holosystolic) or across a PDA. As a general rule, harsh crescendo-decrescendo murmurs heard at birth represent flow across stenotic AV valves. *Many serious cardiac lesions may not present with any murmur at all.* If myocardial function is depressed, a lesion that may be thought to have a murmur upon presentation may have a silent presentation. Do not forget to listen over the head and abdomen for a bruit in a neonate with congestive heart failure; cranial and hepatic AV malformations are infrequent but not rare causes of heart failure, although they may be present without an audible bruit.

The Cyanotic Newborn

Case Study 1

You are called to see a 6-hour-old, 3.8-kg term newborn male, with "blue color" and no dyspnea. On examination, the heart rate is 140 bpm, the respiratory rate is 42, and blood pressure in the right arm is 65/38 mm Hg. There is a generalized cyanotic appearance to the baby. Oxygen saturation readings in the right hand and right leg are 70%. Neither nasal flaring nor retractions are present. The lung fields are clear to auscultation. The cardiac examination reveals an active precordium, normal, equal upper and lower extremity pulses, and no murmur. The liver is not enlarged. The chest radiograph shows normal abdominal situs and a left-sided aortic arch. The lung fields are clear, the heart size is normal, and there is a thymus present. The electrocardiogram reveals normal sinus rhythm and right ventricular hypertrophy appropriate for age.

Exercise 1

QUESTIONS

1. What should be done next?
2. Indicate whether the following statements are true or false.
   a. Peripheral cyanosis in the neonate is never normal.
   b. Central cyanosis in the neonate is normal under certain circumstances.

ANSWERS

1. Give 100% O_2 via nasal cannula at 1.5 L/minute and assess any change in respiratory status.
2. Both statements a and b are false.

Traditionally—now these terms are somewhat outdated—CHD was divided into "cyanotic" and "acyanotic" forms. Prior to describing the presentation and differential diagnosis of "cyanotic" CHD (lesions with a right-to-left intracardiac shunt resulting in arterial hypoxemia), it is useful to review the definition and causes of cyanosis in the newborn.

Cyanosis is a clinical sign manifested by a bluish color of the skin and mucous membranes and caused by the presence of a minimum of 3 to 5 g/dL of deoxygenated hemoglobin in the circulating blood. Cyanosis in the neonate may be "central" (affecting the skin, body organs, and mucous membranes) or "peripheral" (acrocyanosis, affecting the skin of the distal extremities, especially the hands and feet).

Central cyanosis in the neonate is never normal; peripheral cyanosis in the neonate usually is normal in an otherwise healthy-appearing neonate. The unifying feature of all neonates with central cyanosis is an increased level of circulating deoxyhemoglobin and usually a decreased level of circulating oxyhemoglobin. Hypoxemia is the most frequently associated pathologic change and may be due to intracardiac right-to-left shunting ("cyanotic" CHD, or "acyanotic" CHD with elevated pulmonary vascular resistance) or intrapulmonary right-to-left shunting (lung disease, altered control of breathing). Less common etiologies for cyanosis are those without associated hypoxemia and include polycythemia and disorders of hemoglobin/oxygen binding as caused by methemoglobinemia or hemoglobin M disease.

Each gram of hemoglobin maximally binds with 1.34 mL of oxygen. If a neonate's hemoglobin concentration is 18 g/100 mL of blood, at full (100%) saturation, the amount of oxygen carried by the arterial blood is 24.1 mL oxygen/100 mL blood (18 × 1.34). Some oxygen is carried by blood dissolved in plasma, but at usual blood oxygen tensions, this amount of oxygen is negligible. In the preceding example, the oxyhemoglobin concentration is 18 g/100 mL of blood and the deoxyhemoglobin concentration is essentially zero. In this case the oxygen capacity of the blood (the total amount of oxygen that can be bound or taken up by hemoglobin) is 24.1 mL/100 mL blood, the same as the oxygen content (the amount of oxygen actually carried by the blood). However, if the same neonate were hypoxemic, for example, if the hemoglobin saturation of the arterial blood were measured at 60% rather than 100%, the oxygen content of the blood would be 14.5 mL oxygen/100 mL of blood (24.1 × 0.6) and the oxygen capacity would be unchanged at 24.1 mL/100 mL of blood. The oxyhemoglobin concentration would be 10.8 g/100 mL of blood (18.0 × 0.6) and the deoxyhemoglobin concentration would be 7.2 g/100 mL of blood (18.0–10.8). This neonate would appear cyanotic, as there is more than 3 to 5 mg of deoxyhemoglobin in the peripheral circulation. However, this same child might not appear cyanotic in the presence of anemia. For example, if the hemoglobin concentration were 9 g/100 mL of blood and the hemoglobin saturation were 60%, cyanosis would be difficult to detect (9 g/100 mL of blood × 60% saturated = 5.4 g oxyhemoglobin and 3.6 g deoxyhemoglobin/100 mL blood).

Caveat 1

The *presence* of cyanosis typically suggests arterial hypoxemia, but the *absence* of visible cyanosis does not rule out hypoxemia if there is concurrent anemia.

The amount of oxygen carried by hemoglobin is directly related to the partial pressure of oxygen in the blood (Po_2), and to a lesser extent upon blood temperature, pH, and the presence of fetal hemoglobin. Hemoglobin is almost fully (100%) saturated at a Po_2 greater than 70 mm Hg; the hemoglobin saturation does not increase significantly as the Po_2 increases from 70 to 700 mm Hg, although the amount of oxygen dissolved in the plasma does increase. Figure 16-5 depicts the relationship between Pa_{O_2} and hemoglobin saturation of blood. The oxygen content depends upon the hemoglobin concentration and the Pa_{O_2}; the relative contribution of dissolved oxygen can be seen in this figure.

How is partial pressure (gas tension) of individual gases in a mixture determined? Gas tensions are described by Dalton's law, which states that the pressure exerted by gases in a mixture is equal to the sum of the partial pressures of each gas within that mixture. The partial pressure of each gas in a mixture (PA, PB, PC) is the product of the percentage of the gas in that mixture multiplied by the total pressure (PT) of all gases in the mixture.

$$PT = PA(\%A \times PT) + PB(\%B \times PT) + PC(\%C \times PT)$$

For example, PT (barometric pressure) of air at sea level is 760 mm Hg or, as the meteorologist reports, 29.9 inches of mercury (29.9 inches equals 760 mm). The percentage of oxygen in air is approximately 20.9%, that of carbon dioxide is approximately 0.03%, and that of nitrogen is approximately 78.1%, with trace gases composing the remaining 0.97%. Because all gas we breathe is fully humidified, either naturally or artificially, the partial pressure of water vapor (47 mm Hg) must be subtracted from the barometric pressure of air (PT) prior to calculating the partial pressures of each individual gas.

$$PT - PH_2O \text{ vapor} = 760 \text{ mm Hg} - 47 \text{ mm Hg}$$
$$= 713 \text{ mm Hg}$$

Composition of Air

P_{O_2}	713 mm Hg × 0.209	= 150 mm Hg
P_{CO_2}	713 mm Hg × 0.0003	= 0.2 mm Hg
P_{N_2}	713 mm Hg × 0.781	= 556 mm Hg
Other trace gases	713 mm Hg × 0.0097	= 6.9 mm Hg
Total	100%	713 mm Hg

Air enters into the lungs and is distributed to the alveoli by the process of ventilation. In the alveoli, gases diffuse either into or from the blood along concentration gradients (i.e., from regions of higher partial pressures to regions of lower partial pressures) in an attempt to establish equilibrium. Because oxygen is consumed by the body for a vast array of metabolic processes, the blood returning from the systemic circulation and entering the lungs through the pulmonary artery has a lower partial pressure of oxygen than that of fresh alveolar gas. Because carbon dioxide is produced by the body, the blood returning from the systemic circulation and entering the lungs through the pulmonary artery has a higher partial pressure of carbon dioxide than that of fresh alveolar

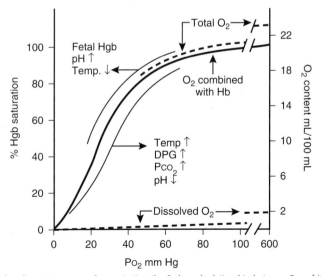

Figure 16-5 Oxyhemoglobin-dissociation curve demonstrating the S-shaped relationship between P_{O_2} of the blood and hemoglobin saturation and the linear relationship between dissolved oxygen and P_{O_2}.

gas. Neither nitrogen nor the trace gases are consumed or produced by the body, so the partial pressure of nitrogen as well as that of the trace gases is the same both in the blood entering the lungs and in the fresh alveolar gas. The percentage of carbon dioxide in alveolar gas under normal conditions of ventilation is 6.5% (P_{CO_2} = 46 mm Hg, 713 mm Hg × 0.065); the percentage of oxygen in alveolar gas is 14.5% (P_{O_2} = 104 mm Hg, 713 mm Hg × 0.145). In the absence of ventilation/perfusion mismatch, hypoventilation or congenital heart lesions in which oxygenated and deoxygenated blood mix in the heart prior to ejection into the aorta, the aortic P_{O_2} should equal pulmonary venous P_{O_2} (approximately 100 mm Hg). The difference between alveolar P_{O_2} (P_{AO_2}) and arterial P_{O_2} (P_{aO_2}), the alveolar-arterial oxygen difference, should be less than 5 mm Hg. This A-a$_{O_2}$ gradient is actually higher in the first few days of life, perhaps 30 to 40 mm Hg, when the lungs transition from the fluid-filled state they had in utero to a gas-filled structure, and pulmonary blood flow is established to 100% of right ventricular output, rather than the 10% of right ventricular output present in utero.

As has been suggested, hypoxemia with resulting cyanosis may be produced by hypoventilation and other forms of lung disease. In these situations, the administration of supplemental oxygen will improve the arterial P_{O_2}. The so-called "hyperoxia test" can typically distinguish CHD with a fixed intracardiac right-to-left shunt from lung disease. When a child with a low measured oxygen saturation is given 100% oxygen to breathe, and the oxygen saturation in the upper and lower extremities does not achieve a value that is greater than 90%, a fixed intracardiac shunt is present and "cyanotic" CHD is likely ("failed" hyperoxia challenge). However, if the oxygen saturation while breathing 100% supplemental oxygen increases to above 95%, it may be necessary to directly measure the arterial P_{O_2}. In the infant without lung disease, breathing 100% oxygen should result in an arterial P_{O_2} greater than 550 mm Hg. In the presence of significant lung disease the P_{O_2} will generally be above 150 mm Hg; an arterial P_{O_2} of 100 mm Hg would be an abnormal response and suggests the possibility of intracardiac right-to-left shunting.

Caveat 2

"Hyperoxia test": If pulse oximetry is less than 90% when breathing both room air and 100% supplemental oxygen, a direct measurement of P_{O_2} is not required to diagnose a fixed intracardiac right-to-left shunt ("cyanotic" CHD); however, if the pulse oximetry reading is less than 90% in room air and increases to more than 95%, direct measurement of P_{O_2} is necessary to help distinguish intrapulmonary from intracardiac right-to-left shunting. A measured P_{O_2} greater than 150 mm Hg is strongly suggestive of intrapulmonary shunting as the cause for the cyanosis.

Newborns that present with cyanotic CHD are usually (though not always) minimally symptomatic with respect to respiratory distress; typically the care team is more distressed than the baby! These children most commonly present within the first hours to days of life and, in general, have structural heart disease on the right side of the heart—resulting in deoxygenated blood being delivered to the systemic circulation without entering the lungs. Examples of "right-sided" lesions include, but are not limited to, tricuspid atresia/stenosis, pulmonary atresia/stenosis, Ebstein's anomaly, transposition of the great arteries, and tetralogy of Fallot with significant subpulmonary stenosis. Other causes of fixed right-to-left shunt include truncus arteriosus, total anomalous pulmonary venous return, and septal defects (e.g., ventricular septal defects, complete atrioventricular canal) with intracardiac mixing or elevated pulmonary vascular resistance. The administration of supplemental oxygen to a neonate with a right-sided obstructive lesion or transposition of the great arteries will minimally (if at all) relieve the hypoxemia. The administration of oxygen to a neonate with a mixing lesion may relieve the hypoxemia somewhat, but usually not to a full hemoglobin saturation and oxygen content. The P_{O_2} measured in these neonates is the result of the quantities of saturated and desaturated blood mixing within the heart, which is ultimately dependent upon the amount of pulmonary blood flow.

Case Study 1 *Continued*

The baby was given 100% oxygen to breathe via nasal cannula at 1.5 L/minute. The respiratory status did not change, and the pulse oximetry readings changed to 82%, suggesting a fixed, intracardiac right-to-left shunt. An arterial blood gas revealed pH of 7.32, P_{CO_2} of 48 mm Hg, P_{O_2} of 42 mm Hg, and bicarbonate of 22 mEq/L. Given the lack of acidosis, normal ventilation, and absence of respiratory distress (with a normal chest radiograph), the child was not intubated or mechanically ventilated. Given the relatively high hemoglobin of the newborn and normal cardiac output, this degree of hypoxemia is well tolerated and provides enough oxygen delivery to prevent acidosis (as manifested by a normal serum bicarbonate). *Supplemental oxygen at 100% was continued until an echocardiogram confirmed transposition of the great arteries with a small 2 mm ductus arteriosus and foramen ovale, but no ventricular septal defect.* Had a septal defect been present, one would have expected a murmur on physical examination, and perhaps less hypoxemia.

The pediatric cardiologist suggests beginning an infusion of prostaglandin E_1 (PGE_1) at 0.02 μg/kg/minute, and decreasing the supplemental oxygen to achieve pulse oximetry reading of 75% to 85%. Although babies with transposition have normal to increased amounts of pulmonary blood flow, that flow is "ineffective," as it represents blood reentering the pulmonary circuit which has already been oxygenated (from the left atrium, to the left

ventricle, and then back to the pulmonary artery). Opening the ductus arteriosus will increase the "effective" pulmonary blood flow as deoxygenated blood will travel from the high resistance systemic circulation (aorta) to the lower resistance pulmonary circulation (pulmonary artery). In return, there will be increased shunting of oxygenated blood from the left to right atrium across the foramen ovale, providing oxygenated blood to the systemic circulation (left atrium to right atrium to right ventricle to aorta). In cases in which there is an inadequate atrial septal defect or foramen ovale, institution of prostaglandin may not result in improvement in systemic oxygenation, and an urgent balloon septostomy or arterial switch operation may be indicated. Note the relationships between the great vessels, semilunar valves, and course of blood flow in the normal heart and in the neonate with d-TGV, as shown in Figure 16-6. The relationship between the great vessels and that of the semilunar valves can be seen by echocardiogram and is one of the findings used by the echocardiographer to diagnose d-TGV.

The Neonate with Circulatory Collapse

Case Study 2

You are called to the well-baby nursery, where a 4-day-old, 38-week gestation, 3.1-kg female neonate has "poor color and grunting respirations."

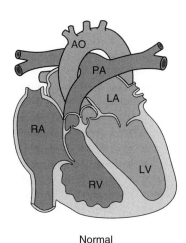 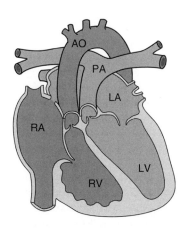

Normal   Transposition of the great vessels

Figure 16-6 Blood flow through a normal heart is compared with a heart in which the great vessels are transposed. AO, aorta; LA, left atrium; LV, left ventricle; PA, pulmonary artery; RA, right atrium; RV, right ventricle.

In the preceding 12 hours her mother noted that she did not seem as interested in nursing. On examination, the baby had a sallow, pale, gray color, with little spontaneous activity and audible grunting upon exhalation. The heart rate is 175 bpm and the respiratory rate is 66, with nasal flaring and subcostal retractions. Peripheral pulses are weak and thready throughout. Neither noninvasive blood pressure measurements nor pulse oximetry measurements can be reliably obtained. The baby responds to stimulation with grimacing and withdrawal. The rectal temperature is 36.5°C. The anterior fontanel is soft, and the baby is mildly jaundiced. There are no petechiae or other skin lesions. The lung fields are clear without rales. The precordium is hyperdynamic, with loud heart tones and a 2/6 harsh systolic regurgitant murmur. The liver edge is palpable 4 to 5 cm below the right costal margin.

Exercise 2

QUESTIONS

1. Which of the following tests would you order next?
   a. Arterial blood gas
   b. Complete blood count
   c. Chest radiograph
   d. All of the above
2. List three left-sided obstructive lesions.

ANSWERS

1. d.
2. a. Coarctation of the aorta
   b. Interruption of the aortic arch
   c. Hypoplastic left heart syndrome

Neonates with "left-sided" obstructions as a manifestation of congenital heart disease (coarctation of the aorta, interruption of the aortic arch, hypoplastic left heart syndrome) typically appear normal at birth, and have a normal physical examination. Systemic blood flow is dependent upon flow from the ductus arteriosus, which may be widely patent at the time of discharge from the well-baby nursery. If there is antegrade flow to the ascending aorta (as in coarctation and interrupted aortic arch), the newborn will not appear cyanotic, as nor-

mally saturated pulmonary venous return is directed to the head and neck. In hypoplastic left heart syndrome, greatly increased pulmonary blood flow may result in relatively high (>85%) oxygen saturations, and visible cyanosis may be absent as well. However, when the ductus arteriosus becomes restrictive, systemic blood flow and oxygen delivery are reduced and circulatory collapse, metabolic acidosis, respiratory distress, and shock ensue; such newborns are frequently misdiagnosed with either bacterial sepsis, viral sepsis, or adrenal insufficiency (secondary to hemorrhage or congenital adrenal hyperplasia).

The diagnosis of congenital heart disease should be considered either before or concurrent with the diagnosis of sepsis or adrenal insufficiency while additional laboratory data are collected and arrangements made for cardiac consultation and echocardiography. Approximately one third of bacteremic neonates have leukopenia and one third have leukocytosis; many have thrombocytopenia. Viral sepsis must be included in the differential diagnosis of a neonate presenting with shock between approximately 2 and 10 days of age. A maternal history of herpesvirus infection or gastrointestinal symptoms secondary to an enteroviral infection may be helpful, but a mother may be asymptomatic if a primary herpes genital infection occurs during gestation. Mothers with a history of previous genital herpes infection may receive chemoprophylaxis to decrease the likelihood of vertically transmitted, perinatally acquired, neonatal herpesvirus disease.

It is important to emphasize that the incidence of congenital heart disease is 8 per 1000 live births; that of sepsis in noninstrumented, term neonates is no greater than 1 per 1000 live births, especially since the introduction and use of chemoprophylaxis to eradicate maternal group B streptococcus colonization of the rectum and genital tract. The incidence of congenital adrenal hyperplasia is 1 in 15,000 live births, making it a much less common diagnosis than either sepsis or CHD. Therefore, the term neonate presenting with acute onset respiratory distress, circulatory insufficiency, or shock must be considered to have left-sided, "ductal-dependent" CHD until proved otherwise. Prostaglandin E_1 should be started while arrangements for definitive diagnosis by echocardiography are being made.

<table>
<tr><td>

Caveat 3

The presence of diminished femoral pulses, brachiofemoral delay, or a higher systolic blood pressure in the upper extremities compared to the lower extremities is highly suggestive of arch obstruction; however, *the absence of a blood pressure gradient does not rule out arch obstruction if the ductus arteriosus is widely patent.*

</td></tr>
</table>

Cardiac Murmurs

Cardiac murmurs are common in the newborn period and are caused by pressure gradients either between the ventricle and the atrium (atrioventricular valve regurgitation), the ventricle and the great artery (pulmonary or aortic stenosis), or the aorta and the pulmonary artery (ductus arteriosus) or between the left and right ventricles once pulmonary vascular resistance has fallen (ventricular septal defect) Thus, murmurs in the newborn may reflect flow patterns that are associated with the normal circulatory transition from fetal life to extrauterine neonatal life, or may be markers of significant congenital heart disease. For example, the murmur of tricuspid regurgitation or that of a closing patent ductus arteriosus may be heard on day 1 and disappear by days 2 to 3. The systolic ejection murmur associated with semilunar valvular stenosis (pulmonary or aortic) is present from birth onward. Murmurs representing left-to-right flow at the ventricular level in neonates with ventricular septal defects may not be present on day 1 but are usually heard later in the first week of life.

<table>
<tr><td>

Caveat 4

A harsh, loud murmur in the delivery room or immediate neonatal period frequently signifies CHD; however, *the absence of a murmur does not rule out CHD.*

</td></tr>
</table>

Case Study 2 *Continued*

The baby was given 100% oxygen to breathe via nasal cannula at 1.5 L/minute. An arterial blood gas revealed a pH of 7.12, P_{CO_2} of 28 mm Hg, P_{O_2} of 56 mm Hg, and bicarbonate of 8 mEq/L. The calculated base deficit was

−18. The serum glucose concentration was 58 mg/dL. Serum sodium, potassium, chloride, and ionized calcium were normal. The white blood cell count was 22,000/mm³ with a hemoglobin of 18 g/dL and platelet count of 242,000/mm³. The differential blood count included 56% polymorphonuclear cells and 4% bands. A chest radiograph showed normal abdominal situs, pulmonary edema versus inflammation, and cardiomegaly. Based upon the postnatal age of the patient, the lack of risk factors or clinical evidence of infection, the severe metabolic acidosis, and poor perfusion, in conjunction with the chest radiographic findings, an infusion of PGE_1 was begun at 0.1 μg/kg/minute (in addition to a blood culture and initiation of broad-spectrum antibiotic therapy). An echocardiogram revealed hypoplastic left heart syndrome with a restrictive, closing ductus arteriosus, moderate tricuspid regurgitation, and normal ventricular function. The cardiologist suggested placing the baby in F_{IO_2} 0.21.

The severe metabolic acidosis represents poor tissue oxygen delivery secondary to low systemic blood flow, rather than secondary to hypoxemia. The single ventricle must supply blood flow to both the lungs and the systemic circulation; in the face of a closing ductus arteriosus, the majority of the cardiac output is recirculated through the lungs, rather than delivering oxygen to the tissues. Pulmonary vasodilators, such as oxygen, and hypocarbia reduce pulmonary vascular resistance and "steal" blood from the systemic circulation; therefore, they should be avoided. In addition, most inotropic agents (e.g., dopamine, dobutamine, epinephrine) will increase systemic vascular resistance and heart rate, but will not improve systemic perfusion until the ductus arteriosus is widely patent. As mentioned in Case Study 1, a systemic oxygen saturation of 75% to 85% is sufficient to provide adequate tissue oxygen delivery, as long as systemic blood flow and hemoglobin concentration are adequate. Supplemental oxygen should be titrated to this target level.

Given the adverse effects on the myocardium of significant metabolic acidosis, cautious administration of sodium bicarbonate via infusion should be performed, with a minimal target pH of 7.3. The acute infusion of bicarbonate generates CO_2 as a by-product, and *adequate ventilation should be assured. In this case, even though there is evidence of good CO_2 elimination (ventilation) on the arterial blood gas, intubation and mechanical ventilation should be considered if the infant's clinical condition does not improve. However, the potential adverse effects of positive pressure ventilation on myocardial preload and variability in pulmonary vascular resistance must be considered; in most cases, spontaneous ventilation is preferred. Central access should be obtained (through the umbilicus if possible). In addition, there should be an evaluation for end-organ injury, especially the brain, kidney, and intestine.*

Congenital Heart Disease Diagnosed Prenatally

Increasingly, complex CHD is being diagnosed in fetal life, with significant advantages to the newborn and family. The baby can be delivered into an expectant team of caregivers. In addition, families can choose location of delivery based upon the expected need of neonatal cardiac surgery, and acquire knowledge about the lesion and anticipated outcomes prior to the stressful postnatal time period. The diagnosis, anticipated course following separation from the placenta, evolution of the physiology during the transitional circulation, and need for prostaglandin should be discussed between the pediatric cardiovascular and perinatal teams. Knowledge of the anticipated oxygen saturation, use of supplemental oxygen, and indications and contraindications for airway management should be anticipated as well.

Caveat 5

A "normal" fetal ultrasound can rule out most, but not all, significant heart disease. Coarctation of the aorta can be particularly difficult or impossible to diagnose in the fetus owing to the patency of the ductus. Transposition of the great arteries may be difficult to exclude in some fetuses with an abnormal lie. *A "normal" prenatal ultrasound should not divert the clinician away from the diagnosis of CHD if other signs or symptoms point to heart disease.*

Initial Management of the Newborn with Suspected or Confirmed Congenital Heart Disease

Management of the neonate with complex CHD needs to be individualized, but a few general principles can be followed. In most cases of critical CHD, patency of the ductus is necessary to provide adequate systemic blood flow (left-sided obstructive lesions) and pulmonary blood flow (right-sided obstructive lesions) and to enhance intercirculatory mixing (transposition of the great arteries). Thus, an infusion of PGE_1 is necessary in many cases. Usual starting doses are 0.05 to 0.1 µg/kg/minute, but this dose may be rapidly decreased to 0.01 µg/kg/minute once patency of the ductus is established by echocardiography. Side effects of prostaglandin are related to higher doses and lower birth weights and include vasodilation with hypotension, apnea, and fever.

In most neonates with CHD, supplemental oxygen will cause a decrease in pulmonary vascular resistance, and in patients with single ventricle heart disease this may result in a "steal" of systemic output into the pulmonary vascular bed. Titration of supplemental oxygen to achieve a systemic oxygen saturation of about 80% is a good guideline in most cases. Following a definitive diagnosis, continued high-dose inotropic support, intubation, and mechanical ventilation are rarely necessary. Sedation may be helpful to reduce oxygen consumption in children with borderline oxygen delivery.

Exercise 3

QUESTIONS

1. Name four categories of lesions that produce CHD.

2. What are the usual presenting signs and symptoms of right-sided obstructive lesions that produce CHD?

3. What are the usual presenting signs and symptoms of left-sided obstructive lesions that produce CHD?

4. What are the usual presenting signs and symptoms of intracardiac mixing lesions without left- or right-sided lesions?

5. What are the usual presenting signs and symptoms of obstruction to pulmonary venous return?

6. Which signs and symptoms should direct thoughts *away* from the diagnosis of CHD and *toward* the diagnosis of early onset sepsis?

7. List the signs and symptoms of systemic viral disease.

ANSWERS

1. Right-sided obstructive lesions, left-sided obstructive lesions, intracardiac mixing lesions without left- or right-sided obstruction, and obstruction to pulmonary venous return.

2. Cyanosis without dyspnea

   Cyanosis not relieved by an increase in the ambient oxygen concentration

   A quiet or active precordium

   Single second heart sound

   Normal heart rate and blood pressure

   A chest radiograph with variable heart size but a decrease in pulmonary vasculature

   Normal gas exchange upon auscultation of the chest

3. Diminished femoral pulses with or without difficulty in feeling axillary pulses

   Hypotension with a sallow appearance, poor capillary refill, and tachycardia

   A quiet or active precordium to palpation

   Single second heart sound

   Respiratory distress usually beginning after a latency period of 12 to 24 hours of age

   Cyanosis relieved somewhat by an increase in ambient oxygen concentration

   A chest radiograph with increased pulmonary vasculature and pulmonary edema with or without cardiomegaly

4. Cyanosis relieved to some extent by increasing ambient oxygen concentration

   Signs of congestive heart failure (tachycardia, tachypnea, dyspnea, cardiomegaly, and hepatomegaly)

   No symptoms for the first few days of postnatal life

5. Cyanosis unresponsive to an increase in the ambient oxygen concentration

   Normal gas exchange upon auscultation of the chest

A normal-sized heart by chest radiograph with lungs that are underaerated and edematous

Air bronchograms could be present on radiograph

Clinically the babies act as if they have surfactant deficiency with pulmonary hypertension

Suspicion for pulmonary venous obstruction should be heightened if the obstetric history is inconsistent with a hostile intrauterine environment and an uncomplicated delivery occurred with reasonably normal Apgar scores

6. Onset of apnea in a term neonate

   Hypothermia or hyperthermia (although most neonates with bacterial sepsis present as normothermic)

   Glucose intolerance (either hypo- or hyperglycemia)

   Acute increase in serum bilirubin concentration with visible jaundice

   Altered state of alertness

   Petechiae

   Hypotension with a sallow appearance and poor capillary refill (although as in Case Study 2, hypotension and poor perfusion may be the presenting signs of left-sided obstructive lesions as well)

   Hypotonia

   A latency period of 12 to 24 hours after birth before onset of symptoms unless associated with premature rupture of membranes (history of chorioamnionitis is frequently absent but if present is helpful)

   Respiratory distress with dyspnea, tachycardia, or hypotension

7. Acute cardiovascular collapse

   Hepatomegaly (a firm liver to palpation rather than the softly enlarged liver seen in congestive heart failure)

   Dyspnea with oxygen dependence

   The presence of petechiae is variable, although the platelet count is frequently decreased

   A bleeding diathesis is usually present

   Cataracts may be present

   Skin vesicles are seen in about one third of neonates with herpesvirus infection

Suggested Readings

Atz AM, Wessel DL: Inhaled nitric oxide in the neonate with cardiac disease. Semin Perinatol 1997;21 (5):441–455.

Castaneda AR, Mayer JE, Jonas RA, et al: The neonate with critical congenital heart disease repair—A surgical challenge. J Thorac Cardiovasc Surg 1989;98 (5):869–875.

Chang AC, Atz AM, Wernovsky G, et al: Milrinone—Systemic and pulmonary hemodynamic effects in neonates after cardiac surgery. Crit Care Med 1995;23(11):1907–1914.

Clancy RR, McGaurn SA, Wernovsky G, et al: Risk of seizures in survivors of newborn heart surgery using deep hypothermic circulatory arrest. Pediatrics 2003;111(3):592–601.

Cua CL, Thiagarajan RR, Gauvreau K, et al: Early postoperative outcomes in a series of infants with hypoplastic left heart syndrome undergoing stage I palliation operation with either modified Blalock-Taussig shunt or right ventricle to pulmonary artery conduit. Pediatr Crit Care Med 2006;7(3):238–244.

Johnson BA, Ades A: Delivery room and early postnatal management of neonates who have prenatally diagnosed congenital heart disease. Clin Perinatol 2005; 32(4):921–946.

Mahle WT, Clancy RR, Moss EM, et al: Neurodevelopmental outcome and lifestyle assessment in school-aged and adolescent children with hypoplastic left heart syndrome. Pediatrics 2000;105(5):1082–1089.

McElhinney DB, Hedrick HL, Bush DM, et al: Necrotizing enterocolitis in neonates with congenital heart disease: Risk factors and outcomes. Pediatrics 2000; 106(5):1080–1087.

Schultz AH, Wernovsky G: Late outcomes in patients with surgically treated congenital heart disease. Semin Thorac Cardiovasc Surg Pediatr Card Surg Ann 2005:8;145–156.

Ward RM, Lugo RA: Cardiovascular drugs for the newborn. Clin Perinatol 2005;32(4):979–998.

Wernovsky G, Rubenstein SD, Spray TL: Cardiac surgery in the low-birth weight neonate—New approaches. Clin Perinatol 2001;28(1):249–264.

Wernovsky G, Chrisant MRK: Long-term follow-up after staged reconstruction or transplantation for patients with functionally univentricular heart. Cardiol Young 2004;14:115–126.

Wernovsky G, Gruber PJ: Common congenital heart disease: Presentation, management and outcomes. In Taeusch HW, Ballard RA, Gleason CA (eds): Avery's Diseases of the Newborn, 8th ed. Philadelphia, WB Saunders, 2004, pp 827–872.

Wernovsky G: Current insights regarding neurological and developmental abnormalities in children and young adults with complex congenital cardiac disease. Cardiol Young 2006;16:92–104.

Wessel DL: Managing low cardiac output syndrome after congenital heart surgery. Crit Care Med 2001;29 (10):S220–S230.

Persistent Pulmonary Hypertension of the Newborn

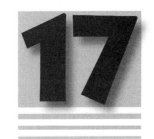

William A. Engle, MD

Persistent pulmonary hypertension of the neonate, historically called persistent fetal circulation, is a potentially life-threatening disorder that may complicate the transition from fetal to postnatal life. This chapter reviews the physiology and pathophysiology, clinical presentation, differential diagnosis, diagnostic evaluation, treatment, and outcomes of neonates with persistent pulmonary hypertension.

This chapter is focused around several case studies, interspersed with exercises followed by discussions.

Pathophysiologic Factors

Case Study 1

A 24-year-old mother presents to the hospital at 39 weeks' gestation for repeat cesarean birth. She has not been in labor. This is her fourth pregnancy; the last two required cesarean section deliveries because the fetus failed to descend during labor. Her last child was critically ill at birth and required intensive care for group B streptococcal sepsis. The mother's prenatal course was complicated by recurrent headaches for which she took large doses of indomethacin daily throughout the third trimester of this pregnancy. There were only two prenatal care visits at 14 and 20 weeks' gestation. Sonography at 20 weeks' gestation was consistent with dating from her last menstrual period, and no gross fetal anomalies were detected. Meconium-stained amniotic fluid (thick and particulate meconium) is noticed when membranes are ruptured at delivery.

Exercise 1

QUESTION

1. Rank the following problems in order of immediate concern in the delivery room for this baby.

   a. Hypothermia

   b. Sepsis

   c. Respiratory distress

   d. Hypoglycemia

ANSWER

1. c, a, d, b. The history of fetal exposure to ibuprofen during the third trimester, a sibling with group B streptococcal sepsis, cesarean section without labor, and the presence of thick and particulate meconium increase the risk for morbidity and death in this infant. Persistent pulmonary hypertension may be associated with a variety of conditions, including transient tachypnea, pneumonia, sepsis, and meconium aspiration syndrome, and may cause severe respiratory failure.[1–6]

Antenatal exposure to inhibitors of prostaglandin synthesis such as ibuprofen and indomethacin can constrict the ductus arteriosus in the fetus. Closure of the ductus arteriosus antenatally forces a greater portion of the fetal cardiac output through the pulmonary vascular bed, resulting in maldevelopment of pulmonary vessels.

Delayed clearance of fetal lung fluid, or transient tachypnea of the newborn, occurs more often in offspring delivered by cesarean section to mothers who have not experienced labor. Although most infants with delayed clearance of fetal lung fluid have mild respiratory distress, this group is at higher risk for persistent pulmonary hypertension than other term infants.

Meconium staining of amniotic fluid occurs in 10% to 20% of all deliveries; meconium aspiration syndrome occurs in 1% to 3% of these cases.[4] The pediatrician's role in managing this infant includes making an immediate decision about whether the infant's trachea should be suctioned for meconium before the first breath. Immediate suctioning of the mouth and nares, followed by visualization of the vocal cords and suctioning of the trachea until it is free of meconium, is indicated for infants born through meconium-stained amniotic fluid who are "not vigorous."[1] "Not vigorous" is defined as having bradycardia (heart rate < 100 bpm), apnea/gasping, or hypotonia. Although thick consistency of meconium is associated with a higher risk for meconium aspiration, immediate tracheal suctioning does not reduce this risk in the vigorous infant.[4,5] The pediatrician's first concern in this case is whether respiratory distress, specifically meconium aspiration syndrome, could be present and whether it might possibly be prevented by suctioning of the trachea before the first breath is taken. Thereafter, drying the infant; assessing respirations, heart rate, and color; and providing further resuscitation are indicated.

Heat loss in the delivery room is usually not an immediate life-threatening problem in a term infant, although it is important to manage the infant in ways to minimize heat loss.[1] Hypothermia is known to increase oxygen consumption, cause release of norepinephrine, and precipitate pulmonary hypertension.[6] Use of a preheated radiant warmer and absorbent towels (for removing wet secretions and amniotic fluid) significantly reduces heat loss.

The infant in this case history is at risk for hypoglycemia. Therefore, attention to glucose homeostasis is important after securing the airway, providing for circulatory adequacy, and ensuring adequate oxygenation.

Although there is no evidence of maternal infection, the risk of chorioamnionitis is increased when a sibling has had group B streptococcal infection. Another risk factor for infection is limited prenatal care. If membranes are ruptured for more than 12 hours (prolonged rupture of membranes), the risk of infection in the neonate is at least 10-fold greater than if membranes are ruptured for less than 12 hours. Concern for infection is appropriate; however, the immediate concern is prompt stabilization and resuscitation.[1] Following stabilization of vital functions, evaluation and treatment for presumptive infection are warranted.

Case Study 1 *Continued*

The baby is "not vigorous" after birth. She is intubated twice and suctioned for a small amount of meconium-stained fluid. Supplemental oxygen (F_{IO_2} 1.0 at 5 L/minute) is administered one-half inch from her nose and mouth to keep the transcutaneous oxygen saturation monitor (on her right hand) reading greater than 95%. The infant is tachypneic and has moderate intercostal retractions. Breath sounds are diminished on the left hemithorax, and a large pneumothorax is confirmed using a transilluminating fiberoptic light. Following thoracentesis, a chest tube is inserted into the fourth left intrapleural space; the tachypnea, retractions, and grunting respirations persist. The transcutaneous oxygen saturation falls to 75% but slowly rises to 91% with administration of 100% oxygen, bag and mask ventilation, and placement on mechanical ventilation. Her right arm, head, and face are pink, but her left arm, trunk, and lower extremities are dusky (Fig. 17-1). The transcutaneous oxygen saturation probe on her right hand reads 90%, and a probe on her foot reads 74%. Hypotension and poor perfusion are treated with an intravenous infusion of normal saline (15 mL/kg) over 15 minutes.

Exercise 2

QUESTIONS

1. What circulatory disturbance is causing the unusual skin color distribution in this infant?

   a. Left-to-right shunting through the foramen ovale

   b. Right-to-left shunting through the foramen ovale

   c. Left-to-right shunting across the patent ductus arteriosus

   d. Right-to-left shunting across the patent ductus arteriosus

2. On Figures 17-2 to 17-4, identify each of the anatomic structures (indicated by lines)

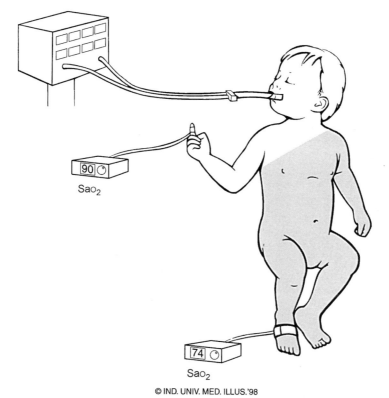

SaO$_2$

SaO$_2$

© IND. UNIV. MED. ILLUS.'98

Figure 17-1 Distribution of cyanosis in the infant in Case Study 1. The clear area represents pink skin color, whereas the gray area indicates cyanosis. This color distribution indicates right-to-left shunting of blood across a patent ductus arteriosus. (Copyright © Indiana University Medical Illustrations, 1998.)

as instructed in the figure legends. Using one line (red) to represent relatively well oxygenated blood and another line (blue) to represent poorly oxygenated blood, trace the expected pathways of blood flow in a fetus, a healthy term neonate (postnatal circulation), and the neonate described in this case study (transitional circulation of persistent pulmonary hypertension). Pay particular attention to the direction of blood flow across the ductus venosus, ductus arteriosus, and foramen ovale in each of the circulations.

ANSWERS

1. d. The presence of pink color in the right arm and head (preductal blood flow distribution) and cyanosis in the left arm, trunk, and lower extremities (postductal blood flow distribution) signifies right-to-left shunting of relatively poorly oxygenated venous blood

across a patent ductus arteriosus (PDA) to the systemic circulation (see Fig. 17-1).[1,3–15] This shunting pattern, which is similar to the fetal circulatory pattern, is maintained because of the presence of increased pulmonary vascular resistance. The presence of this circulatory pattern after birth is termed *persistent pulmonary hypertension of the neonate* (PPHN). Some clinicians prefer the older term *persistent fetal circulation*. Interestingly, only about 50% of patients with PPHN demonstrate right-to-left shunting across the ductus arteriosus. Some of these infants have a bidirectional shunt suggestive of equal pulmonary and systemic arterial pressures. Others exhibit right-to-left shunting across a patent foramen ovale at the atrial level, and those with lung disease also have intrapulmonary shunting; these latter patients are diffusely cyanotic owing to mixing of venous and arterial blood within the left atrium.

2. See Figures 17-5 to 17-7.

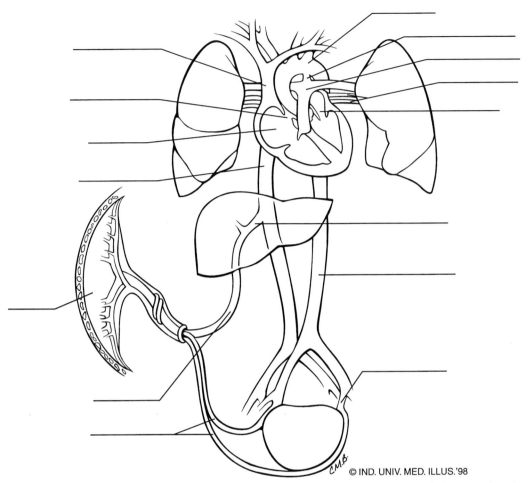

Figure 17-2 Fetal circulation. Identify the aortic arch, superior vena cava, ductus arteriosus, pulmonary trunk, foramen ovale, right atrium, left atrium, pulmonary vein, inferior vena cava, ductus venosus, placenta, internal iliac artery, descending aorta, umbilical vein, and umbilical arteries. Indicate that the blood is well oxygenated by drawing a dotted line and poorly oxygenated by drawing a solid line. Answers are depicted in Figure 17-5. (Copyright © Indiana University Medical Illustrations, 1998.)

Transition from a Fetal Circulation

The transition from a fetal circulatory pattern (see Fig. 17-5) to a postnatal circulatory pattern (see Fig. 17-6) is the result of several simultaneous postnatal events (Table 17-1).[4,10,11,13] Prenatally, the high pulmonary vascular resistance is maintained in the fetus by relative "hypoxemia" (partial pressure of oxygen in umbilical venous blood is approximately 30 mm Hg) and vasoconstrictor dominance of pulmonary vascular tone due to vasoconstricting prostaglandins, leukotrienes, endothelin, and other substances.[7,13,15–25] With the initial respiratory efforts following delivery, air is drawn into the bronchioles and alveolar ducts, and the pulmonary vascular bed is mechanically tethered open; this causes an immediate and significant decrease in pulmonary vascular resistance.[18,26] Pulmonary vascular vasodilatation and increased pulmonary blood flow are further promoted by an increased oxygen tension (especially within the alveolar space), a reduction in carbon dioxide tension, and elevated concentrations of humoral vasodilators such as nitric oxide, prostacyclin, prostaglandin D_2, and bradykinin within the pulmonary circulation.[7,9,11,13,15,27–36] Loss of umbilical venous return from the placenta and closure of the ductus venosus also contribute to a decrease in right atrial pressure (see Fig. 17-7). Furthermore, with

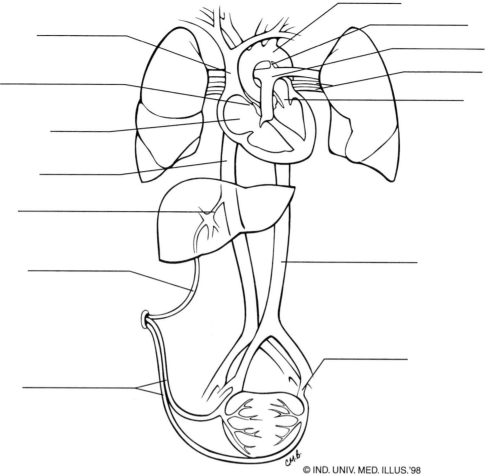

Figure 17-3 Postnatal circulation in a healthy neonate. Identify the superior vena cava, aortic arch, ductus arteriosus, closed foramen ovale, pulmonary trunk, pulmonary vein, right atrium, left atrium, inferior vena cava, ligamentum venosum, descending aorta, ligamentum teres, umbilicus on abdomen, internal iliac arteries, and umbilical ligaments. Using a dotted line for well-oxygenated blood and a solid line for relatively poorly oxygenated blood, indicate the state of oxygenation in the vasculature. Answers are depicted in Figure 17-6. (Copyright © Indiana University Medical Illustrations, 1998.)

loss of the low-reistance placenta and increase in pulmonary venous return to the left side of the heart, systemic vascular resistance increases. The increase in systemic vascular resistance and left atrial pressure and the decrease in pulmonary vascular resistance reverses the right-to-left shunt across the ductus arteriosus and foramen ovale (see Fig. 17-7). The oxygen tension and pressure changes associated with reversal of right-to-left shunting then promote closure of the ductus arteriosus, foramen ovale, and ductus venosus.[37] When these structures close, the transition from the fetal circulation to the postnatal circulation is complete, with the pulmonary vascular tone now dominated by vasodilatory factors (see Fig. 17-6).

Exercise 3

QUESTIONS

1. Which physiologic factors (a through h) are associated with the following four cardiopulmonary transitional events following birth?

   Fall in pulmonary vascular resistance:

   Fall in right atrial pressure:

   Increase in left atrial pressure:

   Increase in systemic vascular resistance:

   Physiologic factors affecting the cardiopulmonary transition after birth:

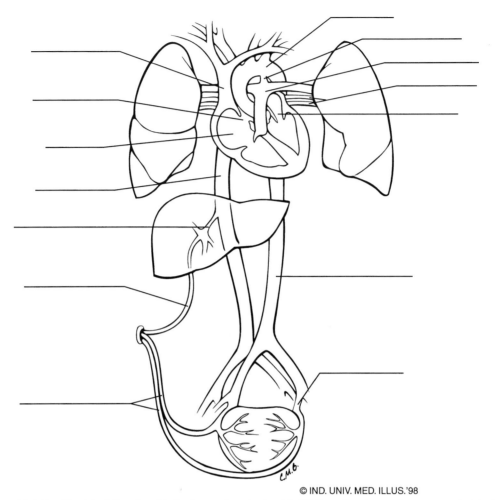

© IND. UNIV. MED. ILLUS.'98

Figure 17-4 Transitional circulation of persistent pulmonary hypertension. Identify the aortic arch, superior vena cava, ductus arteriosus, foramen ovale, pulmonary trunk, right atrium, pulmonary vein, left atrium, inferior vena cava, ligamentum venosum, ligamentum teres, descending aorta, internal iliac arteries, and umbilical ligaments. Indicate the state of oxygenation of the blood by drawing a dotted line for well-oxygenated blood and a solid line for relatively poorly oxygenated blood. Answers are depicted in Figure 17-7. (Copyright © Indiana University Medical Illustrations, 1998.)

a. Initiation of alveolar ventilation

b. Loss of the umbilical circulation

c. Increase in pulmonary venous return

d. Loss of the low resistance placenta

e. Improved oxygenation

f. Closure of the ductus venosus

g. Increase in systemic vascular resistance and left ventricular pressure

h. Change in vasomotor balance due to increased concentrations of vasodilator substances

2. Which of the following factors control pulmonary vascular resistance during the transition of neonates from fetal to neonatal life?

a. Acid-base balance

b. Systemic arterial blood pressure

c. Alveolar distention with inhaled gas

d. Partial pressure of oxygen in arterial blood (Pa_{O_2})

e. Vasodilators (such as nitric oxide, prostacyclin) and vasoconstrictors (such as thromboxanes, leukotrienes, endothelin)

f. Blood viscosity

g. Partial pressure of carbon dioxide in arterial blood (Pa_{CO_2})

ANSWERS

1. Fall in pulmonary vascular resistance: a, e, h.

   Fall in right atrial pressure: b, f.

   Increase in left atrial pressure: c, g.

   Increase in systemic vascular resistance: c, d.

2. a through g.

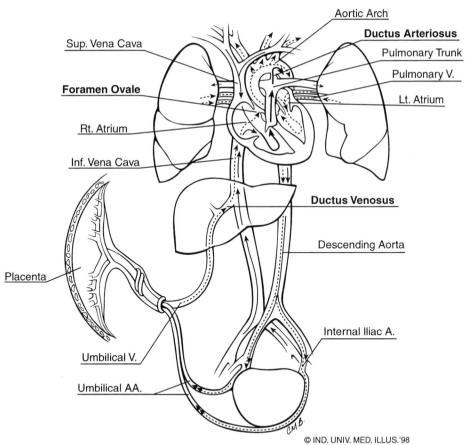

Figure 17-5 Fetal circulation. The three major vascular shunts that maintain the fetal circulatory pattern are the ductus venosus, foramen ovale, and ductus arteriosus. High pulmonary arterial pressure and low systemic vascular resistance play a prominent role in maintaining the shunting of blood from right to left through these shunts during in utero development. (Copyright © Indiana University Medical Illustrations, 1998.)

Postnatal Control of the Pulmonary Vascular Resistance

Neonatal pulmonary vascular resistance and pulmonary blood flow can be altered by an imbalance among the mechanical, humoral, neural, and physical influences that are normally responsible for the decrease in pulmonary vascular tone following delivery (Fig. 17-8).[6,15] Pulmonary hypertension results when an imbalance in these factors occurs. For example, Rudolph and colleagues demonstrated that both hypoxemia and acidosis are potent pulmonary vasoconstrictors that increase pulmonary artery pressure.[26–28] At any given level of oxygen partial pressure in arterial blood (Pao_2), acidosis accentuates hypoxemia-induced pulmonary vasoconstriction.[37] Therefore, any number of neonatal respiratory and cardiac illnesses (Table 17-2) resulting in hypoxemia or acidosis

(respiratory or metabolic acidosis) may precipitate pulmonary vasospasm, decreased pulmonary blood flow, increased right-sided heart strain, and right-to-left shunting through the ductus arteriosus or foramen ovale. Ventilation-perfusion mismatching across diseased lung segments may contribute to intrapulmonary right-to-left shunting. Right-to-left shunting also may be exacerbated further by systemic hypotension. Shunting of relatively poorly oxygenated venous blood into the systemic circulation results in low systemic oxygenation and, if uncompensated by increased cardiac output, reduced oxygen delivery.

The cellular and biochemical events responsible for hypoxic vasoconstriction of the neonatal pulmonary vascular bed are complex and likely due to disruption in the balance between vasodilating and vasoconstricting substances.[6,7,10–13,15] It appears that hypoxia-induced pulmonary

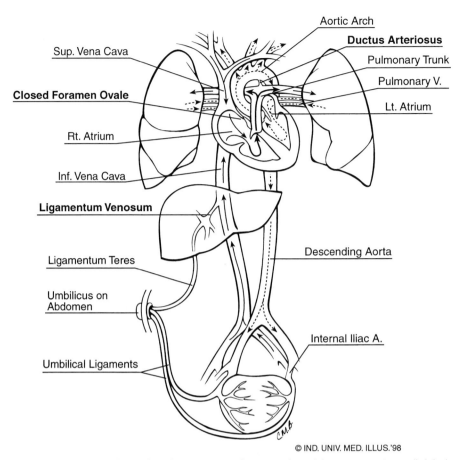

Aortic Arch

Ductus Arteriosus

Pulmonary Trunk

Pulmonary V.

Lt. Atrium

Sup. Vena Cava

Closed Foramen Ovale

Rt. Atrium

Inf. Vena Cava

Ligamentum Venosum

Ligamentum Teres

Umbilicus on Abdomen

Umbilical Ligaments

Descending Aorta

Internal Iliac A.

© IND. UNIV. MED. ILLUS.'98

Figure 17-6 Postnatal circulation. Closure of the ductus arteriosus, foramen ovale, and ductus venosus (now called the ligamentum venosum) characterizes the normal postnatal circulation. Diminished pulmonary arterial pressure, increased arterial oxygen tension, and increased systemic vascular resistance perpetuate the normal flow of blood throughout the pulmonary and systemic circulations. (Copyright © Indiana University Medical Illustrations, 1998)

vasospasm is a *local effect*, because vasoconstriction occurs in experimental preparations in which the nervous system input has been severed.

Decreased concentrations or decreased responsiveness to pulmonary vasodilators (e.g., oxygen, nitric oxide, prostacyclin, potassium-channel activation, or β-receptor activation) may be precipitated by hypoxemia, acidosis, or the underlying disease process.[6,7] Conversely, increased concentrations or increased responsiveness to vasoconstrictors (e.g., leukotrienes C_4 and D_4, thromboxane, endothelin, or α-receptor activation) may be precipitated by similar events.[7] Furthermore, these functional abnormalities may be superimposed on pulmonary vascular maldevelopment (an abnormal distribution of pulmonary vascular smooth muscle and smooth muscle hypertrophy [Figs. 17-9 and 17-10]) and reduction in pulmonary vascular density. Both maldevelopment and reduced

density of the pulmonary vascular tree cause pulmonary hypertension because the portion of cardiac output being pumped through a smaller number of abnormally narrowed vessels is the same or higher than in the normal neonate. Blood flows according to pressure gradients and pressure is proportionate to resistance and blood flow. For example, if resistance increases because the number of pulmonary vessels has decreased without a compensatory reduction in blood flow, pulmonary pressure will increase. Similarly, if pressure in the aorta or the left atrium is lower than the pulmonary artery or right atrium, blood will flow from the pulmonary, or right-sided circulation, across the ductus arteriosus or foramen ovale into the systemic circulation. This abnormal right-to-left shunting of blood flow may be found in a variety of pulmonary and cardiac diseases that cause severe pulmonary hypertension in the newborn.[38–43]

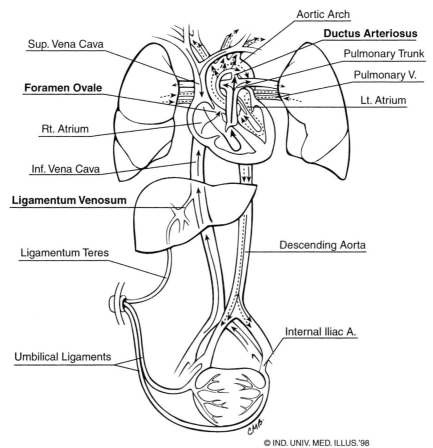

Figure 17-7 Transitional circulation of persistent pulmonary hypertension. Right-to-left shunting of venous blood across the foramen ovale and patent ductus arteriosus due to elevated pulmonary vascular resistance characterizes persistent pulmonary hypertension of the neonate. The poorly oxygenated venous blood mixes with the oxygenated blood exiting the left ventricle, causing systemic cyanosis. (Copyright © Indiana University Medical Illustrations, 1998.)

TABLE 17-1

TRANSITION FROM FETAL TO NEONATAL CIRCULATION

Event	Physiological Consequence	Effect on Cardiovascular System
Alveolar ventilation	Decreased PVR (increased P_{O_2}, prostacyclin, nitric oxide) Increased pulmonary blood flow Increased pulmonary venous return	Increased LA pressure
Placental separation	Decreased IVC return Closure of ductus venosus	Decreased RA pressure Increased SVR
Decreased RA pressure and increased LA pressure		Closure of foramen ovale
Decreased PVR and increased SVR	Reversal of ductal flow Increased P_{O_2} in ductus	Closure of ductus arteriosus

IVC, inferior vena cava; LA, left atrium; PVR, pulmonary vascular resistance; RA, right atrium; SVR, systemic vascular resistance.

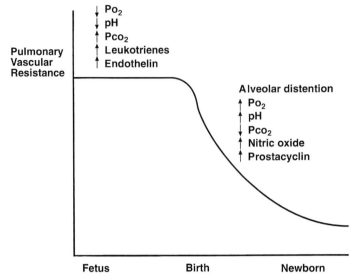

Figure 17-8 Factors that modulate pulmonary vascular resistance in the fetus and newborn infant. Persistent pulmonary hypertension may arise from an imbalance in the factors modulating pulmonary vascular resistance, favoring vasoconstrictive over vasodilatory mediators. (Copyright © Indiana University Medical Illustrations, 1998.)

TABLE 17-2

ILLNESSES ASSOCIATED WITH PERSISTENT PULMONARY HYPERTENSION OF THE NEONATE

Aspiration syndromes: meconium, blood, amniotic fluid
Sepsis/pneumonia
Hyaline membrane disease
Transient tachypnea of the newborn
Idiopathic persistent pulmonary hypertension of the neonate
Air leak phenomena: pneumothorax, pneumomediastinum, pulmonary interstitial emphysema
Pulmonary hypoplasia: congenital diaphragmatic hernia, oligohydramnios sequence
Perinatal asphyxia
Congenital heart disease: total anomalous pulmonary venous return, transposition of great vessels, postoperative cardiovascular surgery

Extracorporeal Membrane Oxygenation

Case Study 2

Baby C, a 2915-g male, is delivered at 37 weeks' gestation to a 33-year-old gravida 1, para 0 woman. The pregnancy was complicated by polyhydramnios. A right-sided diaphragmatic hernia is detected by a fetal sonography at 19 weeks' gestation. Immediately following birth,

baby C is intubated and administered 100% oxygen. An orogastric tube is placed to remove swallowed air. Apgar scores are 6 and 8 at 1 and 5 minutes, respectively. Marked lability in oxygenation is noted with tactile and auditory stimulation. Baby C is mechanically ventilated with 100% oxygen and receives 10 mL/kg normal saline (for poor perfusion) and 0.1 mg/kg midazolam for sedation. Following these interventions, his lability decreases. Umbilical artery and venous catheters are inserted, and an arterial blood gas analysis is performed: pH 7.14, $Paco_2$ 79 mm Hg, Pao_2 49 mm Hg, base excess −2.

Conventional ventilation techniques fail to improve the infant's ventilation and oxygenation, and high-frequency oscillatory ventilation is initiated. Because of worsening hypoxemia (Pao_2 28 mm Hg) despite aggressive medical support (dopamine, dobutamine, intravascular volume expansion, sodium bicarbonate, fentanyl, and inhaled nitric oxide), the family is counseled regarding the risks and benefits of extracorporeal membrane oxygenation (ECMO). After obtaining informed consent, preparations are made for cardiopulmonary bypass. Washed packed red blood cells, platelets, cryoprecipitate, thrombin, and heparin are ordered. Before beginning ECMO, a head ultrasound study and echocardiogram are performed. The head ultrasound is normal, and the echocardiogram reveals changes consistent with pulmonary hypertension. The extracorporeal circuit

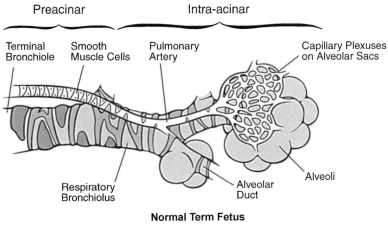

Normal Term Fetus

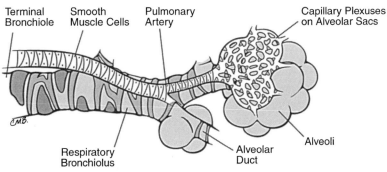

Persistent Pulmonary Hypertension

Figure 17-9 Vascular remodeling occurs in patients with prolonged hypoxia and persistent pulmonary hypertension. The paucity of smooth muscle cells in the arteries within the intra-acinar region of the lung of the normal newborn is replaced by vigorous ingrowth of smooth muscle cells in these arteries in patients with chronic in utero hypoxia or excessive fetal pulmonary blood flow. (Copyright © Indiana University Medical Illustrations, 1998.)

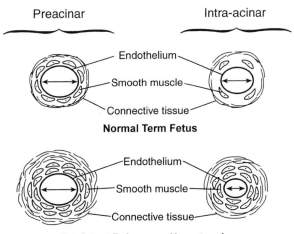

Figure 17-10 Smooth muscle cell mass and mesenchymal connective tissue mass are increased in the intra-acinar pulmonary arteries in patients with prolonged hypoxia or excessive pulmonary blood flow. Vascular remodeling is associated with significantly increased pulmonary vascular resistance, and these patients may be difficult to manage with standard therapeutic strategies. (Copyright © Indiana University Medical Illustrations, 1998.)

is primed, and a double lumen catheter is surgically inserted into the right internal jugular vein. During catheter placement, systemic heparinization is instituted.

Surgical repair of the diaphragmatic hernia is completed at 5 days of age. At 7 days of age, baby C is weaned off ECMO, and at 38 days of age, mechanical ventilation is discontinued. During his postoperative course, baby C is treated with mechanical ventilation and receives therapy for gastroesophageal reflux and intestinal dysmotility. Before discharge at 44 days of age, his neurologic examination is abnormal. At 5 years of age, the child develops a mild pectus excavatum. He is neurologically mildly abnormal with hearing loss in the right ear but appears developmentally normal.

Exercise 4

QUESTIONS

1. Which of the following factors are responsible for the elevated pulmonary vascular resistance in neonates with congenital diaphragmatic hernia?

   a. Pulmonary vasoconstriction

   b. Excess pulmonary blood flow

   c. Pulmonary venous obstruction

   d. Pulmonary vascular hypoplasia

   e. Pulmonary vascular restriction

2. Indicate whether the following statements are true or false.

   a. ECMO allows pulmonary vascular remodeling by providing gas exchange and oxygen delivery while the inherent disease process is treated and the negative effects of high concentrations of oxygen and positive pressure ventilation are reduced.

   b. Venovenous ECMO does not augment cardiac output.

   c. ECMO is associated with an increased risk of intracranial hemorrhage.

   d. Extremely preterm infants (<28 weeks' gestation) are candidates for ECMO.

   e. Neonates with congenital heart disease who are failing medical management despite adequate surgical correction of the defect have a higher survival rate than a neonate with meconium aspiration syndrome failing medical management.

   f. Blood clotting within the ECMO circuit is a relatively common consequence of the need to balance the risk of hemorrhage and the risk of circuit dysfunction due to clot formation.

   g. Hearing loss in critically ill neonates requiring ECMO may not present during the perinatal hospitalization.

ANSWERS

1. a, d, and e. Although *pulmonary vasoconstriction* largely contributes to the increased pulmonary vascular resistance observed in neonates with persistent pulmonary hypertension, *vascular restriction* due to maldevelopment may also contribute to abnormal pulmonary vascular adaptation.[38-41] Extension of pulmonary arterial smooth muscle cells beyond the terminal bronchiolar vessels into the intra-acinar vessels (respiratory bronchiole, alveolar duct, and alveoli) results in a reduction in the internal diameter of these vessels (see Fig. 17-10). Because resistance is inversely proportional to the fourth power of the radius, decreasing the intraluminal diameter increases resistance to pulmonary blood flow substantially. In normal neonates, vascular smooth muscle does not extend beyond the terminal bronchioles. However, in neonates dying from congenital diaphragmatic hernia, persistent pulmonary hypertension, and meconium aspiration syndrome, distal muscular extension into intra-acinar arteriolar vessels occurs.[38,42-44] In addition, neonates with congenital diaphragmatic hernia have *pulmonary arterial hypoplasia* and decreased density of the pulmonary vascular tree because of compression of the lung parenchyma and pulmonary vasculature by intrathoracic bowel or other abdominal organs. If the pulmonary vascular bed is restrictive owing to vascular hypoplasia and distal pulmonary arteriolar muscularization, pulmonary arterial pressure will rise, and right-to-left shunting across the foramen ovale or ductus arteriosus results. In addition, the lung may be hypoplastic.

   An animal model for persistent pulmonary hypertension of the neonate has been developed.[40,41] Ligation of the ductus arteriosus in the fetal lamb 3 to 17 days before delivery causes excessive pulmonary vascular flow and results in increased wall thickness of intra-acinar vessels, elevated pulmonary artery pressure, lower pulmonary blood flow, increased right-to-left shunting, and abnormal pulmonary vascular reactivity. In utero vascular remodeling may be the laboratory correlate for human neonates with extension of pulmonary vascular musculature into intra-acinar locations caused by elevated pulmonary pressure or excessive pulmonary blood. Thus, in utero pulmonary vascular remodeling during human fetal development may signify a preceding in utero stress or a congenital predisposition to neonatal pulmonary vasoreactivity.

2. a, c, f, and g are true; b, d, and e are false.

ECMO is prolonged cardiopulmonary bypass for neonates with respiratory or cardiac failure complicated by pulmonary hypertension or ventricular failure who are unlikely to survive despite maximal medical management.[10,45,46] It is also called extracorporeal life support. During ECMO, oxygen delivery and gas exchange is maintained while the pulmonary and cardiac dysfunction associated with the inherent illness resolve. Pulmonary vascular remodeling and resolution of cardiac dysfunction are the primary events that occur during the ECMO course in those infants who survive. Recovery occurs without the potentially injurious effects of

oxygen toxicity, volutrauma, and barotrauma, which may complicate conventional therapeutic strategies and induce additional pathophysiologic abberations.[47-53]

A diagram of a venovenous (VV) ECMO circuit is depicted in Figure 17-11.[46] Several important observations about the use of prolonged extracorporeal circulation are represented. First, with VV bypass, an extracorporeal circuit is joined to the neonate by a double-lumen internal jugular vein catheter. VV ECMO augments oxygen delivery and partial pressure of oxygen in the right atrium, right ventricle, and pulmonary circulation, thereby effecting a reduction in pulmonary vascular resistance. As a consequence, the flow of well-oxygenated blood increases through the lung and returns to the left atrium, left ventricle, and aortic root. In the aortic root, well-oxygenated blood flows into the coronary circulation and augments cardiac function and output. Therefore, VV ECMO *does* provide support for cardiac function and may be considered in neonates who require high concentrations of vasopressor agents to support blood pressure. However, during insertion of this catheter in the internal jugular vein, the carotid artery is usually identified in the event that cardiac output does not improve on VV ECMO and conversion to venoarterial bypass is required. If the carotid artery must be used for extracorporeal

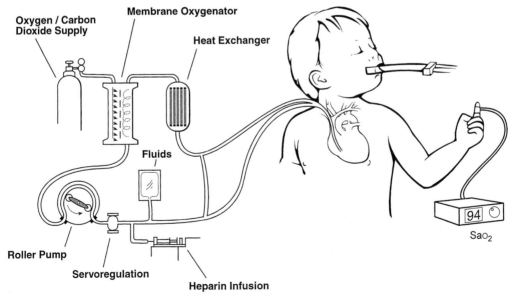

Figure 17-11 Diagram of the circuit used for venovenous extracorporeal membrane oxygenation. Blood drains by gravity from the right atrium into the servoregulating reservoir and is then pumped through a membrane oxygenator for gas exchange and heat exchanger for rewarming before returning to the baby. (Copyright © Indiana University Medical Illustrations, 1998.)

bypass, there is an inherent (but low) risk of cerebral infarction and hemorrhage. The use of VV extracorporeal circulation to avoid carotid artery ligation may reduce this risk.[46,54]

Systemic heparinization to inhibit blood coagulation is necessary because the plastic extracorporeal circuit is thrombogenic.[55-59] In a critically ill, hypoxemic, and acidotic neonate receiving life support with ECMO, there is a moderate risk of intracranial hemorrhage and bleeding.[55] Because of this risk, extracorporeal support is limited to late preterm, term, and post-term infants. Preterm infants are generally excluded from receiving ECMO because of a high inherent risk of severe intracranial hemorrhage. Advances in heparin bonding to the plastic catheters and novel anticoagulation technologies may allow performance of extracorporeal circulation without systemic heparinization in the future.[58,59] Finally, the extracorporeal circuit is a series of mechanical devices, all of which may malfunction.[55] Therefore, specially trained extracorporeal technical specialists must monitor the circuit continuously during treatment to detect and correct equipment malfunction and embolic phenomena (air, fibrin clots).

Candidates for ECMO generally meet specific guidelines (Table 17-3).[10,45,56] To be eligible, neonates are usually older than 34 weeks' gestation (birth weight > 2000 g), have received aggressive mechanical ventilation for less than 10 days (i.e., less likely to have irreversible chronic lung disease), have a reversible pulmonary or cardiac disease, and are at high risk for dying. To predict which infants with respiratory disorders are at highest risk for dying, two indices have been developed to quantitate the degree of respiratory failure.[10,12,45,56] The oxy-genation index (OI) is calculated according to the following formula:

$$OI = \text{Mean airway pressure} \times F_{IO_2} \times 100/Pa_{O_2}$$

An OI greater than 40 (for >2 hours in three of five serial arterial blood gases) is predictive of a 60% to 80% risk of dying.[12,53]

The alveolar-arterial difference in oxygen (AaD_{O_2}) is calculated as follows:

$$AaD_{O_2} = (\text{Atmospheric pressure} \\ -\text{Water vapor pressure})(F_{IO_2}) \\ -\text{Arterial } PO_2 - (Pa_{CO_2}/0.8)$$

A value of 630 or greater for longer than 4 hours is predictive of about an 80% risk of dying.[12]

Many centers that provide extracorporeal support exclude infants with persistent pulmonary hypertension if they have significant intracranial hemorrhage, medically unresponsive bleeding diathesis, irreversible major organ failure, or chromosomal abnormality or syndrome associated with a high mortality rate or extremely poor neurologic prognosis.

When counseling families, it is important to understand that survival outcomes differ depending on the underlying diagnosis. As of July 2004, over 21,000 neonates have received ECMO.[55] Neonates with meconium aspiration syndrome have a 94% survival rate, whereas those with primary persistent pulmonary hypertension and hyaline membrane disease have survival rates of 78% and 84%, respectively. The survival percentages for the other major ECMO patient categories are sepsis, 75%; congenital diaphragmatic hernia, 53%; air leak syndromes, 72%; and congenital heart disease, 36%. Similar to the survival outcomes, the duration of extracorporeal circulation varies with diagnosis. The shortest treatment periods (2 to 5 days) are usually needed for infants with meconium aspiration or primary persistent pulmonary hypertension. Infants with congenital diaphragmatic hernia may require several weeks on ECMO.

The most frequently observed complications in neonates receiving ECMO are intracranial hemorrhage/infarction (15%), cannula site bleeding (6%), surgical site bleeding (6%), seizures (12%), renal insufficiency (9%), hypertension (13%), and hyperbilirubinemia (8%).[10,45,55] Clots within the circuit and cannula problems (11%) represent the most frequent mechanical problems; less frequent problems involve dysfunction of the membrane oxygenator, tubing rupture, cracks in

---

TABLE 17-3

ELIGIBILITY AND EXCLUSION GUIDELINES FOR EXTRACORPOREAL MEMBRANE OXYGENATION

Eligibility
Progressive respiratory or cardiac failure despite maximal medical treatment
≥34 weeks' gestation or birth weight > 2000 g
Reversible pulmonary or cardiac disease

Exclusion
Intracranial hemorrhage (grade II or greater)
Bleeding diathesis unresponsive to medical treatment
Irreversible major organ failure
Chromosomal abnormality or syndrome associated with high mortality or extremely poor neurodevelopmental prognosis

connectors, and air emboli in the circuit. Fortunately, the majority of these mechanical complications are rapidly correctable without adverse outcomes.

Long-term neurodevelopmental outcomes are encouraging for neonates with pulmonary hypertension who are critical enough to receive inhaled nitric oxide or ECMO.[60–74] Nearly 50% to 79% of these children are neurodevelopmentally normal by early school age; 7% to 20% have moderate to severe neurobehavioral problems such as cerebral palsy or low developmental scores on standardized testing.[69–71] However, the incidence of wheezing may be as high as 50% to 75%.[70,72] Neurosensory hearing loss is reported to occur in 3% to 25% of survivors; some infants present with hearing loss during the first one to two years after birth despite passing hearing screening evaluations in the immediate neonatal period. Gastroesophageal reflux and gastrointestinal motility abnormalities frequently occur in neonates with congenital diaphragmatic hernia who survive. These outcomes compare favorably with those neonates with severe persistent pulmonary hypertension who do not receive extracorporeal support or inhaled nitric oxide. The presence of neurodevelopmental and medical disabilities likely reflects the severity of the underlying illnesses experienced by these infants rather than complications of the interventions received.[70,71]

Severe Persistent Pulmonary Hypertension

Case Study 3

Baby H was delivered at 36 weeks' gestation to a 17-year-old gravida 1, para 0 mother who presented to the obstetric clinic because of a decrease in fetal movements. Sonography demonstrated polyhydramnios, absence of a fetal stomach, and fetal hydrops with right pleural effusion, ascites, scalp edema, and anasarca. The fetal heart rate was low at 40 beats per minute, and an emergency cesarean section was performed. Apgar scores were 2 at 1 minute (1 for heart rate of 60, 1 for gasping respiratory efforts) and 5 at 5 minutes (2 for heart rate of 140, 2 for regular respirations, 1 for acrocyanosis, 0 for reflex irritability, and 0 for muscle tone). Immediately after birth, baby H exhibited retractions and grunting respirations. She was diffusely cyanotic

and received supplemental oxygen by mask (F_{IO_2} of 1); 70 mL of clear, yellow fluid was removed from the right hemithorax by thoracentesis. The albumin concentration in the fluid was 2.9 mg/dL and 93% of the white blood cells present were lymphocytes. Owing to persistent respiratory distress and cyanosis, baby H was placed on a mechanical ventilator. Following intubation, the preductal transcutaneous saturation rose to 98%, whereas the postductal transcutaneous saturation remained at 81%. Umbilical arterial and venous catheters were placed under sterile conditions with the tip of the umbilical arterial line in the middle thoracic aorta (postductal). An arterial blood gas from the umbilical arterial line demonstrated pH 7.19, Pa_{O_2} 36 mm Hg, Pa_{CO_2} 45 mm Hg, and base excess −16. During placement of the umbilical lines and suctioning of the endotracheal tube, the preductal oxygen saturation fell to 83% and then gradually returned to 97%. Lability in oxygenation persisted, so minimal stimulation techniques were instituted. In addition, the baby received fentanyl and midazolam. At that time, her physical examination was remarkable for anasarca; diminished breath sounds over the right hemithorax; relative pallor of the left arm, trunk, and lower body; a systolic heart murmur at the left sternal border; a loud second heart sound that split normally; unlabored tachypnea; bilateral transverse palmar creases, flat occiput and facies, epicanthal folds, and hypotonia. The working diagnosis is Down syndrome and congenital chylothorax complicated by hydrops and persistent pulmonary hypertension.

Exercise 5

QUESTION

1. What four clinical findings are indicative of severe persistent pulmonary hypertension in this neonate?

ANSWER

1. a. Cyanosis
   b. Lability in oxygenation
   c. Respiratory distress (tachypnea, retractions, and grunting)
   d. Heart murmur and loud second heart sound

Persistent pulmonary hypertension of the neonate may either be a primary disorder or occur secondary to a variety of underlying pulmonary or cardiac illnesses. Most neonates with pulmonary hypertension are late preterm, term, or post-term.[10,11,53,74] The severity of clinical symptoms associated with persistent pulmonary hypertension varies with the underlying pathology (Table 17-4).

The mildest form of persistent pulmonary hypertension of the neonate is found in infants who present immediately following delivery with cyanosis and unlabored tachypnea. In these infants, the preductal transcutaneous oxygen saturation is usually higher than the postductal saturation due to right-to-left shunting across the ductus arteriosus. This differential in oxygenation usually resolves quickly with administration of oxygen and minimal stimulation. In some cases, intravascular volume expansion and continuous positive airway pressure are required. Chest radiographs are usually clear or may be consistent with retained intraalveolar and interstitial fluid (transient tachypnea). Right-to-left ductal shunting commonly resolves quickly, and normal physiologic stability resumes in less than 24 hours. The terms *delayed transitional circulation* and *transient pulmonary vascular lability* have been used to describe this mild form of persistent pulmonary hypertension of the neonate.[75]

More severe forms of persistent pulmonary hypertension of the neonate are characterized by marked lability in oxygenation, severe cyanosis, and tachypnea. A systolic heart murmur (indicative of tricuspid insufficiency) and hypotension are often observed. Chest radiographs of these patients may be read as normal, may demonstrate mild cardiomegaly, or are consistent with an underlying pulmonary or cardiac disorder. Thrombocytopenia occurs in some infants with persistent pulmonary hypertension. Platelet aggregation within the pulmonary vasculature is thought to occur as a secondary effect of an outpouring of vasoconstrictors (e.g., thromboxanes and endothelin), which induce platelet aggregation and sequestration within the lung.[6,32]

Lability in oxygenation is the hallmark of persistent pulmonary hypertension in neonates. Because this lability is often exacerbated by minimal stresses (e.g., bathing, endotracheal tube suctioning, repositioning), caregiving techniques to minimize these stresses are emphasized. Judicious use of sedatives (e.g., lorazepam, midazolam) and analgesics (e.g., fentanyl, morphine) may be helpful but this is not an evidence-based intervention. Neuromuscular blocking agents (e.g., vecuronium, pancuronium) are occasionally used and generally restricted to infants whose lability in oxygenation is extreme and strict control of ventilation is desired.

Cyanosis and pallor may either be generalized (if right-to-left shunting occurs across the foramen ovale or the diseased lung) or follow a postductal distribution (if right-to-left ductal shunting is present). Differentiating severe persistent pulmonary hypertension from cyanotic congenital heart disease is often difficult when arterial oxygen tensions greater than 100 mm Hg cannot be obtained and the chest x-ray is nondiagnostic. Echocardiography is recommended to help differentiate pulmonary hypertension from other causes of cyanosis in this circumstance (Table 17-5).[76] Echocardiographic features of pulmonary hypertension in neonates include right-to-left or bidirectional shunting across the foramen ovale (or ductus arteriosus), elevated pulmonary artery pressure, bowing of the atrial septum into the left atrium, tricuspid insufficiency, right ventricular enlargement with septal displacement and obstruction of the left ventricular

---

TABLE 17-4

CLINICAL FEATURES OF PERSISTENT PULMONARY HYPERTENSION OF THE NEONATE

Late preterm, term, or post-term gestational age
Onset of symptoms generally within 12 hr of birth or postoperatively
Lability in oxygenation
Intermittent or persistent cyanosis and pallor
Heart murmur
Loud second heart sound
Tachypnea, retractions, or grunting respirations
Variable chest radiograph findings (disease dependent)

TABLE 17-5

EVIDENCE FAVORING THE DIAGNOSIS OF SEVERE PERSISTENT PULMONARY HYPERTENSION OVER THE DIAGNOSIS OF CYANOTIC CONGENITAL HEART DISEASE

Lability in arterial oxygenation or saturation
Pre- and postductal difference in arterial oxygenation or saturation
$Pao_2 > 100$ mm Hg with 100% oxygen inhalation
$Pao_2 > 100$ mm Hg with 100% oxygen and hyperventilation-induced alkalosis
$Pao_2 > 100$ mm Hg with trial of intravenous prostaglandin E_1 administration
Echocardiographic findings of normal cardiac structures and function

outflow tract, and prolongation of the right ventricular pre-ejection phase–right ventricular ejection time ratio.[76] If echocardiography is not available, two simple clinical tests can help differentiate congenital heart disease from pulmonary hypertension (see Table 17-5).[6,10] One is simultaneous measurement of preductal and postductal oxygen saturations or oxygen tension (to detect right-to-left ductal shunting) and the second is placing the infant in 100% oxygen (hyperoxia test) to determine whether an increase in ambient oxygen will significantly increase the partial pressure of oxygen in arterial blood. The presence of a fixed right-to-left shunt as found in congenital heart disease usually precludes an increase in the Pao_2 to 100 mm Hg; an oxygen tension less than 50 mm Hg suggests a diagnosis of cyanotic congenital heart disease. In infants with pulmonary hypertension, oxygen tension usually rises and may exceed 100 mm Hg. If the diagnosis still remains unclear, a hyperoxia-hyperventilation maneuver may be helpful. This test entails lowering the arterial carbon dioxide tension ($Paco_2$ 20 to 35 mm Hg) and elevating the arterial pH to 7.45 to 7.55 by *gently* hyperventilating the infant. An increase in Pao_2 to greater than 100 mm Hg suggests that the patient has persistent pulmonary hypertension rather than cyanotic congenital heart disease. Hyperventilation should not be attempted if it requires raising the ventilator pressures to potentially dangerous levels and should be discontinued as soon as the hyperoxia-hyperventilation maneuver is completed. Some clinicians avoid hyperventilation-induced hypocarbia and alkalosis due to potential for reducing cerebral blood flow.

umbilical arterial blood sample demonstrates pH 7.34, $Paco_2$ 45 mm Hg, Pao_2 33 mm Hg, and base excess −3. The preductal and postductal arterial oxygen saturation concentrations are 82% and 78%, respectively. Additional normal saline (20 mL/kg) is infused, and the rates of administration of dobutamine and dopamine are increased to 20 µg/kg/minute and 15 µg/kg/minute, respectively. In response to these interventions, systolic blood pressure increases to 72 mm Hg. A repeat umbilical arterial blood gas analysis reveals pH 7.35, $Paco_2$ 43 mm Hg, Pao_2 30 mm Hg, and base excess −4. The preductal oxygen saturation is 86% at the time of the blood gas analysis.

High-frequency oscillatory ventilation is initiated at a mean airway pressure of 20 cm H_2O, amplitude of 46 cm H_2O, and frequency of 8 Hz. Surfactant is given through the endotracheal tube. The postductal Pao_2 remains low (38 mm Hg). After a brief trial of conventional ventilation, inhaled nitric oxide is begun at a concentration of 20 parts per million (ppm). A rapid increase in the preductal transcutaneous oxygen saturation to 99% occurs.

Baby H remains stable, and during the next 4 days, she has a significant diuresis and is weaned off the inhaled nitric oxide, vasopressors, and high-frequency oscillatory ventilation. During the subsequent 6 days, she is weaned from mechanical ventilation and supplemental oxygen and advanced to enteral feedings. Karyotype results are compatible with a diagnosis of Down syndrome. Throughout the hospital course, baby H's parents receive support and counseling about their concerns and baby H's medical progress.

Case Study 3 *Continued*

At 12 hours of age, baby H experiences a sudden fall in oxygen saturation while receiving mechanical ventilation at a peak inspiratory pressure (PIP) of 26 cm H_2O, positive end-expiratory pressure (PEEP) of 5 cm H_2O, ventilator rate of 60 breaths per minute, inspiratory time of 0.35 second, and a F_{IO_2} of 1. The PIP is increased, after which the preductal oxygen saturation rises to 96% and the postductal oxygen saturation to 90%. Concurrently, the systemic blood pressure falls from a mean of 52 mm Hg (blood pressure 64/44) to a mean of 36 mm Hg (48/28). Baby H receives 10 mL/kg normal saline, dopamine (5 µg/kg/minute), and dobutamine (10 µg/kg/minute) intravenously. An

Exercise 6

QUESTIONS

Demonstrate your understanding of the treatments for persistent pulmonary hypertension of the neonate by selecting the best answer to the following questions.

1. Treatments to induce alkalinization of the blood may be complicated by which of the following?

   a. Intracellular acidosis

   b. Increased cerebral blood flow

   c. Excessive cardiac output

   d. None of the above

2. Selective pulmonary vasodilation may be achieved with which of the following agents?

    a. Nitric oxide

    b. Nitroprusside

    c. Prostaglandin

    d. Sildenafil

3. Surfactant deficiency may complicate the course of neonates with which of the following?

    a. Meconium aspiration

    b. Sepsis

    c. ECMO therapy

    d. All of the above

ANSWERS

1. a.

2. a.

3. d.

Pulmonary Vasodilation

Alkalinization of the blood with sodium bicarbonate or hyperventilation (to raise the arterial pH to 7.5) is used by some clinicians to induce pulmonary vasodilation in neonates with persistent pulmonary hypertension.[48,77-79] Although the mechanisms by which these therapies effect a decrease in pulmonary vascular resistance are yet to be firmly established, an increase in arterial pH, rather than a decrease in arterial carbon dioxide tension, appears to contribute to this effect.[79,80] Alkalinization with sodium bicarbonate is sometimes used as an adjunct therapy to further increase the arterial pH in an infant who is already being gently hyperventilated. Both sodium bicarbonate infusion and hyperventilation must be used with caution because of potential complications.[49,50,78,81-83] Sodium bicarbonate may aggravate hypercarbia and induce intracellular acidosis.[83] This may result in decreased coronary perfusion pressure, diffuse myocardial ischemia, and diminished cardiac output, thereby compromising cardiac function. Hyperventilation using conventional ventilators may be complicated by barotrauma or volutrauma, with adverse effects on the lung (such as air leak, overdistention, reduced pulmonary blood flow), heart (such as reduced cardiac output), and brain (such as decreased cerebral blood flow).[49,51,60] Alkalinization is not an evidence-based therapy; a gentle-ventilation strategy (e.g., avoidance of hyperventilation) is preferred by many clinicians. High-frequency oscillatory or jet ventilation may be used to minimize some of the risks associated with conventional ventilators when a hyperventilation strategy is used.[74,78,81] Inhaled nitric oxide and ECMO[84] are generally reserved for neonates with severe persistent pulmonary hypertension unresponsive to other supportive therapies (Table 17-6).

Clinician-scientists have investigated a number of agents that dilate the pulmonary circulation.[6,85-93] Inhaled nitric oxide, nitroprusside, prostacyclin, prostaglandins, endothelin, receptor blockers, and inhibitors of phosphodiesterase type five (e.g., sildenafil, dipyridamole, zaprinast) have been administered with variable success.[6,92,93] All of these agents, with the exception of inhaled nitric oxide, unfortunately, dilate both the systemic and the pulmonary beds and may cause systemic hypotension. Only inhaled nitric oxide is a selective pulmonary vasodilator (Fig. 17-12). Inhaled nitric oxide at a concentration of 5 to 20 ppm is safe and effective at reducing risk of dying and decreasing the need for ECMO in neonates with persistent pulmonary hypertension without the need for ECMO.[90,91] Inhaled nitric oxide is particularly

TABLE 17-6

TREATMENT OF PERSISTENT PULMONARY HYPERTENSION OF THE NEONATE

Treat underlying disorder
    Antibiotics
    Surfactant
Monitor arterial oxygenation
Administer oxygen
Attempt to minimize stress in the patient's immediate environment
Administer sedatives and analgesics and, in some cases, induce pharmacological paralysis
Provide mechanical ventilation
Support systemic blood pressure
    Volume expanders
    Vasopressors
Alkalinize the plasma
    Hyperventilation (conventional or high-frequency ventilation)
    Sodium bicarbonate
Administer vasodilator agents
    Selective agents: inhaled nitric oxide
    Less selective agents: nitroprusside, prostacyclin, prostaglandins, tolazoline
Use extracorporeal membrane oxygenation

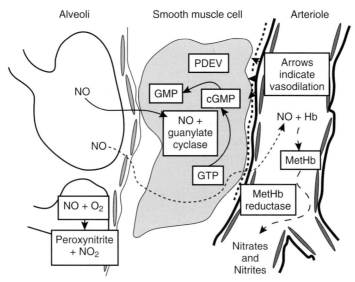

Figure 17-12 Diagram of the nitric oxide (NO) pathway within the lung. Nitric oxide is delivered to the alveolus through the inspiratory limb of the mechanical ventilator and diffuses into the smooth muscle cell surrounding the pulmonary arterioles. Within smooth muscle cells, NO catalyzes the conversion of guanosine triphosphate (GTP) to cyclic guanosine monophosphate (cGMP) by guanylate cyclase. cGMP induces smooth muscle cell relaxation and dilatation of the pulmonary arterioles. cGMP is metabolized by phosphodiesterase V (PDEV). Inhibitors of PDEV act to prolong the presence and vasodilatory effect of cGMP. NO also diffuses into the pulmonary arterioles and combines with hemoglobin (Hb) to form methemoglobin (MetHb). Methemoglobin is metabolized by methemoglobin reductase and excreted as urinary nitrites and nitrates. NO within the alveolus is also converted to peroxynitrites, which are metabolized by superoxide dismutase and nitrogen dioxide (NO_2), which is excreted through the expiratory limb of the mechanical ventilator.

effective when combined with lung recruitment strategies using high-frequency oscillatory ventilation.[91] Although nitric oxide has not been shown to be efficacious in improving survival in neonates with congenital diaphragmatic hernia when used early in their course, some investigators have reported success in stabilizing patients using inhaled nitric oxide until ECMO can be initiated or following treatment with ECMO.

Additional Considerations

Surfactant deficiency in neonates with persistent pulmonary hypertension may complicate meconium aspiration, sepsis or pneumonia, and primary pulmonary hypertension.[94–97] Furthermore, surfactant treatment of neonates with pulmonary hypertension while they are receiving ECMO reduces the duration of extracorporeal support and improves lung compliance, suggesting that secondary surfactant deficiency occurs in these infants.[94–96] Persistent pulmonary hypertension often complicates the pulmonary and cardiac illnesses that affect neonates soon after birth or following cardiovascular surgery. The underlying mechanisms of this physiologic disorder involve an imbalance in positive and negative regulators of pulmonary vascular tone. Resultant cyanosis and hypoxemia further compromise the neonate. Current treatments such as mechanical ventilation, high-frequency ventilation, surfactant replacement, inhaled nitric oxide, and extracorporeal life support have significantly improved morbidity and mortality rates. With increased understanding of the factors that control pulmonary vasomotor tone, we can anticipate the introduction of therapeutic strategies that are more efficacious, carry lower risk, and reduce morbidity.

References

1. Kattwinkel J, Niermeyer S, Denson SE, Zaichkin J (eds): Textbook of Neonatal Resuscitation 4th ed. American Academy of Pediatrics and American Heart Association, 2000, pp 2.1–2.25.
2. Carson BS, Losey RW, Bowes WA, et al: Combined obstetric and pediatric approach to prevent meconium aspiration syndrome. Am J Obstet Gynecol 1976; 126:712–715.
3. Spitzer AR, Davis J, Clark WT, et al: Pulmonary hypertension and persistent fetal circulation in the newborn. Clin Perinatol 1988;15:389–413.
4. Wiswell TE, Gannon CM, Jacob J, et al: Delivery room management of the apparently vigorous meconium-stained neonate: Results of the multicenter, international collaborative trial. Pediatrics 2000;105:1–7.

5. Halliday HL: Endotracheal intubation at birth for preventing morbidity and mortality in vigorous, meconium-stained infants born at term. Cochrane Database Syst Rev 2001;1:CD000500.

6. Ballard RA, Hansen TN, Corbet A: Respiratory failure in the term infant. In Taeusch HW, Ballard RA, Gleason CA (eds): Avery's Diseases of the Newborn, 8th ed. Philadelphia, Elsevier Saunders, 2005, pp 705–712.

7. Soifer SJ, Fineman JR, Heymann MA: Pulmonary circulation. In Gluckman PD, Heymann MA (eds): Pediatrics and Perinatology: The Scientific Basis, 2nd ed. London, Arnold and Oxford Press, 1996, 749–755.

8. Hoffman JIE, Heymann MA: Normal pulmonary circulation. In Scarpelli EM (ed): Normal Pulmonary Physiology. 2nd ed. Philadelphia, Lea & Febiger, 1990, pp 233–256.

9. Heymann MA, Hoffman JIE: Pulmonary circulation in the perinatal period. In Thibeault DW, Gregory GA (eds): Neonatal Pulmonary Care, 2nd ed. Norwalk, CT, Appleton-Century-Crofts, 1986, 149–174.

10. Peters EA, Engle WA, Lemons JA: Persistent pulmonary hypertension of the newborn. Indiana Med 1989;82:13–17.

11. Duara S, Fox WW: Persistent pulmonary hypertension of the neonate. In Thibeault DW, Gregory GA (eds): Neonatal Pulmonary Care. Norwalk, CT, Appleton-Century-Crofts, 1986, pp 461–481.

12. Engle WA, Peters EA, Gunn SK, et al: Mortality prediction in near term and term neonates with respiratory failure and interval until death. J Perinatol 1993;13:368–375.

13. Kinsella JP, Abman SH: Recent developments in the pathophysiology and treatment of persistent pulmonary hypertension of the newborn. J Pediatr 1995; 126:853–864.

14. Kinsella JP, Abman SH: Clinical approach to inhaled nitric oxide therapy in the newborn. J Pediatr 2000;136:717–726.

15. Abman SH: Abnormal vasoreactivity in the pathophysiology of persistent pulmonary hypertension of the newborn. Pediatr Rev 1999;20(11): e103–e109.

16. Ahmed T, Oliver W Jr: Does slow-reacting substance of anaphylaxis mediate hypoxia induced pulmonary vasoconstriction? Am Rev Respir Dis 1983;127:566.

17. Morganroth ML, Reeve JT, Murphy RC, Voelkel NF: Leukotriene synthesis and receptor blockers block hypoxic pulmonary vasoconstriction. J Appl Physiol 1984;56:1340.

18. Enhorning G, Adams FH, Norman A: Effect of lung expansion on the fetal lamb circulation. Acta Paediatr Scand 1966;55:441.

19. Finer NN, Barrington KJ: Nitric oxide in respiratory failure in the newborn infants. Semin Perinatol 1997;21:426–440.

20. Villamor E, LeCras TD, Horan MP, et al: Chronic intrauterine pulmonary hypertension impairs endothelial nitric oxide synthase in the ovine fetus. Am J Physiol 1997;272:L1013–L1020.

21. Galanatowicz ME, Price M, Stolar CJH: Differential effects of alveolar and arterial oxygen tension on pulmonary vasomotor tone in ECMO-perfused isolated piglet lungs. J Pediatr Surg 1991;26: 312–316.

22. Heymann MA: Prostacyclins and leukotrienes in the perinatal period. Clin Perinatol 1987;14:857–880.

23. Duke HN: The site of action of anoxia on the pulmonary blood vessels of the cat. J Physiol 1954;125:373.

24. Leffler CW, Hessler JR, Green RS: Mechanism of stimulation of pulmonary prostaglandins synthesis at birth. Prostaglandins 1984;28:877.

25. Leffler CW, Hessler JR, Green RS: The onset of breathing at birth stimulates pulmonary vascular prostacyclin synthesis. Pediatr Res 1984;18:938.

26. Rudolph AM, Teitel AF, Iwamoto HS, et al: Ventilation is more important than oxygenation in reducing pulmonary vascular resistance at birth. Pediatr Res 1985;20:439.

27. Rudolph AM, Yan S: Response of the pulmonary vasculature to hypoxia and H_2 ion concentration changes. J Clin Invest 1966;45:399.

28. Rudolph AM, Heymann MA: Circulatory changes in fetal lambs. Pediatr Res 1972;6:341.

29. Hauge A: Role of histamine in hypoxic pulmonary hypertension in the rat. I. Blockade or potentiation of endogenous amines, kinins and ATP. Circ Res 1968;22:371.

30. Sada K, Shirai M, Ninomiya I: X-ray TV system for measuring microcirculation in small pulmonary vessels. J Appl Physiol 1985;59:1013.

31. Hammerman C, Lass N, Strates E, et al: Prostanoids in neonates with persistent pulmonary hypertension. J Pediatr 1987;110:470–472.

32. Burhop KE, Zee HFD, Bizios R, et al: Pulmonary vascular response to platelet-activating factor in awake sheep and the role of cyclooxygenase metabolites. Am Rev Respir Dis 1986;134:548–554.

33. Burkov S: Hypoxic pulmonary vasoconstriction in the rat. The necessary role of angiotensin II. Circ Res 1974;35:256.

34. Viles PH, Shepherd JT: Evidence of a dilator action of carbon dioxide on the pulmonary vessels of the cat. Circ Res 1968;22:325.

35. Lyrene RK, Welch KA, Godov G, et al: Alkalosis attenuates hypoxic pulmonary vasoconstriction in neonatal lambs. Pediatr Res 1985;19:1268.

36. Schreiber MD, Heymann MA, Soifer JS: Leukotriene inhibition prevents and reverses hypoxic pulmonary vasoconstriction in newborn lambs. Pediatr Res 1985;19:437–441.

37. Clyman RI: Ontogeny of the ductus arteriosus response to prostaglandin and inhibitors of their synthesis. Semin Perinatol 1980;4:115–124.

38. Reid L: Constrictive and restrictive pulmonary hypertension in the newborn and infant. Am J Cardiovasc Pathol 1987;1:287–299.

39. Murphy JD, Rabinovitch M, Goldstein JD, et al: The structural basis of persistent pulmonary hypertension of the newborn infant. J Pediatr 1981;98: 962–967.

40. Wild LM, Nickerson PA, Morrin FC III: Ligating the ductus arteriosus before birth remodels the pulmonary vasculature of the lamb. Pediatr Res 1989; 25:251–257.

41. Abman SH, Stanley PF, Accurso FJ: Failure of postnatal adaption of the pulmonary circulation after chronic intrauterine pulmonary hypertension in fetal lambs. J Clin Invest 1989;83:1849–1858.

42. Haworth SG: Pulmonary vascular remodeling in neonatal pulmonary hypertension. Chest 1988; 93:1335–1385.

43. Stenmark KR, Orton EC, Reeves JT, et al: Vascular remodeling in neonatal pulmonary hypertension. Chest 1988;93:1275–1325.

44. Glick PL, Leach CL, Besner GE, et al: Pathophysiology of congenital diaphragmatic hernia. III. Exogenous surfactant therapy for the high risk neonate with CDH. J Pediatr Surg 1992;27:866–869.

45. Hirschl RB, Bartlett RH: Extracorporeal membrane oxygenation support in cardiorespiratory failure. Adv Surg 1987;21:189–212.

46. Anderson HL II, Otsu T, Chapman RA, et al: Venovenous extracorporeal life support in neonates using a double lumen catheter. ASAIO Trans 1989;35:650–653.

47. Wung JT, James LS, Kilchevsky E, et al: Management of infants with severe respiratory failure and persistence of the fetal circulation without hyperventilation. Pediatrics 1985;76:488–494.

48. Weigel JT, Hagerman JR: National survey of diagnosis and management of persistent pulmonary hypertension of the newborn. J Perinatol 1990;10:369–375.

49. Hagemann JR, Adams MA, Gardner TH: Pulmonary complications of hyperventilation therapy for persistent pulmonary hypertension. Crit Care Med 1985;31:1013–1014.

50. Cartwright D, Gregory GA, Lou H, et al: The effect of hypocarbia on the cardiovascular system of puppies. Pediatr Res 1984;18:685–690.

51. Bifano EM, Pfannenstiel A: Duration of hyperventilation and outcome in infants with persistent pulmonary hypertension. Pediatrics 1988;81:657–661.

52. Cornish JD, Gertsmann DR, Clark RH, et al: Extracorporeal membrane oxygenation and high-frequency oscillatory ventilation: Potential therapeutic relationship. Crit Care Med 1987;15: 831–834.

53. UK Collaborative ECMO Trial Group: UK collaborative randomized trial of neonatal extracorporeal membrane oxygenation. Lancet 1996;348:75–82.

54. Crombleholme TM, Adzick NIS, deLorimier AA, et al: Carotid artery reconstruction following extracorporeal membrane oxygenation. Am J Dis Child 1990;144:872–874.

55. ECMO Registry of the Extracorporeal Life Support Organization (ELSO), Ann Arbor, MI, July 2004.

56. Bartlett RH, Toomasian J, Roloff D, et al: Extracorporeal membrane oxygenation in neonatal respiratory failure. Ann Surg 1986;204:236–245.

57. VonSegesser K, Turina M: Long term cardiopulmonary bypass without systemic heparinization. Int J Artif Organs 1990;13:687–691.

58. Pasche B, Kodama K, Larm O, et al: Thrombin inactivation on surfaces with covalently bonded heparin. Thromb Res 1986;44:739–748.

59. Larm O, Larson R, Olsson P: A new non-thrombogenic surface prepared by selective covalent binding of heparin via a modified reducing terminal residue. Biomat Med Dev Artif Organs 1983;11:161–163.

60. Ferrara B, Johnson DE, Change P, et al: Efficacy and neurologic outcome of profound hypocapneic alkalosis for treatment of persistent pulmonary hypertension in infancy. J Pediatr 1984;105:457–461.

61. Bernbaum JC, Russell P, Sheridan PH, et al: Long term follow up of newborns with persistent pulmonary hypertension. Crit Care Med 1984;12:579–583.

62. Sell EJ, Gaines JA, Gluckman C, et al: Persistent fetal circulation—Neurodevelopmental outcome. Am J Dis Child 1985;139:25–28.

63. Schumacher RE, Palmer TW, Roloff DW, et al: Follow-up of infants treated with extracorporeal membrane oxygenation for neonatal respiratory failure. Pediatrics 1991;87:451–457.

64. Hofkosh D, Thompson AE, Nozza Jr, et al: Ten years of extracorporeal membrane oxygenation: Neurodevelopmental outcome. Pediatrics 1991;87:549–555.

65. Rosenberg AA, Kennaugh JM, Moreland SG, et al: Longitudinal follow-up of a cohort of newborn infants treated with inhaled nitric oxide for persistent pulmonary hypertension. J Pediatr 1997;131:70–75.

66. Dodge NN, Engle WA, Garg BP, et al: Neurodevelopmental outcomes and respiratory morbidity for extracorporeal membrane oxygenation (ECMO) survivors at age two years: Relations to status at one year. J Perinatol 1996;16:191–196.

67. Towne B, Lott IT, Hicks DA, et al: Long term follow up of infants and children treated with extracorporeal membrane oxygenation: A preliminary report. J Pediatr Surg 1985;20:410–414.

68. Marron MJ, Crisafi MA, Driscoll J, et al: Hearing and developmental outcome in survivors of persistent pulmonary hypertension of the newborn. Pediatrics 1992;90:392–396.

69. Glass P, Wagner AE, Paper PH: Neurodevelopmental status at five years of neonates treated with extracorporeal membrane oxygenation: Neurodevelopmental outcome. Pediatrics 1991;87:549–553.

70. Bennett CC, Johnson A, Field DJ, et al: UK collaborative randomized trial of neonatal extracorporeal membrane oxygenation: Follow-up to age 4 years. Lancet 2001;357:1094–1096.

71. Neonatal Inhaled Nitric Oxide Study Group: Inhaled nitric oxide in term and near-term infants: Neurodevelopmental follow-up of the neonatal inhaled nitric oxide study group (NINOS). J Pediatr 2000;138(2):611–617.

72. Hamutcu R, Nield TA, Garg M, et al: Long-term pulmonary sequelae in children who were treated with extracorporeal membrane oxygenation for neonatal respiratory failure. Pediatrics 2004;114:1292–1296.

73. Lipkin PH, Davidson D, Spivak L, et al: Neurodevelopmental and medical outcomes of persistent pulmonary hypertension in term newborns treated with nitric oxide. J Pediatr 2002;140:306–310.

74. Gupta A, Rastogi S, Sahni R, et al: Inhaled nitric oxide and gentle ventilation in the treatment of pulmonary hypertension of the newborn—A single-center, 5 year experience. J Perinatol 2002;22:435–441.

75. Bonta BW: Transient pulmonary vascular lability: A form of mild pulmonary hypertension of the newborn not requiring mechanical ventilation. J Perinatol 1985;8:19–23.

76. Riggs T, Hirschfield S, Fanaroff A, et al: Persistence of fetal circulation syndrome: An echocardiographic study. J Pediatr 1977;91:626–631.

77. Lloyd TC Jr: Influences of blood pH on hypoxic pulmonary vasoconstriction. J Appl Physiol 1966;21:358–364.

78. Carter JM, Gertsmann DR, Clark RH, et al: High frequency oscillatory ventilation and extracorporeal membrane oxygenation for treatment of acute neonatal respiratory failure. Pediatrics 1990;85:159–164.

79. Schreiber MD, Heymann MA, Soifer SJ: Increased arteriolar pH not decreased $Paco_2$ attenuates hypoxia-induced pulmonary vasoconstriction in newborn lambs. Pediatr Res 1986;20:113–117.

80. Raffestin B, McMurtry IF: Effects of intracellular pH on hypoxic vasoconstriction in rat lungs. J Appl Physiol 1987;63:2524–2531.

81. Carlo WA, Beoglos A, Chatburn RL, et al: High frequency jet ventilation in neonatal pulmonary hypertension. Am J Dis Child 1989;143:233–238.

82. Weisfeldt ML, Geurci AD: Sodium bicarbonate in CPR [editorial]. JAMA 1991;26:2129–2130.

83. Kette J, Weil MH, Gazmuri RJ: Buffer solutions may compromise cardiac resuscitation by reducing coronary perfusion pressure. JAMA 1991;266:2121–2126.

84. Dworetz AR, Moyda FR, Sabo B, et al: Survival of infants with persistent pulmonary hypertension without extracorporeal membrane oxygenation. Pediatrics 1989;84:1–6.

85. Drummond WH, Lock JE: Neonatal pulmonary vasodilator drugs. Dev Pharmacol Ther 1984;7:1–20.

86. Stenmark KR, James SL, Voelkel NF, et al: Leukotrienes C and D in neonates with hypoxemia and pulmonary hypertension. N Engl J Med 1983;309:77–80.

87. Taylor BJ, Fewell JE, Kearns GL, et al: Cromolyn sodium increases the pulmonary vascular response to alveolar hypoxia in lambs. Pediatr Res 1986;20:834–837.

88. Stencenko AA, Lefferts PL, Mitchell JA, et al: Vasodilatory effect of aerosol histamine during pulmonary vasoconstriction in unanesthetized sheep. Pediatr Pulmonol 1987;3:94–100.

89. Roberts JD, Polaner DM, Lang P, et al: Inhaled nitric oxide in persistent pulmonary hypertension of the newborn. Lancet 1992;340:818–819.

90. Kinsella JP, Neish SR, Shaffer E, et al: Low-dose inhalational nitric oxide in persistent pulmonary hypertension of the newborn. Lancet 1992;340:819–820.

91. Kinsella JP, Truog WE, Walsh WF, et al: Randomized, multicenter trial of inhaled nitric oxide and high frequency oscillatory ventilation in severe, persistent pulmonary hypertension of the newborn. J Pediatr 1997;131:55–62.

92. Travadi JN, Patole SK: Phosphodiesterase inhibitors for persistent pulmonary hypertension of the newborn: A review. Pediatr Pulmnol 2003;36:529–535.

93. Kelly LK, Porta NFM, Goodman DM, et al: Inhaled prostacyclin for term infants with persistent pulmonary hypertension refractory to inhaled nitric oxide. J Pediatr 2002;11:830–832.

94. Moses D, Holm BA, Spitale P, et al: Inhibition of pulmonary surfactant function by meconium. Am J Obstet Gynecol 1991;164:477–481.

95. Findlay RD, Taeusch W, Walther FJ: Surfactant replacement therapy for meconium aspiration syndrome. Pediatrics 1996;97:48–52.

96. Lotze A, Knight GR, Martin GR, et al: Improved pulmonary outcome after exogenous surfactant therapy for respiratory failure in term infants requiring extracorporeal membrane oxygenation. J Pediatr 1993;122:261–268.

97. Auten RL, Notter RH, Kendig JW, et al: Surfactant treatment of full term newborns with respiratory failure. Pediatrics 1991;87:101–107.

Suggested Readings

Fox WW, Duara S: Persistent pulmonary hypertension in the neonate: Diagnosis and management. J Pediatr 1983;103:505–514.

Talner NS, Lister G, Fahey JT: Effect of asphyxia on the myocardium of the fetus and newborn. In Polin RA, Fox WW (eds): Fetal and Neonatal Physiology. Philadelphia, WB Saunders, 1991, pp 759–769.

Fiddler GI, Chatrath R, Williams GJ, et al: Dopamine infusion for the treatment of myocardial dysfunction associated with a persistent transitional circulation. Arch Dis Child 1980;55:194–198.

Orchard CH, Kentish JC: Effects of changes of pH on the contractile function of cardiac muscle. Part I. Am J Physiol 1990;258:C967–C981.

Renal Failure in the Newborn Infant

Sharon P. Andreoli, MD

Renal failure in the newborn can result from a number of different causes (Table 18-1). Renal failure may have a prenatal onset in congenital anomalies such as renal dysplasia, cystic kidney disease, and obstructive uropathy, or renal failure may be acquired as a result of a perinatal postnatal insult, such as a hypoxic-ischemic injury, or nephrotoxic insults. Newborns with congenital renal disease associated with oliguria in utero may present with stigmata of Potter's syndrome including pulmonary hypoplasia, flattened nasal bridge, low-set ears, joint contractures, and other orthopedic anomalies due to fetal constraint. Pulmonary hypoplasia associated with Potter's syndrome may range from very mild with only minor respiratory symptoms to lethal respiratory insufficiency. Spontaneous pneumothoraces have been associated with renal disease of prenatal onset.

When caring for the newborn with congenital or acquired renal disease, an understanding of fluid and electrolyte management is critical to preserve renal function and allow for normal renal maturation. Because nephrogenesis proceeds through 34 weeks of gestation, acute insults to the immature developing kidney can result not only in acute renal failure but also in long-term complications associated with "interrupted" nephrogenesis. The medical management of a newborn with acute renal failure requires appropriate diagnostic studies to determine the cause and therapeutic strategies to maintain fluid and electrolyte homeostasis during the period of failure and recovery. In addition, the physician caring for a newborn with acute renal failure must understand when to initiate renal replacement therapy and the indications and contraindi-

cations for the three most common forms of renal replacement therapy: peritoneal dialysis, hemodialysis, and hemofiltration.

Prevention of acute renal failure should always be the physician's primary goal. However, despite optimal management, acute deterioration in renal function is a relatively common occurrence in newborn infants in the intensive care unit. This chapter uses specific case studies to illustrate how to diagnose and manage a newborn with acute renal failure.

Definition

Acute renal failure is characterized by an increase in the blood concentration of creatinine and nitrogenous waste products and by the inability of the kidney to appropriately regulate fluid and electrolyte homeostasis. Most newborn infants with acute renal failure demonstrate oliguria or anuria (urine output <0.5 to 1 mL/kg/hour), but newborns with acute nephrotoxic renal insults, including aminoglycoside nephrotoxicity and contrast nephropathy, are more likely to have acute renal failure with normal urine output (nonoliguric renal failure). The morbidity and mortality rates for nonoliguric acute renal failure are lower than those for oliguric renal failure. Although non-oliguric renal failure is more commonly associated with nephrotoxic insults, the degree of oliguria/anuria is also probably related to the severity of the insult, with less severe insults resulting in a normal or slightly diminished urine output.

TABLE 18-1

CAUSES OF ACUTE RENAL FAILURE IN NEWBORN INFANTS

Prerenal Failure
Decreased true intravascular volume
  Dehydration, gastrointestinal losses
  Salt-wasting renal or adrenal disease
  Central or nephrogenic diabetes insipidus
  Third-space losses (sepsis, traumatized tissues, nephrotic syndrome)
Decreased effective intravascular blood volume
  Congestive heart failure
  Pericarditis, cardiac tamponade

Intrinsic Renal Disease
Acute tubular necrosis
  Hypoxic-ischemic insults
  Drug-induced causes
    Aminoglycosides, intravascular contrast material
    Nonsteroidal anti-inflammatory drugs
  Rhabdomyolysis, hemoglobinuria
Interstitial nephritis
  Drug-induced—antibiotics, anticonvulsants
  Idiopathic
Vascular lesions
  Cortical necrosis
  Renal artery thrombosis
  Renal venous thrombosis
Infectious causes
  Sepsis
  Pyelonephritis

Obstructive Uropathy
Obstruction in a solitary kidney
Bilateral ureteral obstruction
Urethral obstruction

Congenital Lesions
Bilateral renal dysplasia
Cystic kidney diseases
  Autosomal dominant polycystic kidney disease
  Autosomal recessive polycystic kidney disease
  Cystic dysplasia

Causes of Renal Failure

Case Study 1

An 1860-g female infant is born at 30 weeks' gestation following premature rupture of membranes and maternal fever. An ultrasound was normal at 25 weeks' gestation, and the pregnancy had been uncomplicated until the onset of premature labor. She was delivered by emergency cesarean section because of fetal distress with Apgar scores of 6 at 1 minute and 8 at 5 minutes. She required mechanical ventilation, surfactant therapy for respiratory distress, and antibiotic therapy with appropriate doses of gentamicin and ampicillin following an evaluation for sepsis. She is kept NPO (nil per os, nothing by mouth), is given intravenous fluids at a maintenance rate, and on the second day of life is treated with phototherapy for hyperbilirubinemia. On the third day of life her urine output decreases to 0.5 mL/kg/hour, the blood urea nitrogen (BUN) is 26 mg/dL, and the serum creatinine rises to 1.2 mg/dL (compared to 12 mg/dL and 0.7 mg/dL on the second day of life, respectively), and her weight decreases to 1650 g. Her blood pressure is normal; however, she is tachycardic. Her sepsis evaluation is negative to date.

Exercise 1

QUESTION

1. Which of the following acquired or congenital renal abnormalities may be contributing to this newborn infant's oliguria and renal dysfunction?

   a. Polycystic kidney disease

   b. Prerenal azotemia

   c. Intrinsic renal disease

   d. Aminoglycoside nephrotoxicity

   e. Urinary tract obstruction

ANSWER

1. b or possibly c.

A congenital renal disease such as polycystic kidney disease or urinary tract obstruction is not a likely cause of this infant's renal dysfunction, because the ultrasound study at 25 weeks' gestation did not reveal any renal abnormalities. In addition, physical examination did not reveal palpable kidneys or flank masses that can be detected in infants with polycystic kidney disease, ureteropelvic junction obstruction, or lower urinary tract obstruction. Although urinary tract obstruction is not a likely cause of this newborn's renal dysfunction, a renal ultrasound study should be obtained to rule out the possibility, and it will also provide additional important information about renal echogenicity. If Doppler flow studies are obtained, renal blood flow can be estimated.

Acute renal failure due to nephrotoxic insults is not a likely cause of the renal dysfunction, because aminoglycoside antibiotics were administered for only 72 hours, in the recommended doses, and no other nephrotoxic drugs were prescribed. Acute renal failure due to aminoglycoside nephrotoxicity is related to the dose and duration of the antibiotic therapy, as well as to the level of renal function before initiation of therapy. Aminoglycoside-induced renal injury is thought to be related to lysosomal dysfunction of proximal tubules and is reversible once the aminoglycoside antibiotics are discontinued. However, the serum creatinine may continue to increase for several days after the aminoglycoside is discontinued as a result of ongoing tubular injury from residual high renal parenchymal levels of the drug. The half-life of aminoglycosides is substantially longer in the renal parenchyma compared to the serum half-life.

Prerenal azotemia is a strong possibility as a cause of this child's oliguria and acute deterioration of renal function. Prerenal failure results from renal hypoperfusion due to true intravascular volume contraction or a decreased "effective" blood volume. True intravascular volume contraction is observed with hemorrhage, dehydration (caused by gastrointestinal losses), salt-wasting renal or adrenal diseases, central or nephrogenic diabetes insipidus, increased insensible losses (as occurs in extremely low birth weight infants), and disease states associated with third-space losses such as sepsis and capillary leak syndrome. Decreased effective blood volume (when the true blood volume is normal or increased but renal perfusion is decreased) occurs in congestive heart failure, cardiac tamponade, and hepatorenal syndrome. Whether prerenal failure is caused by true intravascular volume depletion or decreased effective blood volume, correction of the underlying disturbance will return renal function to normal. Volume depletion is a distinct possibility due to the tachycardia and weight loss. Intrinsic renal disease secondary to renal hypoperfusion (i.e., prerenal failure that has evolved into acute tubular necrosis [ATN]) is also a possibility in this child. Additional studies of renal function are required to discriminate between prerenal failure and intrinsic renal disease.

Prerenal versus Acute Renal Failure

Exercise 1 *Continued*

QUESTION

2. Indicate how the results of the following tests of renal function can be interpreted to support the diagnosis of prerenal versus ischemic acute renal failure.

a. Urinalysis (normal or abnormal)

b. Urine volume (normal, decreased, or increased)

c. Urine Na^+ (decreased or increased)

d. Urine osmolality (concentrated or isotonic)

e. Fractional excretion of Na^+ (increased or decreased)

ANSWER

2. See the following table.

Renal Function Test	Prerenal Azotemia	Ischemic Acute Kidney Injury
a. Urinalysis	Normal	Normal to mildly abnormal, including granular casts
b. Urine volume	Decreased	Decreased to normal
c. Urine sodium (mEq/L)	<20	>20–30
d. Urine osmolality (mOsm/L)	>350	~300
e. Fractional excretion of sodium (FE_Na)	<2%	>2–3%

The urine osmolality, urine sodium concentration, fractional excretion of sodium, and renal failure index have all been used to help differentiate prerenal failure from hypoxic-ischemic acute renal injury (also called ATN). This differentiation is based on the concept that the tubules are working appropriately in prerenal failure and are, therefore, able to conserve salt and water appropriately. In ATN, the tubules have progressed to irreversible injury and are unable to conserve salt appropriately. During prerenal failure in children and young adults, the tubules are able to respond to decreased renal perfusion by conserving sodium and water, such that the urine osmolality is greater than 300 to 400 mOsm/L, the urine sodium is less than 10 to 20 mEq/L, and the fractional excretion of sodium is less than 1%. The fractional excretion of sodium (FE_Na) is calculated by the formula:

$$FE_{Na\%} = (Urine\ Na/Serum\ Na) \div (Urine\ creatinine/Serum\ creatinine) \times 100$$

Because the renal tubules in newborn and premature infants are relatively immature compared with those of older infants and children, the corresponding values suggestive of renal hypoperfusion are urine osmolality greater than 350 mOsm/L, urine sodium less than 20 to 30 mEq/L, and a fractional excretion of sodium of less than 2% to 3%. When the renal tubules have sustained injury, as occurs in ATN, they cannot appropriately conserve sodium and water, so that the urine osmolality is approximately 300 mOsm/L, the urine sodium is greater than 30 to 40 mEq/L, and the fractional excretion of sodium is greater than 2% to 3%. However, the use of these numbers to differentiate prerenal failure from ATN requires that the patient initially demonstrate normal tubular function before acquiring the injury. For example, fractional excretion of sodium values up to 10% have been described in premature newborns with a gestational age less than 30 weeks with otherwise normal tubular function. In addition, newborn infants with salt-wasting adrenal disease or underlying renal dysplasia may have prerenal failure with urinary and serum indices suggestive of ATN. Therefore, it is essential to consider the effect of gestational age and the state of the function of the tubules preceding the potential insult when interpreting renal function studies.

In prerenal failure the kidneys are intrinsically normal and with restoration of renal perfusion, renal function will return to normal. In ischemic ATN the kidney has suffered anatomic and functional damage, which may evolve from prerenal failure. However, the evolution of prerenal failure to intrinsic renal failure is not sudden, and an understanding of the compensatory mechanisms that maintain renal perfusion in the presence of adverse renal hemodynamics is key to managing patients with prerenal failure.

Intrinsic Acute Renal Failure

Renal hypoperfusion initiates a number of compensatory mechanisms that work to maintain renal perfusion under adverse hemodynamic conditions. When renal perfusion is compromised, the afferent arteriole relaxes its vascular tone to diminish renal vascular resistance and maintain renal blood flow. During renal hypoperfusion, the intrarenal generation of vasodilatory prostaglandins (including prostacyclin) mediates vasodilation of the renal microvasculature to maintain renal perfusion. Administration of aspirin or nonsteroidal anti-inflammatory drugs (e.g., indomethacin) can inhibit this compensatory mechanism and precipitate acute renal insufficiency during renal hypoperfusion states. Similarly, when renal arterial perfusion pressure is low, the intrarenal generation of angiotensin II is increased. Angiotensin increases efferent arteriolar resistance and helps drive glomerular filtration. Administration of angiotensin-converting enzyme inhibitors during renal hypoperfusion states can eliminate the pressure gradient needed to drive filtration and precipitate acute renal failure. Thus, the administration of medications (such as prostaglandin synthetase inhibitors) that interfere with normal compensatory mechanisms can precipitate acute renal failure in certain clinical circumstances.

Case Study 1 *Continued*

The infant's urinalysis is normal, urine sodium low, osmolality high, and fractional excretion of sodium 1.5%. These results are consistent with prerenal failure secondary to renal hypoperfusion due to volume depletion that is probably related to increased insensible losses as a result of phototherapy. She is treated with a fluid bolus of 10 mL/kg of normal saline and intravenous fluids are increased to a higher maintenance rate. Her urine output improves to greater than 1 mL/kg/ hour, her BUN declines to 15 mg/day, and the creatinine declines to 0.8 mg/dL. On the following day, her weight increases to 1780 g and she develops a distended abdomen. An abdominal radiograph demonstrates signs of necrotizing enterocolitis (NEC). She is hypotensive for several hours and requires 40 mL/kg of normal saline to stabilize her blood pressure. Her urine output again decreases to less than 0.5 mL/kg/hour. The urinalysis now demonstrates granular casts, the urine osmolality is 300 mOsm/L, the urine sodium is 55 mEq/L, and the fractional excretion of sodium is now 4.0%.

Exercise 1 *Continued*

QUESTION

3. What is the cause of this infant's acute deterioration in renal function now?
   a. Sepsis
   b. Toxic nephropathy
   c. Prerenal failure

d. Hypoxic-ischemic acute kidney injury (ATN)

e. Obstructive uropathy

ANSWER

3. d and possibly a. This infant has developed intrinsic renal disease with acute renal failure secondary to possible sepsis in association with NEC and hypoxic-ischemic ATN from prolonged hypotension. Her urine studies are now most consistent with ATN.

Over the next 48 hours, she remains oliguric, and her serum creatinine increases to 3.4 mg/dL. Her abdomen is less distended and her blood pressure remains normal. The sodium is 135 mEq/L, potassium 5.9 mEq/L, chloride 90 mEq/L, and bicarbonate 18 mEq/L; the calcium is 7.0 mg/dL and the phosphorus is 8.2 mg/dL. Physical examination demonstrates a liver palpable 1 cm below the left costal margin. In addition, a chest x-ray demonstrates findings consistent with pulmonary edema.

QUESTION

4. What additional diagnostic studies may provide further evidence of the extent of the infant's intrinsic renal disease?

a. Radionucleotide renal scan

b. Renal ultrasound study

c. Abdominal radiograph

ANSWER

4. a and b.

In ATN, the renal ultrasound study demonstrates kidneys of normal size with loss of corticomedullary differentiation. As noted earlier, a renal ultrasound study should be ordered in all infants with significant renal failure to ensure that an obstructive lesion is not present.

The radionucleotide renal scan (with technetium-99-MAG-3 or technetium-99-DTPA) in infants with ATN demonstrates normal or slightly decreased renal blood flow, with poor function and delayed accumulation of the radioisotope in the renal parenchyma and without excretion of the isotope in the collecting system (Fig. 18-1A). The radionucleotide renal scan can also differentiate ATN from cortical necrosis, which may result from ischemic renal injury. The long-term prognosis for return of normal renal function in ATN is substantially better than for cortical necrosis. However, some recent studies suggest that ATN can lead to physiologic and morphologic alterations in the

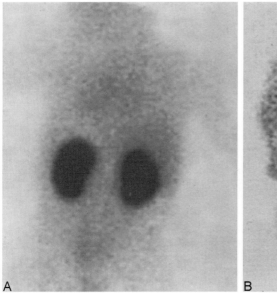
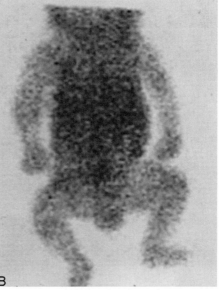

Figure 18-1 Technetium-99-MAG-3 renal scans in a newborn infant with acute tubular necrosis (**A**) and in a newborn with cortical necrosis (**B**). Each scan is taken at 4 hours after injection of isotope. **A**, Delayed uptake of isotope with parenchymal accumulation of isotope and little to no excretion of isotope into the collecting system. **B**, No renal parenchymal uptake of isotope. (From Andreoli SP: Acute renal failure: Clinical evaluation and management. In Avner ED, Harmon WE, Nauidet P [eds]: Pediatric Nephrology. Baltimore, Williams & Wilkins, 2004, pp 1233–1254.)

kidney that may lead to subsequent kidney disease. Recent studies have associated acute renal failure with low Apgar scores and perinatal asphyxia.

In this patient, the renal ultrasound study is normal. The radionucleotide scan reveals near-normal blood flow but delayed excretion of the isotope into the collecting system, consistent with ATN (Fig. 18-1).

The patient begins to have some urine output but remains tachypneic. The chest x-ray findings are consistent with pulmonary edema.

QUESTION

5. What is the best management strategy to improve the urine output and decrease fluid overload?

   a. Dopamine infusion

   b. Diuretic therapy

   c. Mannitol infusion

   d. Renal replacement therapy

ANSWER

5. b.

Drug Therapy

Both dopamine and diuretics have been used extensively in newborn infants and older children with acute renal failure. In this case, however, it is appropriate to begin furosemide (1 to 2 mg/kg/dose), because this baby demonstrates signs and symptoms of intravascular volume expansion. Low-dose dopamine can also be administered if the response to furosemide is poor. Although the effect of these agents in preventing or limiting renal injury is controversial, increasing the urine output helps maintain fluid and electrolyte homeostasis and makes providing adequate calories and protein much easier. However, conversion of oliguric to non-oliguric acute renal failure has not been shown to alter the course of renal failure. Despite widespread use of low-dose (3 to 5 µg/kg/minute) dopamine to improve renal blood flow and stimulate urine output in acute renal failure, there are no definitive studies to demonstrate that such therapy improves survival or reduces the need for dialysis. Controlled studies in adults given lasix and dopamine for acute renal failure have not shown either to alter the course of acute renal failure.

The use of mannitol in infants with acute renal failure can be problematic. For example, a lack of response to therapy can precipitate congestive heart failure, particularly if the child's intravascular volume is already expanded before the mannitol is infused. Furthermore, if mannitol cannot be excreted, it may result in a substantial increase in serum osmolality.

The choice of aggressive diuretic or inotropic therapy to increase urine output needs to be made on an individual basis, with consideration of the risks and benefits. If the infant is unresponsive to diuretic therapy, continued use of high doses is not justified because furosemide therapy has been associated with ototoxicity in patients with renal failure. Therefore, if the patient is unresponsive to diuretic and inotropic agents, consideration of renal replacement therapy is indicated.

Cortical Necrosis

Case Study 2

Full-term male twins were delivered by emergency cesarean section for severe fetal distress during labor. Twin A had Apgar scores of 7 at 1 minute and 9 at 5 minutes and required resuscitation with oxygen. Twin B was delivered several minutes later and twin B's Apgar scores were 1 at 1 minute and 3 at 5 minutes. This twin required vigorous resuscitation, including intubation, mechanical ventilation, and volume expansion for hypotension. At 24 hours of age, he was severely oliguric, and his urine was grossly bloody.

Exercise 2

QUESTION

1. What is the most likely cause of this newborn infant's acute renal failure?

   a. Urinary tract obstruction

   b. Toxic nephropathy

   c. Prerenal azotemia

   d. Intrinsic renal disease

   e. Sepsis

   f. Vascular insult

ANSWER

1. d and f. These findings are suggestive of a vascular insult such as cortical necrosis.

Cortical necrosis as a cause of acute renal failure is much more common in young children, and particularly in neonates. This disorder is generally caused by hypotension accompanied by severe anemia or asphyxia and has been observed in infants experiencing significant blood loss, sepsis, fetomaternal hemorrhage, and severe asphyxia. In each of these disorders, the reduction in blood flow to the kidney is of sufficient severity to cause ischemic tissue necrosis and activation of the blood clotting system.

Newborn infants with cortical necrosis usually have gross or microscopic hematuria and oliguria and occasionally exhibit hypertension. In addition to elevated blood urea nitrogen and creatinine, these infants may demonstrate thrombocytopenia due to the microvascular injury. In the early phase of the disease, renal ultrasound studies are generally normal; in the later phases, the kidney may atrophy and shrink substantially. A radionucleotide renal scan shows decreased or no perfusion with delayed or absent function (see Fig. 18–1B, which is in contrast with the delayed function observed in ATN in Fig. 18–1A).

The prognosis of cortical necrosis is much worse than that of ATN. Children with cortical necrosis may have partial recovery or no recovery at all. Typically, infants with cortical necrosis require some form of dialysis therapy. However, even those infants who recover sufficient renal function to discontinue dialysis are at risk for the late development of chronic renal failure.

Fluid Management

Case Study 2 *Continued*

The infant remains oliguric, and the renal scan demonstrates no flow or function. His BUN and creatinine increase over the next 2 days to 59 mg/dL and 3.9 mg/dL, respectively. His weight increases by 0.4 kg, and he develops respiratory distress. A serum chemistry determination reveals a serum sodium concentration of 125 mEq/L, a potassium concentration of 7.2 mEq/L, a serum bicarbonate concentration
of 13 mEq/L, a calcium concentration of 6.2 mg/dL, and a serum phosphorus level of 10.8 mg/dL.

Exercise 2 *Continued*

QUESTION

2. Which of the following fluid management strategies is appropriate at this time?

   a. Volume expansion with 10 to 20 mL/kg normal saline

   b. Maintenance fluids at 100 mL/kg/24 hours

   c. Restrict fluids to insensible losses (400 to 600 mL/m^2)

   d. Restrict fluids to insensible losses (400 to 600 mL/m^2) and replace other losses milliliter for milliliter

ANSWER

2. c. This is the appropriate fluid management strategy because the newborn is edematous and his weight has increased. The abnormal serum sodium level is most likely due to dilutional hyponatremia. Diuretic therapy as described earlier can be initiated as well. If there is no increase in urine output or improvement with this plan of medical management, renal replacement therapy should be considered.

Newborn infants with acute renal failure may present with hypovolemia, euvolemia, or fluid overload and pulmonary edema. Patients with salt-wasting renal or adrenal disease, diarrhea, or vomiting commonly present with fluid deficits that need correction to a euvolemic state, whereas patients with oliguria or anuria frequently present with hypervolemia and need fluid restriction or acute fluid removal to obtain a euvolemic state. Weight, blood pressure, heart rate, skin turgor, and capillary refill are used to assess the intravascular volume status. In infants whose intravascular volume is depleted, 10 to 20 mL/kg of normal saline can be infused to reestablish a euvolemic state. If urine output does not increase and azotemia does not improve following fluid resuscitation, additional fluid may be administered judiciously. If the child presents with fluid overload that does not respond to diuretic administration, fluid restriction or fluid removal with dialysis or hemofiltration may be necessary. Once normal intravascular volume has been reached, euvolemia can be maintained by providing the child with fluid to replace normal water losses from the skin and the respiratory and gastrointestinal tracts (insensible losses, 400 to 600 mL/m²/24 hours). In a child who is euvolemic, urine losses should be replaced milliliter for milliliter. The composition of the replacement fluid can usually be determined by measuring urine electrolytes. For example, if the urine sodium concentration is 75 mEq/L, the appropriate replacement fluid would be one-half normal saline. Ongoing fluid therapy is guided by obtaining daily weights, blood pressure determinations, and accurate estimates of fluid intake and urine output and by performing a daily physical examination. Those estimates are then modified, based on the nutritional needs of the child.

QUESTION

3. How would you correct the hyponatremia in this patient?

   a. Fluid restriction

   b. Administration of hypertonic saline

   c. Administration of maintenance fluids containing 0.45% sodium chloride

ANSWER

3. a. Restriction of fluid intake alone should correct the hyponatremia, but a lack of increase in urine output or no improvement in serum sodium with this medical therapy may be an indication for the initiation of renal replacement therapy.

   Mild hyponatremia is very common in acute renal failure and often results from an excess of total body free water. If the serum sodium concentration is greater than 120 mEq/L, fluid restriction or water removal by dialysis therapy will correct the hyponatremia. However, if the serum sodium is less than 120 mEq/L, the child is at higher risk for seizures, and correction to a sodium level of approximately 125 mEq/L with hypertonic (3%) saline should be considered. This can be accomplished with the following formula:

   $$125 \text{ mEq/L Na} - \text{Actual serum Na} \times$$
   $$\text{Weight in kg} \times 0.6(\text{volume of distribution of}$$
   $$\text{sodium}) = \text{mEq of Na to be administered}$$
   $$\div 0.5 \text{ mEq/mL to determine milliliters of 3\%}$$
   $$\text{hypertonic saline solution to be administered}$$

   The hypertonic saline is usually infused over several hours to avoid rapid correction of the serum sodium. Although the incidence in infants is unknown, rapid correction of the serum sodium concentration in adults with chronic hyponatremia has been associated with central pontine myelinolysis.

QUESTION

4. Which of the following options should be initiated to evaluate and treat the hyperkalemia in this patient?

   a. Remove potassium from the intravenous fluids

   b. Obtain an electrocardiogram (ECG)

   c. Administer sodium bicarbonate

   d. Administer albuterol

   e. Administer calcium

   f. Administer glucose and insulin

   g. Administer sodium polystyrene sulfonate (Kayexalate)

ANSWER

4. a, b, and possibly c, d, e, f, and g as well. Potassium should immediately be removed from the intravenous fluids. If ECG abnormalities are present, intravenous calcium therapy, intravenous sodium bicarbonate therapy, and (if the potassium does not substantially decrease with these measures) glucose and insulin should be administered to acutely lower the potassium. Kayexalate therapy should also be initiated in this baby. Albuterol can acutely lower the serum potassium by shifting potassium intracellularly and is increasingly becoming a first-line therapy.

   Because the kidney tightly regulates potassium balance and excretes approximately 90% of dietary potassium intake, hyperkalemia is a common and potentially life-threatening electrolyte abnormality in acute renal failure. Hyperkalemia results from decreased renal filtration and impaired tubular secretion of the cation, altered distribution of potassium by acidosis (which shifts potassium from the intracellular to the extracellular compartment), and release of intracellular potassium due to the associated catabolic state. As a general rule, for each 0.1 unit reduction in arterial pH, the serum potassium increases by 0.3 mEq/L. The serum potassium level may be falsely elevated if hemolysis occurs during the blood draw, and the laboratory should note whether any hemolysis is present. "Pseudohyperkalemia" may also occur if the newborn has a high white blood cell or platelet count.

True hyperkalemia results in disturbances of cardiac rhythm by its depolarizing effect on the cardiac conduction pathways. The concentration of serum potassium that results in an arrhythmia is dependent on the acid-base balance and the concentration of other serum electrolytes. Hypocalcemia (which is commonly noted in renal failure) exacerbates the adverse effects of the elevated serum potassium level on cardiac conduction pathways. Tall, peaked T waves are the first manifestation of cardiotoxicity; prolongation of the P-R interval, flattening of P waves, and widening of QRS complexes are later abnormalities. Severe hyperkalemia eventually leads to ventricular tachycardia and fibrillation.

Treatment of hyperkalemia is indicated if cardiac conduction abnormalities are noted or if the serum concentration is greater than 6 to 7 mEq/L; management of hyperkalemia is summarized in Table 18-2. Sodium bicarbonate (0.5 to 1 mEq/kg/dose) transfers potassium into cells, but as described later, this therapy may precipitate seizures and tetany in the presence of hypocalcemia. Intravenous glucose and insulin also shift potassium from the extracellular to the intracellular compartment. Albuterol shifts potassium intracellularly as well. Intravenous calcium gluconate infusion increases the threshold potential of the excitable myocardial cells and counteracts the depolarizing effect of the hyperkalemic state.

Each of these treatments, however, is a temporizing measure and does not remove potassium from the body. Kayexalate given orally, per naso-gastric tube, or per rectum exchanges sodium for potassium in the gastrointestinal tract and results in potassium removal. Complications of Kayexalate therapy include possible hypernatremia, sodium retention, and constipation. In addition, Kayexalate therapy has been associated with intestinal necrosis in postoperative patients and may be hazardous to a patient in whom intestinal perfusion is marginal. Depending on the degree of hyperkalemia and the need for correction of other metabolic derangements in acute renal failure, hyperkalemia frequently requires the initiation of dialysis or hemofiltration.

Acidosis

QUESTION

5. Medical management of the metabolic acidosis in this patient should include which of the following strategies?

   a. Volume expansion with 10 to 20 mL/kg normal saline

   b. Intravenous sodium bicarbonate therapy

   c. Sodium citrate therapy

   d. Increase of the maintenance fluid requirement

   e. Intravenous or oral calcium therapy

ANSWER

5. b or c and possibly e. Either intravenous sodium bicarbonate or sodium citrate by mouth would be acceptable. However, if there are any potential difficulties with gastrointestinal absorption of medications,

TABLE 18-2

TREATMENT OF HYPERKALEMIA

Agent	Mechanism	Dose	Onset	Complications
Sodium bicarbonate	Shifts K^+ into cells	1 mEq/kg IV over 10–30 min	15–30 min	Hypernatremia, change in ionized calcium
Calcium gluconate (10%)	Stabilizes membrane potential	0.5–1 mL/kg IV over 5–15 min	Immediate	Bradycardia, arrhythmias, hypercalcemia
Glucose and insulin	Stimulates cellular uptake of K^+	Glucose 0.5 g/kg Insulin 0.1 U/kg IV over 30 min	30–120 min	Hypoglycemia
Albuterol	Shifts K^+ into cells	400 mg by nebulizer	15–30 min	Hypokalemia
Kayexalate	Exchanges Na^+ for K^+ across the colonic mucosa	1 g/kg PO or PR in sorbitol	30–60 min	Hypernatremia, constipation

IV, intravenous; PO, by mouth; PR, per rectum.

the intravenous route should be used. When treating acidosis, the serum calcium level must be taken into consideration since the serum pH influences the ionized calcium level.

Because the kidney excretes net acids generated by diet and intermediary metabolism, acidosis is very common in acute renal failure. As long as the infant's central nervous system is intact, respiratory compensation will provide partial correction of the acidosis, but if the infant is obtunded, respiratory compensation may be compromised, resulting in severe acidosis. Severe acidosis can be treated with intravenous or oral *sodium bicarbonate*, oral *sodium citrate* solutions, or dialysis therapy.

When considering treatment of acidosis, it is important to consider the serum ionized calcium concentration. Under normal circumstances, approximately half the total calcium is protein bound; the other half is free and in ionized form. It is this ionized form of calcium that determines the transmembrane potential and electrochemical gradient. Hypocalcemia is common in acute renal failure, and acidosis increases the fraction of total calcium present in the ionized form. Treatment of acidosis may shift the ionized calcium to the protein-bound form, decreasing the amount of ionized calcium and precipitating tetany or seizures. Thus, base therapy for acidosis should not be considered without knowledge of the total and ionized calcium concentrations. Because the treatment of acidosis has such widespread effects on electrolyte homeostasis, care should be taken to administer bicarbonate at a safe rate (0.5 to 1 mEq/kg given over approximately 1 hour).

Electrolytes

QUESTION

6. What is the appropriate therapy for this child's hypocalcemia and hyperphosphatemia?
   a. Administer aluminum hydroxide
   b. Administer magnesium hydroxide
   c. Administer calcium carbonate
   d. Administer sodium bicarbonate
   e. Restrict dietary phosphorus

ANSWER

6. c and e.

Because the kidney is the primary route of phosphorus elimination, hyperphosphatemia is a common electrolyte abnormality during acute and chronic renal failure. Hyperphosphatemia should be treated with dietary phosphorus restriction and with oral *calcium carbonate* or other calcium compounds to bind phosphorus and prevent gastrointestinal absorption of phosphorus. *Aluminum*-containing compounds should be avoided, as several studies have demonstrated that oral administration of aluminum-containing phosphorus binders results in substantial aluminum absorption, leading to aluminum intoxication. *Magnesium*-containing antacids may result in hypermagnesemia and are not used in the treatment of hyperphosphatemia in acute renal failure. Dialysis therapy also effectively removes phosphorus, but because phosphorus is a divalent cation, it crosses dialysis membranes less readily than uncharged molecules such as urea or monovalent anions such as potassium.

The cause of hypocalcemia in acute renal failure is multifactorial and may result from hyperphosphatemia, inadequate gastrointestinal calcium absorption due to diminished 1,25-dihydroxyvitamin D production by the kidney, and skeletal resistance to the action of parathyroid hormone. As described earlier, acid-base balance has a profound effect on the ionized calcium concentration, and the degree of acidosis must be considered when selecting a treatment for hypocalcemia. If hypocalcemia is severe or if bicarbonate therapy is necessary for the treatment of hyperkalemia, 10% calcium gluconate (100 mg/kg, up to a maximum of 1 g) should be given over 30 to 60 minutes with continuous ECG monitoring. Hypocalcemia may also be treated by oral administration of calcium carbonate or other calcium salts.

Renal Replacement Therapy

Case Study 2 *Continued*

Over the next few days, the infant remains oliguric and has a progressive rise in serum BUN and creatinine concentrations. In addition, she continues to demonstrate acidemia, hyperphosphatemia, and hypocalcemia. The pediatric nephrologist recommends the initiation of renal replacement therapy.

Exercise 2 *Continued*

QUESTION

7. Which mode of renal replacement therapy is best for this neonate with acute renal failure?

   a. Peritoneal dialysis

   b. Hemodialysis

   c. Continuous venovenous hemofiltration

ANSWER

7. a. Because of the substantial technical difficulties in performing hemodialysis and hemofiltration in newborn infants, most pediatric nephrologists prefer peritoneal dialysis for the treatment of acute renal failure unless contraindications exist.

The purpose of acute renal replacement therapy is to remove endogenous and exogenous toxins and to maintain fluid, electrolyte, and acid-base balance until renal function returns. Renal replacement therapy may be provided by peritoneal dialysis, intermittent hemodialysis, and hemofiltration with or without a dialysis circuit. Many factors, including the age and size of the newborn, the degree of metabolic derangements, the difficulty in maintaining blood pressure control, and nutritional needs, must be considered in deciding whether and when to initiate renal replacement therapy and what therapeutic modality to choose. Table 18-3 highlights the relative advantages and disadvantages of each modality.

The indications for renal replacement therapy are not absolute and take into consideration a number of variables, including the cause of acute renal failure, the rapidity of the onset of renal failure, and the severity of fluid and electrolyte abnormalities. Newborn infants have less muscle mass compared with older children and, therefore, require initiation of renal replacement therapy at lower serum concentrations of creatinine and BUN. The presence of fluid overload unresponsive to diuretic therapy and the need for enteral feedings or hyperalimentation to support nutritional needs are important factors in considering the initiation of renal replacement therapy.

Peritoneal Dialysis

Acute *peritoneal dialysis* (PD) has been the most commonly used modality for acute renal failure, particularly in neonates. PD is frequently used in neonates and small children when vascular access is difficult to maintain. Advantages of PD include the relative ease of performance, lack of requirement for systemic heparinization, and less stringent demands for hemodynamic stability while undergoing the procedure. The

TABLE 18-3

COMPARISON OF RENAL REPLACEMENT THERAPIES

Feature	PD	HD	CVVH(D)
Solute removal	+++	++++	+(++)
Fluid removal	++	+++	+++(+++)
Need for hemodynamic stability	−	+++	−(−)
Effectiveness for treatment of hyperkalemia	++	++++	+(++)
Ease of access	++++	−	−(−)
Continuous	++++	−	++++(++++)
Anticoagulation	−	+++	−/+(−/+)
Hyperglycemia	++	−	−(++)
Potential for respiratory compromise	++	+	−(−)
Peritonitis	++++	−	−(−)
Hypotension	+	++++	+(+)
Disequilibrium	−	+++	−(−)
Specially trained staff	−	++++	+++(+++)

CVVH, continuous venovenous hemofiltration; (D), with dialysis; HD, hemodialysis; PD, peritoneal dialysis.
From Andreoli SP: Clinical aspects and management of acute renal failure in children. In Barratt TM, Avner ED, Harmon WE (eds): Pediatric Nephrology. Baltimore, Lippincott, Williams & Wilkins, 1998.

disadvantages include a slower correction of metabolic parameters and the potential for peritonitis. To maximize the efficiency of PD, frequent exchanges, as often as every hour, and the use of dialysate with high glucose concentrations may be required. Relative contraindications to PD in infants with acute renal failure include recent abdominal surgery and massive organomegaly or intra-abdominal masses. Patients who required ostomy placement following surgical treatment of intestinal dysfunction are also at high risk of peritonitis with PD.

Access to the peritoneal cavity to perform PD is usually gained through placement of a Tenckhoff catheter. PD is initiated in newborn infants with dialysate volumes of 5 to 10 mL/kg body weight. The dialysate volume can be increased to a maximum of 30 to 50 mL/kg, depending on the need for additional solute and fluid removal and the respiratory and nutritional status of the infant.

Hemodialysis

Hemodialysis (HD) has also been used for several years in the treatment of acute renal failure. The advantage of HD is that metabolic abnormalities can be rapidly corrected and hypervolemic states can be rapidly treated with the addition of ultrafiltration. The disadvantages of HD include the requirement for systemic heparinization, the need for maximally purified water by a reverse osmosis system, and the need for skilled personnel. Relative contraindications include hemodynamic instability or ongoing coagulation abnormalities and prior severe hemorrhage. Vascular access in newborn infants can be provided by the umbilical vessels.

Hemofiltration

Over the past several years, renal replacement therapy with *continuous venovenous hemofiltration* (CVVH) or *continuous venovenous hemodialfiltration* (CVVHD) has become increasingly popular in the treatment of acute renal failure in newborn infants. CVVH functions on the principle of removal of large quantities of ultrafiltrate from plasma and replacement with an isosmotic electrolyte solution, and CVVHD includes the addition of a dialysis circuit to the hemofilter and results in solute removal via the added dialysis circuit. The advantages of

hemofiltration (with or without a dialysis circuit) are that it allows for rapid fluid removal and does not require the patient to be hemodynamically stable when a pump is inserted into the circuit. The continuous nature of the filtration avoids rapid solute and fluid shifts, as occurs in hemodialysis. The disadvantages of hemofiltration are that constant heparinization is generally required, and there is a potential for severe fluid and electrolyte abnormalities due to the large volume of fluid removed and subsequently replaced. Hemofiltration is generally used in children who are hemodynamically unstable, have multiorgan dysfunction, and require inotropic support. Given the unstable nature of these patients, it is not surprising that the survival rate of infants with acute renal failure treated with hemofiltration is lower than the survival rate of infants using other modalities. As in hemodialysis, vascular access in newborn infants can be provided by the umbilical vessels.

Nutritional Support

Exercise 2 *Continued*

QUESTION

8. Which of the following statements concerning the nutritional support of infants receiving peritoneal dialysis are true?

    a. Malnutrition develops rapidly in infants with renal failure.

    b. Enteral feedings should be avoided in infants with renal failure.

    c. Caloric intake of at least 120 kcal/kg/day is generally required.

    d. If enteral feedings are chosen, it is best to use a formula with a high phosphorus content.

ANSWER

8. a and c are true.

In many instances, acute renal failure is associated with marked catabolism. Prompt and proper nutrition is essential in the management of a newborn with acute renal failure. If the gastrointestinal tract is intact and functional, enteral feedings with formula (PM 60/40, which is low in phosphorus content) should be instituted as soon as possible. After beginning with diluted formula, feedings can be increased and concentrated to achieve optimal calories. Newborn infants should receive maintenance calories (120 kcal/kg/day), although higher intake may be required to counteract the catabolic state. If enteral feedings are not possible, hyperalimentation, usually though a central line with a high concentration of dextrose (15% to 20%), lipids (2 to 3 g/kg/day), and protein (2 g/kg/day), should be instituted. If the child is oliguric or anuric and sufficient calories cannot be provided while maintaining appropriate fluid balance, dialysis should be instituted.

Prognosis

Exercise 2 *Continued*

QUESTION

9. What prognosis for recovery and long-term morbidity can you offer the parents of this infant with acute renal failure?

ANSWER

9. The prognosis for recovery and the long-term morbidity in newborn patients is highly dependent on the underlying cause of the acute renal failure.

Newborn infants who have acute renal failure as a component of multisystem failure have a much higher mortality rate than children with intrinsic renal disease such as obstructive uropathy or renal dysplasia. Newborn infants with ATN typically recover normal renal function and are at low risk for any late complications. However, neonates who may have suffered a substantial loss of nephrons, as in partial cortical necrosis, are at higher risk for the development of renal failure long after the initial insult. Several studies in animal models of acute renal failure have documented that hyperfiltration of the remnant nephrons may eventually lead to progressive glomerulosclerosis and long-term renal failure. Thus, children who have had cortical necrosis during the neonatal period and recovered partial renal function are clearly at risk for the late development of renal complications. At present, there are few data to accurately predict the long-term outcome of newborn infants with acute renal failure. Such children need lifelong monitoring of renal function, blood pressure,

and urinalysis. Typically, the late development of renal failure first becomes manifest with the development of hypertension, proteinuria, and eventually an elevated BUN and creatinine.

Hypertension

Case Study 3

A female infant weighing 4200 g is delivered at 38 weeks' gestation after a pregnancy complicated by insulin-dependent diabetes mellitus of long-standing duration. Apgar scores are 5 at 1 minute and 8 at 5 minutes. Initially the infant does well with monitoring of blood glucose levels, but on the second day of life the infant has gross hematuria and develops a palpable left flank mass, and the blood pressure is noted to be 132/88 mm Hg. The BUN and creatinine are 17 mg/dL, and 0.7 mg/dL, respectively.

A renal ultrasound study demonstrates two kidneys; however, the left kidney is large, is echogenic, and has loss of corticomedullary differentiation, and there is a clot visualized in the renal vein. A technetium-99-MAG-3 renal scan demonstrates normal flow and function of the right kidney but decreased function of the left kidney.

Exercise 3

QUESTION

1. What is the most likely cause of this neonate's hypertension?
   a. Cortical necrosis
   b. Renal vein thrombosis
   c. Renal artery thrombosis
   d. Acute tubular necrosis

ANSWER

1. b.

Cortical necrosis is an unlikely cause of this child's hypertension, because it typically results in symmetrically decreased blood flow and function on a radionucleotide renal scan. ATN is also unlikely, as the renal scan in these patients demonstrates normal or slightly decreased renal blood flow, with poor function and delayed accumulation of the radioisotope in the renal parenchyma and without excretion of the isotope in the collecting system. Renal artery thrombosis is strongly associated with placement of an umbilical arterial line. In addition to hypertension, newborn infants with renal artery thrombosis may demonstrate gross or microscopic hematuria, thrombocytopenia, and oliguria. In renal artery thrombosis, the initial ultrasound study may appear normal or demonstrate minor abnormalities, and the renal scan demonstrates little to no blood flow to the involved kidney. Therapy should be aimed at limiting extension of the clot by removal of the umbilical arterial catheter and treatment of the hypertension. Anticoagulant or fibrinolytic therapy can be considered, particularly if the clot is large. Because this newborn did not have an umbilical line and because the kidney appeared large, renal artery thrombosis is unlikely.

Renal vein thrombosis is a likely diagnosis. The ultrasound study in infants with renal vein thrombosis demonstrates an enlarged, swollen echogenic kidney, and the renal scan typically demonstrates decreased blood flow and function of the involved kidney. Renal vein thrombosis also occurs more commonly in infants of diabetic mothers.

QUESTION

2. Which of the following antihypertensive medications are appropriate for the neonate with hypertension?

a.   Propranolol

b.   Hydralazine

c.   Captopril

d.   Enalaprilat

e.   Amlopidine

ANSWER

2. b, c, d.

Hypertension in acute renal insufficiency may be related to volume overload or to alterations in vascular tone. If hypertension is related to volume overload, prompt fluid removal with dialysis or hemofiltration is necessary if the patient has not responded to diuretic therapy. Depending on the degree of blood pressure elevation and the cause of the hypertension, antihypertensive therapy may also be indicated. The choice of antihypertensive therapy depends on the degree of blood pressure elevation, the presence of central nervous system symptoms, and the cause of the acute renal failure and hypertension. Drugs commonly used to treat hypertension in newborn infants with renal failure are detailed in Table 18-4.

In the present case, hydralazine or the angiotensin-converting enzyme (ACE) inhibitor captopril would be appropriate choices to treat the hypertension. Hydralazine has been used extensively as an antihypertensive agent in newborn infants. Hydralazine directly relaxes arteriolar smooth muscle tone to decrease vascular resistance. Side effects of hydralazine treatment include tachycardia and fluid retention. These side effects represent the body's attempt to increase the total intravascular volume in the presence of the lowered total vascular resistance. Therefore, as with most direct-acting vasodilating medications, many patients require concomitant treatment with a diuretic.

Captopril, an ACE inhibitor, has also been used extensively to treat hypertension in the newborn. The initial treatment dose of this drug for newborn infants is substantially lower than

TABLE 18-4

DRUGS USED TO TREAT HYPERTENSION IN NEWBORNS

Drug	Starting Dose	Maximum Dose	Mechanism of Action
Hydralazine	0.5–1 mg/kg/day given PO or IV every 4–6 hr	5–6 mg/kg/day given PO or IV every 4–6 hr	Peripheral vasodilator
Captopril	0.03–0.1 mg/kg/day given PO every 8 hr	2–3 mg/kg/day given PO every 8 hr	Competitive inhibitor of ACE
Enalaprilat	0.005–0.01 mg/kg/day given IV every 6 hr	Unknown	Competitive inhibitor of ACE
Propranolol	0.5–1 mg/kg/day given PO every 8–12 hr	Unknown; 5–8 mg/kg/day in older children	β-Blocker
Sodium nitroprusside	0.05–1 µg/kg/min	Unknown; 5–8 µg/kg/min in older children	Peripheral vasodilator, possibly by releasing nitric oxide
Diazoxide	0.5–1 mg/kg/dose	5 mg/kg/dose	Peripheral vasodilator

ACE, angiotensin-converting enzyme; IV, intravenous; PO, by mouth.

doses administered to older children (see Table 18–4). Newborn infants who have received higher treatment doses of captopril have developed severe hypotension, with marked deterioration of renal function. This untoward effect of captopril is exaggerated in the presence of intravascular volume depletion or diuretic use. Captopril must be given orally, but *enalaprilat* is an ACE inhibitor that can be given intravenously. An optimal dose of enalaprilat based on pharmacologic studies in newborn infants has not been reported, and the current dosing recommendations are based on studies performed in older children and adult patients. ACE inhibitors can result in hyperkalemia and acidosis. Therefore, medications that have the potential to cause these metabolic derangements should be used with caution in infants treated with ACE inhibitors.

Calcium-channel blocking drugs are useful antihypertensive agents in older children. These agents inhibit the flux of calcium into cells and result in relaxation of smooth muscle. Amlodipine and nifedipine act primarily on vascular smooth muscle, but may adversely affect cardiac output in patients with preexisting myocardial contractile dysfunction. Use of these agents in newborn infants is hampered by a lack of specific knowledge about the pharmacologic kinetics and optimal doses in newborn infants.

Suggested Readings

Agras PI, Tarcan A, Baskin E, et al: Acute renal failure in the neonatal period. Renal Failure 2004; 26(3): 305–309.

Andreoli SP: Clinical aspects and management of acute renal failure in children. In Avner ED, Harmon WE, Niaudet P (eds): Pediatric Nephrology. Baltimore, Williams & Wilkins, Chapter 64, pages 1233–1254, 2004.

Andreoli SP: Bergstein JM, Sherrard DJ: Aluminum intoxication from aluminum-containing phosphate binders in children with azotemia not undergoing dialysis. N Engl J Med 1984;310:1079–1084.

Andreoli SP: Acute renal failure. Curr Opin Pediatr 2002;14:183–188.

Andreoli SP: Acute renal failure in the newborn. Semin Perinatol 2004;28:112–123.

Australian and New Zealand Intensive Care Society Clinical Trials Group: Low dose dopamine in patients with early renal dysfunction: A placebo controlled trial. Lancet 2000;356:2139–2143.

Badr KF, Ichikawa I: Prerenal failure: A deleterious shift from renal compensation to decompensation. N Engl J Med 1988;319:623–628.

Basile DP, Donohoe D, Roethe K, et al: Renal ischemic injury results in permanent damage to peritubular capillaries and influences long-term outcome. Am J Physiol 2001;281:F887–F889.

Brenner BM, Lawler EV, Mackenzie HS: The hyperfiltration theory: A paradigm shift in nephrology. Kidney Int 1996;49:1774–1777.

Brown CB, Ogg CS, Cameron JS: High dose furosemide in acute renal failure. Clin Nephrol 1981;15:90.

Bunchman TE, Maxvold NJ, Kershaw DB, et al: Continuous venovenous hemodiafiltration in infants and children. Am J Kidney Dis 1995;25:17–21.

Bunchman TE, Wood EG, Schenck MH, et al: Pretreatment of formula with sodium polystyrene sulfonate to reduce dietary potassium intake. Pediatr Nephrol 1991;5:29–32.

Cataldi L, Leone R, Moreti U, et al: Potential risk factors for the development of acute renal failure in preterm infants: A case control study. Arch Dis Child Fetal Neonatal Ed 2005;90:514–519.

Chertow GM, Sayegh MH, Allgren RL, Lazarus JM: Is the administration of dopamine associated with adverse or favorable outcomes in acute renal failure? Am J Med 1996;101:49–53.

Chevalier RL: What treatment do you advise for bilateral or unilateral renal thrombosis in the newborn, with or without thrombosis of the inferior vena cava? Pediatr Nephrol 1991;5:679.

Chevalier RL, Campbell F, Brenbridge ANAG: Prognostic factors in neonatal acute renal failure. Pediatrics 1984;74:265–272.

Denton MD, Chertow GM, Brady HR: "Renal-dose" dopamine for the treatment of acute renal failure: Scientific rationale, experimental studies and clinical trials. Kidney Int 1996;49:4–14.

Drukker A, Guignard JP: Renal aspects of the term and preterm infant: A selective update. Curr Opin Pediatr 2002;14:175–182.

Ellis EN, Arnold WC: Use of urinary indexes in renal failure in the newborn. Am J Dis Child 1982; 136:615–617.

Ellis EN, Pearson D, Belsha CW, Berry PL: Use of pump-assisted hemofiltration in children with acute renal failure. Pediatr Nephrol 1997;11: 196–200.

Gerstman BB, Kirkman R, Platt R: Intestinal necrosis associated with postoperative orally administered sodium polystyrene sulfonate in sorbitol. Am J Kidney Dis 1992;20:159–161.

Gouyon JB, Guignard JP: Management of acute renal failure in newborns. Pediatr Nephrol 2000; 14:1037–1044.

Karlowicz MG, Adelman RD: Nonoliguric and oliguric acute renal failure. Pediatr Nephrol 1995; 9:718–722.

Kellum JA, Decker JM: Use of dopamine in acute renal failure: A meta-analysis. Crit Care Med 2001; 29:1526–1531.

Malone TA: Glucose and insulin versus cation-exchange resin for the treatment of hyperkalemia in very low birth weight infants. J Pediatr 1991; 118:121–123.

Martin-Ancel A, Garcia-Alix A, Gaya F, et al: Multiple organ involvement in perinatal asphyxia. J Pediatr 1995;127:786–793.

Mathew OP, Jones AS, James E, et al: Neonatal renal failure: Usefulness of diagnostic indices. Pediatrics 1980;65:57–60.

Mathews DE, West KW, Rescorla FJ, et al: Peritoneal dialysis in the first 60 days of life. J Pediatr Surg 1990;25:110–116.

O'Dea RF, Mirkin BL, Alward CT, Sinaiko AR: Treatment of neonatal hypertension with captopril. J Pediatr 1988;113:403–405.

Rodriguez-Soriano J: Potassium homeostasis and its disturbances in children. Pediatr Nephrol 1995; 9:364–374.

Ronco C, Brendolan A, Bragantini L, et al: Treatment of acute renal failure in newborns by continuous arterio-venous hemofiltration. Kidney Int 1986; 29:908–915.

Sadowski RH, Harmon WE, Jabs K: Acute hemodialysis of infants weighing less than five kilograms. Kidney Int 1994;45:903–906.

Stapleton FB, Jones DP, Green RS: Acute renal failure in neonates: Incidence, etiology and outcome. Pediatr Nephrol 1987;1:314–320.

Thadhani R, Pascual M, Bonventre JV: Acute renal failure. N Engl J Med 1996;334:1448–1460.

Wells TG, Bunchman TE, Kearns GL: Treatment of neonatal hypertension with enalaprilat. J Pediatr 1990;117:664–668.

Neonatal Seizures

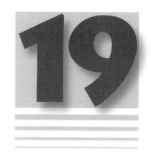

Mark S. Scher, MD

Seizures represent a neurologic emergency but may reflect brain dysfunction or injury either on an acute, subacute, or chronic basis. The clinician caring for a newborn with suspected seizures must promptly formulate diagnostic and therapeutic plans relevant to the history and clinical presentation. The neonate's limited clinical repertoire often hinders the physician's ability to recognize seizures by simple bedside visual inspection. This is compounded by the difficulty in reaching an accurate neurologic assessment of a critically ill infant, confined within an isolette, who may be intubated and receiving multiple pharmacologic agents. These conditions significantly alter arousal and muscle tone and, therefore, limit the clinician's ability to elicit the full complement of clinical neurologic signs.

The first major aim of this chapter is to help the clinician recognize the spectrum of clinical manifestations of seizures in the newborn in order to distinguish normal from abnormal behaviors and epileptic from nonepileptic events. A representative case history is presented that illustrates the diagnostic dilemmas inherent in the description of clinical seizure activities. Additional case histories explore the multiple causes that can be associated with seizures in a newborn infant and provide a framework for a diagnostic evaluation. Consideration for the timing of the brain injury events associated with neonates with seizures is also discussed. This section is followed by a discussion of the treatment modalities available to control neonatal seizures, given that seizures may be a surrogate marker for multiple injurious events during antepartum, peripartum, and postnatal periods. Finally, the chapter concludes with a

discussion of the challenges faced by the clinician in determining the prognosis for an infant with seizures.

Diagnostic Pitfalls

This first case history describes the clinical course of a high-risk newborn infant who exhibits multiple behavioral abnormalities reflective of a neonatal brain disorder that may or may not be epileptic.

Case Study 1

A male infant weighing 1200 g was delivered after a 30-week gestation to a 26-year-old primigravida woman with a history of pyelonephritis. A positive vaginal culture for group B streptococcus was noted and the mother was treated with ampicillin on the day of delivery. The infant was delivered vaginally in vertex presentation. During labor, the mother's temperature rose to 39.4°C (103°F), and she had foul-smelling vaginal fluids. Apgar scores were 4 at 1 minute and 6 at 5 minutes. The infant initially required 100% oxygen in a hood, and at 30 minutes of age an arterial blood gas showed Pao_2 75 mm Hg, Pco_2 53 mm Hg, and pH 7.28. The total serum calcium was 5.1 mg/dL and an ionized calcium was 0.5 mg/dL; all other chemistries were within normal limits.

After intubation and ventilation, the child demonstrated improved activity and color, and vital signs stabilized. Fluids were administered through an umbilical venous catheter, and cultures of blood,

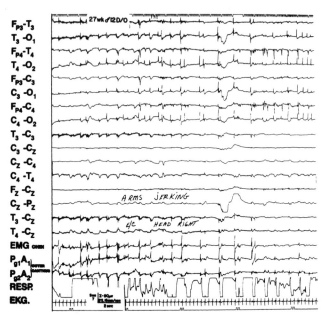

Figure 19-1 Electroencephalogram (EEG) from a 28-week gestation male infant, documenting suppressed EEG activity with myoclonic movements and myogenic potentials in the absence of electrographic seizures.

urine, and cerebrospinal fluid (CSF) were obtained. The child was placed on broad-spectrum antibiotic coverage.

Episode 1. At approximately 12 hours of life, limb tremors were noted, characterized by rapid, rhythmical to-and-fro movements of the extremities that were suppressed by holding or repositioning the affected limb. An electroencephalogram (EEG) was obtained during a period of tremulousness and documented no coincident electrographic seizure activity. While the EEG was being performed, intravenous calcium gluconate was given, which resulted in a rise in the serum calcium concentration from 5.1 to 8.9 mg/dL, and in the ionized calcium from 0.5 mg/dL to 1.3 mg/dL. Following the administration of calcium, the tremors ceased.

Episode 2. On the second day of life, the child began having facial grimacing, episodes of sucking, lateral nystagmoid movements of the eyes, and generalized myoclonic movements. A second EEG was obtained, documenting the above-mentioned behaviors coincident with a continuous admixture of EEG frequencies.

Episode 3. On the third day of life, the child exhibited apnea associated with bradycardia, as well as increased myoclonic movements. The child's overall level of activity decreased, and a lumbar puncture was performed, documenting

cloudy spinal fluid with a protein concentration of 340 mg/dL and a glucose concentration of 30 mg/dL. The serum glucose concentration (obtained immediately before the lumbar puncture) was 110 mg/dL. An EEG was obtained, as illustrated in Figure 19-1, documenting a suppressed EEG background compared with the previously normal EEG study, with numerous myogenic potentials, coincident with myoclonic movements in the absence of electrographic seizures. Both blood and spinal fluid cultures were positive for group B streptococcus.

Episode 4. The child continued to show a depressed sensorium with multifocal myoclonic activity, not suppressed by restraining the affected body part. An EEG again documented myogenic potentials coincident with myoclonus in addition to independently occurring electrographic seizures associated with eye fluttering and tonic horizontal eye deviation.

Because of these four separate episodes, the physicians and nurses had to consider whether the abnormal behaviors were seizures.

Exercise 1

QUESTION

1. In the following table, list the signs occurring in each episode that were suggestive of

seizures. Decide whether the abnormal behaviors were epileptic or nonepileptic, and identify a possible cause for each behavioral abnormality.

Suspicious Clinical Sign	Epileptic Seizure? (Yes or No)	EEG (Normal or Abnormal)	Potential Cause
Episode 1	No	Normal	Hypocalcemia
Episode 2	No	Normal	Sleep behaviors
Episode 3	No	Abnormal	Encephalopathy
Episode 4	Yes	Abnormal	Encephalopathy

ANSWER

Episode 1. Tremulousness or jitteriness is not considered to be an epileptic phenomenon. Tremors are usually provoked by stimulation and suppressed by holding or repositioning the affected body part. The nonepileptic nature of this finding was confirmed by the initial EEG, which showed no evidence of electrographic seizures. The tremulousness may have been related to the low total and ionized serum calcium concentrations.

Episode 2. Rudimentary rapid eye movement (REM) sleep behavior of the preterm neonate consists of periods of rapid eye movements, sucking, and irregular respirations. Neonatal sleep behavior can easily be confused with seizure activity, given rhythmical or isolated motor movements, such as myoclonus. However, coincident neurophysiologic monitoring, preferably with synchronized video, can help distinguish epileptic from nonepileptic behaviors.

Episode 3. The child's episodes of apnea and bradycardia as well as myoclonus are worrisome in the context of a decreasing level of arousal; the third EEG documented a major change in the interictal background rhythm (without seizure activity), which is discussed in a subsequent section. The myoclonic movements, suppressed EEG activity, and abnormal CSF findings suggest an intracerebral inflammatory process, possibly bacterial meningitis.

Episode 4. The tonic eye deviation coincident with electrographic seizure activity on the EEG confirms the diagnosis of seizures in a child with culture-proved bacterial meningitis.

This case study illustrates how a preterm infant may exhibit a wide repertoire of normal sleep behaviors, as well as abnormal seizure and nonseizure clinical movements. Whereas episodic autonomic and motor behaviors can reflect normal sleep activity, nonepileptic abnormal behavior (e.g., myoclonus) may also reflect an evolving encephalopathy.

True epileptic seizure activity may go unrecognized if clinical seizures remain subtle. In those situations, confirmation with an EEG is extremely helpful. The use of synchronized video EEG monitoring can correlate the suspicious behavioral event with the coincident electrographic expression of surface-projected seizure activity. This diagnostic tool will help minimize unnecessary treatment of nonepileptic events.

Types of Seizures

Neonatal seizures are generally brief and subtle and comprise unusual clinical behaviors that sometimes can be difficult to distinguish from normal behavioral patterns. The International Classification of Epileptic Seizures does not specifically define categories that are applicable to neonates; however, novel classification systems are now being recommended.

Although there is no absolute way to behaviorally distinguish seizures from other abnormal behavioral states, the following observations and guidelines can be valuable.

1. Any repetitive stereotypical event should be considered a clinical seizure until proved otherwise.
2. Stereotypical behaviors may be identified as normal neonatal sleep or waking states if documented by polygraphy.
3. Suspicious behavioral phenomena may have an inconsistent relationship with coincident electrographic seizures, suggesting a subcortical seizure focus.
4. Nonepileptic pathologic behaviors can be expressed by a neonate, independently of seizure states.

Subtle or Fragmentary Seizures

The most frequently observed clinical type of suspected neonatal seizures involves an extensive repertoire of activities, including repetitive facial activity, unusual bicycling or pedaling movements, momentary fixation of gaze, or autonomic dysfunction. Repetitive or periodic

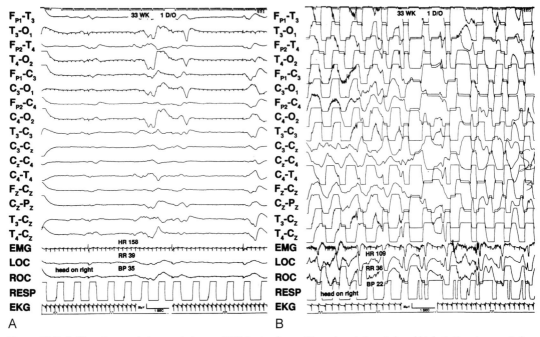

Figure 19-2 A, Discontinuous electroencephalogram (EEG) tracing from a 33-week gestation, 1-day-old infant. No seizures noted. **B,** EEG from the same patient documenting a generalized electrographic seizure, coincident with a drop in heart rate and blood pressure.

changes in blood pressure, heart rate, or oxygenation can also be autonomic manifestations of subtle seizures (Fig. 19-2). Although apnea is observed in newborns with subtle seizures, it is almost never the sole manifestation of seizures. Subtle seizures are difficult to detect but nonetheless may reflect significant brain dysfunction or injury. Subtle seizures are more common in premature than in full-term infants, and are not consistently associated with electrographic abnormalities particularly in full-term infants. Therefore, one must be careful in attributing an epileptic origin to subtle seizures, until an EEG study documents the clinical event coincident with an EEG seizure.

Clonic Seizures

Clonic seizures are commonly described as rhythmic movements of muscle groups in focal or multifocal distributions. Clonic seizures can be distinguished from the symmetrical to-and-fro movements of nonepileptic jitteriness (tremors) and from the quick jerking characteristic of myoclonus by the presence of a rapid phase followed by a slow return movement. In addition, gentle flexion of a body part suppresses tremors, whereas clonic seizures persist. Clonic activity may involve different body parts, including the

pharyngeal and diaphragmatic musculature. Generalized tonic-clonic activity rarely occurs in newborn infants. However, neonates commonly exhibit multifocal clonic seizures that involve several body parts. Focal clonic seizures that involve one body part (face, extremity, neck, or trunk) are more highly associated with localized brain injury in the contralateral hemisphere but may also occur with generalized brain abnormalities. Transient weakness known as Todd's phenomenon can also occur after a focal seizure in a newborn. Clonic seizures are frequently accompanied by abnormal electrographic activity.

Tonic Seizures

A tonic seizure refers to a sustained flexion or extension of an axial or appendicular muscle group. Coincident EEG monitoring is required in any infant with tonic posturing, because the majority of infants demonstrating generalized tonic postures do not have electrographic seizures. Subcortical motor pathways subserve such movements when the inhibitory influences of cortical motor pathways are dysfunctional or injured. Focal tonic seizures are more commonly associated with EEG abnormalities. Significant neocortical damage or dysfunction may be associated with this seizure type.

Myoclonic Seizures

Myoclonic movements may frequently occur in healthy preterm or full-term neonates. Video EEG monitoring helps distinguish normal non-epileptic paroxysmal movements from patho-logic nonepileptic myoclonus or myoclonic epileptic seizures. Generalized myoclonic sei-zures are more likely to be associated with EEG discharges than are focal or multifocal myo-clonic seizures. However, pathologic myoclonus can also occur with or without coincident sei-zure activity. Age-appropriate sleep-related myo-clonic clusters occur during active as well as quiet sleep states and are more commonly noted in preterm than in full-term neonates. Such movements are usually not stimulus sensitive and are suppressed during the waking state. Benign neonatal sleep myoclonus is a variant of normal and can persist for several months. This physiologic entity is discussed later.

Exercise 2

QUESTION

1. Match the following descriptions for the clinical seizure phenomena with these five seizure types: subtle, tonic, focal clonic, multifocal clonic, myoclonic.

    a. Repetitive events of jerking or shaking, limited to one body part or half the body. The jerk may involve a slow followed by a fast phase. The jerk or shake cannot be suppressed by holding or repositioning the involved body part.

    b. Episodes of repetitive jerking or shaking that involve multiple body parts and occur randomly over time; may appear migratory or give the appearance of a generalized clonic seizure event.

    c. Episodes of sudden, brief, shock-like muscle jerks or twitches producing either extension or flexion of limbs or of the midline. They may occur individually or in a brief series of movements.

    d. Episodes of abrupt change in tone characterized by altered body position. These movements can produce the stiffening of a limb or arching of the neck and back.

    e. Episodes of facial movements, including eye movements. Complex automatisms, such as bicycling or autonomic changes that are repetitive, may occur.

ANSWER

1. a. Focal clonic. b. Multifocal clonic. c. Myo-clonic. d. Tonic. e. Subtle.

Nonepileptic Behaviors of the Neonate

Certain neonatal behaviors can be difficult to clas-sify as normal or abnormal activities (Table 19-1). Coincident paper or synchronized video-EEG-polygraphic recordings can accurately document the temporal relationship between electrographic activity and clinical phenomena. Questionable events must be evaluated individually based on the clinician's overall experience. The following are descriptions of normal and abnormal nonepi-leptic neonatal behaviors (see Table 19-1).

Neonatal Sleep-Wake Behaviors

By 30 to 32 weeks postconceptional age (PCA), four rudimentary physiologic states of arousal can be recognized in healthy preterm infants: wakefulness, active or REM sleep, transitional sleep, and quiet or non-REM sleep. Both preterm and full-term infants spend most of their time asleep and regularly alternate between periods of active and quiet sleep. After 36 weeks PCA these EEG sleep rhythms are expressed in a well-developed and predictable manner. During active sleep, paroxysmal clinical behavior such as facial grimacing, rapid horizontal eye move-ments, buccolingual movements (sucking), myoclonic movements of the limbs and trunk, and slower large body movements such as head rolling and squirming are commonly observed. The respiratory pattern can be irregular or even periodic, particularly during REM sleep. EEG activities are continuous with an admixture of various frequencies, corresponding to the child's PCA. Periods of transitional sleep, during which behaviors are not typical of either active or quiet sleep, may be more difficult to classify until after 38 weeks PCA. When REM activity ceases in association with regular bursts of rhythmic sucking movements and regular respirations,

TABLE 19-1

CLINICAL AND LABORATORY FINDINGS THAT DISTINGUISH EPILEPTIC FROM NONEPILEPTIC MOTOR ACTIVITIES IN THE NEONATE

Clinical Event	Duration	Stimulus Sensitive	Lower Extremity	Upper Extremity	Trunk Posture	Respiratory Changes	Ocular/Pupillary Changes	EEG Changes
Tonic seizure	Brief/intermittent	−	Extension	Flexion or extension	Extension	Apnea and/or bradycardia	Blinking, vertical or horizontal deviation, pupillary changes	Yes
Decorticate posturing	Brief/intermittent	+	Extension	Flexed, adducted, internal rotation, fisted	Extension	None	None	No
Decerebrate posturing	Brief/intermittent	+	Extension	Extended, adducted, hyperpronated, fisted	Extension	Tachypnea, irregular respirations, apnea	Pupils enlarged, downward eye deviation	No
Opisthotonos	Prolonged/sustained	+	Extension	Variable; often extended	Prolonged arching	None	None	No
Myoclonic seizures	Brief/intermittent	±	Rapid*	Rapid*	Rapid*	None	None	Yes
Pathologic myoclonus	Brief/intermittent	±	Rapid*	Rapid*	Rapid*	None	None	No
Benign myoclonus	Brief/intermittent during sleep only	−	Rapid*	Rapid*	Rapid*	None	None	No

*Brief, sudden jerk of axial or appendicular musculature.

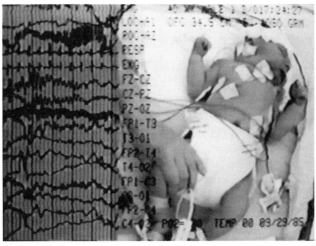

Figure 19-3 Video electroencephalogram (EEG) documenting tremulousness of the upper extremities, coincident with artifact noted on the EEG reflective of the child's tremulous state. No electrographic seizures were noted.

quiet or non-REM sleep can be identified. There is usually a paucity of body movements during quiet sleep. Both preterm and full-term infants younger than 46 weeks PCA characteristically express discontinuous EEG activity during quiet sleep. Paroxysmal motor activities can be observed during quiet or active sleep and may be mistaken for subtle seizure activity. In those situations, subtle seizures should be diagnosed by performing a coincident EEG-video study. In that way, the occurrence of these motor activities can be best correlated with a characteristic EEG polygraphic pattern.

Benign Neonatal Sleep Myoclonus

Myoclonus may occur abundantly during sleep in healthy neonates or infants. Such movements are brief and sudden and may be bilateral and synchronous, but they can also be asymmetrical and asynchronous. Myoclonic activity occurs in clusters, particularly during active sleep, and is expressed predominantly in preterm infants. Physiologic myoclonus is not commonly stimulus sensitive, and no coincident epileptiform activities or interictal EEG sleep-state disturbances are noted. Infants have suppression of this myoclonic activity during the waking state, and a normal, age-appropriate clinical examination supports an exclusionary diagnosis of benign neonatal sleep myoclonus.

Tremulousness or Jitteriness

This motor behavior can be seen with a variety of metabolic or toxin-induced encephalopathies,

including the postasphyxial period, drug withdrawal, and hypoglycemia. Tremulousness has also been observed in infants with intracranial hemorrhage or hypothermia and in those who are small for gestational age (Fig. 19-3).

Stimulus-Evoked Myoclonus

Neonates with severe central nervous system (CNS) dysfunction may present with stimulus-evoked myoclonic activity. CNS infections, cerebrovascular injury, congenital malformations, and rare metabolic or genetic disorders such as glycine encephalopathy may be associated with the expression of pathologic myoclonic activity in an affected infant, independent of seizures. Encephalopathic newborns can manifest stimulus-induced focal, segmental, or generalized myoclonic movements. At times, cortically generated spike or sharp wave discharges on the EEG can be noted, coincident with the myoclonic movements.

Decorticate and Decerebrate Posturing (Including Opisthotonos)

A number of nonepileptic activities can be confused with tonic seizures unless coincident EEG studies are obtained. Decorticate or decerebrate posturing may be stimulus sensitive or spontaneous and is commonly triggered by painful stimulation such as intubation or endotracheal suctioning. With decorticate posturing, the child's lower extremities extend while the arms flex, adduct, and internally rotate (usually with fisting). Decerebrate posturing involves leg and arm extension with hyperpronation and wrist adduction with fisting. Eye findings may include downward deviation of the eyes with pupillary dilatation or constriction. Such clinical activity may be symmetrical or asymmetrical; an asymmetrical clinical sign suggests a pathologic process in the contralateral region of the brain. Infants who exhibit these behaviors are generally neurologically impaired. Decorticate posturing reflects a neurologic syndrome at the level of the diencephalon, midbrain, or upper pontine level of the brain stem. Decerebrate posturing suggests brain stem dysfunction at the pontine or upper medullary level. Lateral and medial subcorticospinal pathways are functionally more dominant with the destruction of corticospinal pathways. The resultant loss of cortical inhibitory input permits the expression of subcortically generated hypertonic movements or postures.

Opisthotonos is a general descriptive term implying abnormal extensor tone of the trunk, which can occur either spontaneously or with stimulation. This posturing indicates dysfunction of pyramidal or extrapyramidal pathways on either an acute or a chronic basis.

Dysautonomia

Autonomic abnormalities can give the appearance of seizures unless careful documentation is performed with coincident EEG studies. Poor temperature regulation (poikilothermy), respiratory disturbances (hypoventilation, hyperapnea, apnea), cardiac rhythm disturbances (tachycardia, bradycardia), and alterations in color (flushing and cyanosis) all may suggest subtle seizures. However, only a small number of neonates will demonstrate coincident electrographic seizure activity unless the events are periodic or repetitive. Table 19-1 lists the clinical and neurophysiologic findings that help distinguish nonepileptic motor activities from seizures.

Electrographic versus Clinical Seizure Criteria

Coincident EEG-video-polygraphic studies are invaluable tools for the verification of suspected seizures, independent of or in the context of a brain disorder. Interpretation of neonatal EEG recordings requires experience. Comparisons of clinical and electrographic behaviors require an appreciation of expected physiologic relationships for the postmenstrual age and state of arousal of the neonate.

There are six clinical circumstances in which neurologically abnormal neonates may be unable to clinically express seizures or mistakenly be assumed to have seizures.

1. *Severe neonatal encephalopathy.* A newborn infant who is comatose may not be able to clinically express seizures because of severe brain dysfunction. In this instance, electrographic seizures are commonly unaccompanied by clinical seizure behaviors. The use of an EEG study can be extremely helpful in such situations (Fig. 19-4).

2. *Pharmacologic paralysis.* This commonly occurs in infants with severe respiratory disease who require pharmacologic paralysis to improve oxygenation or ventilation. In babies who are administered neuromuscular blocking agents, it is impossible to ascertain by clinical criteria the infant's level of arousal, because the paralytic agent suppresses neurologic responses. Serial or continuous EEG tracings should be used during the period of paralysis to provide electrographic documentation of seizures or interictal EEG abnormalities associated with a significant brain disorder (Fig. 19-5). Autonomic findings such as periodic increases in blood pressure or heart rate or a fall in oxygen saturation are unaffected by paralytic medications and may suggest the presence of seizures.

3. *Use of antiepileptic medications (uncoupling phenomena).* Suppression of clinical seizure activities after antiepileptic drug administration (despite the persistence of electrographic seizures) has been termed "uncoupling." This underscores the need for continuous EEG monitoring, particularly after the administration of antiepileptic medications.

4. *Electroclinical disassociation.* It has also been observed that surface-recorded electrographic seizures may have an inconsistent relationship with clinical seizure behaviors, particularly after antiepileptic medications have been administered. This has been referred to as electroclinical disassociation

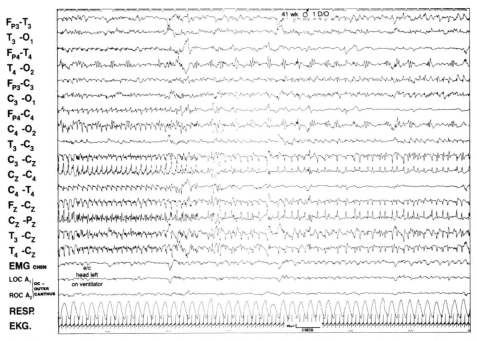

Figure 19-4 Electroencephalogram from a 41-week gestation, 1-day-old male infant with severe asphyxia, demonstrating electrographic seizures with no clinical accompaniments.

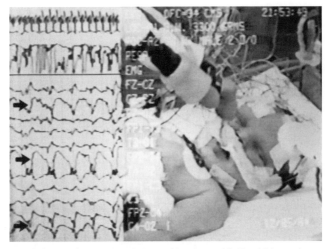

Figure 19-5 Video electroencephalogram documenting electrographic seizure while the child was pharmacologically paralyzed.

(ECD). ECD indicates that repetitive clinical events may occur with or without coincidental electrical seizures, implying that subcortically generated clinical seizures may only intermittently propagate to the cortical surface, at which time electrographic seizures are readily recorded by surface electrodes.

5. *Subcortical release phenomena.* Extrapyramidal and brain stem release phenomena are thought to account for the many nonepileptic motor automatisms (e.g., oral-buccal-lingual movements, ocular signs) as well as tonic posturing seen following a severe injury to the neocortex. Functional decortication following asphyxia-induced brain injury is one example of a clinical situation in which seizure-like behavior can occur without documented electrographic seizures. Subcortical seizures may be differentiated from subcortical release phenomena by continuous video EEG monitoring that

intermittently documents electrographic seizures.

6. *Inadequate duration of monitoring*. Despite one's initial suspicion that clinical behaviors commonly represent seizure activities, electrographic verification is required. Intermittent EEG recordings of 30 to 60 minutes' duration, however, may fail to document all questionable clinical seizure events. Serial or continuous EEG recordings more likely will document the random seizure event. This diagnostic challenge may be particularly problematic for a child who was delivered at an outside institution and has received antiepileptic medications before arrival at the tertiary neonatal intensive care unit (NICU). As noted previously, observable clinical seizure behaviors may be suppressed after drug administration, despite persistent electrographic seizures when an EEG is obtained.

Diagnostic Evaluation

Multiple medical conditions over periods of time can be associated with neonatal seizures (Table 19-2). Seizures are signs of abnormal neurologic function, reflecting systemic or primary nervous system disorders. Combined antepartum, peripartum, and neonatal conditions contribute to the genesis of electrographic seizures. However, these same conditions may also injure the brain, independent of the occurrence of seizures. The next case history illustrates the major etiologic conditions associated with seizure activity in newborn infants.

Case Study 2

A female newborn infant weighing 4800 g was born at 38 weeks postmenstrual age to a 47-year-old primigravida woman who reported loss of fetal movements one day prior to admission. She also began leaking green amniotic fluid approximately 24 hours before entering the hospital. The mother had been followed by the maternal-fetal medicine service because of preeclampsia and insulin-dependent diabetes. The child was delivered in a breech position, after an 8-hour first stage of labor, during which time the mother had a temperature of 38.8°C (102°F). Fetal heart rate monitoring

TABLE 19-2
PEAK ONSET OF CONVULSIONS

24 Hours
Bacterial meningitis
Direct effect of drugs, cocaine
Laceration of tentorium of falx
Perinatal asphyxia encephalopathy
Pyridoxine dependency
Rubella, toxoplasmosis, cytomegalovirus
Sepsis

24 to 72 Hours
Bacterial meningitis
Cerebral contusion with subdural hemorrhage
Cerebral dysgenesis
Drug withdrawal
Intraventricular hemorrhage in a premature infant
Nonketotic hyperglycinemia
Sepsis
Subarachnoid hemorrhage
Urea cycle disturbances

72 Hours
Cerebral dysgenesis
Kernicterus
Ketotic hyperglycinemia
Nutritional hypocalcemia
Smith-Lemli-Opitz syndrome
Urea cycle disturbances

1 Week
Cerebral dysgenesis
Fructose dysmetabolism
Herpes simplex
Ketotic hyperglycinemia
Maple syrup urine disease
Urea cycle disturbances

Modified from Fenichel GM: Neonatal Neurology. New York, Churchill Livingstone, 1980, p 22.

demonstrated intermittent tachycardia with late decelerations and loss of variability in the last hour before delivery. The mother was administered magnesium during labor because of hyperreflexia, intermittent confusion, proteinuria, and hyperlipidemia. Delivery was difficult and required forceps instrumentation. The Apgar score at 1 minute was 4 (heart rate 2, respiration 1, color 1) and at 5 minutes was 7 (−1 each for color, grimace, and tone). With delivery of the cord and placenta, a large area of infarction (estimated to involve 15% of the placental surface) and a true knot in the cord were noted. On microscopic examination, a thrombotic vasculopathy on the maternal side of the placenta was noted, with ischemic changes within the true knot of the umbilical cord without a thrombus. The child was initially pale, with a blood pressure of 60/40 mm Hg and a pulse of 170 beats per minute. The respiratory rate was irregular, and periodic breathing was noted. In the delivery room, the blood glucose concentration was less than

25 mg/dL. At 1 hour of life, an arterial blood sample was obtained and demonstrated pH 7.13, Pco_2 43 mm Hg, Pao_2 79 mm Hg, and base excess −11. Focal clonic seizures were noted in the delivery room involving the right upper and lower extremities. Ten percent dextrose and water, phenobarbital, and antibiotics were administered in the delivery room, following which the infant was transported to the NICU.

On admission to the NICU, the child's pulse remained elevated at 174 bpm. However, the blood pressure decreased to 50/30 mm Hg, and the rectal temperature fell to 33°C (91.4°F). Swelling of the skull that crossed the suture line was noted. Although the child was hypotonic and lethargic, she responded to stimulation. No other abnormalities were noted on examination. Blood was sent to the chemistry laboratory for quantitation of serum electrolytes and specimens of blood and CSF were sent to the microbiology laboratory. Glucose was then administered. Both the serum calcium concentration (total 6.2 mg/dL, ionized fraction 0.49 mg/dL) and serum glucose concentration (12 mg/dL) were abnormal. The serum magnesium concentration was 5.3 mg/dL. A lumbar puncture documented slightly turbid fluid that was xanthochromic, with 15 white blood cells/mm^3, 2000 red blood cells/mm^3, a glucose concentration of 30 mg/dL, and a protein level of 100 mg/dL. A skull x-ray documented a parietal fracture, but a computed tomographic (CT) scan of the brain showed no subdural or intracranial hemorrhage.

A neurologic consultation was obtained immediately upon arrival in the newborn nursery. The neurologist noted the child to be depressed but arousable, with an asymmetrical motor examination; less activity was noted in the right arm and leg. In addition, the withdrawal reflex was asymmetrical, with less extension on the right side despite symmetrical deep tendon reflexes. The Galant reflex was also asymmetrical, with incurvation of the spine to the left but not to the right.

Exercise 3

The case history indicates that multiple causes may contribute to seizure occurrence. The physician's initial evaluation of a child with seizures should be directed toward discovery of the most relevant and remedial causes for the seizures. In conjunction with history, a carefully performed physical examination allows one to decide which tests are most appropriate. For example, although a workup for possible sepsis or meningitis and electrolyte or glucose disturbances is indicated in every infant with seizures, it is inappropriate to send blood or urine routinely for toxicologic studies (unless the history is suggestive). A neuroimaging study is almost always appropriate. In a critically ill infant, this may be limited to the performance of a cranial ultrasound examination. As the child recovers, a magnetic resonance imaging (MRI) scan provides more definitive information, as compared with the CT scan or cranial ultrasound.

QUESTION

1. List six possible causes of the child's seizures. How would you manage each of those possibilities?

ANSWER

Six possible causes of this infant's seizures include the following:

1. Given the history of maternal diabetes, and preeclampsia, loss of fetal movements, elevated fetal heart rate, and abnormal fetal heart rate tracing, *intrauterine asphyxia* (that began during the antepartum period and extended into the intrapartum period) must be considered. The placental findings of vasculopathy on the maternal surface and ischemic changes within the true knot are supportive of more chronic antepartum asphyxial stress to the fetus before the mother's admission to the hospital.

Management: General supportive intensive care, including maintenance of cardiovascular function, ventilation, and metabolic homeostasis, and treatment of seizures should be provided.

2. The pallor of the child and the postnatal fall in blood pressure suggest the possibility of *ischemic brain injury.*

Management: Consider blood transfusion and interventions to support blood pressure (pressors, volume, or both).

3. The infant's generalized neurologic depression and dystonia could be consistent with a *hypoxic-ischemic encephalopathy,* although the elevated serum magnesium constitutes an overlapping rapidly reversible cause.

Management: After documentation of hypermagnesemia, treatment is generally supportive. Although there are theoretical reasons to administer supplemental calcium, a beneficial effect has not been observed in practice. Urine output should be maintained; however, fluids should be administered cautiously in infants who have been asphyxiated.

4. The history of maternal fever and prolonged rupture of membranes suggests *sepsis* or *meningitis* as diagnostic possibilities.

Management: Administer antibiotics and await culture results.

5. Metabolic disturbances such as *hypoglycemia, hypocalcemia,* and other *electrolyte disturbances* should be considered in every infant with seizures.

Management: Correct the hypocalcemia with 10% calcium gluconate and the hypoglycemia with 10% dextrose (see Chapters 3 and 4 for specific details).

6. *Trauma to the CNS* is suggested by the history of a prolonged and difficult labor and the parietal skull fracture. A *subgaleal hematoma* is suggested by swelling of the scalp that crosses the suture line. The presence of red blood cells in the CSF raises the possibility of *intracranial hemorrhage*, although the CT scan did not document hemorrhage. Alternatively, *subarachnoid hemorrhage* may have occurred.

Management: Obtain more definitive neuroimaging studies (i.e., MRI) and consult neurosurgery if a treatable condition is considered. If a subgaleal hematoma is suspected, the hemoglobin concentration should be closely monitored, as some of these infants lose much of their circulating blood volume into the scalp.

History

The history should include a complete survey of the antepartum period, as well as problems that occurred during labor and delivery. Important considerations include the gravidity and parity of the mother, gestational age of the infant, prior history of fetal deaths or stillbirths, presence of maternal illnesses such as diabetes or hypertension, substance abuse and drug exposure during pregnancy, trauma to the mother, and serologic or clinical indicators of possible infection. The results of antepartum fetal testing are particularly important, because they provide data about fetal well-being. Peripartum issues of significance include the presence or absence of risk factors for neonatal sepsis (e.g., prolonged rupture of membranes or signs indicative of chorioamnionitis), abnormal progression of labor, use of local anesthetics or narcotics, abnormal fetal heart rate monitoring, metabolic acidosis, passage of meconium, breech presentation, or difficult delivery. Important postnatal considerations include Apgar scores of the infant, the need for and duration of resuscitation, and the presence and persistence of abnormal antepartum or intrapartum clinical signs after resuscitation.

As listed in Table 19-2, there are many reasons for seizures in newborn infants, and they take on varying significance, depending on the time at which the seizures are noted. Seizures from either antepartum or intrapartum problems commonly occur during the first 48 to 72 hours of life. However, seizures generated from cerebral dysgenesis, inborn metabolic disturbances, or CNS infections can also occur within the same time period. Generally, seizures that occur beyond 3 to 5 days of life suggest metabolic-genetic disorders or brain malformations, once infection, toxin exposure, and intracranial hemorrhage are excluded.

Physical Examination Findings

Every newborn infant requires a thorough physical examination and there are specific features that are particularly important for an infant with a suspected neurologic disease. Vital signs, including respiratory rate, blood pressure, and heart rate, should be initially assessed. The gestational age of the infant should be estimated using one of the standard classification systems (Dubowitz or Ballard). However, in severely depressed infants, such inferences are invalid, because estimations of active and passive tone cannot be assessed. The appropriateness of the infant's growth (head circumference, length, and weight) relative to gestational age should be estimated to assess whether in utero growth restriction has occurred (and if so, whether there has been relative head sparing). Standard growth curves define intrauterine growth restriction. However, more subtle growth compromise can be estimated using the alternate calculations of the ponderal index. Any skin lesions, including rashes, macules, hemangiomas, and hyperpigmented or hypopigmented lesions, should be carefully sought, because their presence may suggest a congenital infection or neurocutaneous syndrome. Consider the use of a Wood's lamp to reveal hypopigmentation that is not visible under natural light; such lesions suggest the diagnosis of a neurogenetic disorder called tuberous sclerosis. A tense or full anterior fontanel or suture separation suggests that intracranial pressure may be increased.

The neurologic examination permits an assessment of the child's level of arousal, cranial nerve function, and motor and reflex capabilities. The child's fundi must be examined to document the presence of hemorrhages, chorioretinitis, or papilledema. Assistance by the pediatric ophthalmologist who applies the skill of using an indirect ophthalmoscope can better document lesions in the posterior portion of the retina. A thorough neurologic evaluation should always include examination of cranial nerves to assess the integrity of brain stem function, particularly with respect to extraocular movements, pupillary equality and light reactivity, corneal response, sucking, swallowing, and phonation. On the motor examination, an assessment should be made of the quality and symmetry of muscle tone and postural and deep tendon reflexes. Primitive reflex testing should include Moro, tonic neck, grasp, trunk incurvation (Galant), and place-step maneuvers. Consideration of the effects of prematurity on the elaboration of specific neurologic signs must be applied.

Specific clinical findings such as joint contractures suggest a long-standing process due to limited movement in utero. Hypertonicity with cortical thumbs in a child who recovers rapidly after a resuscitative effort strongly suggests chronic neurologic compromise. Hypotonia and unresponsiveness are usually expected to persist for at least 4 to 5 days after an intrapartum or peripartum asphyxial stress. However, depressed arousal and hypotonia at birth may reflect an encephalopathy that began well before labor and continued after the onset of labor. Such infants may have preexisting brain injury, despite the appearance of being depressed without muscle tone at the time of birth. Serial examination and the child's response to resuscitative interventions offer clues to the newborn's encephalopathic signs relative to etiology and timing.

Causes of Neonatal Seizures

Asphyxia

Hypoxic-ischemic brain injury traditionally has been considered the most common cause of neonatal seizures. Most neonates suffer asphyxia either before or during parturition; less than 10% of asphyxia cases are the result of postnatal events. The diagnosis of asphyxia must always be verified biochemically by obtaining arterial and venous samples from cord blood. Only a minority of children with suspected asphyxia satisfy a conventional biochemical definition of acute asphyxia (i.e., a pH 7.0 or lower and a base deficit less than or equal to -12 in cord blood on the first postnatal arterial blood gas determination). These values alone, however, do not predict the emergence of a neonatal encephalopathy, describe the severity of brain dysfunction, the presence of brain damage, or the time course over which this process may have occurred. Neonates who are asphyxiated before the onset of labor may have resolution of metabolic acidosis by delivery or, conversely, may demonstrate a worsening acidosis with labor, with or without accompanying brain injury. Resuscitative interventions may include ventilatory assistance, circulatory stabilization inotropic medication support, and bicarbonate administration. However, such measures may not rectify earlier brain injury (remote from the immediate minutes before delivery) or profound acute predominantly subcortical insults. Generally, a neonate's quick adaptation to extrauterine life with stabilization after minimal resuscitative interventions suggests a more remote brain disorder from asphyxia or other possible etiologies.

Intrauterine factors that lead to asphyxia generally compromise gas exchange or nutrient delivery across the placenta to the fetus. Therefore, antepartum or intrapartum asphyxia is often associated with maternal illnesses such as preeclampsia or with uteroplacental abnormalities such as abruptio placentae, cord compression, or placental infarction. Chorioamnionitis also may contribute to the occurrence of intrauterine asphyxia by altering placental circulation and introducing inflammatory mediators (i.e., cytokines) into the infant's bloodstream. Similarly, the passage of meconium into the amniotic fluid may cause vasoconstriction, reduce placental blood flow to the fetus, and increase the potential for asphyxia. If an asphyxial event occurs weeks to months before the time of delivery, brain lesions leading to destruction or dysgenesis may be detected by fetal sonography or cranial imaging before or immediately after birth. Whenever asphyxia is suspected, the placenta should be sent to the pathology laboratory for a detailed analysis. Acute and chronic injury to placental and cord specimens should be compared with the clinical data.

Postnatal complications can also lead to or worsen previously acquired hypoxic-ischemic brain injury. Some examples include persistent pulmonary hypertension (PPHN) of the newborn, cyanotic congenital heart disease, sepsis, and central nervous system infections. However, these postnatal diagnoses may have an antepartum component that contributed to the child's neurologic injury before birth. For example, PPHN is a pathologic condition that promotes increased pulmonary vascular resistance, often after an initial asphyxial event at or after the time of birth. However, in utero events may also contribute to pulmonary hypertension (i.e., remodeling of the pulmonary vasculature) over a period of days to weeks. Infants with PPHN commonly suffer from repeated bouts of asphyxia as their condition worsens during early postnatal life.

Neonatal encephalopathy is a clinical syndrome expressed over days in which seizures may occur. Biochemical sequelae, such as metabolic acidosis at birth, as well as early hypocalcemia, hypoglycemia, and hypomagnesemia, are commonly associated with more acute, presumably intrapartum asphyxial stress. Inflammatory mediators may also contribute to seizure occurrence. Physical examination findings should reflect an acute insult by reduced levels of arousal including coma, hypotonia, brain stem abnormalities, and loss of primitive reflexes. Seizures generally occur within the first three postnatal days after asphyxia but also can occur with neonatal encephalopathies after antepartum rather than intrapartum events. Seizures without accompanying encephalopathic signs require immediate evaluation for metabolic disturbances, CNS infections, hemorrhages, or trauma, after which remote acquired or genetic conditions need to be considered.

Low Apgar scores, as in case study 2, can be noted in infants with or without intrapartum asphyxia. Depressed 1- and 5-minute Apgar scores only indicate the need for continued resuscitation and do not predict long-term outcome. Depressed scores at 10, 15, and 20 minutes of life have greater prognostic significance for neurologic sequelae. Normal Apgar scores, however, do not eliminate the possibility of severe intrauterine brain injury from asphyxia remote from labor and delivery. Intrapartum asphyxia is believed to account for only 4% to 5% of the cerebral palsy observed in older children. As an extension of these observations, the occurrence of neonatal seizures with an accompanying encephalopathy is uncommonly associated with intrapartum asphyxia.

Other clinical and laboratory findings may reflect asphyxial stress, even in the absence of significant metabolic acidosis or brain injury. The passage of meconium in utero is a frequent occurrence in otherwise healthy newborns. However, meconium staining of the child's skin, nails, or umbilical cord may be noted in infants who are also neurologically depressed. Microscopic evidence of meconium-laden macrophages with lymphocytic infiltration may be found within the placenta and suggest chronic stress to the fetus when associated with other abnormalities such as altered villous maturation or placental infarction. These chronic placental abnormalities are significantly more common in infants with seizures with neonatal encephalopathy.

Although endogenous metabolic disturbances usually occur with asphyxia, they can also occur independently. For the present discussion, the findings of hypoglycemia, hypocalcemia, and hyponatremia are included under the general discussion of asphyxia.

Hypoglycemia is discussed in detail in Chapter 4. It should be remembered, however, that there is still no clear consensus concerning the relationship between hypoglycemia and the occurrence of seizures or the possible association with brain injury. Methods of glucose determination (i.e., dextrose stick versus serum sampling) can also affect the accuracy of the measurement. Neonates at highest risk for hypoglycemia include preterm infants, infants of diabetic mothers, small-for-gestational-age infants, large-for-gestational-age infants, and those born following perinatal asphyxia. Tremulousness, apnea, and altered tone are clinical signs that may occur in a child with hypoglycemia with or without the presence of EEG-documented seizures. As with hypoglycemia, the threshold at which hypocalcemic seizures occurs is controversial. Late-onset hypocalcemia has historically been cited as a common cause of seizures, owing to the high phosphate load in cow milk. However, hypocalcemia now occurs more commonly in infants with trauma, hemolytic disease, asphyxia, or congenital heart disease and may coexist with hypoglycemia or hypomagnesemia, after asphyxial stress.

Hyponatremia is an uncommon solitary cause of neonatal seizures and is usually associated with congenital abnormalities of adrenal steroid metabolism or an iatrogenic disturbance of serum sodium balance from intravenous fluid that contains inappropriately low amounts of sodium. Less commonly, hyponatremia may result from inappropriate secretion of antidiuretic hormone following severe brain trauma, infection, or asphyxia.

Infection

CNS infections during the antepartum or postnatal periods have the potential to cause neonatal seizures. Congenital infections, commonly referred to by the acronym TORCH (toxoplasmosis, rubella, cytomegalic inclusion disease, and herpes simplex), can produce severe encephalopathic damage that results in seizures and brain injury. Although the clinical manifestations of antenatal TORCH infections vary with the etiologic agent, affected infants commonly manifest microcephaly, jaundice, body rash, hepatosplenomegaly, and chorioretinitis. Increasing lethargy and obtundation with or without seizures can also suggest a subacute presentation of encephalitis during the postnatal period. Serial spinal fluid analyses can assist by documenting rising protein concentrations or a CSF pleocytosis.

In utero or postnatally acquired bacterial infections are commonly accompanied by neonatal seizures. *Escherichia coli, Streptococcus agalactiae* (group B streptococcus), *Listeria monocytogenes*, and other gram-positive and gram-negative organisms may produce severe leptomeningeal infiltration and inflammation, with abscess formation and subsequent cerebrovascular occlusion. A high percentage of survivors of these infections suffers significant neurologic sequelae.

Blood, urine, and spinal fluid analyses should be obtained for bacterial cultures; broad-spectrum antibiotics should be administered while culture results are pending. Serum titers for toxoplasmosis and rubella, as well as viral cultures for rubella virus, cytomegalovirus, and herpes simplex virus, should be obtained *when the clinical signs suggest a TORCH infection.*

Spinal Fluid Analysis

The following discussion highlights the important ways in which spinal fluid analysis can assist in the differential diagnosis of a neonate with seizures.

Appearance. Normal CSF is colorless and crystal-clear. Yellow discoloration, called xanthochromia, can occur within 12 hours of a cerebral hemorrhage because of the liberation of red blood cell pigments. However, a yellow discoloration of the spinal fluid is most commonly due to bilirubin pigments (small amounts of bilirubin cross the blood-brain barrier in all jaundiced infants) or protein concentrations in excess of 150 mg/dL. It is important to determine the clarity of the CSF, because turbidity or cloudiness suggests an increased cellular or protein content. Total cell counts above $400/mm^3$ increase the turbidity of CSF. Visibly bloody or pink CSF fluid implies a red blood cell count of at least $6000/mm^3$.

Red Blood Cell Count. Spinal fluid obtained by a nontraumatic lumbar puncture in a healthy neonate has a mean red blood cell count of $30/mm^3$. Many pediatricians are willing to accept much higher counts as within the normal range, but counts in excess of $100/mm^3$ should probably be considered significant. A dilemma arises, however, when a spinal tap is thought to be traumatic. In order to distinguish a traumatic tap from a "true" episode of intracranial hemorrhage, the general practice is to use three tubes of CSF and to ascertain the cellular and protein content, particularly in the last tube (after the CSF is cleared of blood) (Table 19-3). It is important to note that the protein content of bloody spinal fluid is increased in the amount of 1 mg/dL for every 1000 red blood cells present. A significant number of red blood cells in a nontraumatic sample of CSF suggests intracerebral hemorrhage, infarction, or hemorrhage secondary to intracranial infection from a bacterial or viral source.

White Blood Cell Count and Protein. Normal values for the white blood cell count and protein concentration in the CSF of healthy term and preterm infants are listed in Table 19-4. The data in the table represent newer studies

DIFFERENTIAL FEATURES OF SUBARACHNOID HEMORRHAGE AND TRAUMATIC PUNCTURE:
THE THREE-TUBE TEST

Cerebrospinal Fluid Finding	Subarachnoid Hemorrhage	Traumatic Puncture
Appearance	Equal amount of blood in all tubes	First or last tube is bloodier; others are clearer
Supernatant fluid color	Pigment in excess of protein level	Clear
Red blood cell (RBC) count and hematocrit	Essentially similar in all tubes	Variable in different tubes
White blood cell count	Proportional to peripheral RBC count in earliest stages, relatively increased later	Proportional to peripheral RBC count
Clot formation	Absent	Occurs rarely
Repeat puncture at higher interspace	Findings similar to those at initial tap	Usually clear

From Fishman RA: Cerebrospinal Fluid in Diseases of the Nervous System. Philadelphia, WB Saunders, 1980, p 172.

in which more sensitive methods were used to exclude neonates with viral illnesses. The white blood cell and protein counts of CSF fall to adult levels over the first 3 months of life. Infants with traumatic spinal taps should not exhibit CSF pleocytosis if the lumbar puncture is repeated within a few days of the initial tap.

The following case history illustrates the method by which a CSF profile can be interpreted.

Case Study 3

A 3-day-old full-term infant is evaluated for seizures. This child's general neurologic examination is remarkable for decreased arousal and hypotonia. Serum electrolyte studies are normal, including serum glucose of 150 mg/dL. The child's hematocrit is 42%, the red blood cell count is $5.13 \times 10^6/mm^3$, and the white blood cell count is $8.1 \times 10^3/mm^3$. Three tubes of spinal fluid are obtained; the first tube is bloody, but the subsequent two are clear. The fluid in the second and third tubes is turbid and slightly xanthochromic after

centrifugation. Analyses of the spinal fluid indicate a red blood cell count in tube 3 of 18,000/mm³, a white blood cell count of 80/mm³, a glucose concentration of 40 mg/dL, and a protein concentration of 270 mg/dL. Inspection of a Gram-stained specimen is negative, and cultures are obtained.

Exercise 4

QUESTIONS

1. What significance do you attribute to the xanthochromia and turbidity after centrifugation?

2. Does the white blood cell count of 80/mm³ suggest a traumatic lumbar puncture or a clinically significant result?

3. Are the concentrations of protein and glucose in the CSF within the range of normal for a term infant?

4. Would you predict that the spinal fluid would be culture-positive for bacterial infection?

CEREBROSPINAL FLUID (CSF) VALUES IN NONINFECTED HIGH-RISK NEONATES

Age	WBC Count	PMNL	Protein	Glucose
Term	7 ± 13* 4†	0.8 ± 6.2* 0†	64 ± 24*	51 ± 13*
Preterm (<1000 g)	4 ± 3* 6†	6 ± 15	150 ± 56	61 ± 34

*Mean ± SD.
†Median.
PMNL, polymorphonuclear neutrophil leukocytes; WBC, white blood cell.
Term values from Ahmed A, Hickey S, Ehrett S, et al: Cerebrospinal fluid values in the term neonate. Pediatr Infect Dis 1996;15(4):298–303; preterm values from Rodriguez AF, Kaplan SL, Mason EO: Cerebrospinal fluid values in the very low birth weight infant. J Pediatr 1990;116:971–974.

ANSWERS

1. The xanthochromia is most probably due to the high protein level of 270 mg/dL and does not necessarily indicate a recent CNS hemorrhage or infection. In addition, the turbidity is due to the presence of an increased CSF red blood cell count of 18,000/mm^3.

2. The ratio of white blood cells to red blood cells in the peripheral blood is 8.1 × 10^3/5.13 × 10^6, or 1.6/1000. Therefore, the 18,000 red blood cells in the spinal fluid can account for 18,000 × 1.6/1000 = 24 white blood cells. The "corrected" white blood cell count is 80 − 24 = 56/mm^3. This is excessively high for any newborn infant.

3. The 18,000 red blood cells can account for 18 mg of protein (18,000 × 1 mg of protein/ 1000 red blood cells). The "corrected" level of protein, 280 − 18 = 262 mg/dL, exceeds the upper limit of normal shown in Table 19-4. Although the level of CSF glucose is in the normal range, the ratio of CSF glucose to blood glucose, 40:150, is abnormally low.

4. One would anticipate that the spinal fluid cultures would be positive.

This child has a heavy growth of Listeria monocytogenes *36 hours following the lumbar puncture.*

Structural Abnormalities of the Brain

Structural lesions of the CNS may give rise to neonatal seizures. These lesions include anomalies that are microscopic or macroscopic, and lesions can be either acquired or congenital. For example, seizures may result from subtle disorganization of neuronal structures, such as isolated pachygyria or heterotopias, or gross developmental brain anomalies, such as lissencephaly and holoprosencephaly. Seizures may also occur secondary to acquired lesions such as neuronal necrosis and edema following asphyxia or infection, or after more localized destruction resulting from occlusion of a major intracerebral artery or intraparenchymal hemorrhage. Cranial imaging (in addition to lumbar puncture) is an invaluable laboratory tool to help establish the diagnosis. The preferred method of neuroimaging is MRI. However, with medically unstable neonates, preliminary studies should begin with a cranial ultrasound study at the bedside, or cranial computed tomography. Unfortunately, treatment for most of these conditions is nonspecific and supportive.

Cerebrovascular Lesions

Hemorrhagic or ischemic cerebrovascular lesions can be associated with neonatal seizures. Intraventricular or periventricular hemorrhage (IVH or PVH) is the most common intracranial hemorrhage of preterm infants and is associated with neonatal seizures in as many as 45% of affected premature infants. Intracranial hemorrhage usually occurs within the first 72 hours of life in a preterm infant. IVH is uncommon in full-term infants, and in that population, IVH usually originates from the choroid plexus or the thalamus, possibly secondary to venous stasis with elevated hydrostatic pressure. See Chapter 20—for a more complete discussion.

Subarachnoid hemorrhage (SAH) can be a cause of neonatal seizures, particularly if SAH is excessive. Fortunately, for most neonates, seizures after SAH are generally associated with a more favorable outcome. Posthemorrhagic hydrocephalus, however, may result after massive SAH.

Subdural hemorrhage is a less common cause of neonatal seizures and is usually associated with a traumatic delivery. Whenever there is focal trauma to the face, scalp, or head in an encephalopathic infant, an area of subdural bleeding should be considered. Subdural hematoma is a treatable cause of neonatal seizures but may be fatal if unrecognized. Traumatic brain injury producing a subdural hematoma may occur after a precipitious, prolonged, or difficult delivery or even following trauma to the mother's abdomen during the antepartum period. When the amount of bleeding is excessive, a craniotomy may be needed to remove the blood clot from the overlying brain. With extracranial bleeding from a cephalhematoma or subgaleal hematoma, intracranial injury should be suspected.

Cerebral infarction has been described in neonates with seizures and can result from events that occur during the antepartum, intrapartum, or neonatal period. The use of cranial imaging before birth or during the first day or two after birth may help document older brain lesions (Fig. 19-6A). Destructive cystic lesions such as porencephaly require at least 5 to 7 days before becoming radiographically visible by cerebral CT studies. Specific MRI images (diffusion-weighted images) can approximate lesions that may have occurred within 48 hours. Cerebral infarctions originating in the postnatal period may be associated with asphyxia, polycythemia, dehydration, coagulopathy, or infection (Fig. 19-6B).

Cerebral infarctions also result from occlusions in either the venous or arterial systems. Lateral or sagittal sinus thromboses can occur secondary to systemic infection, polycythemia, or dehydration; there is an increased risk in an infant with an underlying genetic thrombophilia. Seizures occur in approximately two thirds of the infants with major sinus thromboses. Venous stasis leading to infarction within the deep white matter of a preterm infant can also contribute to the development of IVH that is frequently accompanied by parenchymal involvement. Magnetic resonance venography with subtraction imaging yield optimal images to document a thrombus.

Seizures are the most common presenting sign of an arterial or venous occlusion. Motor abnormalities may not be readily observed during the neonatal period, even when major vessels are occluded. The most common site of arterial occlusion is the middle cerebral artery; occlusion of the carotid artery or segments within the circle of Willis are seen less frequently. However, a significant percentage of neonates with stroke events do not present clinically at birth and only later express motor asymmetries or seizures during infancy.

The anatomic site of injury within the nervous system determines the spectrum of neurologic findings an infant displays. Supratentorial lesions, particularly those that involve a localized area of the cerebral cortex, may produce contralateral hemiparesis and focal seizures in the same body distribution. If cerebral edema and herniation coexist, ipsilateral pupillary dilatation and lateral eye deviation (indicative of third cranial nerve weakness) may also be noted. Conversely, infratentorial brain lesions within the posterior fossa may precipitate a more abrupt change in level of arousal and include coma, respiratory abnormalities, autonomic abnormalities, quadriparesis, and bilateral pupillary and oculomotor abnormalities.

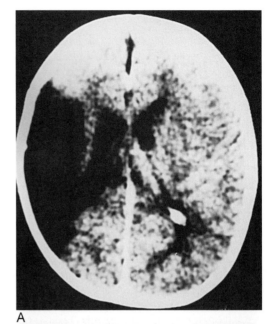

A

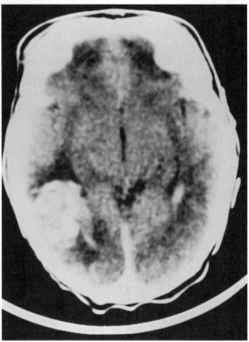

B

Figure 19-6 A, Computed tomography (CT) scan from a full-term infant who had seizures during the first 24 hours of life, documenting a cerebral infarction that occurred at least 1 week before labor and delivery, based on the appearance of porencephaly in the distribution of the right middle cerebral artery. **B,** CT scan from a full-term infant with severe asphyxia and persistent pulmonary hypotension of the newborn. A hemorrhagic infarction was documented on the second day of life, with radiographic features suggesting a more acute onset, possibly at or after the time of delivery.

Central Nervous System Malformations

Disorders of induction, segmentation, proliferation, migration, dendritic arborization, synaptogenesis, and myelination all have the potential to contribute to seizures in newborn infants. Some malformations such as holoprosencephaly may be associated with facial anomalies (midfacial hypoplasia, cleft lip and palate) that lead to a rapid diagnosis initially by fetal sonography. Most infants, however, lack stigmata to suggest a brain malformation. An MRI study, therefore, should be obtained in an otherwise healthy neonate with persistent seizures after the third day of life, or in any newborn infant with seizures for which a cause is not evident (Fig. 19-7). In general, focal or regional brain malformations are uncommon causes of severe early onset epilepsy in neonates and infants. Functional imaging studies, including single-photon emission computed tomography (SPECT), positron emission tomography (PET), and magnetic resonance spectroscopy (MRS), can also help localize areas of altered brain metabolism in children with dysplastic brain who express persistent or intractable seizures.

Inborn Errors of Metabolism

Inherited metabolic abnormalities are uncommon causes of neonatal seizures, but need to be considered when (1) the onset of seizures is

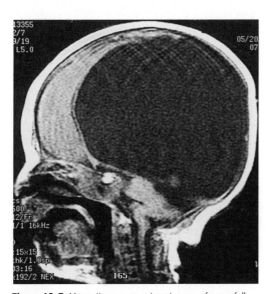

Figure 19-7 Magnetic resonance imaging scan from a full-term infant with neonatal seizures, showing severe lissencephaly and hypoplasia of the cerebellum and brain stem.

beyond day 1 of life (an exception is pyridoxine dependency), (2) an infant becomes symptomatic following the introduction of enteral or parenteral nutrition, and (3) seizures are intractable and do not respond to conventional antiepileptic medications. Infants with inborn errors of metabolism commonly have uncomplicated birth histories. The presence of a dysplastic brain lesion on a neuroimaging study does not eliminate the possibility of an inborn error of metabolism, because some biochemical defects such as a glycine encephalopathy are associated with either dysplastic or destructive gray or white matter lesions.

Food intolerance within a few days of birth associated with altered arousal and seizures may be an early indicator of a specific inborn error affecting protein, carbohydrate, or lipid metabolism. For example, the urea cycle defect carbamoyl phosphate synthetase deficiency may present with coma and seizures after introduction of formula feedings, resulting in marked elevations in plasma ammonia levels. Such infants require aggressive treatment with exchange transfusion, dialysis, and specialized diets. It is important to make a specific and rapid diagnosis in all suspected disorders of metabolism, because some of them may respond to vitamin supplementation.

Vitamin B_6 or pyridoxine dependency is a rare cause of neonatal seizures. Pyridoxine acts as a cofactor for synthesis of γ-aminobutyric acid (GABA), and its absence or paucity promotes seizures. Mothers carrying an affected infant may report paroxysmal fetal movements that reflect an in utero fetal seizure state. An infant without an obvious cause for seizures who is unresponsive to conventional antiepileptic medications should initially receive 50 to 100 mg of pyridoxine intravenously. The EEG should be monitored before and after the pyridoxine is administered. Additional doses of pyridoxine up to a total of 300 to 500 mg have been suggested. Termination of seizures with coincidental improvement of the EEG background rhythm disturbances after infusion of vitamin B_6, supports the clinical diagnosis of a pyridoxine-dependent seizure state. The diagnosis must then be verified biochemically, including appropriate spinal fluid studies. Prophylactic doses of pyridoxine may be administered to improve seizure control. In addition to pyridoxine, other cofactor deficiencies should be considered for reversible encephalopathies (e.g., folinic acid deficiency).

Inborn errors of metabolism presenting with seizures during the neonatal period include the aminoacidopathies (e.g., homocystinuria), organic acidopathies (e.g., methylmalonic acidemia), urea cycle defects (e.g., ornithine transcarbamoylase deficiency), fatty acid oxidation disorders, mitochondrial disorders (e.g., Leigh disease), carbohydrate disorders (e.g., glycogen storage diseases), peroxisomal disorders (e.g., Zellweger syndrome), and lysosomal storage diseases (e.g., Krabbe disease). Specific metabolic defects may mimic hypoxic-ischemic encephalopathy (e.g., sulfide oxidase deficiency).

When an inborn error of metabolism is suspected, the anion gap should be calculated from a serum electrolyte determination: anion gap = $[Na] + [K] - ([Cl] + [HCO_{3^-}])$. Normal values range from 8 to 16 mEq/L. Blood should be sent routinely for glucose determination, ammonia levels, and pH. If there is evidence of metabolic acidosis, blood should be sent for lactate and pyruvate concentrations. In addition, a complete blood count should be obtained (neutropenia and thrombocytopenia are associated with a number of organic acidemias). All infants with seizures should have a lumbar puncture; CSF should be sent for lactate, pyruvate, glycine, and glucose (in addition to the routine tests). Hypoglycorrhachia in a CSF specimen in association with a normal serum glucose concentration suggests the diagnosis of a glucose transporter defect. In addition, brain-specific defects of mitochondrial metabolism may result in normal levels of pyruvate and lactate in blood but abnormal CSF levels. The same is true for nonketotic hyperglycinemia, in which the most consistent elevation of glycine is found in the CSF. In any child with a suspected inborn error of metabolism, serum amino acids should be quantified, and urine should be sent for amino acid and organic acid determinations. Rarely, tissue sampling for ultrastructural electromicroscopy, as well as biochemical studies for respiratory chain enzyme deficiencies, may be required.

Drug Withdrawal and Intoxication

Neonates born to mothers with prenatal substance abuse are at an increased risk for seizures. Exposure to barbiturates, alcohol, marijuana, cocaine, or methadone may present with neurologic findings in the newborn period consisting of tremors, irritability, muscle tone abnormalities, and other signs of withdrawal. Symptoms may continue for as long as 4 to 6 weeks after birth for specific substances such as barbiturates. Prenatal exposure to cocaine may result in an irritable, hypertonic infant. Seizures may occur directly after cocaine withdrawal but may also be indirectly associated with uteroplacental insufficiency induced by chronic substance use, poor prenatal health care of the mother, or placental abnormalities such as abruptio placentae. The child may appear growth-restricted with associated signs of chronic neurologic injury (i.e., dysmorphia, hypertonia, contractures). Certain substances such as short-acting barbiturates are associated with seizures in the immediate postnatal period. Electroencephalographic confirmation of suspected clinical seizures is strongly recommended before initiating an antiepileptic medication.

More recently, maternal use of serotonin reuptake inhibitors for mood disorders, including depression and anxiety, has also been reported to result in neonatal withdrawal signs suggestive of seizures. Characteristically these nonepileptic signs persist for up to the first week of life, with resolution. Coincident EEG recordings fail to document coincident electrographic seizures.

The inadvertent injection of the fetal scalp with a local anesthetic during delivery may induce intoxication. During the first several hours of life, these neonates present with seizures, apnea, bradycardia, and hypotonia. They are frequently comatose and have absent brain stem reflexes. A puncture site on the scalp can usually be identified in symptomatic infants. Determination of plasma levels of the suspected anesthetic agent establishes the diagnosis. Treatment generally consists of supportive care and interventions that accelerate drug clearance, such as forced diuresis and urinary acidification. In rarer situations, exchange transfusion may be needed. Antiepileptic medications are rarely needed.

Diagnostic Approach to Seizures

Following a careful review of the medical histories of the mother, fetus, and newborn (and in the absence of a known cause), blood should be sent for determination of glucose, electrolytes, ammonia, lactate, pyruvate, magnesium, and calcium levels. A complete family history should include relatives with epilepsy or neonatal seizures. A lumbar puncture should routinely be done and fluid sent for cell count, protein, glucose, and culture. Additional spinal fluid should be set aside for pyruvate, lactate, glycine determinations, or other metabolic studies (see earlier). The presence of multiorgan dysfunction should alert the clinician to the possibility of a postasphyxial syndrome. The presence of intrauterine growth restriction, early muscle hypertonicity, or an elevated nucleated red blood cell value are clinical/laboratory data that cumulatively may suggest that the fetus was stressed during the antepartum period. Careful review of the placental and cord specimens is imperative to help distinguish antepartum from more acute disease processes. A neuroimaging study is mandatory, preferably with MRI. Serial use of EEG-polygraphy can document the persistence or resolution of seizures with or without encephalopathic patterns, especially in infants receiving paralytic or antiepileptic medications or who are profoundly comatose. Finally, a comprehensive workup for inborn errors of metabolism may need to be performed, if warranted by the clinical history, examination findings, and laboratory data.

Treatment of Neonatal Seizures

With the development of rapid methods to assess serum glucose and electrolyte abnormalities, prompt infusions of glucose or other electrolytes are rarely given without documentation of a specific disturbance. When hypoglycemia is associated with seizures, it should be corrected by intravenous administration of 2 mL/kg of a 10% dextrose solution followed by a constant infusion supplying 4 to 6 mL/kg/minute. Persistent hypoglycemia may require hypertonic glucose solutions. See Chapter 2—for a discussion of other management strategies.

Hypocalcemia-induced seizures should be treated with intravenous administration of calcium gluconate (100 to 200 mg/kg). This dosage may need to be repeated every 4 to 6 hours over the first 24 hours. In any infant with hypocalcemic seizures, a serum magnesium concentration also should also be measured, because hypomagnesemia may accompany hypocalcemia or occur independently of it. Hypomagnesemia is defined as a serum magnesium level less than 1.6 mg/dL. However, clinical signs are uncommon with serum levels greater than 1.2 mg/dL. Hypomagnesemia may be treated by administering magnesium sulfate (MgSO$_4$) intramuscularly or intravenously. See Table 19-5 for the recommended doses.

A depressed serum sodium concentration is a rare cause of neonatal seizures. In such cases, either fluid restriction or replacement with hypertonic saline is appropriate.

As mentioned earlier, pyridoxine dependency is confirmed by the cessation of electrographic seizures following the administration of 50 to 100 mg of pyridoxine during a seizure. A beneficial effect may be seen immediately or occur within several hours. If the response is positive, prophylactic treatment with pyridoxine (50 to 100 mg/day) is recommended.

If the decision to treat a neonate with antiepileptic medications is reached, important questions must be addressed.

1. When should antiepileptic medications be used?
2. What is the drug of choice?
3. How long should the medications be continued?

Some suggest that only neonates with clinical seizures should receive medications, and that electrographic seizures need not be treated. However, most clinicians advocate more aggressive treatment of all seizure manifestations, including electrographic seizures without clinical signs, because of the possible association of uncontrolled seizures and brain injury.

A pediatrician who is considering using an antiepileptic medication to treat neonatal seizures should consider several issues:

1. Clinical seizure activity may be subtle or unrecognized, particularly with pharmacologic paralysis, coma, or antiepileptic drug treatment. The clinician must consider the possibility that the true frequency of seizures has been underestimated and obtain an EEG study. Alternatively, suspicious clinical behavior may be normal or abnormal but nonepileptic; therefore, drug treatment may be avoided unless EEG-documented seizures are observed.
2. Although the clinical manifestations of the seizure appear to be brief, more prolonged electrographic seizures may be documented

TABLE 19-5

RECOGNITION AND TREATMENT OF METABOLIC DEFICIENCY STATES

Deficiency State	Blood Level	Replacement Solution	Delivery Route	Loading Dose	Maintenance Dose	Comment
Hypoglycemia	<40 mg/dL	10% dextrose (100 mg/mL)	IV	2 mL/kg (200 mg/kg)	4–6 kg/min IV, depending on blood glucose levels	Keep blood glucose in normal range if frequent, recurring seizures are present
Hypocalcemia	<7 mg/dL	5% calcium gluconate (50 mg/mL)	IV	4 mL/kg (200 mg/kg)	250 mg/kg/day PO or IV, as needed	Monitor cardiac rate by ECG during loading dose
Hypomagnesemia	<1.5 mg/dL	50% MgSO$_4$ (500 mg/mL) 2–3% MgSO$_4$ (20–30 mg/mL)	IM IV	0.2 mL/kg (100 mg/kg) 2–6 mL/kg	0.2 mL/kg IM as needed —	Infusion of MgSO$_4$ may produce hypotonia and weakness due to curare-like neuromuscular blockade
Pyridoxine dependency	Diagnosis rests on family history and cessation of seizures after administration of vitamin B$_6$	Pyridoxine hydrochloride	IV	100 mg	10–40 mg/day	Administer with EEG monitoring if possible

ECG, electrocardiogram; EEG, electroencephalogram; IM, intramuscular; IV, intravenous; MgSO$_4$, magnesium sulfate; PO, by mouth.
From Clancy R: Neonatal seizures. In Polin RA, Yoder MC, Burg FD (eds): Workbook in Practical Neonatology, 2nd ed. Philadelphia, WB Saunders, 1993, p 349.

by EEG, particularly after antiepileptic drug use.

3. Physiologic consequences of neonatal seizures may include compromise of cerebral blood flow with disturbances of cerebral perfusion and cellular metabolism.

4. Depletion of intracellular substances required for energy expenditure of the neuron may occur if seizures go unrecognized. The use of an EEG both before and after treatment is imperative to assess the true severity of the seizure state.

5. Prolonged or frequent seizures may reduce glucose levels within neuronal cells and raise intracellular lactate concentrations.

6. In the rodent, persistent seizures result in a reduction in brain weight and the neuronal content of DNA, RNA, and protein.

Given these caveats, it is important to consider (at least initially) a short-term course of antiepileptic medications.

The following case study illustrates the decision pathway to follow in a rational approach to treatment of neonatal seizures.

Case Study 4

Baby M is a female infant weighing 4020 g, delivered after a 42-week gestation to a healthy, 24-year-old, primigravida mother. Following spontaneous rupture of membranes, there was sudden onset of profuse vaginal bleeding in the delivery room. An emergency cesarean section was performed, documenting a uterine rupture as the cause of the exsanguination. The infant's Apgar scores were 1 at 1 minute, 3 at 5 minutes, and 7 at 10 minutes. Following resuscitation, the child was taken to the NICU, where she required mechanical ventilation. Tremors were noted at 1 hour of life, unassociated with electrographic abnormalities. However, buccolingual and nystagmoid movements began within the first 24 hours of life and were accompanied by seizure activity. Her general physical examination was significant for pallor, hyperirritability, and tremors. A neurologic examination demonstrated depressed mental status consistent with stupor. She responded to painful stimulation. The child's pupillary light reactions were normal, and extraocular movements were full. Sucking and swallowing were present but diminished. A gag reflex was also present. Spontaneous motor activity was observed, but the child had moderate generalized hypotonia without any focality. Glucose, electrolyte, and CSF studies were normal. A cranial ultrasound examination was read as normal. Given the EEG confirmation of seizures, the decision to begin antiepileptic medications was made.

Exercise 5

QUESTIONS

1. Which antiepileptic medication would you choose in this case?

2. What are the side effects associated with the drug you have chosen?

3. What are the optimal serum concentrations required to stop seizures?

4. What are the initial loading doses and the maintenance doses for phenobarbital and phenytoin?

5. How should antiepileptic medications be administered?

6. How quickly can antiepileptic medications be administered?

7. What other drug options are there if the first antiepileptic medication fails?

ANSWERS

Answers to Questions 1 to 7 are given in the following discussions of each drug.

Antiepileptic Medications

Phenobarbital, phenytoin, and benzodiazepines (lorazepam or diazepam) remain the most widely used antiepileptic medications (Table 19-6).

Phenobarbital

Phenobarbital is currently the drug of choice for managing neonatal seizures. This drug is administered intravenously, intramuscularly, or orally to produce blood levels in the therapeutic range of 10 to 40 µg/mL. The initial loading dose in a preterm or full-term infant should be 20 mg/kg. In an infant with seizures, it should be administered intravenously over 20 minutes to achieve a blood level of 20 µg/mL. Excessively rapid administration may lead to

TABLE 19-6

GENERAL PHARMACOLOGIC PROPERTIES OF PHENOBARBITAL, PHENYTOIN, DIAZEPAM, AND LORAZEPAM

Drug Feature	Phenobarbital	Phenytoin	Diazepam	Lorazepam
Delivery route	IV, IM, PO	IV	IV	IV
Initial loading dose	20 mg/kg	20 mg/kg	0.25 mg/kg	0.05–0.1 mg/kg
Rate of administration	Give IV dose over 20 min	Give IV dose no faster than 1 mg/kg/min with ECG monitoring	Give IV dose over 2 min	Give IV dose over 2 min
Maintenance dosage	3–4 mg/kg/day divided every 12 hr	3–4 mg/kg/day divided every 12 hr	0.25 mg/kg every 15–30 min after loading	0.05–0.1 mg/kg prn (after loading dose)
Timing of first maintenance dose	12–24 hr after loading	12–24 hr after loading	15–30 min after loading	Up to 12 hr
Therapeutic level	20–40 μg/mL	10–20 μg/mL	—	—
Serum half-life	Varies from 40–100 hr, depending on age and duration of drug usage	Newborn: approximately 104 hr; by 1 mo, 2–7 hr	31–75 hr, but seizure control may be much shorter	12 hr
Possible adverse effects	Respiratory depression, hypotension, lethargy if given in excess or too rapidly	Heart block, hypotension if given too rapidly	Respiratory depression, hypotension	Respiratory depression, hypotension

ECG, electrocardiogram; IM, intramuscular; IV, intravenous; PO, by mouth; prn, as needed.

depression of respiration, blood pressure, and alertness, particularly in the context of previous benzodiazepine use. Conversely, phenobarbital is eliminated slowly from the bloodstream, with a serum half-life ranging from 45 to 173 hours. Twelve to 24 hours after the initial loading dose, the first maintenance dose (3 to 4 mg/kg/day divided every 12 hours) should be given. Subsequent changes in the maintenance dose will result in a new steady-state blood level within five half-lives. Because electrographic seizures may persist after suppression of clinical seizure behaviors, the dose of phenobarbital needed to stop seizures may be difficult to predict. Therefore, the use of continuous EEG monitoring is suggested. The time course for the treatment of seizures, particularly after an acute asphyxial illness as seen in Case Study 4, is also debatable. Most children with seizures secondary to perinatal asphyxia have resolution of the seizures with or without antiepileptic medications. Therefore, it is reasonable to consider treatment for only a short period (several days), until clinical signs and EEG studies suggest that the medication can be slowly withdrawn. Some children will require preventive treatment after discharge.

Phenytoin

Phenytoin (Dilantin) is another common antiepileptic medication for the treatment of seizures in newborn infants. It is not well absorbed when administered orally or intramuscularly and should be administered intravenously. A water-soluble form, fosphenytoin, may be used to avoid the harmful effects of subcutaneous infusion or leakage of phenytoin. The therapeutic range is 10 to 20 μg/mL. In a term or preterm infant, the initial loading dose of 20 mg/kg is administered at a rate of 1 mg/kg/minute to achieve an average serum level of 15 μg/mL. Excessively rapid administration may produce heart block and hypotension. Therefore, electrocardiographic monitoring during the initial loading dose is recommended. Maintenance doses of phenytoin (3 to 4 mg/kg/day divided every 12 hours) are begun 12 to 24 hours following the first loading dose. The serum half-life of phenytoin is also age dependent and may fall during the immediate neonatal period. Therefore, frequent blood levels are necessary to guide dosage adjustments. Early discontinuation of phenytoin is generally recommended during the convalescent period in the second week of life.

Diazepam

Diazepam (Valium) may be needed to control seizures in neonates with status epilepticus. The therapeutic dose of diazepam (0.1 to 0.25 mg/kg intravenously) is very close to the toxic dose that causes respiratory depression. Therefore, diazepam should be administered slowly (0.1 mg/kg/minute). The clinical response to diazepam is short-lived because of its rapid clearance from the brain. In contrast, the elimination half-life of diazepam is much slower (25 hours in preterm infants, and 30 to 35 hours in full-term infants). Because of the short-term antiepileptic effect, it is often necessary to administer diazepam every 15 minutes to 2 hours.

Lorazepam

Lorazepam (Ativan) is an alternative to diazepam. A standard dose of 0.05 to 0.1 mg/kg is administered intravenously over 2 to 3 minutes. The clinical response may be significantly prolonged, up to 12 hours, compared with the short duration of diazepam. Like diazepam, lorazepam may cause hypotension and respiratory depression, particularly when phenobarbital has also been administered.

Efficacy of Treatment

The maximal dose of antiepileptic drugs that can be safely administered is controversial. Some clinicians have suggested that a much higher loading dose (up to 40 mg/kg) of phenobarbital is needed for the acute treatment of neonatal seizures. Unfortunately, there is no consensus supporting 40 mg/kg as more efficacious than 20 mg/kg for resolution of *electrographic seizures*, relative to the brain disorder causing the seizures. Furthermore, more recent studies have challenged the efficacy of treating neonatal seizures with either phenobarbital or phenytoin.

Several investigators have suggested that quantitation of free and protein-bound fractions is a better way to assess the efficacy and toxicity of antiepileptic medications in children. Unfortunately, the partitioning of free and protein-bound fractions for the commonly used antiepileptic medications has only recently been reported. Serum binding can be dramatically altered in a sick neonate. At a constant total serum concentration, an increase in the free fraction of the drug may be associated with an increase in untoward side effects, without any improvement in seizure control. It may be necessary in the future to evaluate antiepileptic drugs more critically, by considering total as well as free and bound fractions.

Prophylactic Treatment Beyond the Newborn Period

After the clinician has initiated one or more antiepileptic medications, the more problematic issue is how long to treat a child who has had neonatal seizures. Long-term treatment usually involves the administration of a single oral antiepileptic medication after the acute phase of the seizure disorder has subsided. The following caveats may be helpful in reaching a decision regarding the use of prophylactic antiepileptic medications after discharge from the newborn nursery.

1. Specific drugs such as phenobarbital may disturb the child's level of arousal and behavior and may contribute to long-term changes in brain development.
2. There is no indication that the continued treatment of seizures during infancy prevents the development of epilepsy in later years.
3. The incidence of epilepsy in childhood following the appearance of neonatal seizures is 20% to 56%. Studies suggest that the onset of seizures can occur as long as a decade or more after birth. The incidence of epilepsy in the general population is 0.5%.
4. Seizure disorders that occur at older ages may require the use of antiepileptic medications other than those used in the newborn period. For example, infants with infantile spasms or myoclonic seizures are treated with adrenocorticotropic hormone (ACTH) or valproic acid, respectively.
5. Antiepileptic medications should be maintained beyond the newborn period if a child has ongoing seizures, persistent neurologic abnormalities, or evidence of brain injury or malformations on neuroimaging studies.
6. It is reasonable to consider stopping an antiepileptic medication as early as the time of discharge from the nursery if the child is seizure free, appears developmentally and

neurologically normal, has a convalescent EEG without major abnormalities, and has no major destructive or congenital lesions on a neuroimaging study.

Estimating Prognosis

The prognosis of neonates who have suffered neonatal seizures can be difficult to determine. Anxious parents and families anticipate that the physician will offer precise estimates of the likelihood for neurologic deficits. Unfortunately the clinician may not be able to provide that kind of information.

Several general guidelines may be helpful when considering the prognosis of children with neonatal seizures. The mortality rate of infants who present with neonatal seizures has declined over the last four decades, from 40% to 15%. However, the incidence of adverse neurologic sequelae remains high, particularly for children with a history of meningitis, severe asphyxia, or congenital anomalies.

Prediction of outcome should be considered in the context of the postmenstrual age, the cause of seizures, the intractable nature of the seizures, and interictal EEG patterns. The neurologist can estimate a general outcome based on three possible neurodevelopmental scenarios: (1) a favorable outcome in which there is an 85% to 90% likelihood of survival with a normal outcome, (2) an unfavorable prognosis indicating an 85% to 90% likelihood of death or serious handicap in the survivor, and (3) an intermediate or mixed category with an uncertain prognosis (Table 19-7). The last scenario remains the most problematic one.

The Immature Central Nervous System

The incidence of seizures during the neonatal period exceeds that seen in all other stages of life except for the most elderly. The high incidence of seizures in neonates most likely reflects the vulnerability of the immature brain to neuropathologic processes. Unlike the mature brain, the immature nervous system responds to injury in a manner that preserves neuronal integrity, although the neuronal-glial populations may be altered with negative consequences. Aberrant circuitry due to altered membrane receptors among multiple neuronal networks can be the result of injury to the immature brain. These maladaptive changes increase susceptibility for neurologic sequelae at older ages, which include cognitive and behavioral problems as well as intractable seizure disorders. Premature infants are comparably more resistant to neonatal seizures than term infants but are also more vulnerable to greater morbidities and even death, in part because of the type of neurologic deficits that accompany injury to the very immature brain.

TABLE 19-7

INFLUENCE OF ETIOLOGY ON PROGNOSIS FOR INFANTS WITH NEONATAL SEIZURES

Etiology	Favorable Outcome	Mixed Outcome	Unfavorable Outcome
Toxic-metabolic	Simple late-onset hypocalcemia Hypomagnesemia Hyponatremia Mepivacaine toxicity	Hypoglycemia Early-onset complicated hypocalcemia Pyridoxine dependency	Some aminoacidurias
Asphyxia	—	Mild hypoxic-ischemic encephalopathy	Severe hypoxic-ischemic encephalopathy
Hemorrhage	Uncomplicated subarachnoid hemorrhage	Subdural hematoma Intraventricular hemorrhage (grades I and II)*	Intraventricular hemorrhage (grades III and IV)*
Infection	—	Aseptic meningoencephalitis; some bacterial meningitides	Herpes simplex encephalitis; some bacterial meningitides
Structural	—	Simple traumatic contusion	Malformations of central nervous system

*Grade I, hemorrhage confined to the germinal matrix; grade II, hemorrhage involves the germinal matrix and the ventricle, but the ventricle is normal in size; grade III, hemorrhage involves the germinal matrix and the ventricle, which is enlarged and distended with blood; grade IV, hemorrhage has extended beyond the germinal matrix and the ventricle into the parenchyma of the brain.

Cause of Neonatal Seizures

The underlying cause of neonatal seizures plays a central role in the estimation of prognosis. For example, at one end of the spectrum, infants who suffer neonatal seizures from an electrolyte abnormality (e.g., hypocalcemia or hypomagnesemia) or limited subarachnoid hemorrhage, have a more favorable outcome and respond quickly to the simple administration of the deficient electrolyte or nutrient. At the other end of the diagnostic spectrum are infants with inborn errors of metabolism or cerebral dysgenesis, or those who have seizures following severe in utero asphyxia, for whom the outcome is far worse.

Intractable Nature of Seizures

Based on studies in which the EEG was monitored continuously, it has been estimated that as many as one third of full-term infants present with intractable seizures, which satisfy one definition for status epilepticus. The intractable nature of a seizure condition both underscores the underlying cause, which is primarily responsible for brain damage, and epileptic-induced brain damage. Both conditions substantially increase risk for death or long-term neurologic sequelae.

Interictal EEG-Sleep Studies

The use of an EEG-sleep study provides useful prognostic information, based on the interictal or "between seizure" EEG background activities, as well as assessment of state organization and cyclicity. Although a normal interictal EEG-sleep study cannot assure a normal outcome, there is a higher probability for functionally appropriate development. Conversely, severely abnormal EEG patterns such as a burst suppression background, low amplitude, or isoelectric background without sleep state organization carry a higher predictive value for either a fatal outcome or severe neurologic sequelae. Serial EEG-sleep studies implemented during the first several days to a week or two of life more accurately document the persistence or resolution of neurophysiologic EEG abnormalities. Beyond this time, nonspecific normalization of the EEG may occur, even with the presence of significant neurologic damage.

Therefore, neurologic prognostication should rely strongly on EEG findings, particularly bridging the acute and subacute phases of the illness, when the most abnormal EEG findings may be documented. Persistence of EEG abnormalities over the first week or two of life suggests a worse prognosis.

Case Study 5

A 1350-g female infant, 32 weeks postmenstrual age, was born small for gestational age. She demonstrated intractable seizures during the first day of life following sepsis and a hematologic syndrome of disseminated intravascular coagulation. She suffered from severe fatal anemia noted at birth secondarily to massive fetomaternal hemorrhage. As a result of her bleeding disorder, IVH with parenchymal extension was documented by cranial sonography. An interictal EEG on day 2 of life was obtained following the diagnosis of the intracranial hemorrhage, documenting a low-voltage pattern with no recognizable background activity for the child's postmenstrual age.
By the second and third weeks of life, repeat EEG studies documented moderate to markedly abnormal EEG-polygraphic disorganization during sleep.

Case Study 6

A 4-week-old full-term infant demonstrated lethargy and poor feeding on the second day of life and had several episodes of apnea with bradycardia. An evaluation for sepsis included spinal fluid studies, and the diagnosis of group B streptococcal meningitis was made. The child was treated with appropriate antibiotic medications. An EEG study on day 3 was read as mildly abnormal, with a normal study on day 10 of life.

Case Study 7

A 36-week-gestation male infant had an isolated seizure at 4 days of age after an uneventful pregnancy, labor, and delivery. On physical examination, microcephaly and hypotonia were noted in the absence of other general and neurologic abnormalities. Infectious and metabolic evaluations were negative, but the EEG demonstrated major disorganization of both the left and right hemispheres. MRI of the head revealed the presence of a major brain malformation termed lissencephaly.

Case Study 8

A 37-week-gestation female infant was born with the assistance of forceps after a prolonged and difficult labor. The child's Apgar scores at 1 and 5 minutes were 7 and 9, respectively. Approximately 12 hours after birth, the child began to have seizures, confirmed by coincident EEG recording. Infectious and metabolic evaluations were negative, and a CT scan documented subarachnoid blood in the interhemispheric fissure and within the tentorium. The child suffered three brief isolated seizures, and no antiepileptic medications were given. Her neurologic examination at the time of discharge was normal.

Exercise 6

QUESTION

For Case Studies 5 to 8, classify the infant's prognosis as favorable, unfavorable, or mixed.

ANSWER

Case 5: unfavorable. Case 6: mixed. Case 7: unfavorable. Case 8: favorable.

Conclusion

Neonates with seizures require careful diagnostic and therapeutic considerations that differ from older infants and children. A neurophysiologic evaluation, preferably with coincident EEG-video-polygraphic monitoring, is required for the accurate detection and classification of clinical behaviors. Fetal as well as neonatal disease states contribute to the seizure occurrence, with or without accompanying encephalopathic signs. A child may experience "multiple-hits" to the brain, both in utero and at birth that contribute to the continuum of injury expressed by neonatal seizures. Therapeutic management should be tailored for short-term acute care, with careful consideration of medication options and dosages. The underlying causes for the neonatal seizures ultimately determine long-term outcome pertaining to neurodevelopmental and epilepsy risks.

Suggested Readings

Diagnostic Dilemmas

Berger A, Shar B, Winter ST: Pronounced tremors in newborn infants: Their meaning and prognostic significance. Clin Pediatr 1975;14:834–837.

Brown JK, Ingram TTS, Seshia SS: Patterns of decerebration in infants and children: Defects in homeostasis and sequelae. J Neurol Neurosurg Psychiatry 1973;36:431–437.

Clancy R, Legido A: The exact ictal and interictal duration of electroencephalographic neonatal seizures. Epilepsia 1987;28:537–541.

Coulter DL, Allen RJ: Benign neonatal sleep myoclonus. Arch Neurol 1982;39:191–192.

Fenichel GM, Olson BJ, Fitzpatrick JE: Heart rate changes in convulsive and nonconvulsive apnea. Ann Neurol 1979;6:171.

Hakamada S, Watanabe K, Hara K, et al: Development of motor behavior during sleep in newborn infants. Brain Dev 1981;3:345–350.

Kellaway P, Hrachovy RA: Status epilepticus in newborns: A perspective on neonatal seizures. In Delgado-Escueta AV, Wasterlain CG, Treiman DM, et al (eds): Status Epilepticus: Mechanisms of Brain Damage and Treatment. New York, Raven Press, 1983, pp 93–99.

Levy SR, Abroms IF, Marshall PC, et al: Seizures and cerebral infarction in the full-term newborn. Ann Neurol 1985;17:366–370.

Mizrahi EM, Kellaway P: Diagnosis and Management of Neonatal Seizures. Philadelphia, Lippincott-Raven, 1998, pp 1–155.

Monod N, Pajot N, Guidasci S: The neonatal EEG: Statistical studies and prognostic value in full term and preterm babies. Electroencephalogr Clin Neurophysiol 1972;32:529.

Resnick TJ, Moshé SL, Perotta L, et al: Benign neonatal sleep myoclonus: Relationship to sleep states. Arch Neurol 1986;43:266–268.

Rose AL, Lombroso CT: Neonatal seizure states. Pediatrics 1970;45:404.

Sarnat M: Pathogenesis of decerebrate "seizures" in the premature infant with intraventricular hemorrhage. J Pediatr 1975;87:154–162.

Scher MS: Neonatal EEG-sleep, normal and abnormal features. In Neidermeyer E, daSilva L (eds): Electroencephalography, 5th ed. Baltimore, Lippincott, Williams & Wilkins, 2004, pp 896–946.

Scher MS: Neonatal seizures and brain damage. Pediatr Neurol 2003;29:381–390.

Scher MS: Pathological myoclonus of the newborn: Electrographic and clinical correlations. Pediatr Neurol 1985;1:342–348.

Scher MS, Alvin J, Painter MJ: Uncoupling of clinical and EEG seizures after antiepileptic drug use in neonates. Pediatr Neurol 2003;28:277–280.

Tharp BR, Cukier F, Monod H: The prognostic value of the electroencephalogram in premature infants. Electroencephalogr Clin Neurophysiol 1981;51:219.

Weiner SP, Painter MJ, Scher MS: Neonatal seizures: Electroclinical disassociation. Pediatr Neurol 1991;7:363–368.

Clinical Correlation

Escobedo M, Barton LL, Volby J: Cerebrospinal fluid studies in the intensive care nursery. J Perinat Med 1975;3:204–208.

Hillman LS, Hillman RE, Dodson WE: Diagnosis, treatment, and follow-up of neonatal mepivacaine intoxication secondary to paracervical and pudendal blocks during labor. J Pediatr 1979;94:472–477.

Kairam R, DeVivo DC: Neurologic manifestations of congenital infection. Clin Perinatol 1981;8:455–465.

Palmini A, Andermann E, Andermann F: Prenatal events and genetic factors in epileptic patients with neuronal migration disorders. Epilepsia 1994;35:965–973.

Scher MS: Neonatal seizures: An expression of fetal or neonatal brain disorders. In Stevenson DK, Sunshine P (eds): Fetal and Neonatal Brain Injury. Cambridge, Cambridge University Press, 2003, pp 735–784.

Schreiner RL, Kleinman MB: Incidence and effective traumatic lumbar puncture in the neonate. Dev Med Child Neurol 1981;21:483–487.

Antiepileptic Drug Treatment

Carmo KB, Barr P: Drug treatment of neonatal seizures by neonatologists and paediatric neurologists. J Pediatr Child Health 2005;4:313–316.

Holmes GL: Effects of seizures on brain development: lessons from the laboratory. Pediatr Neurol 2005;33:1–11.

Painter MJ, Minnigh B, Mollica L, et al: Binding profiles of anticonvulsants in neonates with seizures. Ann Neurol 1987;22:413–420.

Painter MJ, Pippenger C, Wasterlain C, et al: Phenobarbital and phenytoin in neonatal seizures, metabolism, and tissue distribution. Neurology 1981;31:1107–1112.

Painter MJ, Scher MS, Stein AD, et al: Phenobarbital compared with phenytoin for the treatment of neonatal seizures. N Engl J Med 1999;341:485–489.

Smith BI, Misoh RE: Intravenous diazepam in the treatment of prolonged seizure activity in neonates and infants. Dev Med Child Neurol 1971;13:630–634.

Estimating Prognosis

Caravale B, Allemand F, Libenson MH: Factors predictive of seizures and neurologic outcome in perinatal depression. Pediatr Neurol 2003;29:18–25.

Clancy RR, Legido A: Postnatal epilepsy after EEG-confirmed neonatal seizures. Epilepsia 1991;32:69–76.

Holden KR, Mellits ED, Freeman JM: Neonatal seizures. I. Correlation in prenatal and perinatal events with outcomes. Pediatrics 1982;70:165–176.

McBride M, Laroia N, Guillet R: Electrographic seizures in neonates correlate with poor neurodevelopmental outcome. Neurology 2000;55:506–514.

Monod N, Pajot N, Guidasci S: The neonatal EEG: Statistical studies and prognostic value in full-term and preterm babies. Electroencephalogr Clin Neurophysiol 1972;32:529–544.

Scher MS, Aso K, Beggarly ME, et al: Electrographic seizures in preterm and full-term neonates: Clinical correlates, associated brain lesions, and risk for neurological sequelae. Pediatrics 1993;91:128–134.

Temple CM, Dennis J, Carney R, et al: Neonatal seizures: Long-term outcome and cognitive development among "normal" survivors. Dev Med Child Neurol 1995;37:109–118.

Tharp BR, Cukier F, Monod N: The prognostic value of the electroencephalogram in premature infants. Electroencephalogr Clin Neurophysiol 1981;51:219.

Intraventricular Hemorrhage

Jeffrey M. Perlman, MB

The premature infant is at high risk for the development of hemorrhagic and ischemic cerebral injury, which contributes significantly to neonatal mortality as well as long-term neurodevelopmental deficits. Periventricular-intraventricular hemorrhage (PV-IVH) remains the most common lesion, particularly in the very low birth weight infant (<1000 g birth weight). In the mildest form, hemorrhage is confined to the germinal matrix, and in more severe cases there is extension of bleeding into the adjacent ventricular system or periventricular white matter. Periventricular leukomalacia (PVL), the principal ischemic lesion, is characterized by symmetrical periventricular white matter injury, invariably in the absence of hemorrhage. The advent of cranial ultrasound imaging in the late 1970s greatly enhanced the understanding of both conditions. This is highly relevant because, in most cases, the evolution of hemorrhagic-ischemic cerebral injury in the premature infant occurs in the absence of clinical symptoms. The case studies in this chapter will highlight PV-IVH and PVL in terms of pathophysiology, diagnosis, treatment, and outcome.

Periventricular-Intraventricular Hemorrhage

Case Study 1

BE, a 720-g, 26-week, appropriate for gestational age, white female was born to a 26-year-old primigravida mother whose pregnancy was complicated by periodic spotting and the premature onset of labor. Upon arrival in the labor and delivery unit, the cervix of the mother was noted to be dilated 6 cm with the infant in the breech position and the cord prolapsed. An emergent cesarean section was performed. The infant was delivered with minimal tone at birth and with a heart rate of 60 beats per minute. Resuscitation included bag and mask ventilation and intubation. The Apgar scores were 3 and 7 at 1 minute and 5 minutes, respectively. The infant developed progressive respiratory distress and received a dose of surfactant replacement therapy within the first 60 minutes of life. The ventilatory support and oxygen requirements initially decreased, but by 6 hours of life there was a deterioration in the clinical status with an F_{IO_2} requirement of 0.60, an assisted rate of 35 breaths/minute utilizing a synchronous mode of ventilation, a peak inflating pressure of 20 cm H_2O, and a peak end-expiratory pressure of 5 cm H_2O. An umbilical arterial blood gas revealed the following: Pao_2 48 mm Hg, $Paco_2$ 62 mm Hg, pH 7.24. A second dose of surfactant was given. The initial mean arterial blood pressure (BP) was 27 mm Hg with a capillary refill time of 2 to 3 seconds and the infant was given a 10 mL/kg bolus of normal saline. Subsequent blood pressure measurements were considered appropriate for age. Over the subsequent 24 hours, the infant continued to exhibit moderate costal retractions, and the F_{IO_2} requirement gradually decreased to 0.45; the infant remained on unchanged ventilator support. A third dose of surfactant was administered at 18 hours of age. Over the course of the day, the infant was noted to be extremely

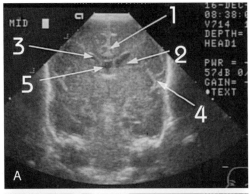

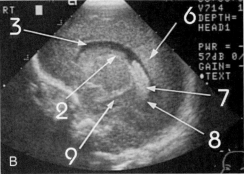

Figure 20-1 A, Coronal section of brain. The right side of the photograph represents the left side of the infant. All coronal films are shown in this convention. **B,** Sagittal scan. The infant is looking to the left and the occipital horn is on the right. All sagittal scans are shown in this convention. The important structures are numbered and depicted in Table 20-1.

irritable. Additional ancillary information revealed the following: the weight was 740 g; the urine output for the initial 24 hours was 0.8 mL/kg/ hour; a serum K^+ was 7.2 mEq/L, and the hematocrit had fallen from 45% to 32%. A cranial ultrasound scan was obtained at 24 hours of age because of the irritability and fall in hematocrit to exclude a bleed and is shown in Figure 20-1.

Exercise 1

QUESTIONS

1. Identify each of the numbered structures in Figure 20-1. Are these cranial ultrasound scans normal or abnormal?

2. What is the risk for hemorrhage in this infant?

3. What is the source of bleeding in premature infants?

4. Why do the blood vessels rupture?

5. Are clinical signs common in premature infants with intraventricular hemorrhage?

6. When should the next cranial ultrasound be obtained in this infant?

7. How would you counsel the parents at this stage?

ANSWERS

1. A series of coronal and sagittal images are utilized to image the brain. The pertinent structures are indicated in Table 20-1. Specifically, there was no evidence of increased echogenicity within the germinal matrix, ventricular system, or adjacent white matter. If such echoes are noted within the germinal matrix or ventricular system, this would be consistent with hemorrhage. However, the presence of increased echogenicity within the white matter may represent edema, ischemia, hemorrhage, or artifact. Serial imaging is necessary to fully evaluate the significance of this finding. The ventricular system was in addition not enlarged. The scan was interpreted as being normal for gestational age.

2. The routine use of cranial ultrasonography in the early 1980s to readily visualize the intracranial contents defined the magnitude of the problem of PV-IVH in the premature infant. Thus, several large series reported the incidence of PV-IVH to range between 30% and 40% for infants less than 1500 g, with the incidence as high as 50% to 60% for infants less than 1000 g and approximately 10% to 15% for infants between 1001 and 1500 g.[1] However, in recent years there has been a declining overall incidence of PV-IVH, which appears to be related to both

TABLE 20-1

NOTABLE AREAS ON CORONAL AND SAGITTAL SCANS

Structure	Number*
Intrahemisphere fissure	1
Germinal matrix region	2
Frontal horn of lateral ventricle	3
Sylvian fissure	4
Cavum septum pellucidum	5
Periventricular white matter	6
Choroid plexus	7
Occipital horn of lateral ventricle	8
Temporal horn of lateral ventricle	9

*Numbers on Figure 20-1.

intrapartum and postpartum factors.[2] However, for infants less than 1000 g, the incidence still remains substantial, and up to 40% may experience any form of hemorrhage and 10% to 15% will experience severe hemorrhage[3,4] (Table 20-2).

3. The primary lesion in PV-IVH is bleeding from small vessels in the subependymal germinal matrix. The hemorrhage may be confined to the germinal matrix region or it may extend and rupture into the adjacent ventricular system or into the periventricular white matter (Fig. 20-2). The germinal matrix, a source of neurons and glia for the developing brain, is a transitional gelatinous region, which provides limited support for the luxurious blood vessels that course through it. The rich arterial supply feeds an extensive and immature capillary bed within the matrix; these are irregular vessels that cannot be categorized as arterioles, capillaries, or venules.[5] With increasing gestational age, this matrix region becomes less prominent, and by term it is essentially absent. The capillaries drain into a well-developed venous system. The peculiarity of the venous anatomy appears to be important in the genesis of bleeding. Thus, the venous drainage of this region and the cerebral white matter is via the terminal, choroidal, and thalamostriate veins. These vessels course anteriorly to a point of confluence at the level of the head of the caudate nucleus and the foramen of Monro to form the internal cerebral vein that traverses directly posteriorly to join the vein of Galen. At the usual site of hemorrhage, the blood flow takes a peculiar U-turn, suggesting that increases in venous pressure may also be important in the genesis of hemorrhage.

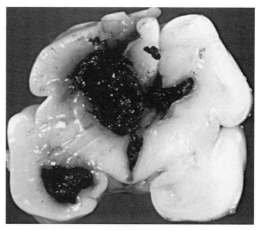

Figure 20-2 Neuropathologic specimen, coronal view. The right side of the photograph represents the left side of the brain. Note the large right-sided germinal matrix hemorrhage, blood in the adjacent right lateral ventricle with marked dilation of the frontal horn. Note blood in the frontal horn of the left lateral ventricle. Also note blood in the temporal horn of the right ventricle as well as blood in the third ventricle.

4. It is unclear why capillaries within the germinal matrix rupture and bleed in certain premature infants and not in others. The fragility of the germinal matrix vessels, as noted earlier, coupled with intravascular, vascular, and extravascular influences, is likely to be very important and will vary as a function of factors such as gestational age (Fig. 20-3). Based on experimental studies and clinical observations, perturbations in cerebral blood flow (CBF) appear to be of particular importance in the pathogenesis of hemorrhage. First, it has been shown that the cerebral circulation of the sick infant is pressure passive, because CBF varies directly with changes in systemic blood pressure changes.[6,7] Second, in a beagle puppy model, germinal matrix hemorrhage was produced by systemic

---

TABLE 20-2

FREQUENCY OF SEVERE INTRAVENTRICULAR HEMORRHAGE (IVH) IN LOW-BIRTH-WEIGHT INFANTS* **(1995–1996)**

Grade of IVH	501–750 g $n = 1002$	751–1000 g $n = 1084$	1001–1250 g $n = 1053$	1251–1500 g $n = 1299$
Intraventricular hemorrhage III	13%	6%	5%	2%
III + IPE	13%	6%	3%	1%
Total	26%	12%	8%	3%

*500 to 1500 g. IPE, intraparenchymal echodensity or grade IV hemorrhage.
Adapted from Lemons JA, Bauer CR, Oh W, et al; Very low birth weight outcomes of the National Institute of Child Health and Human Development, Neonatal Research Network, January 1995 through December 1996. Pediatrics 2001;107:e1.

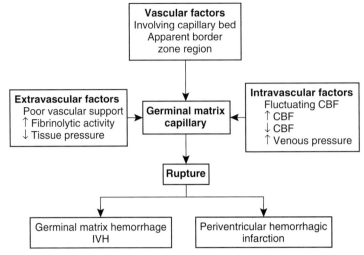

Figure 20-3 Factors important in pathogensis of periventricular-intraventricular hemorrhage. CBF, cerebral blood flow.

hypertension with or without prior hypotension.[8,9] Third, clinical studies indicate important associations between fluctuations in systemic blood pressure and CBF that may occur in the ventilated premature infant with respiratory distress syndrome or increases in CBF that may occur with rapid volume expansion or a pneumothorax and PV-IVH.[10–12] Conversely, decreases in CBF secondary to systemic hypotension, which may occur prior to delivery or postnatally, may play an important role in the genesis of PV-IVH in certain infants.[13,14] A major consequence of a decrease in CBF is injury of germinal matrix vessels that may rupture subsequent to reperfusion. Fourth, elevations in venous pressure may also contribute to the occurrence of PV-IVH. Elevations in venous pressure at the U-shaped junction mentioned

previously increase the likelihood of venous distention with obstruction of the terminal and medullary veins and hemorrhage or ischemia. Indeed, simultaneous elevations in venous pressure have been observed in those infants who exhibit changes in arterial blood pressure, as with respiratory distress syndrome with or without its associated complications, such as pneumothorax or pulmonary interstitial emphysema, or with mechanical or high-frequency ventilation[16–18] (Fig. 20-4). Thus, it is likely that both arterial and venous pertubation contribute to the IVH. In addition to these intravascular factors, vascular and extravascular influences, such as the poorly supported blood vessels, excessive fibrinolytic activity noted within the matrix region, and a prominent postnatal decrease in tissue pressure, are all additional risk factors for hemorrhage[1] (see Fig 20-4).

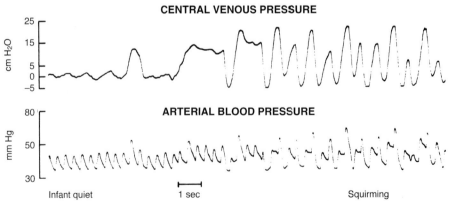

Figure 20-4 Simultaneous central venous tracing and arterial blood pressure from an intubated infant with respiratory distress syndrome. Note the fairly stable tracings when the infant is quiet, and the marked variability in both the venous as well as the arterial tracing when the infant is irritable and squirming.

5. Screening protocols for PV-IVH have been developed because up to 70% of infants do not exhibit overt clinical signs. Infants with more extensive hemorrhage usually exhibit a gradual deterioration over several hours characterized by irritability, increasing respiratory distress accompanied by a respiratory or metabolic acidosis, and occasionally, pulmonary hemorrhage and hyperglycemia. Rarely, infants exhibit a catastrophic deterioration characterized by acute apnea, hypotonia, brain stem dysfunction, seizures, bulging fontanel, and a fall in hematocrit.[1,4] The majority of cases of PV-IVH (>90%) occur within the first 72 postnatal hours. In the smallest premature infants, the onset tends to be early, within the first 24 hours, whereas in "larger" premature infants, the onset is later, from 25 to 72 hours.[19] However, recent reports suggest a later onset in the smallest, sickest infants who often require more prolonged and intensive medical support.[20] PV-IVH is most likely to occur in the intubated premature infant and in particular in those infants with respiratory distress syndrome (RDS). By contrast, in the nonintubated infant, the risk for PV-IVH is below 10%.[21]

6. Because most cases of PV-IVH are asymptomatic, screening protocols have evolved to evaluate premature infants.[20] These protocols vary among institutions. We screen premature infants who weigh less than 1500 g as follows: initial scan on day 3 to 5 (should capture >90% PV-IVH), second scan on day 10 to 14 (should capture the remaining cases of PV-IVH and detect early complications, i.e., post-hemorrhage hydrocephalus), and a third scan on day 28 (will identify the occasional late hemorrhage and complications). A fourth scan is obtained prior to discharge (to assess ventricular size and identify any other complications). When clinically indicated, scans should be obtained more frequently.

7. The parents should be informed that there is at least a 30% risk of their infant developing any hemorrhage, even though the initial scan is negative. They should also be informed that the RDS will likely worsen prior to improvement over the subsequent 48 to 72 hours. As the RDS progresses or worsens, the risk for bleeding increases. A repeat sonogram will usually not be obtained for at least 2 or 3 days unless there is a change in the clinical condition.

Case Study 1 *Continued*

The infant continued to exhibit respiratory distress with a worsening respiratory acidosis. An arterial blood gas at 30 hours revealed Pao_2 58 mm Hg, $Paco_2$ 68 mm Hg, and pH 7.15. There was a suggestion of pulmonary interstitial emphysema (PIE) on a chest radiograph, while the lung fields appeared well expanded. The infant was switched to a high-frequency oscillator utilizing the following parameters: Fio_2 0.50, 1200 Hz, amplitude 30, mean airway pressure 14 cm H_2O. There was clinical, biochemical, and radiologic improvement over the subsequent 12 hours. Thus, the $Paco_2$ decreased to 52 mm Hg, the pH increased to 7.28, and lungs were less expanded and the PIE had resolved. However, at approximately 40 hours of life, bloody secretions were noted within the endotracheal tube. Upon suctioning of the airway, copious bloody secretions were removed. A repeat chest radiograph revealed bilateral opacified lung fields. The hematocrit had fallen from 36% to 23% and the infant received a blood transfusion. An arterial blood gas revealed the following: Pao_2 50 mm Hg, $Paco_2$ 72 mm Hg, pH 7.10. The ventilator support was accordingly increased to amplitude of 38 and mean airway pressure of 16 cm H_2O. The blood gases gradually corrected over the next 8 hours. A repeat sonogram was performed at 48 hours (See Fig. 20–2).

Exercise 1 *Continued*

QUESTIONS

8. What do the coronal and sagittal ultrasound scans demonstrate that was not present in the scan obtained 24 hours earlier?

9. How are hemorrhages graded?

10. What is the relationship of grade of hemorrhage to outcome?

11. Why is white matter injury associated with a poor outcome?

12. What clinical events may have contributed to the PV-IVH in this case?

13. How would you counsel the family at this stage?

ANSWERS

8. The repeat scan (Fig. 20-5A, coronal view) reveals a large left-sided germinal matrix hemorrhage (GMH) with extension of blood into the left lateral ventricle. There are increased periventricular echoes fanning out into adjacent frontal matter of the lateral ventricle (arrow). On the sagittal view (Fig. 20-5B), there is a large GMH distending into the ventricle (long arrow). The left lateral ventricle appears to be at least 50% filled with blood (curved arrow), and there is associated ventricular dilation.

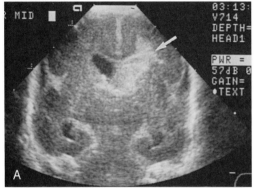

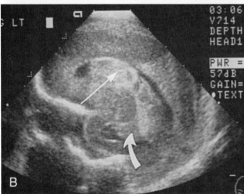

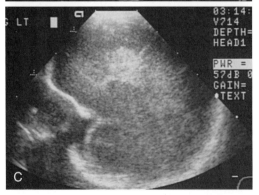

Figure 20-5 A, Coronal image on day 2 in Case Study 1; **B** and **C,** left sagittal view on day 2 from Case Study 1. See text for further discussion.

In Figure 20-5C, note the increased periventricular echogenicity within the white matter. This may represent ischemia or hemorrhage and will need to be evaluated with serial sonograms. The findings are consistent with a grade III IVH with an associated small intraparenchymal echodensity (IPE). This is also referred to as a grade IV IVH.

9. Cranial ultrasonography has provided a simple method of defining the severity of PV-IVH. This is of particular relevance because outcome is related to the severity of the bleed. The sonographic grading system we use to assess PV-IVH is based on the presence of blood in the germinal matrix and the amount of blood in the lateral ventricles[1,4] (Table 20-3).

10. The findings on cranial ultrasound have been used as a marker of both short-term outcome (i.e., death) and long-term outcome (i.e., neurodevelopmental sequelae). In the *short term*, PV-IVH, when severe, still contributes significantly to the mortality risk of the very low birth weight infant. In recent years, it is the tiniest of premature infants (i.e., <750 g) who are most vulnerable to large hemorrhage and death (see Table 20-1).[3] The most critical determinant of *long-term outcome* is the degree of parenchymal injury.[1,22] Of particular importance is the size and location of the parenchymal lesion.[1,4] Thus, when an IPE is large, more than 1 cm in diameter, and extensive (i.e., involves frontoparietal-occipital region) (Fig. 20-6A and B), mortality rate is highest

TABLE 20-3

GRADING OF SEVERITY OF PERIVENTRICULAR-INTRAVENTRICULAR HEMORRHAGE (PV-IVH) BY CRANIAL ULTRASOUND SCAN

Grade	Description
Grade I	Germinal matrix blood only
Grade II	Intraventricular blood (filling <50% of lateral ventricular area on sagittal view)
Grade III	Intraventricular blood (filling >50% of lateral ventricular area or sagittal view; the ventricular system is unusually dilated)
IPE*	Periventricular echodensity (indicate location and size)

*IPE (intraparenchymal echodensity) refers to periventricular white matter involvement, also referred to as grade IV by others.

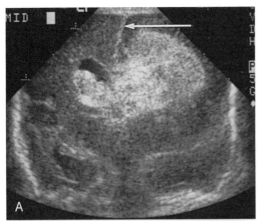

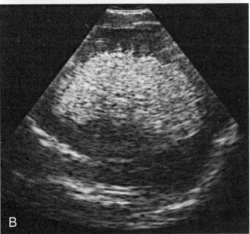

Figure 20-6 A, Coronal image of an infant demonstrating a left-sided grade III IVH with a large intraparenchymal echodensity involving frontoparietal-occipital cortex. Note the midline shift (*arrow*). **B,** Sagittal image from same infant, left-sided. Note the diffuse involvement of the white matter.

TABLE 20-4

RELATIONSHIP OF GRADE OF PERIVENTRICULAR-INTRAVENTRICULAR (PV-IVH) HEMORRHAGE TO OUTCOME

Grade of PV-IVH	Incidence of Definite Neurologic Sequelae
I	10%
II	20%
III	35%
III and periventricular hemorrhagic infarction	
Extensive	100%
Localized	80%

Adapted from Volpe JJ: Neuroloy of the Newborn, 3rd ed. Philadelphia, WB Saunders, 2001; Perlman JM, Rollins N: Surveillance protocol for the detection of intracranial abnormalities in premature neonates. Arch Pediatr Adolesc Med 2000;154(8):822–826; and Perlman JM: Intraventricular hemorrhage. Pediatrics 1989;84:913–914.

(80%) and long-term outcome is invariably poor (Table 20-4). With a smaller lesion (i.e., <1 cm) that is localized (i.e., to either frontal, parietal, or occipital region; see Fig. 20-5A and C), the outcome is less precise and likely to be more favorable. However, almost 80% of such infants will still have an abnormal outcome.[1] Thus, if the term grade IV hemorrhage is utilized, it does not indicate the extent of white matter involvement, which may have significant clinical implications when discussing outcome issues with the family.

11. The substrate for the white matter injury appears to be a venous infarction with bleeding occurring as a secondary phenomenon.[1,23,24] Thus, the white matter lesion visualized by cranial ultrasound imaging likely represents a small component of a much larger lesion. The timing and the pathogenesis of the primary ischemic event remain unclear. Two possibilities exist. A direct relationship to the ipsilateral IVH is suggested from the following: (a) the IPE is always noted with or following a large PV-IVH, (b) rarely is it observed prior to PV-IVH, and (c) the IPE is ipsilateral to the side of the larger PV-IVH when there is bilateral involvement. This relationship between the PV-IVH and the IPE may in part be explained by the venous drainage of the deep white matter as discussed in Exercise 1 (Fig. 20-7A and B). An alternative explanation is that the germinal matrix and periventricular white matter are both border zone regions, which increases the risk for ischemic injury during periods of cerebral hypoperfusion. Hemorrhage then occurs as a secondary phenomenon, reperfusion injury. The fairly consistent observation of the simultaneous detection of PV-IVH and IPE supports this theory. Moreover, elevated hypoxanthine and increased uric acid levels (which may be markers of reperfusion injury) have been observed on the first day of life in infants who subsequently develop white matter injury.[25,26]

Understanding the mechanisms contributing to the white matter necrosis is crucial in order to prevent the lesion. For example, if there is a direct crucial link to PV-IVH, then prevention of PV-IVH should reduce the occurrence of the white matter injury. However, if the two

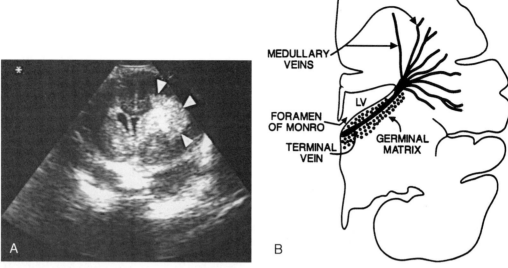

Figure 20-7 **A,** Coronal image from an 800-g 25-week infant. Note the left large germinal matrix hemorrhage and intraventricular hemorrhage. Note the large fan-shaped intraparenchymal echogenicity (*arrowheads*). **B,** Schematic diagram of the venous drainage of the cerebral white matter showing the medullary veins (arranged in a fan-shaped distribution) that drain blood from the cerebral blood matter into the terminal vein, which comes through the germinal matrix. (From Volpe JJ: Neurology of the Newborn, 3rd ed. Philadelphia, WB Saunders, 2001, p 408.)

conditions occur concurrently, as a consequence of a primary ischemic event, then prevention of secondary hemorrhage may not have an impact upon the primary ischemia. A recent follow-up study suggests that this may occur clinically. Thus, in a prospective study designed to prevent "grade IV" IVH utilizing indomethacin, outcomes at 18 months revealed a similar occurrence of cerebral palsy in both groups while there was a significant decrease in the incidence of severe hemorrhage in the treated group (Table 20-5).[27]

12. The infant exhibited several clinical characteristics that increased the risk for PV-IVH. First, the respiratory disease was associated with progressive hypercarbia.

Although permissive hypercapnia is being accepted more readily in the management of infants with RDS, increases in $Paco_2$ levels are associated with increases in CBF. Second, the infant appeared irritable, which most likely was associated with arterial and venous perturbations. Third, the infant developed pulmonary interstitial emphysema, which may compromise venous return and as a consequence give rise to an increase in venous pressure. Fourth, the high mean airway pressures generated by the high-frequency oscillator also increase the risk of impeding venous return. Finally, the appearance of pulmonary hemorrhage during the acute phase of RDS has also been associated with

TABLE 20-5

SHORT- AND LONG-TERM NEUROLOGIC OUTCOME IN INFANTS WHO RECEIVED INDOMETHACIN AND INFANTS WHO RECEIVED A PLACEBO

Outcome	Indomethacin Group (*n* = 574)	Placebo Group (*n* = 569)	Adjusted Odds Ratio (95%CI)	*P* Value
Severe IVH	52/569(9%)	75/567(13%)	0.6(0.4–0.9)	0.02
Cerebral palsy	58/467(12%)	56/477(12%)	1.1(0.7–1.6)	0.64
Cognitive delay (MDI < 70)	118/444(27%)	117/457(26%)	1.0(0.8–1.4)	0.86

CI, confidence interval; IVH, intraventricular hemorrhage; MDI, mental development index.
Adapted from Schmidt B, Damis P, et al: Long-term effects of indomethacin prophylaxis in extremely low birth weight infants. N Engl J Med 2001;344(26):1966–1972.

PV-IVH.[4] The mechanism(s) that links these two lesions remains unclear.

13. The parents should be informed that the infant has had a bleed within the brain. It is important to describe the location of the bleed (we often use a schematic drawing to illustrate this point) to stress that the infant is not actively bleeding at the current time, and that in most cases if the infant remains stable, there should be no further hemorrhage. It is also important to explain that there is a large amount of blood within the ventricular system, and this may cause complications for the following reason. Spinal fluid, which nourishes and protects the brain, is continuously being produced within the ventricular system. Within certain areas, the ventricular system narrows, and the blood may obstruct the system at these locations. As a consequence, the spinal fluid will back up and distend the ventricles, a condition known as hydrocephalus. This is best assessed utilizing serial sonograms. It is also critical to explain to the parents that with time the blood will be reabsorbed. Finally, it is important to raise the issue of potential neurodevelopmental deficits, although the full expression of these problems will most likely only become clear with time.

Case Study 1 *Continued*

The clinical course was as follows: there was gradual improvement in the respiratory status and the infant was weaned to low supplemental oxygen and off the ventilator by the third week of life (day of life [DOL] 21). The neurologic examination remained essentially nonfocal; the anterior fontanel appeared soft, and the head circumference was increasing appropriately. Follow-up cranial sonograms were obtained on DOL 10 and 28 (Figs. 20-8 and 20-9).

Exercise 1 *Continued*

QUESTIONS

14. Which complications of PV-IVH are evident on these serial sonograms?

15. What is the structure indicated by the arrow in Figure 20-9A?

16. What is the treatment of the observed complication?

17. Could the hemorrhage have been prevented in this case?

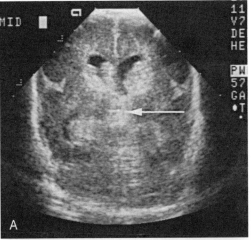

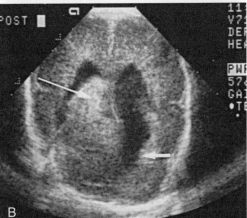

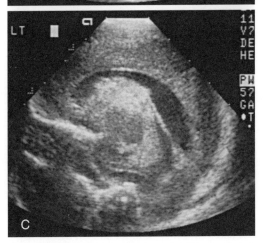

Figure 20-8 A and B, Coronal image on day 10 in Case Study 1. C, Left sagittal image on day 10 in Case Study 1. See text for further discussion.

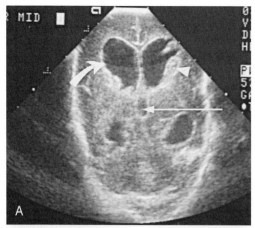

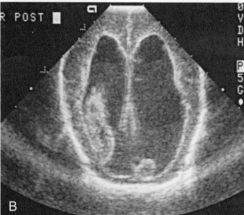

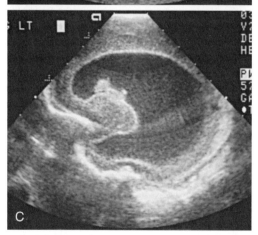

Figure 20-9 A and **B,** Coronal images on day 28 in Case Study 1. **C,** Left sagittal image on day 10 in Case Study 1. See text for further discussion.

ANSWERS

14. The images obtained on day 10 (see Fig. 20-8A to C) demonstrate bilateral germinal matrix and bilateral intraventricular hemorrhage (see Fig. 20-8B, *arrows*) as well as blood in the third

ventricle (see Fig. 20-8A, *arrow*). There is interval bilateral enlargement of the lateral ventricles. The IPE noted previously on the left is now not apparent.

15. On the follow-up scan obtained on day 28 (see Fig. 20-9A and C), there has been progressive ventriculomegaly involving the occipital and temporal lobes of the lateral ventricles. The arrow in the coronal section (see Fig. 20-8B) indicates a dilated third ventricle. There is cystic degeneration of the blood within the left germinal matrix region (*arrowhead* in Fig. 20-9A). The ventricular lining is very echogenic, suggestive of a ventriculitis (*curved arrow* in Fig. 20-9A).

16. Post-hemorrhagic hydrocephalus (PHH) complicates approximately 40% to 50% of cases of severe IVH.[1] The progression of hydrocephalus may be rapid, over days, and in such cases, it is usually associated with an elevation in intracranial pressure. The obstruction under such circumstances is often secondary to an obstruction of cerebrospinal fluid caused by particulate clot either at the foramen of Monro or the aqueduct of Sylvius. If the obstruction is at the former level, the lateral ventricles are enlarged with a normal sized third ventricle. Blockage at the level of the aqueduct will result in dilatation of the lateral and third ventricles. Treatment is usually immediate, via external drainage above the site of observation. More commonly, as in this case, a communicating hydrocephalus evolves from 1 to 4 weeks following the diagnosis of hemorrhage. The hydrocephalus is commonly secondary to an obliterative arachnoiditis in the posterior fossa distal to the outflow of the fourth ventricle. The clinical criteria of evolving hydrocephalus—full anterior fontanel and rapid head growth—do not appear for days or weeks after ventricular dilation is already present. Indeed, in this case, the head circumference was "growing" normally. Possible explanations for this discrepancy include (1) the relative excess of water in the centrum semiovale, (2) the relatively large subarachnoid space, and (3) the lack of cerebral myelin. Thus, serial scans are critical to follow the evolution of PHH.

    Understanding the natural history of PHH is essential for developing a treatment strategy. The natural tendency is to intervene immediately. However, in most cases, the ventricular dilation is under normal pressure and progresses slowly.[28] In approximately half of the cases, the progression ceases without intervention, usually within the first month. In the remaining 50% the ventriculomegaly is progressive and under increased pressure necessitating intervention. Thus, we prefer to observe the infant over the first month, provided that the PV-IVH progression is not rapid and the intracranial pressure is normal. We always recommend obtaining a pressure measurement when a lumbar puncture or ventricular tap is performed. The ventricular fluid under such circumstances will invariably reveal many red blood cells, an elevated white blood cell count, a high protein, and low glucose.

The management of PHH will depend on the size of the infant, the amount of blood in the ventricles, and the intracranial pressure. Many neurosurgeons prefer not to place a ventriculoperitoneal shunt until the infant's weight is at least above 1500 g. In the smallest premature infants, temporizing diversion techniques to control ventricular size have evolved and include the placement of an external ventricular drain or subgaleal shunt, serial lumbar punctures, and the use of drugs, namely acetazolamide and isosorbide.[28-30]

17. The key to prevention of PV-IVH would be the prevention of prematurity. Until then we must focus on potential perinatal and postnatal strategies (Table 20-6). Perinatal pharmacologic interventions have included the administration of phenobarbital and vitamin K. The largest study to date has failed to demonstrate a beneficial effect of phenobarbital, and the data regarding vitamin K are conflicting with regard to benefit, suggesting no role for either agent in the prevention of IVH.[31-34] The antenatal administration of glucocorticoids to augment pulmonary maturation has had the positive, unanticipated benefit of a significant reduction in the incidence of severe IVH.[35-37] From a review of several large observational databases, the unadjusted odds ratio for severe IVH following any antenatal glucocorticoid exposure ranged from 0.49 to 0.79.[38-41] We have demonstrated a significant beneficial effect

TABLE 20-6

CURRENT POTENTIAL STRATEGIES IN THE PREVENTION OF PERIVENTRICULAR-INTRAVENTRICULAR HEMORRHAGE

Perinatal interventions
   Prevention of premature birth
   Pharmacologic interventions: glucocorticoids
   Optimal labor and delivery management
Postnatal interventions
   Correction or prevention of major hemodynamic disturbances
   Pharmacologic interventions: indomethacin

of antenatal steroids; however, the effect is dose dependent[41] (Table 20-7). The mechanism(s) whereby glucocorticoids reduce severe IVH remains unclear, but may relate to less severe distress syndrome, higher blood pressure, or accelerated maturation of the germinal matrix region.[43,44]

Maternal events associated with a lower incidence of IVH include pregnancy-induced hypertension (PIH). We reported a lower incidence of severe PV-IVH in infants born to mothers with PIH than in those without PIH, 8.2% versus 14% with an odds ratio estimate of 0.43 (95% confidence intervals 0.30 to 0.61),[45] a finding consistent with other reports.[46,47] The mechanism(s) whereby PIH may influence IVH remain unclear, but may relate to accelerated brain maturation in such infants, or the use of medications, specifically magnesium sulfate, to treat the mother.[48,49] However, recent retrospective data suggest that magnesium sulfate is not associated with a reduction in PV-IVH or subsequent cerebral palsy.[50-53] Moreover, tocolytic agents in general, including magnesium sulfate, are associated with an increased risk for IVH.[54,55]

There is conflicting data regarding the route of delivery and subsequent IVH.[47,56-60] Interpreting the data is difficult because some of it is retrospective. However, this does not exclude the possibility that under certain circumstances, intrapartum events may contribute to the pathogenesis of severe IVH. Thus, in some studies there is an increased risk for IVH with increasing duration of the active phase of labor, and a lower risk in those infants delivered via cesarean section prior to the active phase of labor.[47,56] Many of these studies were analyzed prior to the more frequent use of antenatal glucocorticoids.[59] More recent evidence would

TABLE 20-7

MULTIVARIATE PREDICTION OF SEVERE INTRAVENTRICULAR HEMORRHAGE (IVH) FOR PRETERM INFANTS LESS THAN 1250 G BIRTH WEIGHT*,†

Predictor	P Value	Odds Ratio Estimate	95% Confidence Limits
Antenatal glucocorticoid administration	<0.01	0.16	0.03, 0.73
Pregnancy-induced hypertension	<0.03	0.10	0.01, 0.83
Intubation	<0.02	4.24	1.17, 15.31
Cesarean section	<0.62	0.83	0.40, 1.71
Gestational age	<0.0001	1.58	1.30, 1.92

*Delivered at Parkland Memorial Hospital in Dallas, Texas, between January 1993 and November 1995.
†For each week decrease in gestational age, there is 1.58-fold increased risk for severe IVH.

suggest that placental evidence of inflammation and in particular funisitis obviates the effect of cesarean section.[60]

Postnatal strategies to prevent severe IVH have been studied without much success. Intervention strategies should incorporate several important recent observations: (1) in most neonatal intensive care units, the incidence of all grades of IVH appears to be declining in the absence of specific intervention[2]; (2) severe IVH in most cases occurs predominantly in the smallest premature infant, under 1000 g[3]; and (3) the condition of the infant at delivery (influenced in part by perinatal events) significantly impacts upon the likelihood of severe IVH. Future postnatal strategies, therefore, should focus on the premature infant at highest risk for developing severe IVH and IPE (see Table 20-7). For example, the risk for severe IVH in the nonintubated infant is low, less than 10%.[21] Factors associated with an increased risk include decreasing gestational age, lower birth weight (<1000 g), male sex, intubation, and respiratory distress syndrome (see Table 20-7). For infants with respiratory distress syndrome, the risk for IVH is even greater when there are associated perturbations in arterial and venous pressures (see Fig. 20-4).[10,18] These vascular perturbations are in part related to the infant's breathing patterns usually being out of synchrony with the ventilator breath.[61] The perturbations can be minimized with careful ventilator management, including the use of synchronized mechanical ventilation, sedation, or in more difficult cases with paralysis.[62] Interestingly, surfactant administration with improved respiratory function has not been associated with a significant reduction in the incidence of IVH.[63] It should be noted that the infant in our case received two doses of surfactant.

Postnatal administration of medications to reduce severe IVH has included the use of phenobarbital,[64–66] vitamin E,[67] ethamsylate,[68] and indomethacin.[27,69,70] The initial enthusiasm for the use of these medications in the prevention of IVH has not been borne out over time. Indeed, in one study, infants who received phenobarbital exhibited a higher incidence of severe IVH when compared to control infants.[67] Currently, indomethacin appears to hold the most promise in the prevention of severe hemorrhage. Ment and associates, in a randomized placebo controlled study, demonstrated a significant reduction in the incidence of severe IVH plus IPE in infants who received indomethacin versus a large group of control infants.[70] In a subsequent multicenter randomized study, indomethacin was shown to reduce the incidence of severe IVH in the treated versus control group from 13% to 9%. However, at 18-month follow-up, the incidence of cerebral palsy was comparable between groups.[27] This observation coupled with the known reduction in cerebral blood flow that accompanies indomethacin administration warrants cautious use of this agent.[71,72]

Case Study 1 *Continued*

Serial lumbar punctures were initially attempted to treat the hydrocephalus.[29] However, because the amount of fluid removed was low, less than 5 mL/kg (to be effective at least 10 mL/kg of CSF should be removed), the neurosurgeons proceeded to placement of a subgaleal shunt. The ventricular size stabilized. When the infant was approximately 35 weeks postconceptual age and weighing 1900 g, a ventriculoperitoneal shunt was placed. A cranial ultrasound prior to discharge still demonstrated moderate ventriculomegaly. However, there was no evidence of a porencephalic cyst. Additional clinical problems included the evolution to chronic lung disease, recurrent apnea and bradycardia, retinopathy of prematurity (stage 3), and sensorineural hearing loss. At 18 months follow-up, the infant has evidence of a spastic quadriplegia, with the right side more affected than the left. In addition, he has a moderate to severe cognitive deficit.

The outcome is perhaps more severe than some may have anticipated from the final appearance of the cranial ultrasound scan in the absence of overt white matter injury. Recent data indicate that magnetic resonance imaging (MRI) performed at the time of discharge is more sensitive in identifying injury to white matter than head ultrasound scan (HUS).[73] Several important points should be made from this case. Although the IPE resolved without cyst formation, this was likely a marker of underlying white matter injury. In support of this concept is the persistent moderate ventriculomegaly noted at the time of discharge. This finding may be indirect evidence of injury to white matter with the ventriculomegaly representing an ex vacuo phenomenon. The presence of ventriculomegaly is associated with a three- to fivefold increased likelihood of neurodevelopmental abnormalities.[20] Moreover, coexisting medical problems (chronic lung disease, apnea of prematurity) as well as medications used to treat these conditions (theophylline) all have the potential for adversely affecting neurodevelopmental outcome.

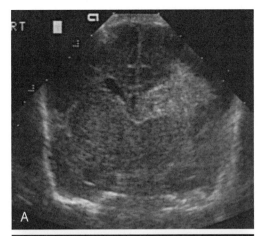

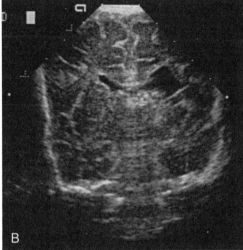

Figure 20-10 **A,** Coronal image on day 3 in Case Study 2. **B,** Coronal image on day 10 in Case Study 2.

Case Study 2

BH was a 1100-g 28-week premature infant born to a 17-year-old gravida 1 para 0 black mother. The infant was delivered vaginally and breathed spontaneously at birth. Because of retraction the infant was placed on CPAP; the Apgar scores were 6 at 1 minute and 8 at 5 minutes. The postnatal course was characterized by severe RDS treated with surfactant replacement therapy. A screening cranial sonogram was performed on DOL 3 (Fig. 20-10A). The infant's subsequent course was complicated by the development of chronic lung disease, medically treated necrotizing enterocolitis (Bell stage 2), and Staphylococcus epidermidis infection. The infant underwent serial ultrasound scans. The final scan is depicted in Figure 20-10B.

Exercise 2

QUESTIONS

1. Where has the hemorrhage occurred on the coronal image?

2. What is the name of the cystic structure located in the left hemisphere in Figure 20-10B?

3. What is the long-term neurodevelopmental outcome likely to be?

ANSWERS

1. The coronal image in Figure 20-10A indicates a large germinal matrix hemorrhage with intraventricular extension into the frontal horn of the lateral ventricle. There is a fan-shaped IPE localized to left frontal white matter.

2. A porencephalic cyst is apparent in the left hemisphere. By definition, porencephalic cysts are single large space(s) that usually communicate with the lateral ventricle. This is a characteristic response of the newborn brain in which areas of infarction are replaced by a cystic cavity, which is usually well defined. One should note that there is asymmetry to the ventricular size with the left greater than the right. This is in contrast to Case Study 1, in which the IPE did not evolve to cyst formation.

3. This infant has neurodevelopmental abnormalities at 18 months chronologic age: notably, a contralateral spastic hemiplegia, a seizure disorder, as well as moderate cognitive delay. This outcome is not unanticipated, given the final ultrasound appearance.

Periventricular Leukomalacia

Case Study 3

PP was a 1350-g 29-week, appropriate for gestational age, Hispanic male born to a 22-year-old gravida 4 para 2 mother. There was premature rupture of the membranes at 27 weeks' estimated gestational age. The mother received a complete course of glucocorticoids immediately prior to delivery. Approximately 18 hours prior to delivery, the mother developed a fever with some uterine tenderness. Antibiotics were started. The infant delivered vaginally in the cephalic position and cried at birth. Resuscitation included some supplemented oxygen. The Apgar scores were 7 at 1 minute and 8 at 5 minutes. The infant exhibited minimal respiratory distress and received supplemental oxygen for 2 days. A sepsis workup was performed and the infant was treated with antibiotics for 7 days. The blood cultures were negative; the chest radiograph initially was interpreted as being consistent with retained lung fluid. The only pertinent clinical findings were feeding difficulties and recurrent apnea and bradycardia requiring theophylline therapy. The infant was never hypotensive. Placental pathology was consistent with acute chorioamnionitis and funisitis. Serial screening cranial ultrasound scans were obtained on days 5, 14, and 28. The first and third scans are depicted in Figure 20-11.

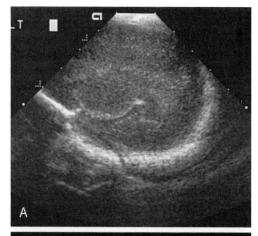

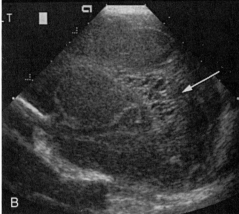

Figure 20-11 A, Sagittal image on day 3 in Case Study 3. **B,** Sagittal image on day 28 in Case Study 3.

Exercise 3

QUESTIONS

1. What do the serial scans demonstrate?
2. What causes this lesion in general?
3. What may have caused the lesion in this case?
4. Are clinical signs common with this lesion?
5. What are associated risk factors?
6. Can the lesion be prevented?
7. What is the significance of the sonographic findings?
8. Why are these infants so vulnerable to neurodevelopmental abnormalities?

ANSWERS

1. The sagittal image obtained on the third day is normal. A second scan obtained on day

10 was also normal (not shown). However, the third scan obtained on day 28 indicated diffuse cystic changes within periventricular white matter, predominantly involving posterior white matter (see Fig. 20-11B, *arrow*). These findings are consistent with the diagnosis of periventricular leukomalacia (PVL). PVL refers to necrosis of white matter adjacent to the external angle of the lateral ventricles. The incidence of bilateral cystic PVL approximates 3% to 4% of infants weighing less than 1500 g.[74,75] Such cysts within periventricular white matter may be present at birth, which would be consistent with an antepartum injury, or evolve postnatally usually within the first 2 or 3 weeks of life, although later-appearing lesions are also noted.[76,77]

The pathologic features of PVL include focal periventricular involvement commonly observed at the level of the occipital radiation at the trigone of the lateral ventricles, and at the level of the cerebral white matter around the foramen of Monro, as well as more diffuse cerebral white matter involvement. The latter is more commonly noted in the small premature infant requiring prolonged ventilator support. The histologic changes are characterized by coagulation necrosis, microglial infiltration, astrocytic proliferation, and eventual cyst formation.[78–82] It is these cysts that are readily detected by cranial ultrasonography when they are approximately 0.5 cm or greater. These cavities usually diminish in size over time secondary to progression of gliosis. Myelin loss and focal ventricular dilation in the region of the trigone of the lateral ventricles are long-term sequelae. The ventricular dilation is more prominent with more diffuse involvement of the white matter. The presumed sonographic correlates of the preceding pathologic findings of PVL include (1) bilateral increased periventricular echogenicity; (2) evolution to cyst formation usually over a period of 7 to 21 days; (3) resolution of the cysts over the ensuing 1 to 2 months; and (4) a final appearance of ventriculomegaly.

Several important clinical points regarding sonography and PVL need to be made. Many infants with increased periventricular echogenicity resolve without cyst formation or the development of ventriculomegaly.

The significance of this observation remains unclear. Conversely, there are more and more infants identified who progress to cyst formation in the absence of prior increased echogenicity.[20]

2. The pathogenesis of PVL, similar to IVH, is complex and likely multifactorial. Based on experimental and clinical observations, two basic factors appear to be operative in the genesis of the injury: (1) vascular factors that increase the risk for cerebral hypoperfusion and (2) the intrinsic vulnerability of the oligodendroglia within white matter. The developmental features of the blood supply to the white matter may help explain the propensity for injury in this patient population.[83–86] Thus, the penetrating branches of the anterior, middle, and posterior cerebral arteries end in border zones, areas that are most vulnerable to decreases in cerebral blood flow. Such decreases in cerebral blood flow are likely to occur during episodes of systemic hypotension, particularly in the sick infant with a pressure passive circulation.[6] It is within these border zones or "watershed" area that the focal necrosis of PVL typically occurs. Moreover, the penetrating cerebral vessels, which include long branches that terminate in the deep periventricular white matter and short branches that terminate in the subcortical white matter, vary as a function of gestational age. Thus, at approximately 24 to 30 weeks of gestation, the long penetrators have few side branches and intraparenchymal anastomosis with the short branches, resulting in border zones in white matter beyond the periventricular region. This may account for the more diffuse lesion noted in the small premature infant. From 32 weeks on, there is a marked increase in vascular supply as a result of increase in vessel length and anastomosis, decreasing the likelihood of injury to this region in the larger infant.

There is increasing evidence that differentiating oligodendroglia in the process of myelination are vulnerable to injury. Potential pathogenetic factors include free radicals, excess extracellular glutamate and cytokine/inflammatory cells.[1,2,87,88] The role for free radical–induced damage triggering the death of the early differentiating oligodendrocyte is supported by the cryoprotection provided by free radical scavengers (superoxide dismutase, deferoxamine, and vitamin E).[1] Glutamate can lead to the death of oligodendroglial precursors via mechanisms that involve both receptor and nonreceptor mechanisms. The nonreceptor mechanism involves glutamate intracellular entry in exchange for cystine via activation of a glutamine-cystine exchange transporter, resulting in a decrease in intracellular cystine and thereby glutathione synthesis.[1,2] The result is glutathione depletion and free radical mediated cell death. The latter can be totally prevented by the addition of free radical scavengers such as vitamin E.[1]

An important mechanism for oligodendroglial precursor cell death may be mediated via cytokines. It is well established in animals that a paradigm of ischemic/reperfusion is accompanied by a rapid activation of microglia, secretion of cytokines, and migration of inflammatory cells.[1,2,89] Moreover, cytokines and inflammatory cells are also a consistent feature of the response to infection. There is both experimental and clinical evidence demonstrating an association between maternal infection/inflammation of the chorion or amnion with or without fetal vascular involvement (i.e., funisitis) and white matter injury. Thus, intraperitoneal injection of lipopolysaccharides into kittens, and exposing pregnant rabbits intrauterine infection results in white matter injury, similar to that observed in human.[90] Several clinical studies have demonstrated an association between chorioamnionitis and PVL.[74,91] Akin to intraventricular hemorrhage, this association appears to be accentuated in the presence of funisitis.[60,92] The link between chorioamnionitis may be mediated via cytokines. Thus, high levels of cytokines (IL-6 and

IL-1β)? have been found in the amniotic fluid,[93] in cord blood (IL-6), and in neonatal blood (IL-1, IL-6, and interferons) of preterm infants who develop PVL or cerebral palsy. Finally, microglial expression of tumor necrosis factor-alpha (TNF-α) and interleukin 6 immunoreactivity is found twice as often in the white matter of infants with PVL than in the absence of injury to the region.[94] Not all cytokines injure the CNS; the pattern of injury may depend on the regional production of neurotoxic and neuroprotective cytokines. For example, in a murine model of hypoxia ischemia lacking TNF-α, focal cerebral ischemia was exacerbated. In contrast, injury-induced microglial activation was suppressed in the TNF-α knock-out mice.[95] These latter observations point to the complex interrelationships between cytokines and white matter injury. Cytokines may be released in response to hypoxia-ischemia or to infection (Fig. 20-12).

3. In this case, there were no obvious perinatal or postnatal hypotensive events. One potential cause for the white matter injury may relate to infection, as the mother's clinical and pathologic findings were consistent with chorioamnionitis and funisitis. However, it remains unclear how an infection at the time of delivery can be linked to the appearance of diffuse cystic white matter injury beyond the first postnatal month. Because apnea with associated bradycardia creates the potential for cerebral perfusion,[96] it is possible that the recurrent episodes noted in this infant contributed to the white matter injury.

4. There are no neurologic signs that are specific to this condition. During the sonographic evolution of the disease, infants are often noted to have severe and persistent

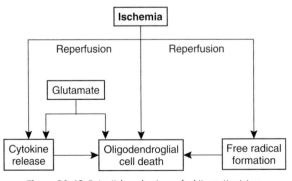

Figure 20-12 Potential mechanisms of white matter injury.

apneic and bradycardic episodes.[74] It is unclear whether these episodes are a consequence of the brain injury, or if the episodes of bradycardia contribute to the white matter injury (see previous discussion). Electrophysiologic studies indicate a high incidence of disturbance of visual evoked potentials, which is consistent with the frequent involvement of the optic radiation with cystic PVL.[97,98]

5. The diagnosis of cystic PVL is invariably made by cranial ultrasonography.[20] More recent evidence suggests that MRI is more sensitive in detecting diffuse noncystic white matter injury.[73] Perinatal events associated with postnatal cystic PVL include a history of chorioamnionitis, prolonged rupture of membranes, peripartum hemorrhage, asphyxia, hypovolemia, sepsis, hypocarbia, symptomatic patent ductus arteriosus, and recurrent apnea and bradycardia.[99–108] Many of these associations have in common a reduction in systemic blood pressure. However, in a recent study of 14 infants who developed PVL, only four (30%) had overt evidence of postnatal systemic hypotension and asphyxia was an uncommon finding.[74] Others have also failed to demonstrate a consistent association with hypotension and PVL.[106,107]

6. Prevention of PVL is likely to be difficult for several reasons. First, it is a relatively uncommon condition; second, the pathogenesis of PVL (as noted earlier) is complex; and third, the presentation is often subtle. As an example, there is increasing evidence pointing to an association between perinatal infection (i.e., chorioamnionitis) and PVL.[74,91,92] However, the mechanism(s) of injury linking these two events remain unclear; the positive predictive value of a history of chorioamnionitis and subsequent PVL is low (10%), and many cases of infection are asymptomatic with the diagnosis only established upon histologic examination of the placenta. The now almost routine administration of antibiotics to mothers in preterm labor may have some indirect benefit in this regard. More specific potential strategies include (1) the appropriate treatment of infants with low blood pressure for a given gestational age with volume replacement therapy or inotropic support as clinically indicated; (2) the careful ventilatory management of infants with respiratory distress so as to avoid hypocarbia; and (3) the use of antioxidant therapy to counter the free radical injury demonstrated in experimental models. However, antioxidant therapy has not been successful in the treatment of other neonatal conditions presumed to be related in part to free radical injury.[109]

7. Although the sonographic diagnosis of cystic PVL affects only a small percentage of preterm infants (∼ 3%), the condition poses a significant problem in that the vast majority of infants have major long-term neurodevelopmental problems. The most commonly described long-term motor sequela of PVL is a spastic diplegia.[1] It should be apparent from the anatomic course of the corticospinal tracts that traverse from the motor cortex in close proximity to the periventricular region into the internal capsule (Fig. 20-13) that the most medial of these fibers subserve the lower extremities and are more likely to be affected than the more lateral fibers supplying the upper extremities and face. This automatic arrangement accounts for the propensity to develop

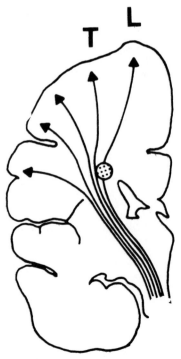

Figure 20-13 Schematic drawing depicting the anatomic cause of the corticospinal tracts. L refers to those fibers that subserve the lower extremities; T refers to those fibers that subserve the trunk.

spastic diplegia. However, recent reports describe a more severe deficit with involvement of all four extremities as well as visual and cognitive deficits.[110–114] This more severe outcome is consistent with the diffuse white matter injury noted on neuropathology in preterm infants who die with PVL.[80,81,115,116] The genesis of the cognitive deficits with PVL remains unclear. It has been speculated that the injury may secondarily affect neuronal cortical organization due to injury to subplate neurons or late migrating astrocytes.[117] Indeed, an MRI study of infants with PVL studied at term showed smaller cortical gray matter as compared to preterm infants without PVL and normal term infants.[118]

8. Injury to periventricular white matter remains the most significant problem contributing to adverse neurodevelopmental outcome in premature infants. A clearer understanding of pathogenesis is critical in order to provide targeted intervention to those infants at highest risk.

References

1. Volpe JJ: Neurology of the Newborn. 3rd ed. Philadelphia, WB Saunders, 2001.
2. Shalak L, Perlman JM: Hemorrhagic-ischemic cerebral injury in the premature infant: Curr Concepts Clin Perinatol 2002;29:745–763.
3. Lemons JA, Bauer CR, Oh W, Korones SB, et al: Very low birth weight outcomes of the National Institute of Child Health and Human Development, Neonatal Research Network, January 1995 through December 1996. Pediatrics 2001;107:e1.
4. Perlman JM, Rollins N, Burns D, et al: Relationship between periventricular intraparenchymal echodensities and germinal matrix-intraventricular hemorrhage in the very low birth weight neonate. Pediatrics 1993;91:474–480.
5. Hambleton G, Wiggelsworth JS: Origin of intraventricular hemorrhage in the preterm infant. Arch Dis Child 1976;57:651–655.
6. Lou CH, Lassen NA, Friis-Hansen B: Impaired autoregulation of cerebral blood flow in the distressed newborn infant. J Pediatr 1979;94: 118–125.
7. Pryds O, Griesen G, Lou H, et al: heterogeneity of cerebral vasoreactivity in preterm infants supported by mechanical ventilation. J Pediatr 1989; 115:638–645.
8. Goddard-Finegold J, Armstrong D, Zeller RS: Intraventricular hemorrhage following volume expansion after hypovolemic hypotension in the newborn beagle. J Pediatr 1982;100:796–799.
9. Ment LR, Stewart WB, Duncan CC, et al: Beagle puppy model of intraventricular hemorrhage. J Neurosurg 1982;57:219–223.
10. Perlman JM, McMenamin JB, Volpe JJ: Fluctuating cerebral blood flow velocity in respiratory distress syndrome. Relation to the development of intraventricular hemorrhage. N Engl J Med 1983; 309: 204–209.
11. Goldberg RN, Chung D, Goldman SL, et al: The associations of rapid volume expansion and intraventricular hemorrhage in the preterm infant. J Pediatr 1980;96:1060–1063.
12. Hill A, Perlman JM, Volpe JJ: Relationship of pneumothorax to the occurrence of intraventricular hemorrhage in the premature newborn. Pediatrics 1982;69:144–149.
13. Miall-Allen VM, DeVries LS, Whitelaw AG: Mean arterial blood pressure and neonatal cerebral lesions. Arch Dis Child 1987;62:1068–1069.
14. Tsuji M, Saul JP, du Plessis A, et al: Cerebral intravascular oxygenation correlates with mean arterial pressure in critically ill premature infants. Pediatrics 2000;106:625–632.
15. Bada HS, Korones SB, Perry EH, et al: Mean arterial blood pressure changes in premature infants and those at risk for intraventricular hemorrhage. J Pediatr 1990;117:607–614.
16. Mirro R, Buslta D, Green R, et al: Relationship between mean airway pressure, cardiac output and organ blood flow with normal and decreased respiratory compliance. J Pediatr 1987;111: 101–106.
17. Vert P, Monin P, Sibout M: Intracranial venous pressure in newborns: Variations in physiologic and neurologic disorders. In Stern L, Friis-Hansen B, Kildeberg P (eds): Intensive Care of Newborns. New York, Masson, 1975, p 185.
18. Perlman JM, Volpe JJ: Are venous circulatory changes important in the pathogenesis of hemorrhagic and/or ischemic cerebral injury? Pediatrics 1987;80:705–711.
19. Perlman JM, Volpe JJ: Intraventricular hemorrhage in the extremely small premature infant. Am J Dis Child 1986;140:1122–1124.
20. Perlman JM, Rollins N: Surveillance protocol for the detection of intracranial abnormalities in premature neonates. Arch Pediatr Adolesc Med 2000;154(8):822–826.
21. Perlman JM: Intraventricular hemorrhage. Pediatrics 1989;84:913–914.
22. Stewart AL, Reynolds EOR, Hope RL, et al: Probability of neurodevelopmental disorders estimated from ultrasound appearance of brains of very preterm infants. Dev Med Child Neurol 1987; 29:3–11.
23. Guzzetta F, Schackelford GD, Volpe S, et al: Periventricular intraparenchymal echodensities in the premature newborn: Critical determinant of neurologic outcome. Pediatrics 1986;78: 945–1006.
24. Gould SJ, Howard S, Hope PL, et al: Periventricular intraparenchymal cerebral hemorrhage in preterm infants: The role of venous infarction. J Pathol 1987;151:197–202.
25. Russell GAB, Jeffers G, Cook RWI: Plasma hypoxanthine: A marker for hypoxic-ischemic induced periventricular leukomalacia? Arch Dis Child 1992;67:388–392.
26. Perlman JM, Risser R: Relationship of uric acid concentrations and severe intraventricular hemorrhage/leukomalacia in the premature infant. J Pediatr 1998;132:436–439.
27. Schmidt B, Davis P, Moddemann D, et al: Long-term effects of indomethacin prophylaxis in extremely-low-birth-weight infants. N Engl J Med 2001;344(26):1966–1972.

28. Hill A, Volpe JJ: Normal pressure hydrocephalus in the newborn. Pediatrics 1981;68:623.

29. Ventriculomegaly Trial Group: Randomized trial of early tapping in neonatal post-hemorrhagic ventricular dilation. Arch Dis Child, 114:611.

30. Shinnar S, Gammar K, Bergman EW, et al: Management of hydrocephalus, use of acetazolamide and furosemide to avoid cerebrospinal fluid shunts. J Pediatr 1985;107:31.

31. Shankaran S, Papile LA, Wright LL, et al: The effect of antenatal phenobarbital therapy on neonatal intracranial hemorrhage in preterm infants. N Engl J Med 1997;337:466–471.

32. Pomerance JJ, Teal JG, Gogolok JF, et al: Maternally administered antenatal vitamin K: Effect on neonatal prothrombin activity, partial prothrombin time and intraventricular hemorrhage. Obstet Gynecol 1987;70:235–241.

33. Kazzi N, Llagan NB, Liang KC, et al: Maternal administration of vitamin K does not improve the coagulation profile of preterm infants. Pediatrics 1989;84:1045–1050.

34. Garite TJ, Rumney PJ, Briggs GC, et al: A randomized placebo controlled trial of betamethasone for the prevention of respiratory distress syndrome at 24–28 weeks gestation. Am J Obstet Gynecol 1992;166:646–651.

35. Kari MA, Hallman M, Gronen M, et al: Prenatal dexamethasone treatment in conjunction with rescue therapy of human surfactant: A randomized placebo-controlled multicenter study. Pediatrics 1994;93:730–736.

36. Jobe AH, Mitchell BR, Gunkel JH: Beneficial effects of combined use of prenatal steroids and postnatal surfactant on preterm infants. Am J Obstet Gynecol 1993;168:508–513.

37. Crowley P, Chalmers I, Keirse MJ NC: The effects of corticosteroid administration before preterm delivery: An overview of the evidence from clinical trials. Br J Obstet Gynecol 1990;97:11–25.

38. Shankaran S, Bauer CR, Bain R: Prenatal and perinatal risk factors and protective factors for neonatal intracranial hemorrhage. Arch Pediatr Adolesc Med 1996;150:491–497.

39. Maher JE, Cliver SP, Goldenberg RL, et al: March of Dimes Multicenter Study Group. The effect of glucocorticoid therapy in the very premature infant. Am J Obstet Gynecol 1994;170:869–873.

40. Wright LL, Homar JD, Gunkel H: Evidence from multicenter networks on the current use and effectiveness of antenatal corticosteroids in low birthweight infants. Am J Obstet Gynecol 1995;173:263–269.

41. Salhab W, Hyman L, Perlman JM: Partial or complete antenatal steroids treatment and neonatal outcome in extremely low birth weight infants {less than or equal to1000 grams: Is there a dose dependent effect? J Perinatol 2004;23:668–672.

42. Garland JS, Buck R, Leviton A: Effect of maternal glucocorticoid exposure on risk of severe intraventricular hemorrhage in surfactant-treated preterm infants. J Pediatr 1995;126:272–279.

43. Perlman JM, Nissen PD: Glial fibrillary acidic protein in RNA gene expression in human astroglial cells is modulated by dexamethasone. Ann Neurol 1995;38:495. (abstract)

44. Perlman JM, Risser RC, Gee JB: Pregnancy induced hypertension and reduced intraventricular hemorrhage in preterm infants. Pediatr Neurol 1997;17:29–33.

45. Kuban KCK, Leviton A, Pagano M, et al: Maternal toxemia is associated with a reduced incidence of germinal matrix hemorrhage in premature babies. J Child Neurol 1992;7:70–76.

46. Leviton A, Pagano M, Kuban KCK, et al: The epidemiology of germinal matrix hemorrhage during the first half of life. Dev Med Child Neurol 1988;33:138–145.

47. Hadi HA: fetal cerebral maturation in hypertension disorder in pregnancy. Obstet Gynecol 1984; 63:214–219.

48. Gould JB, Gluck L, Kulovich MV: The relationship between accelerated pulmonary maturity and accelerated neurologic maturity in certain chronically stressed pregnancies. Am J Obstet Gynecol 1997;127:181–186.

49. Nelson KB, Grether JK: Can magnesium sulfate reduce the risk of cerebral palsy in very low birthweight infants? Pediatrics 1995;95:263–269.

50. Crowther CA, Hillier JE, Doyle LW, et al: Effect of magnesium sulfate given for neuroprotection before preterm birth: A randomized controlled study. JAMA 2003;290:2669–2776.

51. Leviton A, Paneth N, Susser MW, et al: Magnesium receipt does not appear to reduce the risk of neonatal white matter damage. Pediatrics 1997;99:4.E2.

52. Paneth N, Jettan J, Pinto-Martron J, et al: Magnesium sulfate and risk of neonatal brain lesions and cerebral palsy in low birthweight infants. Pediatrics 1997;99:5.1–5.7.

53. Groome LJ, Goldenberg RL, Cliver SP, et al: March of Dimes Multicenter Study Group: Neonatal periventricular-intraventricular hemorrhage after maternal β-sympathomimetic tocolysis. Am J Obstet Gynecol 1992;167:873–879.

54. Atkinson MW, Goldenberg RL, Gaudier FL, et al: Maternal corticosteroid and tocolytic treatment and morbidity and mortality in very low birthweight infants. Am J Obstet Gynecol 1995;173:299–304.

55. Anderson GD, Bada HS, Shaver BM, et al: The effect of cesarean section on intraventricular hemorrhage in the premature infant. Am J Obstet Gynecol 1992;166:1091–1101.

56. Low JA, Galbraith RS, Sauerbrei EE, et al: Maternal fetal and newborn complications associated with newborn intracranial hemorrhage. Am J Obstet Gynecol 1986;154:345–352.

57. Strauss A, Kirz D, Mandalou HD, et al: Perinatal events and intraventricular/ependymal hemorrhage in the very low birthweight infant. Am J Obstet Gynecol 1985;151:1022–1027.

58. Ment LR, Oh W, Ehrenkrantz R, et al: Antenatal steroids, delivery mode and intraventricular hemorrhage in preterm infants. Am J Obstet Gynecol 1995;172:795–800.

59. Shankaran S, Bauer CR, Bain R, et al: Prenatal and perinatal risk and protective factors for neonatal intracranial hemorrhage. Arch Pediatr Adoles Med 1996;150:491–497.

60. Hansen A, Leviton A: Labor and delivery characteristics and risks of cranial ultrasonographic abnormalities among very-low-birth-weight infants. The Developmental Epidemiology Network Investigators. Am J Obstet Gynecol 1999;181(4):997–1006.

61. Perlman JM, Thack BT: Respiratory origin of fluctuations in arterial blood pressure in premature infants with respiratory distress syndrome. Pediatrics 1988;81:399–403.

62. Perlman JM, Goodman S, Kreusser KL, et al: Reduction of intraventricular hemorrhage by elimination of fluctuating cerebral blood flow velocity in preterm infants with respiratory distress syndrome. N Engl J Med 1985;312:1253–1257.

63. Jobe AH: Pulmonary surfactant therapy. N Engl J Med 1993;328:861–868.

64. Donn S, Roloff DW, Goldstein GW: Prevention of intraventricular hemorrhage in preterm infants by phenobarbitone: A controlled trial. Lancet 1981;ii:215–217.

65. Bedard MP, Shankaran S, Slovis TL, et al: Effect of prophylactic phenobarbital on intraventricular hemorrhage in high risk infants. Pediatrics 1984; 73:435–439.

66. Kuban KC, Leviton A, Krishnamoorthy KS, et al: Neonatal intracranial hemorrhage and phenobarbital. Pediatrics 1986;77:443–450.

67. Sinha S, Davis J, Tonger N, et al: Vitamin E supplementation reduces frequency of periventricular hemorrhage in very preterm infants. Lancet 1987;11:466–471.

68. Morgan ME, Benson JT, Cooke RW: Ethamsylate reduces the incidence of periventricular haemorrhage in very low birthweight babies. Lancet 1981;1:830–831.

69. Bada HS, Green RS, Pourcyrous M, et al: Indomethacin reduces the risk of severe intraventricular hemorrhage. J Pediatr 1989;115:631–637.

70. Ment LR, Oh W, Ehrenkranz RA, et al: Low-dose indomethacin and prevention of intraventricular hemorrhage: A multicenter randomized trial. Pediatrics 1994;94:543–550.

71. Pryds O, Griesen G, Johansen KH: Indomethacin and cerebral blood flow in preterm infants treated for patent ductus arterious. J Pediatr 1988;147: 315–316.

72. Edwards AD, Wyatt JS, Richardson C, et al: Effects of indomethacin on cerebral hemodynamics in very preterm infants. Lancet 1990;335:491–495.

73. Inder TEM, Anderson NJ, Spencer C, et al: White matter injury in the premature infant. A comparison between serial cranial sonographic and MR findings at term. Am J Neuroradiol 2003;24: 805–809.

74. Perlman JM, Risser R, Broyles RS: Bilateral cystic periventricular leukomalacia in the premature infant: Associated Risk Factors. Pediatrics 1996; 97:822–827.

75. De Vries LS, Regev R, Dubowitz LMS, et al: Perinatal risk factors for the development of extensive cystic leukomalacia. Am J Dis Child 1988;142:732–735.

76. Leviton A, Paneth N: White matter damage in preterm newborns—An epidemiologic perspective. Early Hum Dev 1990;24:1–22.

77. De Vries LS, Regev R, Dubowitz LMS: Late onset cystic leukomalacia. Arch Dis.Child 1986;61:298–299.

78. Banker BQ, Larroche JC: Periventricular leukolalacia of infancy: A form of neonatal anoxic encephalopathy. Arch Neurol 1962;7:386–410.

79. De Reuck J, Chatta AS, Richardson EPJr: Pathogenesis and evolution of periventricular leukomalacia in infancy. Arch Neurol 1972;27:229–236.

80. Armstrong D, Norman MG: Periventricular leukomalacia in neonates: Complications and sequelae. Arch Dis Child 1974;49:367–375.

81. Paneth N, Rudelli R, Monte W, et al: White matter necrosis in the very low birth weight infants: Neuropathologic and ultrasonographic findings in infants surviving six days or longer. J Pediatr 1990;116:975–984.

82. De Reuck J: The human periventricular arterial blood supply and the anatomy of cerebral infarctions. Euro Neurol 1971;5:321–334.

83. Takashima S, Tanaka K: Development of cerebrovascular architecture and its relationship to periventricular leukomalacia. Arch Neurol 1978;35: 11–16.

84. De Reuck J: Cerebral angioarchitecture and perinatal brain lesions in premature and full term infants. Acta Neurol Scand 1984;70:391–395.

85. Rorke LB: Anatomic features of the developing brain implicated to hypoxic-ischemic injury. Brain Pathol 1992;2:211–221.

86. Larroche JC: Developmental Pathology of the Neonate. Amsterdam, Excerpta Medica, 1977.

87. Oka O, Belliveau I, Rosenberg PA: Vulnerability of oligodendroglia to glutamate: Pharmacology, mechanisms and prevention. J Neurosci 1993;13: 1331–1453.

88. Leviton A, Gilles FH: Acquired perinatal leukoencephalopathy. Ann Neurol 1984;16:1.

89. Adinolfi M: Infectious diseases in pregnancy, cytokines and neurologic impairment: A hypothesis. Dev Med Child Neurol 1993;35:549–553.

90. Yoon BH, Kim CJ, Romero CJ: Experimentally induced intrauterine infection causes fetal brain white matter lesions in rabbits. Am J Obstet Gynecol 1997;177:797–802.

91. Zupman V, Gonzalez P, Lacaze-Masmontiel T, et al: Periventricular leukomalacia: Risk factors revisited. Dev Med Child Neurol 1996;38:1066–1067.

92. Leviton A, Pareth N, Reuss L, et al: Maternal infection, fetal inflammatory response and brain damage in very low birth weight infants. Pediatr Res 1999;46:566–575.

93. Hillier SL, Witkin SS, Krohn MA, et al: The relationship of amniotic fluid cytokines and preterm delivery, amniotic fluid infection, histologic chorioamnionitis and chorioamnion infection. Obstet Gynecol 1996;174:330–334.

94. Yoon BH, Romero R, Kim CJ, Namkoo J, et al: High expression of tumor necrosis factor α and interleukin 6 in periventricular leukomalacia. Am J Obstet Gynecol 1997;177:406–411.

95. Bonce AJ, Boling W, Kindy MS, et al: Altered neuronal and microglial response to excitotoxic and ischemic brain injury in mice lacking TNF receptor. Nat Med 1996;2:788–794.

96. Perlman JM, Volpe JJ: Episodes of apnea and bradycardia in the preterm newborn: Impact on cerebral circulation. Pediatrics 1985;76:333–338.

97. De Vries LS, Connell JA, Dubowitz LMS, et al: Neurological, electrophysiological and MRI abnormalities in infants with extensive cystic leukomalacia. Neuropediatrics 1987;18:61–66.

98. Jacobson LK, Dutton GN: Periventricular leukomalacia: An important cause of visual and ocular motility dysfunction in children. Surv Ophthalmol 2000;45(1):1–13.

99. Low JA, Froese AF, Galbraith RS, et al: The association of fetal and newborn acidosis with severe periventricular leukomalacia in the preterm infant. Am J Obstet Gynecol 190;162:977–982.

100. Baud O, Foix-L'Helias L, Kaminski M, et al: Antenatal glucocorticoid treatment and cystic periventricular leukomalacia in very premature infants. N Engl J Med 1999;341(16):1190–1196.

101. Faix RG, Donn SM: Association of septic shock caused by early onset group B streptococcal sepsis and periventricular leukomalacia in the preterm infant. Pediatrics 1985;76:415–419.

102. Greisen G, Munck H, Lou H: Severe hypocarbia in preterm infants and neurodevelopmental deficit. Acta Paediatr Scand 1986;76:401–404.

103. Fujimoto S, Togari H, Yamaguchi N, et al: Hypocarbia and cystic periventricular leukomalacia in premature infants. Arch Dis Child 1994;71: F107–F110.

104. Wiswell TE, Graziani LJ, Kornhauser MS: Effects of hypocarbia on the development of cystic periventricular leukomalacia in premature infants treated with high frequency jet ventilation. Pediatrics 1996;98:918–924.

105. Perlman JM, Hill A, Volpe JJ: The effect of patent ductus arteriosus on flow velocity in the anterior cerebral arteries: Ductal steal in the premature newborn infant. J Pediatr 1981;99:767–771.

106. Weindling AM, Wilkinson AR, Cook F, et al: Perinatal events which precede periventricular hemorrhage and leukomalacia in the newborn. Br J Obstet Gynecol 1985;92:1218–1223.

107. Trounce JQ, Shaw DE, Levene MI, et al: Clinical risk factors and periventricular leukomalacia. Arch Dis Child 1988;63:17–22.

108. Graziani LJ, Spitzer AR, Mitchell DG, et al: Mechanical ventilation in preterm infants: Neurosonographic and developmental studies. Pediatrics 1992;90: 515–522.

109. Phelps DL, Rosenbaum AL, Isenberg SJ, et al: Tocopherol efficacy and safety for preventing retinopathy of prematurity: A randomized controlled, double-masked trial. Pediatrics 1987;79:489–500.

110. Fazzi E, Lanzi G, Gerardo A, et al: Neurodevelopmental outcome in very low birth weight infants with or without periventricular hemorrhage and/or leukomalacia. Acta Paediatr 1992;81:808–811.

111. Roger B, Msall M, Owens T, et al: Cystic periventricular leukomalacia and type of cerebral palsy in preterm infants. J Pediatr 1994;125:51–58.

112. De Vries LS, Eken P, Groenendaal F, et al: Correlation between the degree of periventricular leukomalacia using cranial ultrasound and MRI in infancy in children with cerebral palsy. Neuropediatrics 1993;24:263–268.

113. Scher MS, Dobson V, Carpenter NA, et al: Visual and neurological outcome of infants with periventricular leukomalacia. Dev Med Child Neurol 1989;31:353–365.

114. Dambska M, Laure-Kamionowska M, Schmidt-Sidor B: Early and late neuropathological change sin perinatal white matter damage. J Child Neurol 1989;4:291–298.

115. De Vries L, Wiggelsworth JS, Regev R, et al: Evaluation of periventricular leukomalacia during the neonatal period and infancy: correlation of imaging and postmortem findings. Early Hum Dev 1988;17:205–219.

116. Van der Bor M, den Ouden L, Guit GL: Value of cranial ultrasound and magnetic resonance imaging in predicting neurodevelopmental outcome in preterm infants. Pediatrics 1992;90:196–199.

117. Evrard P, Gressens P, Volpe JJ: New concepts to understand the neurologic consequences of subcortical lesions in the premature brain. Biol Neonate 1992;61:1–3.

118. Inder TE, Huppi PS, Warfield S, et al: Periventricular white matter injury in the premature infants is followed by reduced cerebral cortical gray matter volume at term. Ann Neurol 1999;46:755–760.

Birth Defects and Genetic Disorders

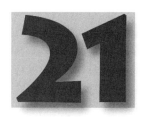

David D. Weaver, MS, MD

Birth defects and genetic disorders in newborns are common, frequently cause major disability, and can often be lethal. For example, major structural defects occur in 2% to 3% of live-borns.[1] Furthermore, 20% to 40% of neonates admitted to tertiary neonatal intensive care facilities have major birth defects, significant genetic disorders, or related problems.[2,3] Because of the high incidence of birth defects and genetic disorders, and the disabilities associated with them, neonatologists and other neonatal care providers need an extensive understanding of human genetics and genetic disorders, and a systematic approach to the evaluation and care of involved children. The purpose of this chapter is to review basic genetic principles, discuss the evaluation of common neonatal genetic conditions, and provide guidelines for the appropriate treatment and counseling of patients and their families with these problems. This chapter also provides information on how to obtain up-to-date information on genetic conditions, the names and locations of laboratories doing genetic testing, and resources for families with neonates who have genetic anomalies.

Note to reader: This chapter is relatively long and may be difficult to complete in one sitting. Listed here are the various chapter segments to help guide you through the work.

Frequency and Importance of Birth Defects and Genetic Disorders

Causes of Birth Defects

Genomic and Molecular Medicine

Significance of Prenatal Development on Neonatal Function and Survival

Dysmorphology

Approach to Specific Neonatal Genetic Disorders and Birth Defects

> Hypotonia
>
> Robin Sequence
>
> Hydrops Fetalis, Edema, and Cystic Hygroma
>
> Chromosomal Anomalies
>
> Intrauterine Growth Retardation/Small for Gestational Age
>
> Large for Gestational Age/Overgrowth Syndromes
>
> Fractures at Birth and in the Neonatal Period
>
> Bone Dysplasias
>
> Neuronal Migrational Disorders
>
> Teratogens

Inborn Errors of Metabolism

Information on Genetic Disorders and Laboratories Doing Specialized Genetic Testing

Frequency and Importance of Birth Defects and Genetic Disorders

Birth defects and genetic disorders are relatively common not only in neonates but in persons of all ages. Major birth defects are physical abnormalities that require medical or surgical intervention; they are life-threatening, cause long-term disability, or are of major cosmetic concern. Chromosomal abnormalities occur in 0.6% of all neonates and in about 12% of newborns with multiple congenital anomalies who die in the perinatal period. By 1 year of age, 3% to 5% of children will be found to have major congenital anomalies. Over half of all admissions to pediatric hospitals are directly or indirectly related to genetic disorders.[4] For example, leukemia occurs in about 1% of children with Down syndrome. If a child with Down syndrome were admitted to the hospital for leukemia, the admitting diagnosis would be leukemia, but Down syndrome would be the underlying cause of the leukemia. In addition, leukemia is now considered a genetic condition, because all leukemias are thought to be caused by gene mutations. Furthermore, children admitted with genetic disorders or complications of such disorders have, on average, more admissions and longer hospital stays than children without genetic conditions.[4] Birth defects and genetic disorders are the leading causes of infant deaths in the United States.

Causes of Birth Defects

It is safe to say that all birth defects have a cause, but all the causes for birth defects have not been established. The traditional causes of birth defects and genetic disorders (i.e., those mechanisms recognized for decades) include single gene defects, multifactorial inheritance, chromosomal aberrations, and environmental or teratogenic agents. Single gene disorders involve changes (*mutations*) in normal genes and are produced when there is either a single mutated gene or a pair of mutated genes present in an individual. If a single mutated gene produces a genetic disorder, the gene is considered to be a *dominant* gene, and if that gene is located on one of the nonsex chromosomes, an *autosome*, the gene is considered to be an *autosomal dominant* gene. The inheritance pattern resulting from such a gene would be an autosomal dominant pattern. If a dominant gene is located on the X chromosome, the gene would be an *X-linked dominant* gene. Although autosomal dominant genes are relatively common, X-linked dominant genes are rare, with hypophosphatemic rickets being the most common disorder caused by the latter mechanism. If a mutant gene is not expressed when matched with a normal paired gene (*allelic gene*), the gene is classified as a *recessive* gene. If a recessive gene is located on an autosome, the gene is an *autosomal recessive* gene; if

situated on the X chromosome, it is an *X-linked recessive* gene. *Gene carriers* for autosomal recessive conditions are individuals who possess one recessive gene and one normal allelic gene and are phenotypically normal. This is because under normal circumstances, both allelic genes in an autosomal recessive disorder must be mutated to result in an affected individual. In contrast, males who possesses an X-linked recessive gene are typically affected, such as in classic hemophilia (factor VIII deficiency). Because males normally have only one X chromosome in each of their cells, the majority of the genes on the X chromosome are not paired with an allelic gene, and are expressed whether the genes are recessive or dominant in the female. In contrast to autosomal recessive genes, the female who "carries" an X-linked recessive gene may manifest some or all of the traits seen in affected males. Usually females are not as severely affected as males with the condition.[5] The main reason for this expression in female carriers is the percentage of her X chromosomes carrying the mutated gene that is inactivated. In general, the lower the percentage of X chromosomes carrying the mutant gene that are inactivated, the greater the expression of the condition in the female.

The normal pattern of X-linked inheritance is that half of the sons of an unaffected carrier mother are affected. This pattern of inheritance occurs because a mother passes on the mutated X-linked gene to 50% of her sons, who then will be affected. The other 50% of her sons receiving the normal X-linked allele will be normal. With autosomal recessive inheritance, one fourth of the children of carrier parents are affected; these parents are phenotypically normal. If a parent has an autosomal dominant condition, his or her chance of passing on the mutant gene to each offspring is 50%, and in most situations, the offspring receiving the gene will have or will develop the disorder.

Over the last few decades, nontraditional causes of birth defects and genetic disorders have been discovered. These nontraditional mechanisms include genetic imprinting, uniparental disomy, contiguous gene deletions, microscopic and submicroscopic microdeletions, germline mosaicism, confined placental mosaicism, trinucleotide repeats, and mutations located at various locations in a gene. Case reports and explanations of some of these mechanisms are presented later.

Genomic and Molecular Medicine

In 1953, James Watson and Francis Crick discovered the structure of DNA and proposed the mechanisms through which DNA functions as the inherited genetic material.[6] In 1961, the genetic code—the combination of DNA bases that determine the sequence of amino acids in proteins—was unraveled. Since then, tremendous effort has been put forth to understand the structure, function, and regulation of human genes; to develop techniques to identify and sequence these genes; and to detect gene mutations. This effort has been so productive that since the late 1970s, researchers have found and sequenced thousands of human genes, identified mutations in these genes that result in genetic disorders, and sequenced most of the genetic material in humans, the latter project called the human genome project.

Advances in molecular genetics are occurring so quickly that it is now impossible to keep abreast of all the new discoveries. For example, over the last decade, approximately two new genes or new genetic disorders have been reported *per day*. Many of these newly discovered genes represent previously unrecognized biochemical mechanisms and this new knowledge has allowed further insights into the structure and functioning of the human body.

What do all these advances in molecular genetics mean to the daily practice of medicine and neonatology? How will these discoveries impact the future of medicine? To begin with, inherent in the discovery and sequencing of most new genes is the discovery of new biochemical pathways that have allowed greater insight into the biology and pathogenesis of disease. Second, the identification of new mutations has made it easier to confirm the diagnosis of suspected genetic disorders, classify specific subtypes of a single genetic condition, identify carriers of genetic conditions, and provide reliable genetic counseling and prenatal testing of at-risk fetuses. Third, these discoveries have increased our understanding of the structure and function of genes and how genes are regulated. Fourth, molecular genetic technology is being used in a variety of other disciplines, including forensic medicine, paternity testing, and infectious diseases. Finally, the technology is being used to produce a variety of gene products for the treatment of human diseases (e.g., human insulin and human growth hormone).

Exercise 1

QUESTION

1. Figure 21-1A is an illustration of a typical normal human gene and some gene products. The names of the anatomic portions of the gene or gene products are listed here in the left column, and the locations of these anatomic regions or products are labeled on the figure and listed here in the right column. Draw a line to connect each gene structure or product with the letter corresponding to the correct location.

Cap site	A
TATA box	B
Transcription	C
Stop codon	D
Intron	E
Initiation codon	F
Mature mRNA	G
CCAAT box	H
Exon	I
Immature mRNA	J

ANSWER

1. Answers are found in Figure 21-1B.

The basic structure of a human gene is now well understood (see Fig. 21-1B).[7] The coding regions of nuclear genes are the *exons*. Located between the exons are intervening nucleotide sequences called *introns*. Just before the first exon, a leader sequence is located, and is where *transcription* (production of messenger RNA [mRNA]) begins. This leader sequence, often called a *cap site*, is not translated into the protein, however. Preceding the cap site are two DNA base sequences, referred to as *TATA* and *CCAAT* sequences, or TATA and CAT boxes. All three of these sequences are important in the transcription of DNA. These segments promote the attachment of the enzyme RNA polymerase II to the DNA, and this enzyme then moves along the DNA to produce mRNA. The mRNA produced by this process is called *immature mRNA* and contains both exons and introns; the introns, however, are subsequently

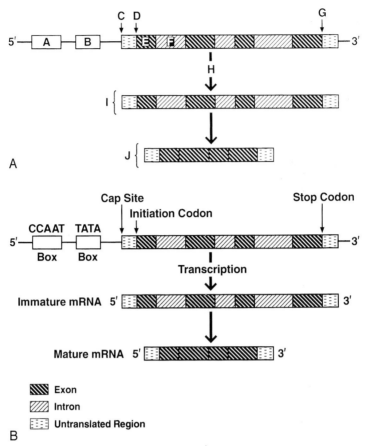

Figure 21-1 **A,** Stylized human gene. **B,** Transcription begins from the 5′ end of the DNA (represented by the straight line). CCAAT and TATA boxes and the cap site enhance the attachment of RNA polymerase II to the gene and the production of immature mRNA. The introns are split out of the immature mRNA to produce the mature mRNA.

spliced out from the mRNA. The resulting mRNA is referred to as *mature mRNA*. This mRNA moves to the cytoplasm, where ribosomes read the genetic code encrypted in the mRNA, and produce a polypeptide or protein with the amino acids arranged according to the code in the original DNA. For most genes, translation of the genetic code of the DNA into proteins begins with the mRNA derived from the first exon.

A mutation, defined here as a permanent transmissible change in the DNA, may occur in the leader sequence, in either of the TATA or CCAAT boxes, in the introns or exons. Mutations in these sequences may result in lack of transcription of the gene, as often happens with the thalassemias, or in a decreased rate of transcription. A mutation in an intron may have no effect, because the intron is not incorporated into the mature mRNA; alternatively, a mutation here may lead to a premature stop code, a sequence of three DNA bases that stops transcription of RNA before the RNA polymerase II reaches the

end of the gene. A mutation also may cause a shift in the reading frame, which results in an abnormal amino acid sequence in the developing protein. When mutations occur within an exon, all the preceding consequences can occur. In addition, a change in a single DNA base in an exon may result in a change in one or more amino acids, which in turn may lead to the formation of an abnormal protein or enzyme. The production of an abnormal protein or enzyme ultimately may result in a genetic disease in the affected individual. An example is sickle cell anemia, in which a valine is substituted for a glutamic acid in the sixth amino acid position in β-globin. The amino acid substitution is caused by a change in a single DNA base. Deletion of one or more DNA bases may also occur, resulting in a frameshift reading of the DNA or deletion of one or more amino acids. For instance, approximately 60% of all cases of Duchenne muscular dystrophy are produced by deletions of sizable portions of the gene. Such deletions result in the absence of multiple amino acids from dystrophin, the normal protein produced by this gene, or even to total absence of dystrophin. In cystic fibrosis, the most common mutation is del-taF508, which causes a deletion of three nucleotides that, in turn, translates into a deletion of one amino acid.

Significance of Prenatal Development on Neonatal Function and Survival

The development of a human being is a continuous and carefully orchestrated process that begins with conception and is not completed until late adolescence. Shortly after conception, the embryo is represented by a *blastocyst*, a hollow ball of cells. The blastocyst consists of an outer layer, the trophoblast, that ultimately forms the placenta and the outer fetal membrane, the chorion, and an inner cell mass that eventually forms the definitive embryo. By the beginning of the third week following conception, the embryo begins forming the three basic embryonic tissue types. These tissue types are (1) the *ectoderm*, which eventually forms the epidermis, central nervous system, and ectodermal derivatives, including hair, teeth, sweat glands, and nails; (2) the *endoderm*, which forms the gut and its derivatives, such as the lungs, liver, and pancreas; and (3) the *mesoderm*, which forms muscles, bones, connective tissue, blood vessels, dermis, and other structures. Organs begin forming from the third through the eighth weeks of development, and this process of organ formation is known as *organogenesis*. The *embryonic stage* of development extends from the first division of the conceptus (the *zygote*) through the end of the eighth week. During the *fetal period*, from the beginning of the 9th week (11th week after the last menstrual period) until birth, primary growth and maturation of the organs of the fetus occur.

Most organs and organ systems of the fetus function before birth. If they do not, then they will probably not function adequately postnatally. The following case study illustrates this point.

Case Study 1

Baby I is a 2350-g term neonate born to a 25-year-old gravida 3 para 3 woman. Her prenatal history was significant for severe oligohydramnios detected at 32 weeks. The oligohydramnios was so severe that amniotic fluid could not be obtained for a chromosomal analysis. An ultrasonographic assessment of the fetus at the time failed to detect any other significant problems. The mother reported little fetal movement during the last trimester of the pregnancy.

Immediately following his birth, Baby I developed severe respiratory distress, and was intubated and treated with ventilatory support at high settings. During the first 6 hours after birth, a pneumothorax developed that required placement of chest tubes. Despite all efforts, Baby I died from respiratory insufficiency at 11 hours of age. Other significant findings included a rounded forehead and nose (Fig. 21-2), flattened and hypoplastic ears, micrognathia, and mildly limited motion of the wrists, elbows, hips, and knees.

Exercise 2

QUESTION

1. What is the most likely cause of the severe oligohydramnios?

   a. Renal agenesis

   b. Urinary tract obstruction

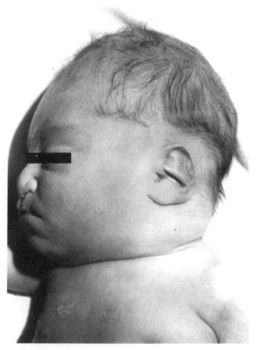

Figure 21-2 Postmortem view of baby I with Potter sequence secondary to bilateral renal agenesis. Note the rounded forehead, flattened nose, all secondary effects of uterine compression because of the oligohydramnios.

c. Amniotic fluid leak

d. Placental dysfunction

ANSWER

1. a.

After about the fourth month of pregnancy, most of the amniotic fluid is fetal urine produced by the fetal kidneys. Oligohydramnios after the fourth month generally is caused by a lack of urine production due to dysplastic or absent kidneys, obstruction of the urinary tract at any place from the kidneys to the urethra, leakage of fluid from the amniotic cavity because of ruptured or leaky fetal membranes, or placental dysfunction. Other than the oligohydramnios, the ultrasound evaluation of this pregnancy was normal. Because prenatal ultrasound assessments are not totally reliable, this did not mean that Baby I's kidneys were present and functioning. If kidneys had been identified and had appeared normal, then absent or dysplastic kidneys would have been unlikely. Because the kidneys apparently were not identified, a postnatal ultrasound evaluation or an autopsy in this situation was indicated.

If a urinary tract obstruction in Baby I had been the cause of the oligohydramnios, then distention of some part of the urinary system should have been observed. If a leak in the fetal membranes had been present, there should have been a history of excessive vaginal discharge or a positive Nitrazine paper test on the vaginal fluid. Placental dysfunction generally does not lead to severe oligohydramnios, and when oligohydramnios is present, the dysfunction normally is associated with intrauterine growth restriction of the fetus.

The autopsy on Baby I found absence of kidneys, and severe hypoplasia of the lungs, as was suspected from his postnatal course.

Most evidence for the association between lung hypoplasia and oligohydramnios suggests an indirect effect of the oligohydramnios. For proper lung development, intrauterine breathing must occur. Restriction of the chest by direct uterine compression limits expansion of the chest wall and results in the lungs being underdeveloped or hypoplastic at birth. If this hypothesis is true, then hypoplastic lungs will develop with any process that leads to oligohydramnios; from any mechanism that reduces respiratory effort, such as prenatal muscle weakness; from any situation that elevates the diaphragm, such as large polycystic kidneys or extensive accumulation of ascitic fluid, as seen in the prune belly syndrome; or from any other mechanism that causes intrathoracic lung compression, such as bowel within the chest cavity secondary to diaphragmatic hernia.

Exercise 2 *Continued*

QUESTIONS

2. If the condition in Baby I proved to be an autosomal dominant disorder, what should the parents be told regarding the potential recurrence of this condition in subsequent children?

   a. The recurrence risk for affected siblings would most likely be less than 1%. If the parents are normal and if the baby's condition is dominant, then he would most likely represent a new dominant mutation in the egg or sperm.

   b. 3% to 5%

   c. 25%

   d. 50%

   e. 50% but the expression of the condition could vary considerably and subsequent affected children might have kidney abnormalities but not necessarily bilateral renal agenesis

3. If the condition in Baby I proved to be an autosomal recessive condition, how would you modify the information on recurrence risk for the parents?

   a. Less than 1% recurrence risk in subsequent offspring

   b. 3% to 5%

   c. 25% with similar severity as in baby I

   d. 25% with marked variation in severity expected

   e. 50% with dysplastic kidneys in one of the parents

ANSWERS

2. e. 50% but the expression of the condition could vary considerably and subsequent affected children might have kidney abnormalities but not necessarily bilateral renal agenesis

3. c. 25% with similar severity as in baby I.

Although the cause of the renal agenesis in most neonates is never determined, the condition can be inherited, and if so, there may be a significant risk of recurrence in subsequent children.[8] When one encounters a newborn with renal agenesis, both parents need abdominal ultrasound examinations to determine the status of their kidneys. These procedures are needed to diagnose hereditary renal adysplasia, an autosomal dominant condition with extensive variation in expression of renal disease. In hereditary renal adysplasia, one or both kidneys may be dysplastic in some individuals; others in the same family may have unilateral renal agenesis. Occasionally, an individual with this condition has bilateral renal agenesis, which is fatal in the neonatal period. If hereditary renal adysplasia were the cause of baby I's bilateral renal agenesis, there would be a significant chance that one of his parents had the gene and a 50% chance that any full sibling of his would have some type of renal abnormality. Bilateral renal agenesis is rarely inherited in an autosomal recessive manner, with both parents being carriers and both having normal kidneys. In this situation, the recurrence risk for affected siblings would be 25% and the severity probably would be about the same. This is the case because as a general rule, autosomal recessive conditions normally do not vary greatly in severity from one affected sibling to the next, while with autosomal dominant disorders, variation in the severity is the rule rather than the exception.

The parents of baby I should have genetic counseling. If kidney abnormalities were detected in one of them, they should be told that the recurrence risk for renal abnormalities in future offspring could be as high as 50%. If their kidneys are normal, the recurrence risk probably would be less than 1% but could be as high as 25%, if the cause of the renal agenesis were an autosomal recessive condition. Further, one should counsel the parents that prenatal diagnosis is possible by detecting a recurrence of oligohydramnios, or by finding dysplastic or absent kidneys. However, if the quantity of amniotic fluid were normal and if fetal renal ultrasound examinations were normal, the fetus still could have dysplastic kidneys and be affected.

This case illustrates the significance of proper organ function prenatally with regard to the ultimate development and function of multiple organ systems postnatally. In this case, the child did not die from uremia (renal failure) but from pulmonary failure secondary to lung hypoplasia (secondary to diminished amniotic fluid and inadequate fetal breathing). Other examples of this phenomenon include hypoplastic left or right side of the heart (secondary to abnormal valvular or vessel development), microcolon (secondary to a more proximal aganglionic segment), and arthrogryposis (congenital joint contractures secondary to decreased movement).

Dysmorphology

In 1966, Dr. David W. Smith delineated dysmorphology, the study of abnormal morphology or shape (birth defects), as a separate pediatric discipline.[9] Smith defined dysmorphology as the study of all aspects of birth defects, including etiology, pathogenesis, complications, prevention, treatment, and associated long-term disabilities. Research in this area has led to the recognition of a number of mechanisms that produce birth defects.

Exercise 3

QUESTIONS

1. Match the physical findings listed here to the patient displaying those features shown in Figures 21-3 through 21-8.

   a. Constriction bands, distal digit amputation, and pseudosyndactyly

   b. Torticollis and plagiocephaly

   c. Oligodactyly

   d. Midfacial hypoplasia, short limbs, small thorax

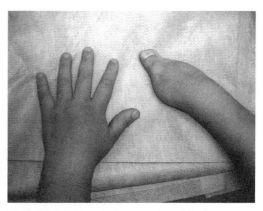

Figure 21-3 See Exercise 3, answers 1c and 2c.

2. Match the diagnosis or classification of defects listed here with Figures 21-3 through 21-8.

   a. Thanatophoric dysplasia

   b. Extrinsic deformation

   c. Limb reduction malformation

   d. Amniotic band disruption sequence

ANSWERS

1. a. Constriction bands, distal digit amputation, and pseudosyndactyly (Fig. 21-4). The characteristic aberrations in the hand shown in this photo are the cutaneous fusion of the distal parts of the second through the fifth fingers, distal amputation of the fourth and fifth fingers, and the grooves around the fused fingers. The skin between the proximal portions of the second to the fifth fingers is not fused, and it was possible to pass a probe between these fingers. This latter finding implies that at one time during development, all four fingers were separated and they subsequently became fused distally. The term for this finding is pseudosyndactyly. Amniotic bands, which are strands of amnion that float freely in the amniotic fluid and can wrap around digits and limbs, caused this patient's defects. In this case, an amniotic band apparently wrapped around the four fingers and, with subsequent growth, caused the grooves (constriction bands) to form, the fingers to fuse distally, and amputation of the distal portion of the fourth and fifth fingers secondary to loss of blood supply that led to necrosis.

   b. Torticollis and plagiocephaly (Figs. 21-5 and 21-6). The 2-month-old female infant pictured in these figures was born with torticollis, marked plagiocephaly (asymmetrical skull shape), and bowing of the tibia and fibula bilaterally. Her twin sister is completely normal. The pregnancy was complicated by left lateral chest wall pain and heartburn, necessitating small, frequent meals. The mother also reported that one twin appeared to be fixed in a single position. At 37 weeks of gestation, spontaneous labor began and the first twin was delivered without difficulty. However, labor did not continue, and with further assessment, the second twin (the twin shown here) was found to be located ex utero. She then was delivered by cesarean section. The surgeon found that the patient's head was lodged under the left rib cage and that the placenta was attached to the outside of the uterus. On examination following delivery, she had major limitation of neck movement, marked asymmetry of the skull, and more than usual bowing of the lower legs.

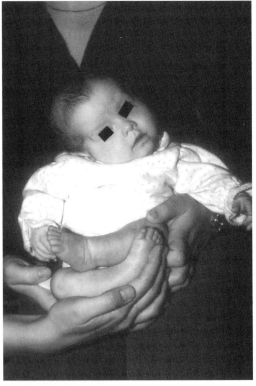

Figure 21-5 See Exercise 3, answers 1b and 2b.

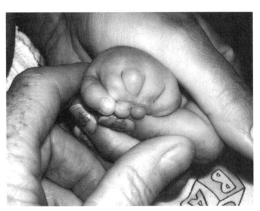

Figure 21-4 See Exercise 3, answers 1a and 2d.

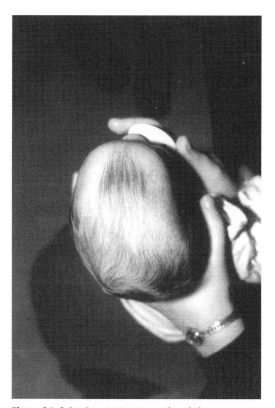

Figure 21-6 See Exercise 3, answers 1b and 2b.

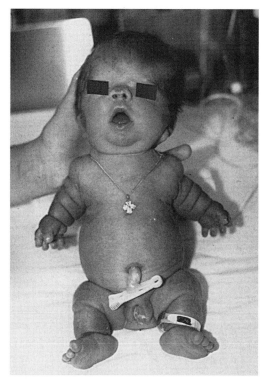

Figure 21-7 Typical presentation of a newborn with thanatophoric dysplasia. Note the midfacial hypoplasia, short and upturned nose, short arms and legs with extra skin creases, small chest, and prominent abdomen.

c. Oligodactyly (Fig. 21-3). The hand shown here is that of a 5-year-old female child who is completely normal physically and developmentally except for her hand and unexplained mild hypotonia. The hand defect was a congenital defect, which consists of absence of the thumb and fourth and fifth fingers on the right hand and fusion of the second and third fingers. When there is complete fusion of the skin between two fingers, the term syndactyly is applied. In this case, there is total lack of separation of the fingers, so much so that they appear to be one finger (monodactyly). Note, however, that there is a longitudinal ridge running down the nail indicating duplication of the finger. The etiology of this defect is not known, and commonly the defect is not inherited.

d. Midfacial hypoplasia, short limbs, small thorax (Figs. 21-7 and 21-8). The most striking feature of the neonate in Figure 21-7 is her short limbs. In addition, she has midfacial hypoplasia, depressed nasal bridge, small thorax, prominent abdomen, and extra skinfolds on her extremities. On radiographic evaluation,

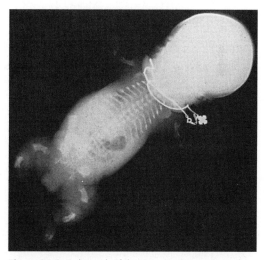

Figure 21-8 Radiograph of the patient in Figure 21-7 with thanatophoric dysplasia. Observe the bowing and shortening of the long bones of the extremities, thin and short ribs, U-shaped and flat vertebral bodies, and small, poorly aerated lungs.

there was shortening of all long bones, including the ribs; abnormal curvature of all long bones; and U-shaped and flattened vertebrae (Fig. 21-8). The child died within hours after birth from respiratory insufficiency secondary to lung hypoplasia resulting from short ribs and a small rib cage (Fig. 21-8).

2. a. Thanatophoric dysplasia (Figs. 21-7 and 21-8). Thanatophoric dysplasia is a lethal skeletal dysplasia caused by a mutation in the fibroblast growth factor receptor 3 (*FGFR3*) gene. Essentially all the problems seen in this neonate are the result of abnormal bone growth secondary to a mutation in this gene. This type of bone disorder is classified as a *dysplasia*. By definition, a dysplasia occurs when there is abnormal tissue formation. In the case of thanatophoric dysplasia, the abnormal tissue is the bone.

   Even though thanatophoric dysplasia is the result of a mutation in the *FGFR3* gene, the recurrence risk for subsequent siblings is normally less than 1%. This is the case because the mutation is an autosomal dominant one, and all affected individuals die in the neonatal period or during the first year or two of life. As a result, an affected individual never passes on the mutant gene to descendants. With thanatophoric dysplasia and other similar dominant lethal situations, there is occasionally a recurrence in siblings. The recurrence usually is due to *germline mosaicism* involving the same mutation. When germline mosaicism is present, one parent possesses a clone of cells containing the mutation in one or both gonads. In most of these cases, the parent does not have the mutation in his or her somatic cells and therefore is phenotypically normal. But because of the mosaicism, there is an increased risk of recurrence in subsequent offspring. The recurrence risk depends on the percentage of germ cells that have the mutation; empirical observations in these situations indicate a risk of recurrence of between 5% and 10% in most cases. When providing genetic counseling to parents in dominantly inherited situations, one needs to raise the possibility of germline mosaicism. Prenatal testing is available to test for a recurrence.

   b. Extrinsic deformation (Figs. 21-5 and 21-6). This child's defects resulted from her being confined in a fixed position with her head lodged beneath her mother's rib cage for much of the latter part of the pregnancy. These types of defects are classified as a *deformation*, an abnormality resulting from abnormal extrinsic (outside) or intrinsic (internal) forces applied to the fetus or parts of the fetus. Most extrinsic deformations are the result of abnormal fetal compression by the uterus because of oligohydramnios, uterine abnormalities, or abnormal positioning of the fetus. In this case, the limited intra-abdominal space secondary to the size of the uterus, the intra-abdominal pregnancy and abdominal organs, and the abdominal wall musculature produced the abnormal forces. Because of this pressure, the head molded to the rib cage producing plagiocephaly, flexion contracture of the neck resulting in torticollis, and bowing of the lower legs as they were fixed in position and overlapping.

   Intrinsic deformations may result from such forces as hypertonia, distention of an organ, or abnormally large organs. An example is clubfoot deformities in patients with meningomyeloceles. These deformities result from spasticity of the muscles of the legs secondary to lost or decreased innervation caused by the meningomyeloceles.

   c. Limb reduction malformation (Fig. 21-3). In this case, the defective fingers did not form in a normal fashion from the beginning of their development. The thumb and fourth and fifth fingers never developed, and the second and third digits formed together and never separated in the normal manner. Because the fingers failed to form in a normal fashion from the beginning, one would classify these defects as *malformations*.

   d. Amniotic band disruption sequence (Fig. 21-4). A *disruption* is a defect produced when an organ or region of the body begins development in a normal fashion, and is subsequently destroyed. In the case presented here, presumably the fingers formed in a normal manner but then were damaged by an amniotic band. The distal tips of fingers 4 and 5 are missing, presumably because the blood supply was compromised and the tips became necrotic and fell off. Pseudosyndactyly developed because the fingers were held together, and the tissue between them fused. A *sequence* occurs when a single defect leads to other secondary and tertiary defects. In this case, the initial defect was the amniotic band, which secondarily caused the pseudosyndactyly, the constriction bands, and the vascular compromise, leading to the amputation of the fingers.

Approach to Specific Neonatal Genetic Disorders and Birth Defects

In this section, several case studies depict genetic problems that may be encountered in the daily practice of neonatology. Because advances in genetics are occurring so rapidly, the recommendations presented here may no longer be the latest approach. One should always review the current literature or consult a clinical geneticist or other specialist for the current testing, evaluations, and treatments of genetic conditions. However, the scenarios that follow illustrate frameworks from which the evaluation of neonates with these problems can be approached.

Hypotonia

Hypotonia is not an uncommon finding in neonates and may portend a dire outcome. Hypotonia may be caused by a central nervous system birth defect, a peripheral nerve problem, a muscle disorder, a metabolic error, or a perinatal or postnatal event affecting the nervous system. Often the underlying problem is found to be genetically determined.

Case Study 2

Baby M (Fig. 21-9) was born to a 23-year-old primigravida white mother. The pregnancy was complicated by polyhydramnios and preterm labor. The delivery occurred at 37 weeks' gestation, but because of fetal distress and breech presentation, a

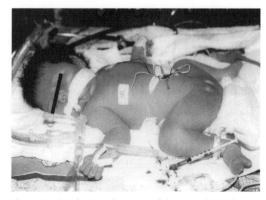

Figure 21-9 Baby M with congenital myotonic dystrophy. Observe the positioning of the arms and legs. She also had very little movement, mild contractures of the limbs, and marked hypotonia.

cesarean section was necessary. Birth length, weight, and head circumference were 53.5 cm (95th percentile), 3880 g (80th percentile), and 39 cm (>97th percentile), respectively. Following birth, she had no respiratory effort, and required mechanical ventilation. Subsequent physical examination found a large-appearing neonate who was cyanotic and hydropic, moved little, and had marked lateral extension of her legs. Other findings included a large anterior fontanel (4 × 3 cm), bitemporal narrowing, broad nasal bridge, mild micrognathia, adducted thumbs, and marked hypotonia. After a prolonged hospital stay (37 days), her respiratory status improved, and she was taken off assisted ventilation. At discharge, she still had considerable hypotonia.

Exercise 4

QUESTIONS

1. Indicate whether the following statements are true or false.

   a. The diagnosis of hypotonia is based on electromyographic results.

   b. Hypotonia may be the first presenting feature of an inborn error of metabolism.

   c. Genetic testing is available to diagnose some causes of hypotonia in neonates.

   d. In some patients, neonatal hypotonia may be a transient, benign condition.

2. Which of the following steps should be taken next to determine a diagnosis for Baby M?

   a. Start an evaluation of the child to determine the etiology of her condition.

   b. Obtain more information about the health of the mother and other family members.

   c. Consult a pediatric neurologist or clinical geneticist for his or her input into the evaluation of the child.

   d. All of the above.

ANSWERS

True: b, c, d. False: a.

1. 2. All of the above.

Hypotonia is a significant decrease in muscle tone. This abnormality is a clinical finding, and the severity generally is not quantified beyond stating that it is mild, moderate, or profound.

Environmental factors causing hypotonia in neonates and infants include perinatal or postnatal hypoxic ischemic brain injury, medications or illicit drugs, intracranial or spinal cord infections, cerebral hemorrhage, and cerebral or spinal trauma. In any neonate with hypotonia, one needs to consider these possibilities because treatment is available for some of these conditions. In many other neonates, the etiology is not environmental but hypotonia is caused by anomalies of the brain or spinal cord that may or may not be genetically determined, or by genetic conditions adversely affecting the central or peripheral nervous system or muscles. Table 21-1 lists some of the known congenital and genetic causes of hypotonia.

TABLE 21-1

CAUSES OF NEONATAL HYPOTONIA

Central Nervous System Conditions
Angelman syndrome
Congenital hypothyroidism
Down syndrome
Gangliosidoses
Joubert syndrome
Malformation or disruption of the brain
Miller-Dieker syndrome
Möbius syndrome
Rett syndrome
Trisomy 13 syndrome
Trisomy 20p syndrome
Zellweger syndrome (cerebrohepatorenal syndrome)
4p- syndrome
5p- syndrome
9p- syndrome
18q- syndrome

Spinal Cord Abnormalities
Arthrogryposis (amyoplasia)
Spinal dysraphism (meningomyelocele, rachischisis)
Spinal muscular atrophy type I (Werdnig-Hoffman syndrome)

Peripheral Nerve Disorders
Acetylcholine receptor defect
Charcot-Marie-Tooth disease type 1A
Familial dysautonomia (Riley-Day syndrome)
Natal neonatal radiculoneuropathy

Neuromuscular Junction Disorders
Familial infantile myasthenia gravis
Transient myasthenia gravis

Muscle Disorders
Congenital myopathies
Congenital myotonic dystrophy
Duchenne muscular dystrophy
Mitochondrial disorders
Myotubular myopathy
Nemaline myopathy

Miscellaneous Disorders
Achondroplasia
Biotinidase deficiency
Blepharophimosis syndrome
Camptomelic dysplasia
Carbohydrate-deficient glycoprotein syndrome type Ia
Coffin-Lowry syndrome
Complex I mitochondrial respiratory chain deficiency
Complex IV mitochondrial respiratory chain deficiency
Congenital Marfan disease
Cri du chat syndrome
Cutis laxa (X-linked)
Ehlers-Danlos syndrome type VI
Fabry syndrome
Fetal hyperthermia
Fetal warfarin syndrome
Fragile X syndrome
Glutaricaciduria
Glycogen storage diseases
Hyperglycinemia
Hypophosphatasia
Langer-Giedion syndrome
Leigh syndrome
Long QT syndrome type 1
Lowe syndrome
Mannosidosis
Maple syrup urine disease
Medium chain acyl-CoA dehydrogenase deficiency
Menkes' syndrome
3-Methylcrotonylglycinuria I
Methyltetrahydrofolate:1-homocysteine S-methyltransferase deficiency
Neuraminidase deficiency
Osteogenesis imperfecta type II
Peroxisome disorders
Phenylketonuria II (dihydropterine reductase deficiency)
Prader-Willi syndrome
Propionicacidemia type I
Pseudovitamin D deficiency rickets
Pyruvate carboxylase deficiency
Pyruvate dehydrogenase complex, component X defect
Pyruvate dehydrogenase complex, E1-alpha polypeptide 1 defect
Refsum disease (infantile form)
Rieger syndrome
Severe primary neonatal hyperparathyroidism
Short chain acyl-CoA dehydrogenase deficiency
Shprintzen omphalocele syndrome
Sotos' syndrome
Stickler syndrome
Thanatophoric dysplasia
Toriello-Carey syndrome
Trichorhinophalangeal syndrome
Velocardiofacial syndrome
Walker-Warburg syndrome
Weaver syndrome
Williams syndrome
XXXXY syndrome

Adapted from Jones KL: Smith's Recognizable Patterns of Human Malformation, 5th ed. Philadelphia, WB Saunders, 1997; McKusick VA: Online Mendelian Inheritance in Man, 2005, accessed at www3.ncbi.nlm.nih.gov/Omim/.

In question 2 we must determine not only the tests but the sequence that will likely yield the diagnosis. The choice rests on discerning the clues present in the child, and the experience of the attending physician.

Metabolic disorders should be high on the list of possibilities. For instance, Zellweger syndrome is a metabolic disorder involving the absence of peroxisomes and peroxisomal enzymes. These deficiencies result in medium- and long-chain dicarboxylic aciduria, decreased synthesis of plasmalogens, accumulation of very long chain fatty acids and trihydroxycoprostanic acid in the blood, and increased levels of pipecolic acid in the blood and urine.[10–12] One of the enzymes missing in Zellweger syndrome is dihydroxyacetone phosphate acyltransferase, an enzyme involved in lipid synthesis in the peroxisomes. The course of the disease is rapidly progressive, with severe failure to thrive, developmental delay, and death usually by 1 year of age. The diagnosis is established first by detecting elevated serum levels of very long chain fatty acids and then by finding elevations and deficiencies of other peroxisomal metabolites and enzymes. Conditions related to Zellweger syndrome include hyperpipecolic acidemia, infantile Refsum disease, neonatal adrenoleukodystrophy, rhizomelic chondrodysplasia punctata, and pseudo-Zellweger syndrome. One also needs to consider these conditions in the differential diagnosis in Baby M.

To diagnose other conditions listed in Table 21-2, the following additional evaluations should be made: a serum thyroxine and thyroid-stimulating hormone evaluation to eliminate the possibility of congenital hypothyroidism, a computed tomographic (CT) or magnetic resonance imaging (MRI) scan of the head to uncover many of the central nervous system problems resulting in hypotonia, and a standard chromosomal analysis to diagnose many of the chromosomal problems associated with hypotonia. Specific cytogenetic testing for suspected microdeletion syndromes such as Miller-Dieker syndrome should also be done. The specific fluorescence in situ hybridization (FISH) test should be dictated by the history, physical examination, and other findings. For instance, one should consider doing the Miller-Dieker FISH probe if the characteristic facial features associated with this syndrome are present or there is lissencephaly present on the CT or MRI scan. Prader-Willi syndrome (PWS), another disorder in the differential diagnosis, is diagnosed by assessing methylation patterns in a specific gene region; testing for PWS should be done in patients with hypotonia when the diagnosis of another condition is not immediately apparent. Furthermore, specific gene testing can now be used to diagnose many causes of hypotonia. For instance, gene testing can make or confirm the diagnosis of achondroplasia, congenital myotonic dystrophy, fragile X syndrome, many mitochondrial disorders, and spinal muscular atrophies.

Other dysmorphic or neurologic syndromes can be diagnosed solely on the patient's physical and neurologic findings. For example, Möbius syndrome is diagnosed by the presence of unilateral or bilateral sixth and seventh nerve palsies that result in the absence of lateral gaze and an expressionless face. Other conditions such as spinal muscular atrophy can be diagnosed by specific tests such as an electromyography, nerve conduction studies, and muscle biopsy, but the more accurate diagnosis is established by specific gene testing. When one is considering congenital myotonic dystrophy as a diagnosis, one needs to evaluate the mother of the child for myoclonus and other features of the adult form of this disease. Five of the six types of Ehlers-Danlos syndrome can be diagnosed either by gene testing or enzyme assay, the exception being type III, the familial hypermobility type. The likelihood of transient myasthenia gravis is increased by a positive response to an intramuscular injection of neostigmine. With this condition there should be significant and immediate improvement in the patient's strength following the injection.

A physician can diagnose many muscular dystrophies such as Duchenne muscular dystrophy by finding elevated serum creatine kinase (CK) levels, characteristic anatomic findings, and specific test results on muscle tissue. Therefore, the evaluation of hypotonia should also include a serum CK determination, appropriate gene testing, and in some cases, a muscle biopsy. The timing of the biopsy will be dictated by the physical size and condition of the patient, and by a previous negative workup. One can suspect mitochondrial disorders by detecting elevated levels of serum or cerebrospinal fluid lactic and pyruvic acids (lactate or pyruvate levels). On muscle biopsy, mitochondrial disorders typically have "ragged red fibers" histologic pattern. Specific mitochondrial enzyme and gene testing to determine the exact mitochondrial condition is available for many disorders. A neurologist or clinical geneticist can be consulted for more specific information on mitochondrial testing.

TABLE 21-2

CONDITIONS IN WHICH HYDROPS MAY BE PRESENT IN THE NEWBORN

Cardiovascular Defects

Absence of atrioventricular node
Absence of ductus venosus
Acardia
Aortic coarctation
Aortic valve atresia
Aortic valvular stenosis
Atrial flutter
Complete heart block
Endocardial fibroelastosis
Hypoplastic ventricle
Iliofemoral arterial thrombosis
Persistent truncus arteriosus
Pulmonary valve atresia
Rhabdomyoma
Sinus bradycardia
Supraventricular tachycardia
Tetralogy of Fallot
Twin-to-twin transfusion syndrome
Vascular tumors
Wolff-Parkinson-White syndrome

Chromosomal Aberrations

Chromosome XXXXY syndrome
Tetraploidy
Tetrasomy 12q
Trisomy 18 syndrome
Turner syndrome

Gastrointestinal Problems

Bowel atresias
Duplication of the gut
Peritonitis
Volvulus of small bowel

Hematologic Disorders

Anemia
Erythroblastosis fetalis (Rh hemolytic disease of the newborn)
Maternal use of chloramphenicol
Pyruvate kinase deficiency of erythrocyte
Spherocytosis type I
α-Thalassemia
β-Thalassemia

Intrauterine Infections

Cytomegalovirus
Listeriosis
Parvovirus
Rubella
Syphilis
Toxoplasmosis

Metabolic Disorders

Carbohydrate-deficient glycoprotein syndrome type Ia
Gaucher disease type I
Glucose-6-phosphate isomerase deficiency

Metabolic Disorders—cont'd

Morquio disease type A
Neuraminidase deficiencies
Smith-Lemli-Opitz syndrome

Miscellaneous Conditions

Arthrogryposis
Cystic hygroma (neck)
Hemangioendothelioma (metastatic)
Hemochromatosis (neonatal)
Hydrops fetalis (idiopathic)
Lupus erythematosus
Neuroblastoma (neck, with metastatic spread)
Nuchal bleb (familial)
Teratoma (brain, mediastinum, thyroid)

Placental/Umbilical Cord Problems

Chorioangioma
Fetomaternal transfusion
Torsion of the cord
Umbilical cord stricture
Umbilical vein thrombosis

Recognized Syndromes

Achondrogenesis type II
Congenital intrauterine infection–like syndrome
Down syndrome
Elejalde syndrome
Fetal akinesia-hypokinesia sequence
Fryns' syndrome
Holoprosencephaly
Klippel-Trénaunay-Weber syndrome
Microcephaly-lymphedema syndrome (autosomal recessive type)
Myotonic dystrophy
Neu-Laxova syndrome
Noonan syndrome
Short rib–polydactyly syndrome (Beemer-Langer type)
Simpson-Golabi-Behmel syndrome (infantile lethal variant)
Sly syndrome
Thanatophoric dysplasia
Williams syndrome

Respiratory Conditions

Congenital bronchial cyst
Congenital chylothorax
Cystic adenomatoid malformation of lung
Diaphragmatic hernia
Hydrothorax (idiopathic)
Laryngeal atresia
Sequestration of the lung

Urinary/Renal Abnormalities

Polycystic kidney disease (autosomal dominant)
Urethral atresia/obstruction

Adapted from McGillivray BC, Hall JG: Nonimmune hydrops fetalis. Pediatr Rev 1987;9:197–202; McKusick VA: Online Mendelian Inheritance in Man, 2005, accessed at www3.ncbi.nlm.nih.gov/Omim/; Weaver D: Catalog of Prenatally Diagnosed Conditions. Baltimore, Johns Hopkins University Press, 1999.

Exercise 4 *Continued*

QUESTIONS

3. Which tests would you likely order to further evaluate and to establish the diagnosis at this point?

   a. Serum very long chain fatty acids levels

   b. Serum pipecolic acid level

   c. Serum free T_4 and TSH levels

   d. Serum creatine kinase level

   e. Serum lactate level

   f. Standard chromosomal analysis

   g. CT scan/MRI of the head

   h. Prader-Willi methylation study

   i. Spinal muscular atrophy type 1 gene testing

   j. Myotonic dystrophy gene testing

4. Which of the following conditions would be likely in Baby M?

   a. Duchenne muscular dystrophy

   b. Spinal muscular atrophy type 1

   c. Congenital myotonic dystrophy

   d. Prader-Willi syndrome

ANSWERS

3. In many such situations, all of the above tests would be warranted. In the further evaluation of baby M, the family history was significant. The mother, a maternal uncle, the maternal grandmother, and three maternal grand aunts and uncles had some type of muscle disorder. The mother was also mentally impaired.

4. a. No. Duchenne muscular dystrophy is not likely because it generally is not as severe in the neonatal period as seen in this case and it normally only affects males because it is inherited as an X-linked disorder. Also, the muscle problem in baby M's family appears to be inherited in an autosomal or X-linked dominant mode.

   b. No. Although spinal muscular atrophy can be as severe as in Baby M, the disorder is inherited in an autosomal recessive fashion, which does not fix the inheritance in Baby M's family.

   c. Most likely. Because of the presentation and the family history, congenital myotonic dystrophy is highly likely.

   d. Unlikely. On occasion, Prader-Willi syndrome can present with this severity but generally is not inherited. It is possible that Baby M's condition is totally unrelated to the family's condition.

Myotonic dystrophy is an autosomal dominant condition caused by a trinucleotide repeat defect affecting the function of the dystrophia myotonica protein kinase gene (*DMPK*). The severity of the disease varies widely with mild, classic, childhood, and congenital forms delineated. Individuals with mild and classic forms of myotonic dystrophy usually are completely normal and disease free as children and teenagers. Various features of myotonic dystrophy then develop during the teenage years and adulthood; disabilities become worse with age, and some individuals are considerably incapacitated. Features of mild and classic myotonic dystrophy include myotonia (delayed muscle relaxation), muscle weakness, muscle wasting (particularly noticeable in the temporal muscles, leading to temporal hollowness), myopathic or expressionless face, cataracts, retinal degeneration, droopy eyelids, difficulty swallowing (which can lead to aspiration), problems with intestinal motility, conduction defects of the heart (that can cause sudden death), hypoventilation, testicular atrophy, diabetes, and progressive loss of mental function. The congenital form of myotonic dystrophy is the severe form and often is fatal. Another characteristic feature of myotonic dystrophy is that those affected in the first generations of a family are generally less severely affected than the succeeding generations. This phenomenon (the condition worsening with succeeding generations) is called *anticipation*. For myotonic dystrophy, we now understand the mechanism producing the disease and anticipation. The disorder is produced by an abnormal expansion of the number of the DNA bases, cytosine, thymine, and guanine (trinucleotide repeats) in the *DMPK* gene. In normal individuals, the number of triple repeats of CTG in this gene ranges from 5 to 49. In myotonic dystrophy, however, affected individuals have an increased number of CTG repeats, and the number of repeats roughly correlates with the severity of the disease. In mildly affected individuals, there are between 50 and about 150, in the classic form between about 100 and 1000, for the childhood type between about 350 and 1500, and in the congenital form more than 1000 CTG trinucleotide units. With few exceptions, the neonate with congenital myotonic dystrophy inherits the abnormal kinase gene from his or her mother who usually has the classic form of myotonic dystrophy. Why this excessive expansion occurs only when the gene is passed through the mother is unknown. Anticipation occurs because the size of the repeat increases with succeeding generations, leading to more severely affected individuals.

Gene testing was done on Baby M and she had an estimated 1200 copies of the CTG repeats, thus confirming the diagnosis of congenital myotonic dystrophy. Subsequently the mother was tested and found to have 658 repeats.

Robin Sequence

A relatively common birth defect is Robin sequence (also frequently referred to as Pierre Robin sequence) with an estimated incidence of 1 in 8500. The sequence is named after the person who first reported this condition in 1923. Pierre was the first name of Dr. Robin and by convention, we normally do not use first names of those for whom syndromes are named; thus, the preferred term is Robin sequence. The following case study illustrates the complexities of this sequence.

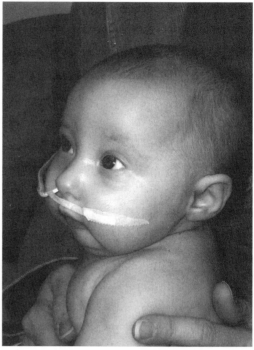

Figure 21-10 Baby O with Robin sequence. Apparent is the moderate micrognathia and prominent left ear. Because of her posterior placed tongue and cleft palate, most of her feedings were by nasogastric tube.

Case Study 3

At 6 days of age, Baby O (Figs. 21-10 and 21-11) was admitted to the pulmonary service of the neonatal intensive care unit because of noisy breathing and feeding difficulty. She was born at 38 weeks' gestation to a 30-year-old white para 1 gravida 2 woman. The mother was diagnosed with heterozygous factor V Lieden deficiency at 33 weeks' gestation, and she subsequently received low-molecular-weight heparin until delivery. Labor and delivery were unremarkable; birth length, weight, and occipitofrontal circumference (OFC) (48.8 cm, 2.23 kg, and 34 cm, respectively) were all normal for gestational age. Following birth, physical examination revealed moderate micrognathia and a large U-shaped cleft palate. She also had a few minor dysmorphic features. Her noisy breathing began around the second day of life and the parents noted it to be worse when she was lying on her back. The family history was negative for other children with micrognathia or cleft palate, severe vision problems or blindness, hearing loss, congenital heart defects, and short stature. The pulmonary physician at this point diagnosed Baby O with Robin sequence.

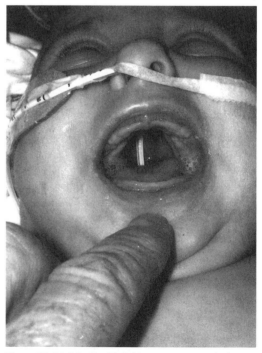

Figure 21-11 Baby O with Robin sequence. Note the large cleft of the palate, which was U-shaped.

Exercise 5

QUESTIONS

1. Which of the following explains why Robin sequence is considered a sequence and not a syndrome?

   a. The micrognathia, cleft palate, and glossoptosis all are produced by the same etiology.

   b. The micrognathia produces an elevation of the tongue, which in turn prevents the palate from closing.

   c. The tongue was elevated because it was enlarged and it in turn caused a deformity of the palate.

2. Which of the following evaluations should be done at this point to determine the etiology of Baby O's Robin sequence?

   a. Ask if alcohol or unusual medications were consumed during the pregnancy.

   b. Perform a careful dysmorphologic examination.

   c. Obtain a FISH analysis for 22 q11 deletion.

   d. Obtain an ophthalmologic evaluation.

   e. Do a hearing evaluation.

   f. Order standard chromosomal assessment.

   g. Order gene testing for Stickler syndrome.

3. Of the following precautions and actions, which ones should be taken with Baby O during her hospital stay and following her discharge?

   a. Admit the child to a regular nursery.

   b. Keep the child on her back following the "Back to sleep" campaign.

   c. Order vital signs taken every 6 hours.

   d. Obtain an oral surgery consult.

   e. Arrange a polysomnography and swallow study.

   f. Schedule full-time nursing care after discharge.

ANSWERS

1. b.

2. All of the above should be considered in the evaluation of a neonate with Robin sequence.

3. d and e.

The classification of Robin sequence as a *sequence* is based on the initiating event being the micrognathia. According to the most prevalent hypothesis, the mandible lags behind in its development during the embryologic period. This in turn causes the tongue to be elevated, which interferes with the growth of the lateral palatine shelves and fusion with the nasal septum. The lateral palatine shelves normally form the bony portion of the palate. Additionally, the micrognathia causes the tongue to be positioned posteriorly, and following birth, to obstruct the oral pharynx. In some cases, this obstruction can result in severe hypoxia and death. The Robin sequence is a sequence because one defect, namely micrognathia, results in a secondary defect, the elevation and posterior placement of the tongue that then blocks the closure of the palatal shelves. In other words, there is a cascading of events initiated by the micrognathia.

Robin sequence is a feature in at least 70 syndromes. When evaluating a newborn with this sequence, one should attempt to determine if any of these syndromes is present. The two most commonly diagnosed conditions are Stickler syndrome and velocardiofacial syndrome (VCF, or Shprintzen syndrome). Stickler syndrome is an autosomal dominant condition characterized by eye abnormalities, including severe myopia, cataracts, and a characteristic vitreous abnormality that can lead to retinal detachment and blindness; flat midface; sensorineural deafness; and early onset arthritis associated with a mild spondyloepiphyseal dysplasia. Newborns may have no features other than Robin sequence. Stickler syndrome is a collagenopathy produced by abnormalities in either type 2 or 11 collagen, and testing is now available for the genes involved in this condition. Patients with VCF have oropharyngeal insufficiency resulting in a nasal voice, congenital heart defects, and a characteristic face. This syndrome is also associated with a microdeletion involving 22 q11. The etiology of Robin sequence is unknown in roughly two thirds of patients that do not have an apparent syndrome.

An evaluation of a newborn or neonate with Robin sequence should include a careful prenatal history for alcohol and medication use, a thorough dysmorphologic examination, an ophthalmologic examnation, standard chromosomal assessment, FISH probe for 22 q11 deletion (DiGeorge FISH probe), and hearing testing; one should also consider Stickler gene testing. If there appears to be a relative with VCF or Stickler syndrome, one also should evaluate and test that individual for these conditions. If the caring physician suspects other dysmorphic conditions, he or she may also want to consult a clinical geneticist.

Left untreated, approximately 50% of infants with Robin sequence will die from the disorder. Physicians taking care of newborns with this sequence often underestimate its seriousness because typically the respiratory distress does not occur or is minimal during the first two days following birth. Regardless, one should immediately initiate the following precautions with any affected newborn. First, the child should be admitted to the NICU. Second, the patient should be kept on her or his stomach, except for brief periods of time. Third, cardiac and oxygen monitoring should be done while the patient is in the hospital, and cardiac monitoring continued following discharge. Other measures should include consulting an oral, plastic, or ear, nose, and throat surgeon in reference to airway management. In severe cases, tracheostomies may be considered to circumvent the respiratory problems produced by the glossoptosis. Tongue-tying procedures, which are designed to keep the tongue forward, are rarely used. Severely affected infants are increasingly being treated with a new surgical procedure termed mandibular distraction. The technique involves cutting the mandible on both sides, attaching an instrument to each side of the mandible, and then gradually spreading the instrument and mandible daily. A developmental pediatrician or similarly trained person should instruct the parents on oral feeding techniques. If there is any indication that aspiration may be occurring, the patient needs polysomnography and a swallow study. And finally, a clinical geneticist should provide genetics counseling to the parents with regard to possible genetic conditions and possible recurrence risk in subsequent offspring. If the child has an inherited syndrome, the recurrence risk would be related to the inheritance pattern of the disorder. In nonsyndromic Robin sequence, the recurrence appears to be less than 1%. However, there have been several reports in which nonsyndromic Robin sequence is inherited as an autosomal recessive trait in which case the recurrence risk for the parents would be 25%.

Hydrops Fetalis, Edema, and Cystic Hygroma

Generalized edema or anasarca in a fetus is termed hydrops fetalis. Although most fetuses with hydrops fetalis do not survive to the age of viability, it is not an uncommon problem. Prior to the effective prevention of erythroblastosis fetalis, that condition was the most common cause of hydrops fetalis. As erythroblastosis fetalis is, by and large, preventable, most cases of hydrops fetalis are the result of nonimmune causes. The estimated incidence of nonimmune hydrops fetalis is 1 in 2000 to 3000 pregnancies. When a newborn has hydrops fetalis, the neonatologist needs to undertake an appropriate evaluation and initiate any indicated treatment. The following case illustrates these points.

Case Study 4

Baby S was delivered from a 22-year-old gravida 2 para 2 white female at 37 weeks +6 days gestational age by spontaneous vaginal delivery with the use of forceps. A prenatal ultrasound evaluation detected generalized hydrops fetalis, a cystic hygroma, and possible coarctation of the aorta. Following birth, Baby S had numerous physical abnormalities, but the most striking findings were the generalized edema (Figs. 21-12 and 21-13) and the marked excessive nuchal skin (Fig. 21-14). Other physical findings included reversed epicanthal folds, depressed nasal bridge, smooth philtrum, long upper lip, micrognathia, prominent and hypoplastic ears, lateral webbing of the neck, and small fingernails. An echocardiogram revealed a borderline small left ventricle and aortic arch, bicuspid aortic valves, and a small patent ductus arteriosus. An ultrasound demonstrated a horseshoe kidney. The attending cardiologist thought that the smallish left ventricle and aortic arch did not require treatment. Baby S had no other problems and she was discharged from the neonatal unit at age 13 days. At follow-up at 19 months, she was developing normally, had adequate growth (height, weight, and head circumference were 15th percentile, 5th percentile, and 50th percentile, respectively) and was having no major problems. She still had edema on the back of her hands and feet.

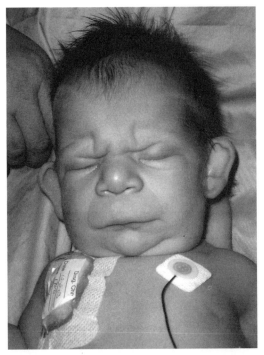

Figure 21-12 Baby S, who has Turner syndrome, in the newborn period. Note the redundant skin of the face, edematous facial appearance, long and smooth upper lip, and hypoplastic and cupped ears.

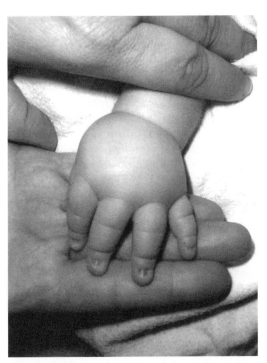

Figure 21-13 Hand of Baby S with Turner syndrome. Observe the marked edema of the dorsum of the hand and the fingers, and the small fingernails.

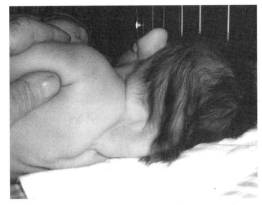

Figure 21-14 Posterior neck of Baby S with Turner syndrome, also shown in Figure 21-12. There is marked redundancy of the skin, indicating that she had a large cystic hygroma at one time during fetal life. The cystic hygroma was so large that it caused the ears to be pushed forward.

Exercise 6

QUESTIONS

1. Indicate whether the following statements are true or false.

   a. The prognosis of an infant with hydrops fetalis is generally good.

   b. The earlier the diagnosis of hydrops fetalis is made in the pregnancy, the better the prognosis is for the fetus.

   c. Polyhydramnios frequently accompanies pregnancies complicated by hydrops fetalis.

2. Which of the following pathophysiologic derangements contribute to the edema observed in fetuses and infants with hydrops fetalis? Choose all that apply.

   a. Increased capillary pressure

   b. Decreased capillary permeability

   c. Lymphatic obstruction

   d. Absent lymphatic vessels

ANSWERS

1. a and b: false. c: true.

2. a, c, and d.

The prognosis for a fetus with hydrops fetalis is generally poor, particularly if the edema becomes worse over time. The survival rate is lower if the hydrops fetalis has an onset before 24 weeks' gestation. In one study of nonimmune hydrops fetalis,[13] the overall survival rate was only 4% when hydrops was present before 24 weeks, but 28% after this age. The combined survival rate was 19%. The postnatal survival rate is equally poor, with the fatality rate in the neonatal period being 80%.[14]

Fetuses and neonates with hydrops fetalis often have pleural and pericardial effusions, ascites, placental thickening, and polyhydramnios. The exact cause for the relationship between hydrops fetalis and polyhydramnios is not known, but polyhydramnios is present in 75% of nonimmune hydrops fetalis cases. The pathogenesis for the development of the edema in hydrops fetalis includes increased intravascular hydrostatic pressure, decreased plasma osmolality, increased capillary permeability, absent or hypoplastic lymphatic structures, and obstruction of lymphatic flow.[15,16]

Table 21-2 lists the etiologic categories of hydrops fetalis in the neonate and a number of disorders associated with this condition. These categories can be used to direct the evaluation of patients with this finding. To rule out cardiac problems, a chest radiograph, electrocardiogram, and echocardiogram should be obtained. Vascular malformations with significant arteriovenous shunting should be sought. In most cases, a chromosomal analysis needs to be performed unless such an analysis was done prenatally and established the diagnosis. The quality of prenatal cytogenetic analysis normally is not greater than the 500-band level. This is an important consideration because the higher the band level, the greater is the quality of the chromosome study. At a 500-band level or less, there is a significantly increased risk of small chromosomal deletions and duplications going undetected. Postnatally, leukocyte studies usually are of higher quality, and for an acceptable study, the band level needs to be at least 550. The patency of the gastrointestinal tract should be established. Severe anemia (an important cause of hydrops fetalis) should be considered and evaluated with appropriate blood testing. One also needs to evaluate the patient for prenatal infections, particularly those listed in Table 21-2. The possibility of autoimmune disease in the mother or child should be assessed by testing for various autoimmune antibodies in both. Tumors or cysts located in the brain, chest, or mediastinum should be ruled out by doing a CT scan or MRI of the head and by radiographs of the chest. If the radiographs are suggestive of intrathoracic pathology, one should also consider an MRI of the chest. The placenta needs to be located and

carefully examined for vascular and other pathologic changes. Further, the placenta should be submitted to the pathology service for more detailed assessment, including histologic examination. If significant pleural fluid is present, a thoracocentesis needs to be performed to determine the makeup of the fluid (in particular to rule out chylothorax) and to improve pulmonary function. A renal ultrasound study also needs to be done. The medical staff should obtain a detailed family history to determine the possibility of familial hydrops and other inherited causes of the hydrops fetalis. A clinical geneticist should be asked to conduct a dysmorphologic evaluation to determine if a syndrome is present. In addition, other consultants need to be involved as dictated by the patient's problems. Finally, as medical problems are discovered, treatment needs to be initiated. If one discovers a lethal disorder, a decision needs to be made whether to continue support.

Exercise 6 *Continued*

QUESTION

3. Of the following conditions, which one does Baby S most likely have?

    a. Down syndrome

    b. Turner syndrome

    c. Noonan syndrome

    d. α-Thalassemia

ANSWER

3. b.

Although generalized hydrops fetalis can be observed in infants with Noonan syndrome and α-thalassemia, and infants with Down syndrome frequently have excessive nuchal skin, the size of the cystic hygroma and the amount of edema in Baby S is more typical for Turner syndrome. However, in Baby S's case, the edema and redundant nuchal skin are more marked than usual. The redundant nuchal skin is related to an abnormally large jugular lymph sac during uterine development. The jugular lymph sac, which is located in the posterior neck, normally connects to the inferior vena cava at about 40 days of development, and doing so allows the lymphatic fluid to return to the circulatory system. If this connection does not occur, there is distention of the jugular lymph sac, which stretches the skin over the back of the neck. If subsequently the jugular lymph sac makes the vascular connection, the fluid drains and the sac collapses, leaving behind redundant skin at the sides and back of the neck. In some cases, the excessive skin produces webbing of the neck. In the case of Baby S, the distention of the jugular lymph sac was so marked that it pushed the ears forward, and at birth both ears were quite prominent (Fig. 21-14).

Chromosomal analysis on Baby S was done and she was missing one sex chromosome from all 50 cells analyzed (45,X).

Chromosomal Anomalies

Chromosomal anomalies often produce serious congenital birth defects, and affected infants constitute a significant proportion of the neonatal intensive care population.

Exercise 7

QUESTION

1. Listed here are the most commonly encountered chromosomal problems in newborns and neonates. Match the types of chromosomal abnormalities with their definitions.

Chromosomal Abnormalities l

1. Numerical aberration
2. Translocation
3. Mosaicism
4. Segmental deletion
5. Segmental duplication
6. Subtelomeric abnormality

Definitions of Chromosomal Abnormalities

a. The presence of a duplicated segment of chromosomal material resulting in segmental trisomy.

b. The occurrence of two cell lines in an individual, each with a different chromosomal complement. An example is Down syndrome mosaicism, which occurs in about 2% to 3% of children with this syndrome.

c. An instance when two different chromosomes have exchanged chromosomal material.

d. An instance when a segment of chromosomal material is missing, resulting in segmental monosomy. Deletions are classified into macroscopic deletions (i.e., deletions that can be detected by standard chromosomal analyzes, e.g., cri du chat syndrome, in which a portion of the short arm of chromosome 5 is missing) and microdeletions (i.e., deletions that cannot be recognized without using molecular techniques, e.g., DiGeorge syndrome, in which a segment is missing from the long arm of chromosome 22 located at q11).

e. A situation in which there is an entire extra chromosome present or missing in each of the cells of the individual. Examples are trisomy 18 and Turner syndrome (monosomy X).

f. A deletion and duplication at the end of a chromosome. These abnormalities are typically not detectable by standard chromosomal testing and occur at the ends of all but the short arms of the acrocentric chromosomes.

ANSWERS

1. a. Segmental duplication.

   b. Mosaicism.

   c. Translocation.

   d. Segmental deletion.

   e. Numerical aberration.

   f. Subtelomeric abnormality.

The following four cases illustrate some of these chromosomal aberrations.

Translocations

Case Study 5

After a pregnancy complicated by decreased fetal movements, Baby V was delivered vaginally at term without difficulty. He was small for gestational age, with his weight well below the 5th percentile (−4 SD). He also had microcephaly, a prominent glabella (the point in the midline between the eyebrows), nevus flammeus, ocular hypertelorism, telecanthus, bilateral epicanthal folds, down-slanting palpebral fissures, bilateral partial cleft lip and complete cleft palate, natal tooth, downturning of the corners of the mouth, micrognathia, hypoplastic and cupped ears (Fig. 2-15), first-degree hypospadias, and hypotonia.

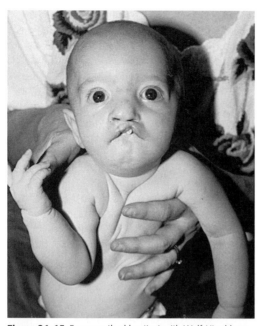

Figure 21-15 Four-month-old patient with Wolf-Hirschhorn syndrome (Baby V). Observe his nevus flammeus, telecanthus, ocular hypertelorism, strabismus, partial bilateral cleft lip, natal tooth and down-turned mouth. (From Wheeler PG, Weaver DD, Palmer CG: Familial translocation resulting in Wolf-Hirschhorn syndrome in two related unbalanced individuals: Clinical evaluation of a 39-year-old man with Wolf-Hirschhorn syndrome. Am J Med Genet 1995;55:462–465.)

Other than a feeding difficulty, Baby V had no significant problems in the immediate newborn period. His feeding problems primarily were related to his cleft lip and palate. The mother denied use of unusual medications, illicit drugs, tobacco, or ethanol during the pregnancy. She had had no fevers, skin rashes, accidents, or other problems during the pregnancy. The family history was significant for a 39-year-old paternal great-uncle who was dysmorphic and mentally retarded.

Exercise 8

QUESTION

1. What would be the neonatologist's first priority for this patient?

   a. Focus on the stabilization and overall care of the infant

   b. Consult the clinical geneticist

   c. Prepare for the long-term care of the patient

ANSWER

1. a. When a child is born with multiple congenital anomalies, the first priority of the neonatologist is to assess and treat any life-threatening problems. In the case of Baby V, there were no such problems, so the focus should be on managing his feeding difficulty and determining the cause of his syndrome.

There are now over 3000 recognized dysmorphic syndromes. Based on his multiple birth defects, Baby V appears to have a dysmorphic syndrome. The problem facing the neonatologist in such cases is to identify what syndrome is present.

QUESTION

2. Which of the following approaches would you use to identify the syndrome in a dysmorphic neonate?

   a. Immediately recognize the syndrome based on past experience with the syndrome (i.e., Down syndrome).

   b. Identify the unique features in the neonate and then consult a dysmorphology syndrome book.

   c. Enter the features of the neonate into a syndrome database such as POSSUM.

   d. Do appropriate and indicated laboratory testing such as a chromosomal analysis.

   e. Consult a clinical geneticist.

ANSWER

2. All of the above.

Some syndromes are common, have unique features, are recognized easily and immediately, and are familiar to most physicians. An example is Down syndrome. With others, one may not immediately recognize the disorder but because of unique features and with a review of the literature, one can often identify the condition. For instance, Meckel-Gruber syndrome is characterized by occipital encephalocele, polycystic kidneys, and polydactyly. These features are nearly pathognomonic for the disorder, because there are only a few recognized syndromes that share these three features. Conversely, one may not easily recognize other syndromes because the associated abnormalities are found in many disorders. To aid in the diagnosis of dysmorphic conditions, a number of computer databases have been developed (Table 21-3). For example, upon entering 11 findings from Baby V in the POSSUM database, 24 conditions were identified that have 9 or more of these features (Table 21-4). An alternative method of identifying dysmorphic syndromes is to use syndrome identification books that provide information and pictures of various dysmorphic conditions (Table 21-5). Yet another approach is to consult a clinical geneticist who has considerable experience with the recognition and diagnosis of dysmorphic syndromes and has access to syndrome databases.

In Baby V's case, a diagnosis was not immediately recognized. As such, his condition could have been a single gene defect, chromosomal abnormality, or teratogenic dysmorphic syndrome. His condition was unlikely to be multifactorial, because multifactorial conditions typically result in only single defects, such as a congenital heart defect, neural tube defect, pyloric stenosis, or cleft lip. A teratogenic agent could have produced his multiple anomalies. Table 21-6 lists the recognized human teratogens; however, none of these teratogenic agents produces a pattern of defects similar to that seen in Baby V. Furthermore, the pregnancy history was unremarkable for exposure to any known potential teratogenic agents. A chromosomal abnormality could also explain Baby V's abnormalities. The only way to prove that a chromosomal abnormality exists is to perform a chromosomal analysis. In addition to the classic chromosomal abnormalities such as trisomy 13, trisomy 18, Down syndrome, Klinefelter syndrome (47,XXY), and Turner syndrome (45,X), in which entire extra chromosomes are present or missing, and large partial trisomy and deletion conditions, we now recognize a number of microdeletion syndromes (Table 21-7). The ones that have the most

TABLE 21-3

GENETIC AND NEUROGENETIC DATABASES

Subscription Databases

London Cytogenetic Database	Has data and references for many cytogenetic disorders.
London Medical Database—Dysmorphology	Contains a large number of dysmorphic syndromes and pictures of these conditions; does not list many chromosomal abnormalities.
London Medical Database—Neurogenetic	Lists many of the genetically determined neurologic syndromes.
Pictures of Standard Syndromes and Undiagnosed Malformations (POSSUM)	Contains a large number of dysmorphic syndromes and pictures of these conditions. This database also includes chromosomal syndromes and bone dysplasias.
Reproductive Toxicology (REPROTOX)	Provides information about human teratogens.
Teratogen Information Service (TERIS)	Provides information about human teratogens.

Internet Databases

Alliance of Genetic Support Groups (www.geneticalliance.org)	Lists information on genetic support groups.
Family Village (www.familyvillage.wisc.edu)	Resources for lay and professional audiences regarding genetic conditions and support services.
GeneReviews (www.geneclinics.org/profiles/all.htm)	Provides a large number of review articles on genetic disorders.
GeneTests (www.genetests.org)	Provides information on molecular testing for human genetic disorders.
Genetic Disorders and Birth Defects Information Center (geneinfo.medlib.iupui.edu)	Website that provides a large number of links to other databases on genetic disorders and birth defects.
March of Dimes (MOD) (www.marchofdimes.com)	Information on birth defects for the general public and professionals.
Mitochondrial Map (www.mitomap.org)	Database that provides up-to-date information on mitochondrial diseases.
Mothers United for Moral Support National Parent-to-Parent Network (MUMS) (www.netnet.net/mums)	Parent organization that matches families with genetic disorders to other families with the same condition.
Neuromuscular Disease Center (www.neuro.wustl.edu/neuromuscular)	Database with extensive data and differential diagnoses on neurologic and muscular disorders.
NIH Office of Rare Diseases (www.rarediseases.info.nih.gov)	Index of support groups, clinical research, databases, investigators, and glossary.
Online Mendelian Inheritance in Man (OMIM) (www3.ncbi.nlm.nih.gov/Omin)	Contains a large amount of information on recognized human genetic disorders and human genes.

Organizations printed in **bold** are the major resources for clinical genetic information for physicians.

TABLE 21-4

DIFFERENTIAL DIAGNOSIS OF BABY V (POSSUM ANALYSIS)

Traits Entered in the POSSUM Database
Small for gestation age (intrauterine growth retardation)
Microcephaly
Hypertelorism
Down-slanting palpebral fissures
Micrognathia/agnathia total/retrognathia
Epicanthal folds
Paramedian/lateral cleft lip (unilateral/bilateral)
Cleft hard palate
Abnormal ear shape/structure
Hypospadias/epispadias
Hypotonia

Match Syndromes	Number of Features Matched*
Chromosome 4, partial del 4p	11
Chromosome 3, del 3p(p25->pter)	10
Chromosome 5, partial del 5p	10
Chromosome 9, trisomy 9	10
Chromosome 16, interstitial del 16q	10
Chromosome 21, monosomy 21	10
Chromosome 22, partial dup 22q	10
Chromosome 22, trisomy 22	10
Baller-Gerold syndrome	9
Chromosome 2, terminal del 2q	9
Chromosome 3, partial dup 3q	9
Chromosome 4, partial del 4q	9
Chromosome 6, distal del 6q	9
Chromosome 7, partial dup 7q	9
Chromosome 9, partial tetrasomy 9p	9
Chromosome 10, partial del 10p	9
Chromosome 10, terminal del 10q	9
Chromosome 13, del 13q(q22or31->qter)	9
Chromosome 17, del 17p(p11.2p11.2)	9
Chromosome 17, partial dup 17q	9
Craniocerebellocardiac syndrome	9
Fetal aminopterin syndrome	9
Hypertelorism-hypospadias syndrome	9
Madokoro-Ohodo syndrome	9

*Syndromes that matched at least 9 of the 11 traits.

TABLE 21-5

SYNDROME BOOKS

Cohen MM Jr (ed): Craniosynostosis: Diagnosis, Evaluation, and Management. New York, Raven Press, 1986.

Gorlin RJ, Cohen MM Jr, Levin LS: Syndromes of the Head and Neck, 3rd ed. New York, Oxford University Press, 1990.

Graham JM Jr: Smith's Recognizable Patterns of Human Deformation, 2nd ed. Philadelphia, WB Saunders, 1988.

Jones KL: Smith's Recognizable Patterns of Human Malformation, 6th ed. Philadelphia, WB Saunders, 2005.

Norman MG, McGillivray BC, Kalousek DK, et al: Congenital Malformations of the Brain: Pathological, Embryological, Clinical, Radiological and Genetic Aspects. New York, Oxford University Press, 1995.

Nyhan WL, Barshop BA, Ozand PR (eds): Atlas of Metabolic Diseases, 2nd ed. London, Hodder Arnold, 2005.

Scriver CR, Beaudet AL, Sly WS, et al (eds): The Metabolic and Molecular Basis of Inherited Disease. New York, McGraw-Hill, 2001.

Stevenson RE, Hall JG (eds): Human Malformations and Related Anomalies, 2nd ed. New York, Oxford University Press, 2005.

Temtamy SA, McKusick VA: The Genetics of Hand Malformations. New York, AR Liss, 1978.

Tewfik TL, der Kaloustian VM: Congenital Anomalies of the Ear, Nose, and Throat. New York, Oxford University Press, 1997.

notoriety include Angelman, DiGeorge, Miller-Dieker, Prader-Willi, velocardiofacial, and Williams syndromes. In each of these microdeletion syndromes, a microscopic or submicroscopic piece of chromosomal material from a specific chromosomal location is deleted. For the most part, the deletions producing these conditions are located on different chromosomes. When the deletion is submicroscopic, the deleted material is not detectable by standard chromosomal analysis. Rather, a molecular technique called FISH (fluorescence in situ hybridization) analysis is used. This is a process whereby a unique DNA segment (probe) is tagged with a fluorescent substance. The probe, which normally attaches to the specific chromosomal segment of interest, fails to attach because that region is missing. The problem with FISH analysis, however, is that the clinician must first suspect the diagnosis and then order the specific FISH analysis for the suspected disorder. Baby V's findings did not fit any of the recognized microdeletion syndromes, and the consulting geneticist did not recommend any of these studies.

We also know that a number of syndromes are caused by an aberration called *uniparental disomy*. Uniparental disomy occurs when both pairs of paired (homologous) chromosomes come from the same parent. For instance, in 20% of patients with Prader-Willi syndrome, the syndrome results from maternal uniparental disomy for chromosome 15. The mechanism that produces the syndrome is called *genomic imprinting*, and the phenomenon is the result of a gene being turned on or off, depending on whether the gene is transmitted through the father or mother. Again, none of the recognized uniparental—disomy–caused syndromes appeared to fit Baby V's condition.

Finally, Baby V's findings could result from a mitochondrial disorder. Mitochondrial condi-

TABLE 21-6

KNOWN HUMAN TERATOGENS

Chemicals
Carbon monoxide (toxic levels)
Gasoline fumes (recreational abuse)
Polychlorinated biphenyls (PCBs)
Toluene (recreational abuse)
Drugs
Alcohol (ethanol)
Aminoglycosides (gentamicin, kanamycin, streptomycin)
Aminopterin, amethopterin, methotrexate
Androgenic hormones
Angiotensin I–converting enzyme (ACE) inhibitors (captopril, enalapril)
Barbiturates (phenobarbital and primidone)
Busulfan
Carbamazepine
Chlorambucil
Cocaine
Cyclophosphamide
Diethylstilbestrol (DES)
Iodide (deficiency or excess)
Lithium
Methimazole
Misoprostol
Penicillamine
Phenytoin (hydantoin)
Propylthiouracil
Tetracyclines
Thalidomide
Trimethadione, paramethadione
Valproic acid
Vitamin A congeners (etretinate, isotretinoin [13-*cis*-retinoic acid])
Warfarin
Heavy Metals
Lead
Mercury, organic
Maternal Conditions
Cigarette smoking
Folic acid deficiency
Hyperthermia
Immune-mediated thrombocytopenia
Insulin-dependent diabetes mellitus
Marijuana smoking

Maternal Conditions—cont'd
Maternal phenylketonuria
Myasthenia gravis
Sjögren's syndrome
Systemic lupus erythematosus
Virilizing tumors
Intrauterine Infections
Cytomegalovirus
Herpes simplex virus
Lymphocytic choriomeningitis virus
Mycoplasmas
Parvovirus
Rubella virus
Toxoplasma gondii (toxoplasmosis)
Treponema pallidum (syphilis)
Varicella-zoster virus
Venezuelan equine encephalitis virus
Others
Amniotic bands
Chorionic villus sampling (early)
Hypoxia
Monozygotic twinning
Multiple gestation
Oligohydramnios
Radiation
Uterine malformations and tumors
Unlikely Human Teratogens
Agent orange
Anesthetics
Aspartame
Aspirin
Bendectin
Birth control pills (oral contraceptives)
Caffeine (moderate doses)
Corticosteroids
Diagnostic x-rays
Electromagnetic radiation
Imipramine
Lysergic acid diethylamide (LSD)
Rubella vaccine
Spermicides
Ultrasonography (diagnostic levels)
Video display screens

TABLE 21-7

WELL-KNOWN MICRODELETION SYNDROMES

Name of the Condition	Chromosome Location
Angelman syndrome	15 q11-q13
DiGeorge syndrome	22 q11
Langer-Giedion syndrome	8 q24.11-24.13
Prader-Willi syndrome	15 q11-q13
Smith-Magenis syndrome	17 p11.2
Velocardiofacial syndrome (Shprintzen)	22 q11
WAGR syndrome (Wilms' tumor, aniridia, genital anomalies, and mental retardation)	11 p13
Williams syndrome	7 q11.23

tions generally result from decreased energy production at the cellular level, and as a result, normally lead to hypotonia and muscle weakness. However, brain abnormalities, vision problems, hearing loss, endocrine dysfunctions, and neurologic abnormalities may all be present either singly or in combination in an affected individual. Because of this wide range of defects, one could not rule out a mitochondrial problem in Baby V.

At this point, Baby V needed to be evaluated further. A clinical geneticist was consulted, a chromosomal assessment ordered, and a computer database analysis done. Additionally, a pediatric neurologist evaluated the child because of his hypotonia. Several other consultations were obtained, including a plastic surgeon (because of the cleft lip and palate), a pediatric urologist (because of the hypospadias), and a developmental pediatrician (to coach the parents on feeding techniques). Finally, because of the microcephaly, an MRI scan of the brain was done to rule out structural abnormalities of the brain.

Based on the physical characteristics in Baby V, the consulting clinical geneticist suspected Wolf-Hirschhorn syndrome, a chromosomal condition caused by partial deletion of the short arm of chromosome 4.[17] A POSSUM analysis supported this, as 11 of 11 features entered into the computer matched the features of Wolf-Hirschhorn syndrome (see Table 21-4). A chromosomal analysis confirmed the suspicion of a partial deletion of the short arm of chromosome 4. However, the study also demonstrated that Baby V had an unbalanced chromosomal translocation between chromosomes 4 and 8. The chromosomal formula was 46,XY,der(4;8) (p15.32p22). The chromosomal aberration in him involved not only a deletion of the terminal portion of chromosome 4 from band p15.32 to the end but also a small portion of the short arm of chromosome 8 attached to the deleted end of chromosome 4. His chromosomal constitution was unbalanced because he had two normal chromosome 8s, an extra portion of the short arm of chromosome 8 attached to chromosome 4, and a missing terminal part of the short arm of chromosome 4.

Because chromosomal translocations can be inherited, it is important to do chromosomal analyzes on parents whose children have unbalanced chromosomal problems. Commonly in these situations, one parent carries a balanced translocation, a chromosomal inversion, or an unbalanced translocation that has led to their offspring's chromosomal problem. In Baby V's family, the father, grandfather, great-grandfather, and great-great-grandfather each carried a balanced translocation involving chromosomes 4 and 8 [t(4;8)(p15.32p22)]. These individuals were phenotypically normal because they had neither a gain nor a loss of chromosomal material. Rather, they had rearrangement of their chromosomal material. Further investigation found that the mentally retarded paternal great-uncle of the proband had the identical unbalanced translocation as Baby V. When the great-uncle was later examined, he, too, clearly had Wolf-Hirschhorn syndrome.

The parents of Baby V need to be informed fully of the chromosomal situation in their son and their family, and counseled with regard to their chances of having other children with unbalanced chromosomal problems in any subsequent pregnancy. In addition to Baby V's chromosomal abnormality, any future offspring of his parents could have a partial deletion of chromosome 8, partial trisomy of chromosome 4, balanced 4;8 translocation (as was present in the father), or normal chromosomes. These chromosomal possibilities can occur with most familial balanced translocations. Because any two chromosomes can be involved in translocations and because different sizes of chromosomes can be translocated, the chances of a balanced translocation carrier producing chromosomally unbalanced offspring or having miscarriages differ with different translocations. The probabilities of having abnormal offspring, miscarriages, and normal children with various translocations have been tabulated and can be provided by most clinical geneticists.

The prognosis for Baby V is poor. Approximately a third of children with Wolf-Hirschhorn syndrome die during the first 2 years of life, and those that survive typically have profound retardation and seizures. The prognosis for children with other unbalanced translocations varies according to the size of chromosomal pieces and the chromosomes involved.

Chromosomal Mosaicism

Exercise 9

QUESTION

1. Which of the following statements are true about patients with chromosomal mosaicisms?

    a. Chromosomal mosaicism exists when there are two or more different cell lines with different chromosomal constitutions in an individual.

    b. Chromosomal mosaicism can involve any chromosome.

    c. Trisomy rescue can result in a viable fetus, chromosomal mosaicism, and uniparental disomy in the disomic cell line.

    d. When one cell line is trisomic, the individual is dysmorphic.

ANSWER

1. a. True. One defines chromosomal mosaicism as the presence of two or more cell lines with different chromosomal makeup in an individual. Mosaicism can arise in two ways. First, the fertilized egg can have a normal chromosomal constitution (i.e., XY,46 or XX,46). At some point during intrauterine development, however, an error in the separation of chromosomes during cell division (nondisjunction) occurs. As a result, one daughter cell ends up with one missing chromosome (monosomy) and the other with an extra chromosome (trisomy). The rest of the cells in the embryo or fetus will be disomy and have the normal complement of chromosomes. If both monosomic and trisomic cell lines persist, the individual will have three separate cell lines at birth. If either the monosomic or the trisomic cell line dies out, then the newborn will possess only two cell lines. Because humans tolerate monosomies more poorly than trisomies, the individual with a mosaic condition normally ends up with disomy/trisomy cell lines.

   The second mechanism that may result in mosaicism is when the fertilized egg (zygote) has a trisomy constitution. Most trisomies result in early embryonic deaths (e.g., trisomy 3); thus, if an embryo with a trisomy is to survive, some cell in this embryo must convert to a disomy. If this situation arises, then the embryo and the resulting neonate is a disomic/trisomic mosaic for the chromosome involved.

   b. True. Chromosomal mosaicism can involve any of the 24 different chromosomes. Because complete trisomies for our larger chromosomes are normally lethal, the only way an embryo or fetus with a trisomy for one of the larger chromosomes can survive is for chromosomal mosaicism to develop. There are rare exceptions to this generalization; however, mosaicism for all of the different chromosomes has been observed.

   c. True. As stated earlier, trisomy rescue can lead to a viable embryo/fetus. If trisomy rescue occurs in the cell that forms the definitive embryo, then the embryo and resulting offspring will be disomic and have a normal-appearing chromosome constitution. On the other hand, if trisomy rescue happens after the formation of the definitive embryo, the embryo and child can be a mosaic. In either case, trisomy rescue may result in uniparental disomy (UPD). Normally in the formation of the egg or sperm, the chromosome number is reduced from 46 to 23, and one of each of the 22 paired chromosomes plus one of the sex chromosomes is transmitted to the egg or sperm. However, when a nondisjunction event occurs, both paired chromosomes can go to the same egg or sperm. If this egg or sperm is involved in conception, then the zygote is trisomic for the chromosomes involved in nondisjunction. If trisomy rescue occurs, and if the two remaining chromosomes both came from the egg or sperm, then uniparental disomy is present. Because of genomic imprinting, uniparental disomy in turn can lead to physical and neurologic abnormalities in the child.

   d. False. Not all chromosomal mosaicisms produce dysmorphic features in the child. If dysmorphic features are present, these features are most likely related to the percentage of trisomic/disomic cells present in various tissues or organs, and the chromosomes involved. One of the most extensively studied mosaicisms is trisomy 18 mosaicism, which occurs in about 10% of the cases of trisomy 18. In this disorder, affected individuals may have all of the features normally seen in full trisomy 18, may have only a few features and mild psychomotor delay, or may have no physical features and be intellectually normal. In the third situation, these individuals may discover that they have trisomy 18 mosaicism by producing a child with complete trisomy 18.

Case Study 6

Baby R was 14 months old when last evaluated by a clinical geneticist. She was the offspring of a 21-year-old gravida 1 para 1 black woman. The pregnancy was unremarkable except for the discovery of a two-vessel umbilical cord on a

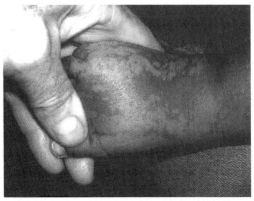

Figure 21-16 Irregular pigmentation over the dorsum and wrist of Baby R, a black infant with a robertsonian 14;14 translocation mosaicism.

prenatal ultrasound examination. Delivery occurred at term and was uncomplicated. Baby R, however, became cyanotic immediately following birth. In addition, she was slightly dysmorphic, had moderately severe hypotonia, and possessed multiple, irregular areas of hyperpigmentation over her limbs, trunk, and face (Fig. 21-16). She later was found to have a submucous cleft palate. An echocardiogram revealed that she had tetralogy of Fallot. The family history was unremarkable for other children with birth defects, mental retardation, or hyperpigmentation.

Exercise 10

QUESTION

1. In order to determine the etiology of her condition, which of the following evaluations would be appropriate to undertake initially?

   a. Serum lactate, carnitine, and acylcarnitine levels

   b. Prader-Willi FISH analysis

   c. Urine metabolic screen

   d. CT scan of her brain

   e. Standard chromosomal analysis

   f. Skin biopsy for fibroblast chromosomal analysis

ANSWER

1. a, d, and e.

Because Baby R has hypotonia, it is reasonable to evaluate her for mitochondrial disorders and carnitine deficiency. The lactate, carnitine, and acylcarnitine levels were determined and were within normal limits. Therefore, it is less likely that she has a mitochondrial disorder or a deficiency of carnitine. Individuals with Prader-Willi syndrome normally do not have congenital heart disease, so doing Prader-Willi FISH testing at this time is not indicated. However, it is reasonable to consider the diagnosis because typically neonates with Prader-Willi syndrome have moderate to severe hypotonia. The urine metabolic screen analyzes urine for abnormal metabolic products and detects many inborn errors of metabolism. However, most newborns with metabolic disorders normally are not dysmorphic and do not have major birth defects. As such, doing a urine metabolic screen on Baby R is not likely to detect an abnormality. Hypotonia would be an indication for doing an MRI or CT scan of her head. A CT scan was normal in her. In most dysmorphic newborns in whom the etiology of the features is unknown, a standard chromosome analysis is indicated. This test was done and the cytogenetic result was abnormal: 46,XX,+14,der (14;14)(q10;q10)[1]/46,XX[19].

QUESTION

2. Match the parts of the chromosome formula on the right with the explanation listed here at left.

a. Marker dividing the two cell lines	1. 46
b. Denotes the structurally abnormal and derived chromosome (translocated chromosome)	2. XX
c. Break points of the derived chromosome	3. +14
d. Number of cells in the second cell line	4. der(14;14)
e. The number of chromosomes in the first cell line	5. (q10;q10)
f. The type of sex chromosomes in the different cell lines	6. [1]
g. The number of chromosomes in the first cell line	7. /
h. Indicates an extra number 14 chromosome present in the cells of the first cell line	8. [19]

ANSWER

a. 7

b. 4

c. 5

d. 8

e. 1

f. 2

g. 6

h. 3

The number 46 in the karyotype indicates the total number of chromosomes present per cell. XX indicates that two X chromosomes were present. +14 means that there is an extra chromosome 14 present in each of the cells of the first cell line. The *der* stands for derived chromosomes, der(14;14) indicates that the two number 14 chromosomes are attached to each other. (q10;q10) states that the derived 14 chromosomes are attached to each other at the 10 regions of each chromosome 14, the centromeric regions, and that the long arms (q) of these chromosomes are present. This type of translocation (when two long arms of two acrocentric chromosomes fuse) is called a robertsonian translocation. Acrocentric chromosomes (13, 14, 15, 21, and 22) are the chromosomes in which the centromere is near the end, and all five acrocentric chromosomes engage in robertsonian translocations. The [1] denotes that there was only one derived chromosome present in the 20 cells evaluated. The slash (/) indicates that there are two cell lines present. The other cell line contained 46 chromosomes with two X chromosomes and there were 19 cells [19] that the cytogenetic technician counted with this chromosome constitution.

What is the significance of this chromosomal result? It is not unusual to observe random loss of a whole chromosome in one or a few cells when doing chromosomal analyzes. This loss is an artifact introduced during the processing of the cells in preparation for chromosomal staining and analyzes. In Baby R's case, however, finding the derived (14;14) chromosome probably was not related to an artifact, but represented a real chromosomal abnormality. In effect, she had three number 14 chromosomes, or effectively, trisomy 14 mosaicism. In addition, she was missing the two short arms (p arms) of the derived chromosome 14s. However, loss of these two arms is not a significant loss because the genes on these p arms are duplicated elsewhere and losing them has no phenotypic impact.

To further clarify Baby R's chromosome status, another peripheral blood chromosomal analysis was performed; the identification of additional derived chromosomes would confirm the diagnosis. The derived chromosome was discovered in three out of 30 cells, confirming the diagnosis.

Because of the hyperpigmented skin lesions and the peripheral blood chromosome results, it was highly likely that Baby R also had chromosomal mosaicism in her skin. Empirically, many children with these types of skin lesions (i.e., blotchy or swirled or linear pigmentation patterns) have chromosome mosaic conditions. A skin biopsy and subsequent fibroblast analysis indeed did show that Baby R had a mosaic pattern in her skin fibroblasts: 46,XX,+14,der (14;14)(q10;q10)[2]/46,XX[40].

As noted, the child had mosaic trisomy 14, although the trisomy was the result a robertsonian translocation. Most conceptuses with full trisomy 14 spontaneously abort during the first trimester of pregnancy. However, a number of mosaic trisomy 14 individuals, produced by trisomy rescue or who have a robertsonian 14;14 translocation, have been reported in the literature. Typically, these individuals have multiple congenital anomalies and varying degrees of mental retardation. Among the frequently seen anomalies are cleft palate, congenital heart defects, and genitourinary anomalies.

At 1 year of age, Baby R successfully had repair of her tetralogy of Fallot. At 14 months, her development was assessed to be at the 9-month level. At 19 months, she was doing well except for her developmental delay. A single umbilical artery (i.e., two vessel umbilical cord) is an important indication of possible major birth defects in the newborn. Normally, a single umbilical artery does not affect the viability of a fetus, but at birth there is a 21% chance that the affected neonate has at least one major malformation as compared to 3% to 5% when there are two umbilical arteries. The reason for this increased incidence of birth defects is not known.

Microdeletion

A third category of chromosomal abnormalities is the microdeletion. As noted earlier, some microdeletions are large enough that they can be detected on standard chromosomal analyzes. However, smaller deletions may not be visualized by standard cytogenetic analysis and are detected using FISH probes. Deletions can be quite small, involving only a portion of a gene. For instance, in Duchenne muscular dystrophy, 60% of cases have a deletion of part of the gene. In other situations, the deletion may encompass a larger segment, including not only a whole gene but neighboring genes as well. The situation in which two or more proximally located genes are deleted, resulting in an abnormal child, is called a contiguous gene deletion syndrome. An example is Williams syndrome. The consistently deleted gene in this syndrome is the elastin gene found on chromosome 7 at q11.23. Deletion of this gene accounts for some features seen in this condition. Deletions of genes located near the elastin gene account for the other features. The variation in the findings in Williams syndrome is related to the extent to which genes have been deleted in the individual; the fewer the number of contiguous genes deleted, the milder the disorder.

Exercise 11

QUESTION

1. Which of the following conditions are considered to be microdeletion syndromes?

    a. DiGeorge syndrome

    b. Beckwith-Wiedemann syndrome

    c. Cri du chat syndrome

    d. Prader-Willi syndrome

ANSWER

1. a and d. Beckwith-Wiedemann syndrome is an overgrowth syndrome that results from mutations or imprint errors in a number of different genes. Cri du chat syndrome is a deletion syndrome (partial deletion of the short arm of chromosome 5), but the deletion is large enough so that one can detect the abnormality by standard chromosomal analyzes. Table 21-7 lists the well-characterized microdeletion/contiguous gene deletion syndromes.

The following case study illustrates some of the features of microdeletions.

Case Study 7

Baby C (Figs. 21-17 and 21-18) was born at 38 weeks' gestation to a gravida 1 para 1 mother. The only significant prenatal problem was a cystic hygroma detected at 11 weeks, which remained relatively small throughout the rest of the pregnancy. Following birth, she had some dysmorphic findings including lateral fullness of her

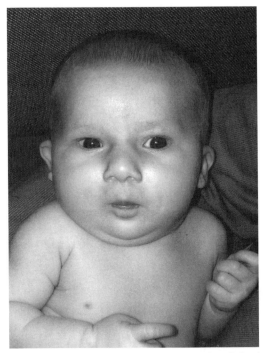

Figure 21-17 One-month-old Baby C with the velocardiofacial syndrome (22 q11 deletion syndrome). Note the lateral fullness of the nose and prominent ears.

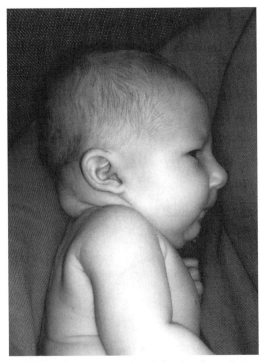

Figure 21-18 Baby C with velocardiofacial syndrome. Note the posteriorly rotated right ear, the moderate micrognathia, and the excessive nuchal skin.

nose, posteriorly rotated and prominent ears, and tetralogy of Fallot with pulmonary valve atresia and a hypoplastic pulmonary artery. Because of her dysmorphic features, conventional G-banded chromosomal analysis and DiGeorge/velocardiofacial FISH probe were done. The standard chromosomal analysis at the 610 band level was normal, but the FISH study indicated that she had a microdeletion in chromosome 22 (22 q11 deletion). Additional studies included normal serum calcium levels and normal T-cell function by immunologic evaluation.

At the age of 1 month, when she was last evaluated by a clinical geneticist, her weight and occipitofrontal circumference (OFC) were 3.5 kg (>97th percentile) and 34.7 cm (5th percentile), respectively. She appeared essentially the same as in the neonatal period. The parents appeared to be normal and they denied consanguinity. The rest of the family history was noncontributory.

Exercise 12

QUESTION

1. Behind each of the features listed here, indicate with a "D" if the feature predominately is found in individuals with DiGeorge syndrome, a "V" for features predominately found in velocardiofacial syndrome, and a "B" when the feature frequently is found in both conditions.

   a. Downslanting palpebral fissures

   b. Unusually shaped nose

   c. Abnormal speech

   d. Hypocalcemia

   e. Recurrent infections

   f. Congenital heart disease

   g. Deletion of 22 q11

ANSWER

1. a. D
   b. V
   c. B
   d. D
   e. D
   f. B
   g. B

Facial features in DiGeorge syndrome include ocular hypertelorism, downslanting palpebral fissures, cleft palate or bifid uvula, micrognathia, and low-set and malformed ears. Often not all of these features are present in one individual and the facial appearance may not be significantly abnormal. Congenital heart defects in DiGeorge syndrome often involve defects of the aorta and pulmonary arteries secondary to abnormal septation of the truncus arteriosus, the common embryonic vessel that when divided becomes the aorta and pulmonary artery. Abnormalities in these vessels occur in about 75% of cases. Other defects include absence or hypoplasia of the parathyroid glands, and deficiency of parathyroid hormone leading to hypocalcemia; abnormalities in T-cell function leading to recurrent infections; mild to moderate learning difficulties, hypernasal speech, and seizures. The condition is associated with a microdeletion at 22 q11. Velocardiofacial syndrome (VCF), also known as Shprintzen syndrome, is characterized by microcephaly, narrow palpebral fissures, prominent tubular nose with hypoplastic nasal alae and bulbous nasal tip, cleft palate with velopharyngeal insufficiency, mildly dysmorphic ears, congenital heart defect (aortic problems of various types), slender hands and fingers, learning difficulties or frank mental retardation, and behavioral and psychological problems. Affected individuals often have a nasal voice, and occasionally will have "neonatal" hypocalcemia and an increased incidence of T-cell related infections. Like those with DiGeorge syndrome, affected individuals also have deletion of 22 q11. In some families, VCF syndrome is inherited in an autosomal dominant fashion; typically DiGeorge syndrome is sporadic.

DiGeorge syndrome and VCF syndromes represent a spectrum disorder with many overlapping features. As such, there is no pattern of defects that clearly separates these two disorders.[18] However, based on clinical findings, clinical geneticists often will categorize a child with thymic, parathyroid, and heart-related problems into DiGeorge syndrome and those with velopharyngeal insufficiency and the more typical VCF facial features into the VCF syndrome. Alternatively, the designation of 22 q11 deletion syndrome to include both conditions can be used.

The neonatologist should consider DiGeorge or VCF syndrome in any patient who has congenital heart defects or aortic abnormalities, hypocalcemia, and a mildly dysmorphic facial appearance. In those neonates suspected to have these syndromes, it is appropriate to obtain a

FISH probe testing for deletion of 22 q11. When a deletion is detected, the attending physician or clinical geneticist should provide appropriate counseling to the parents and recommend deletion testing in both parents unless one parent clearly is affected. In that situation, the suspect parent should be tested first. The serum calcium levels of the neonate should be checked periodically until it is clear that he or she does not have hypocalcemia. The adequacy of T-cell function also needs to be determined.

Ambiguous Genitalia

Case Study 8

Baby B was born following an uncomplicated 42-week gestation to a gravida 2 para 2 29-year-old woman. The delivery was induced because of postmaturity and complicated by shoulder dystocia. Birth length, weight, and OFC were 45 cm (<3rd percentile), 3.26 kg (50th percentile), and 33.5 cm (40th percentile), respectively. Following birth Baby B had slight molding of the head and ambiguous genitalia. There was a phallic-like structure that was 2 cm in length, a chordee, third-degree hypospadias, and scrotal-like sac that was fused in the midline (Fig. 21-19). No gonads were palpable. Routine serum laboratory values including a serum sodium (136 mEq/L) were normal. Subsequently, she developed hyperbilirubinemia with a peak value of 13.5 mg/dL at 4 days of age. An abdominal ultrasound demonstrated a structure that appeared to be a uterus. Subsequently, a voiding cystourethrogram and urogram indicated a vagina that communicated to a posterior urethra, a normal bladder with reflux into the ureters, and normal kidneys. A rapid chromosomal analysis indicated normal female constitution (46,XX). A serum 17-hydroxyprogesterone at age 2 days was elevated at 1924 ng/dL. On day 7 she developed hyponatremia and hyperkalemia. At age 10 days, she developed a right-sided inguinal hernia and at 2 weeks of age had bilateral inguinal herniorrhaphies. During this operation, the surgeon found a fallopian tube and ovary on the right.

Exercise 13

QUESTION

1. Which of the following conditions is the most likely diagnosis in this patient?

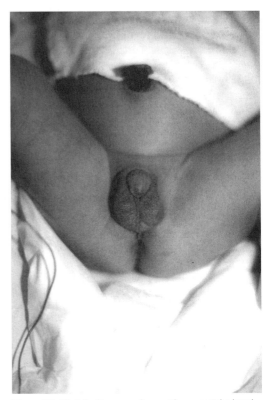

Figure 21-19 Baby B as a newborn with congenital adrenal hyperplasia. Note marked masculinization of the external genitalia, so much so that the genitalia look like male genitalia and rugation of the scrotum.

a. Smith-Lemli-Opitz syndrome

b. Urorectal septum malformation sequence

c. Complete androgen insensitivity syndrome (testicular feminization syndrome)

d. Congenital adrenal hyperplasia

e. Mixed gonadal dysgenesis

ANSWER

1. d.

By definition, ambiguous genitalia in the newborn means that the sex of the individual cannot be determined with certainty based solely on the appearance of the external genitalia. In rare cases, such as complete androgen insensitivity (testicular feminization), the external genitalia are unequivocally female but the gonads and chromosomal sex are male. In Baby B's case, she had significant masculinization of the external genitalia but because of the chordee and severe hypospadias, these genitalia were not those of a normal male. Her chromosomal analysis determined that her chromosomal sex was female. Consistent with the chromosomal result were the findings of a uterus on ultrasound and a fallopian tube and ovary at surgery.

In any newborn with ambiguous genitalia, the evaluation must proceed in a timely fashion. First, one needs to formulate a plan to evaluate the neonate and establish the diagnosis. Second, the neonatologist and the consulting team caring for the child must discuss the issue of sex assignment with the parents. Input from a urologist, endocrinologist, clinical geneticist, pediatric surgeon, and pediatric psychiatrist is crucial at this time. Male sex assignment depends in part on the anticipated adequacy of penile sexual function as an adult. Third, the physicians involved with the case need to develop a treatment plan for the immediate and long-term care of the patient. Finally, one must be concerned about the development of hyponatremia and hyperkalemia due to salt-wasting congenital adrenal hyperplasia (CAH), which if severe enough can lead to vascular collapse and death. However, with salt-wasting CAH, the hyponatremia and hyperkalemia normally do not develop before 1 week of age. Thus, daily sodium and potassium levels should be tested starting at about day 5 or 6.

Exercise 13 *Continued*

QUESTION

2. Indicate if the following statements about congenital adrenal hyperplasia are true or false.

   a. CAH only affects females.

   b. CAH is caused by an impaired synthesis of cortisol in the mineralocorticoid or glucocorticoid metabolic pathways.

   c. The ambiguous genitalia seen in CAH are related to excessive testosterone levels in females.

   d. CAH most frequently is inherited in an autosomal recessive fashion.

   e. If there is a deficiency of aldosterone production in an affected individual, that individual normally will be a "salt waster."

   f. Most cases of CAH are caused by a mutation in the *CYP21A2* gene that codes for the production of 21-hydroxylase.

ANSWER

2. True: b, d, e, f. False: a, c.

Congenital adrenal hyperplasia is the most common cause of ambiguous genitalia in females with an incidence in both sexes of approximately 1 in 15,000 live births. The condition is the result of impaired synthesis of cortisol in the mineralocorticoid or glucocorticoid pathway in the adrenal cortex. As a result, there is a deficiency of cortisol and an excess of cortisol precursors. The excessive cortisol precursors result from high levels of adrenocorticotropic hormone (ACTH) that drive the system in an attempt to produce more cortisol. The elevation of ACTH is due to the lack of feedback inhibition from cortisol. Because the cortisol precursors typically have an androgenic effect, they are the basis for the partial masculinization of the external genitalia in females. In about 75% of CAH cases, there also is a deficiency of aldosterone. This deficiency in turn leads to salt wasting from excessive urinary sodium loss. Salt-wasting CAH normally occurs when there is a total lack of the enzyme; if some activity is present, there is normally no salt wasting.

In classic CAH, females are generally born with partial masculinization of the external genitalia and clitorimegaly. If they are not started on hormone treatment, children with the non–salt-wasting classic CAH often will experience excessive growth. In addition, they will exhibit an advanced bone age and develop precocious puberty. Growth cessation will occur at that point, and the affected individual will be of short stature as an adult. In males with CAH, the testes produce adequate amounts of testosterone and there is usually normal masculinization of the external genitalia. Because these males have normal genitalia, the diagnosis normally is not made in the neonatal period. If they are also salt wasters, they may experience vascular collapse and die from their condition at 1 to 2 weeks of age. Affected males who are treated immediately and vigorously may survive. Owing to the difficulty of diagnosing such males, many states in the United States now have mandatory newborn screening for CAH.

In 90% of cases of CAH, the cause is a mutation in the *CYP21A2* gene, which codes for the production of 21-hydroxylase. Molecular testing of the gene is available to confirm the diagnosis, to provide carrier detection of at-risk relatives, and to allow for prenatal testing. A molecular panel that includes nine of the most common *CYP21A2* mutations causing CAH currently is available for gene testing. For mutations not included in this panel, there is also the availability of complete gene sequencing.

Mutations in other genes that code for enzymes in the adrenal steroid biosynthesis pathway also result in CAH. One can find a listing of these latter genes, and the enzymes they produce, in any standard pediatric or endocrine textbook. However, no commercial laboratory currently offers sequencing of the other genes that produce CAH. With regard to Baby B, CAH is likely because of her marked masculinization of the external genitalia, presence of fallopian tube and ovary, and normal female karyotype. She also had the salt-wasting type of CAH.

Exercise 13 *Continued*

QUESTION

3. Which of the following should be done on newborns/neonates who have ambiguous genitalia?

    a. A complete history

    b. A complete physical examination

    c. An ultrasound examination of the pelvis and adrenal glands

    d. A chromosomal analysis

    e. Consultation with an endocrinologist, pediatric urologist, a clinical geneticist, and a psychiatrist.

    f. Serum concentration of 17-hydroxyprogesterone

    g. ACTH stimulation test or molecular testing for the genes causing CAH (currently 21-hydroxylase)

    h. Testing serum sodium levels daily starting on day 5 or 6

ANSWER

3. a through h.

Normally one would do all the above items unless a specific diagnosis is established that negates the necessity for doing some of these items. For example, if the diagnosis is clearly CAH, then one does not need to do the ACTH stimulation test. Molecular testing for CAH is indicated for reasons stated earlier. Because CAH is an endocrine disorder, one normally establishes the diagnosis by demonstrating abnormal hormone levels (specifically a defi-ciency of cortisol, and marked elevations in one or more of the cortisol precursors, e.g., 17-hydroxyprogesterone) or by finding a significant mutation in the *CYP21A2* gene.

The treatment of CAH normally begins with hydrocortisone; dexamethasone is too potent to safely use in neonates. In the treatment of CAH, there is a narrow line between excessive corticosteroid dosage and insufficient treatment. In addition, neonates also need additional oral sodium chloride because breast milk and formula are relatively low in sodium chloride and even "non–salt wasters" lose more than the normal amounts of sodium in the urine. Further, if the affected neonate turns out to be a salt waster, then one should initiate fludrocortisone acetate (Florinef) therapy. In addition to these actions, an endocrinologist, pediatric urologist, clinical geneticist, and psychiatrist should be consulted to handle the other facets of this disorder. In neonates with vascular collapse, the treatment should include intravenous saline and glucose, correction of the hyperkalemia, and intravenous hydrocortisone at three times the normal calculated physiologic dose.

Neonatologists and other physicians caring for newborns also need to be familiar with other causes of ambiguous genitalia. One such condition is the urorectal septum malformation sequence. Although this condition is not well known, it appears to be the most common cause of ambiguous genitalia in males. The major characteristics of the condition include unusual external genitalia (Fig. 21-20), absence of urethral and vaginal openings, imperforate anus (see Fig. 21-20), vesicorectal fistula, distal colonic atresia, dysplastic or absent kidneys, and sacral agenesis.[19] Both sexes are affected about equally. However, because some affected females possess a phallic-like structure, these newborns often are mistakenly identified as males. The fully expressed condition is usually fatal in the neonatal period, secondary to lung hypoplasia. If the neonate survives the respiratory problems, unfortunately, he or she will usually die during infancy from renal failure secondary to dysplastic or absent kidneys. A partial urorectal septum malformation sequence has recently been recognized that is less severe and in which survival is common. These children almost always require extensive reconstructive surgery.

A number of other syndromes also have ambiguous genitalia as a feature, but they occur less frequently than CAH and the urorectal septum malformation sequence. For exam-

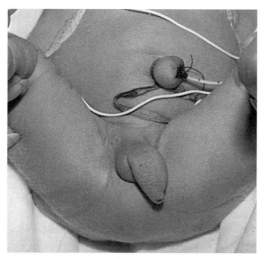

Figure 21-20 Female neonate with the urorectal septum malformation sequence. Note the phallic-like structure, hypoplastic "scrotum," and imperforate anus. The phallic-like structure did not contain a urethra. The chromosomes were 46,XX. (From Wheeler PG, Weaver DD, Obeime MO, et al: Urorectal septum malformation sequence: Report of thirteen additional cases and review of the literature. Am J Med Genet 1997;73:456–462.)

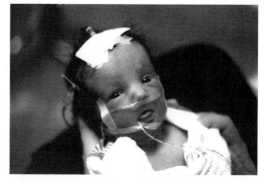

Figure 21-21 Baby T with mosaic trisomy 7 and the Russell-Silver syndrome. Note her petite face with a mildly triangular shape, broad forehead, large-appearing eyes, prominent nasal bridge, lateral nasal prominence, short nose, and mild micrognathia.

ple, Smith-Lemli-Opitz syndrome, a defect in cholesterol biosynthesis, has a frequency of 1 in 20,000 births. The genital abnormalities in males include cryptorchidism and hypospadias. The features in Baby B are more severe than those normally seen in Smith-Lemli-Opitz syndrome, and she does not possess the other characteristics usually seen in Smith-Lemli-Opitz syndrome. As a gauge of the number of dysmorphic syndromes with ambiguous genitalia, the syndrome database, POSSUM, lists 91 such syndromes.

Intrauterine Growth Restriction/Small for Gestational Age

Case Study 9

Baby T (Fig. 21-21) was born at term gestation to a 33-year-old gravida 3 para 3 mother by elective cesarean section at 38 weeks' gestation. The pregnancy was complicated by an abnormal maternal serum triple screen done at 18 weeks' gestation when there was low human chorionic gonadotropin (hCG) level (0.11 multiples of the median). Because of the abnormal screening result, the mother elected to have an amniocentesis, which was done at 19 weeks. A chromosomal analysis of the amniotic fluid cells revealed mosaic trisomy 7 (47,XX,+7[13]/46,XX[19]). Because of the

possibility of imprinting problems in the fetus secondary to the disomic cell line, testing for uniparental disomy (UPD) was undertaken. This analysis indeed demonstrated maternal uniparental disomy in the disomic cell line. Subsequent ultrasounds indicated a normal placenta and normal amniotic fluid volume, a two-vessel umbilical cord, and cardiomegaly. The delivery was uncomplicated. Birth length was 45 cm (15th percentile), the weight was 2.05 kg (−3 SD), and the head circumference was 34.5 cm (80th percentile). Postnatal karyotyping of various tissues gave the following results: cord blood—normal chromosomal complement (46,XX), chorionic villus tissue—complete trisomy 7 (47,XX,+7[19]), and skin fibroblasts from a hyperpigmented swirled area—mosaic trisomy 7 (47,XX,+7[9]/46,XX[20]). On the newborn physical examination, she had a mildly triangular face, broad forehead, large-appearing eyes, prominent nasal bridge, lateral nasal prominence, short nose, mild micrognathia, broad and low-set ears, clinodactyly of the fifth fingers, and little subcutaneous fat. Following birth, she had mild respiratory distress and hypoglycemia, and developed a small right pneumothorax. An echocardiogram demonstrated a patent foramen ovale and PDA. She initially required supplemental nasal oxygen and nasogastric feeding, but improved quickly and was discharged.

Exercise 14

QUESTION

1. Which of the following diagnoses is most likely the cause of Baby T's low birth weight?

a. Placental dysfunction

b. Intrauterine infection

c. Chromosomal abnormality

d. A dysmorphic syndrome, which is associated with intrauterine growth restriction

ANSWER

1. Probably a, c, and d.

As indicated by the complete trisomy 7 constitution of the placenta, placental dysfunction could have played a role in the growth deficiency of Baby T. It is now well recognized that chromosomally abnormal placentas may function poorly. In fact, 1% to 2% of intrauterine growth restriction (IUGR) is due to confined placental mosaicism. This mosaicism exists when a chromosomal abnormality is present in the placenta but not in the fetus. In this situation, all placental cells may possess the same chromosomal abnormality, or some placental cells may have a chromosomal abnormality, while others have a normal chromosomal complement—placental mosaicism. The presence of a chromosomal abnormality in the placenta results in a dysfunctional placenta, which may then lead to growth deficiency in the fetus, even though the chromosomal constitution of the fetus is normal. Therefore, a chromosomal analysis of the placenta needs to be performed whenever the cause of IUGR cannot be determined. In order to detect placental chromosomal abnormalities in IUGR, however, one must obtain placental tissue for chromosomal analysis soon after placenta delivery. If the placenta and fetus both have a chromosomal aberration, the growth deficiency is often more severe than if the aberration is confined to the placenta. Furthermore, fetuses with chromosomal abnormalities often have growth deficiency at birth. For instance, the POSSUM database lists 566 syndromes associated with intrauterine growth restriction (IUGR)/small for gestational age (SGA). Of these 566 conditions, 117 (21%) are caused by chromosomal abnormalities.

Trisomy 7 mosaicism has been occasionally reported prenatally. Most of the resulting children have been normal. However, when trisomy 7 mosaicism has been diagnosed postnatally, these children have had renal dysplasia, congenital heart defects, and other defects. Several have died soon after birth.

By visually inspecting the placenta postnatally, one often can detect placental abnormalities, while pathologic examination of the placenta frequently is even more informative. However, because placentas are routinely discarded after visual inspection by the delivering physicians, it is imperative in a case of IUGR that the delivering physician or the neonatologist make an immediate and specific request for pathologic examination of the placenta. Placental dysfunction may also occur with maternal autoimmune diseases such as lupus erythematosus and in diabetes associated with advanced vascular disease. Therefore, one should check the mothers of neonates with growth deficiency for these disorders.

Intrauterine infections are recognized causes of IUGR. Chorioretinitis and calcification in the brain are suggestive of a prenatal infection. Brain calcifications can be detected by skull radiographs or CT scans of the head. Common agents responsible for intrauterine infections include *Toxoplasmosis gondii*, *cytomegalovirus*, *herpes simplex*, and *Treponema pallidum* (syphilis) (the so-called TORCH infections), and these infections need to be ruled out in undiagnosed cases of IUGR. Rubella virus can also cause IUGR but is an uncommon cause in developed countries because of vaccinations.

Case Study 9 *Continued*

At 5 months of age, Baby T had persistent growth deficiency of height and weight, and developed recurrent hypoglycemia. Further studies demonstrated that she had growth hormone deficiency. At 1 year, she was started on growth hormone replacement therapy and demonstrated some improvement. At 14 months, she still had the previously noted physical findings plus she had developed hyperpigmented swirled skin lesions. Her height and weight were still significantly below the 3rd percentile but her head size was normal (90th percentile). Developmental testing at 29 months using a Bayley Scales of Infant Development indicated a developmental index of 59. Further extensive testing for her growth deficiency failed to uncover any other abnormalities.

Exercise 14 *Continued*

QUESTION

2. Given that Baby T has a chromosomal abnormality and is dysmorphic, which of the

following syndromes does she most likely have?

a. Down syndrome

b. Russell-Silver syndrome

c. de Lange syndrome (Cornelia de Lange syndrome)

d. Fetal alcohol syndrome

e. Thanatophoric dysplasia

ANSWER

2. b.

Baby T has many of the physical features of Russell-Silver syndrome, including pre- and postnatal growth deficiency, normal head size, triangular face, micrognathia, fifth finger clinodactyly, hypoglycemia, and growth hormone deficiency. Other characteristics that are also seen in this syndrome include down-turned corners of the mouth, body asymmetry, café au lait spots, and developmental delay. This diagnosis in Baby T is even more likely as 10% of cases of Russell-Silver syndrome have uniparental disomy for chromosome 7 (which she has).

The other choices are unlikely. Down syndrome is caused by trisomy 21, which she does not have. In addition, she does not have the phenotypic features seen in Down syndrome. Similarly, de Lange syndrome is not likely, because the features seen in Baby T are not those seen in this syndrome. In de Lange syndrome, there normally is pre- and postnatal growth deficiency, microcephaly, eyebrows that extend across the brow (synophrys), thin upper lip with down-turned corners of the mouth, congenital heart defect, upper limb deficiencies, marked cutis marmorata, and a low-pitched, growling cry. In the full fetal alcohol syndrome (FAS), IUGR is normally present, a direct result of the teratogenic effects of prenatal alcohol exposure. However, Baby T did not have the facial features normally seen in FAS and the mother vehemently denied drinking during the pregnancy. Finally, thanatophoric dysplasia is also an unlikely diagnosis, for this dysplasia normally is fatal within the first few hours or days following birth and has marked midfacial hypoplasia and moderately short limbs.

Table 21-8 lists other common causes for IUGR and SGA. The most common cause of mild IUGR is maternal smoking, which gener-

ally does not lead to structural defects observed in this child. The degree of growth restriction is dose related. The mother of Baby T did not smoke during the pregnancy, and therefore, prenatal smoking was not a contributing factor to her growth deficiency.

When caring for newborns with IUGR, one should consider each of the conditions listed in Table 21-8. Establishing an etiology is important since some disorders causing IUGR can be treated. Determining the diagnosis is also helpful in counseling parents with regard to long-term prognosis and to recurrence of the condition in subsequent offspring.

TABLE 21-8

COMMON CONDITIONS ASSOCIATED WITH INTRAUTERINE GROWTH RETARDATION*

Maternal medical conditions
  Hypertension, chronic
  Diabetes mellitus
  Hypoxic lung disease, severe
  Inflammatory bowel disease
  Preeclampsia early in gestation
  Renal disease, chronic
  Malnutrition, severe
  Systemic lupus erythematosus
Teratogens
  Alcohol
  Cocaine
  Phenytoin (Dilantin)
  Smoking
  Warfarin (Coumadin, Panwarfin)
Infections
  Cytomegalovirus infection
  Hepatitis B
  Herpes simplex virus (HSV-1 or HSV-2) infection
  Human immunodeficiency virus (HIV-1) infection
  Rubella
  Syphilis
  Toxoplasmosis
Chromosomal abnormalities
  Trisomy 13
  Trisomy 18
  Trisomy 21
  Turner syndrome
Miscellaneous
  Prior history of pregnancy with intrauterine growth retardation
  Residing at altitude above 5000 ft

---

*There are over 560 syndromes listed in the POSSUM database that have Intrauterine growth retardation as a feature. For a complete list of these syndromes, contact your local clinical geneticist.
Modified from Vanderbosche RC, Kirchner JF: Intrauterine growth retardation. Am Fam Physician 1998;58:1384–1390, 1393–1394.

Large for Gestational Age/Overgrowth Syndromes

Excessive intrauterine growth is a common feature in neonates with overgrowth syndromes, certain chromosomal disorders, a number of dysmorphic syndromes, and infants born to women with diabetes mellitus. Being large for gestational age (LGA) is not as common as growth restriction. However, the LGA group of disorders represents an important category of disorders because LGA babies are more likely to have dystocia and postnatal problems such as hypoglycemia. The following case exemplifies some of the problems seen in neonates with overgrowth syndromes.

Case Study 10

Baby D (Fig. 21-22) was born to a 30-year-old gravida 3 para 3 white mother. The pregnancy was complicated by preeclampsia and then HELLP syndrome. During her pregnancy the mother took Aldomet, Prozac, and Singulair for preeclampsia, depression, and allergies, respectively. In addition, an omphalocele was detected prenatally by ultrasound. The infant was delivered by cesarean section at 30 weeks; length, weight, and OFC were 37 cm (25th percentile), 1.51 kg (50th percentile), and 29 cm (80th percentile), respectively.

Following birth, he was noted to have a prominent nevus flammeus over the forehead, eyelids, and nose; macroglossia; small shallow pits on the back of the ears; and a moderately large omphalocele. There were no palpable abdominal organs or body asymmetry. Subsequently, an echocardiogram demonstrated a patent ductus arteriosus and a patent foramen ovale/atrial septal defect secondum. His blood glucose levels were in the normal range. An ultrasound of the abdomen was normal except for bilateral mild hydronephrosis. Standard and subtelomeric FISH chromosomal studies were also normal. Serum alpha-fetoprotein (AFP) level at age 2 weeks was normal. On the second day following birth, Baby D had his omphalocele successfully repaired by a primary closure. Throughout the latter part of his hospital stay, one of his major difficulties was oral feedings because of the size of his tongue. The family history was unremarkable for large babies, childhood tumors, mental retardation, omphaloceles, or other birth defects.

He was discharged from the hospital at a postnatal age of 3 months. At a 7-month follow-up

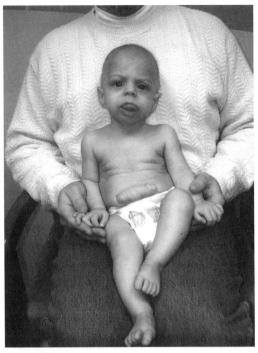

Figure 21-22 Seven-month-old male (Baby D) with Beckwith-Wiedemann syndrome. Observe the macroglossia and abdominal wall hernia, the residual defect from his omphalocele repair.

outpatient visit, his height, weight, and OFC all were at the 5th percentile. The tongue was still large and he still was having some feeding difficulties because of the macroglossia. The tongue, however, was not causing any respiratory difficulties.

Exercise 15

QUESTIONS

1. What is the most likely diagnosis for Baby D?
   a. Congenital hypothyroidism
   b. Down syndrome
   c. Sotos syndrome
   d. Infant of diabetic mother
   e. Beckwith-Wiedemann syndrome (BWS)

2. Which of the following are common problems in neonates with BWS?
   a. Hypoglycemia
   b. Seizures
   c. Respiratory difficulties
   d. Neoplasias
   e. Feeding problems

3. Which of the following would be helpful in making the diagnosis of BWS?

   a. Prenatal history of elevated maternal or amniotic fluid AFP level

   b. Prenatal diagnosis of an omphalocele

   c. Postnatal finding of large for gestational age (LGA), macroglossia, and visceromegaly in a newborn

   d. Family history of Beckwith-Wiedemann syndrome

   e. Gene testing

ANSWERS

1. e. Prominent nevus flammeus over the forehead, eyelids, and nose; macroglossia; congenital heart disease; and omphalocele are commonly seen in BWS, and these features make this diagnosis likely in Baby D. Furthermore, the ear pits, which are almost unique to BWS, make the diagnosis even more likely. Other features often found in neonates with BWS include ear creases; umbilical hernia; visceromegaly involving the liver, pancreas, and kidneys; hemihypertrophy; macrosomia; and hypoglycemia. The reason why Baby D was not macrosomic is unknown.

2. a, c, and e. Neonatal hypoglycemia occurs in 30% to 50% of cases of BWS as a result of hyperinsulinemia and islet cell hyperplasia. The hypoglycemia usually is transitory, lasting not more than 3 or 4 days, and responds well to medical management. Seizures normally are not part of BWS. Respiratory problems commonly occur owing to the obstruction of the posterior pharynx by a large tongue. If this is the case, keeping the neonate on his or her stomach may relieve the respiratory distress. Neoplasias occur in an estimated 7% of cases. Commonly reported tumors in BWS include Wilms' tumor, neuroblastoma, hepatoblastoma, adrenocortical carcinoma, rhabdomyosarcoma, and gonadoblastoma. These tumors, generally, are not present at birth, nor are they seen in the neonatal period. They can arise during infancy, however. Feeding problems result from the macroglossia, which may be so massive that the tongue fills the entire mouth, making feeding difficult, if not impossible.

3. b, c, d, and e.

For diagnostic purposes, the features of BWS have been divided into major and minor characteristics. To make the diagnosis, there must be at least two major features and one minor feature (for a listing of the major and minor features, see the review article on BWS in GeneReviews at http://www.genetests.org, or consult a clinical geneticist). Alternatively, one can establish the diagnosis by molecular testing. We now know that BWS results from abnormal transcription and gene regulation in an imprinted region at chromosome 11p15.5. Such an error may arise from a chromosome aberration (translocation or inversion) leading to 11p15 duplication (1% to 2% of cases), the presence of paternal uniparental disomy (10% to 20%), abnormal methylation of the genes *KCNQ1OT1* (50% to 60%) or *H19* (2% to 7%), or a *CDKN1C* (5% to 10%) gene mutation. If other individuals in a family are affected, the chance of finding a mutation in the *CDKN1C* gene increases to about 40%. In practice, one normally orders a standard chromosomal analysis, followed by methylation analysis of *KCNQ1OT1* and *H19* genes, UPD assessment, and then sequencing of the entire coding region of *CDKN1C*. The latter three tests can be ordered together from commercial molecular biology laboratories. A positive finding from one of these tests normally confirms the diagnosis. Baby D did have gene testing at age 6 months and had lack of maternal methylation of *KCNQ1OT1*. This imprinting error means that the recurrence risk for the parents of Baby D and for his children is probably less than 1%.

Elevated AFP levels in maternal serum and amniotic fluid normally are found in fetuses who have an omphalocele because AFP readily diffuses across the membrane covering the herniated viscera. However, there are over 100 conditions that will elevate AFP levels, and BWS is only one of them. On the other hand, one should put BWS high on the differential diagnosis list of any fetus with an omphalocele.

Fractures at Birth and the Neonatal Period

Fractures in a newborn result from dystocia in an LGA fetus delivered vaginally, from weaker than normal bones caused by a primary bone disorder (e.g., osteogenesis imperfecta), or from a fetal disorder leading to decreased or no fetal movement. Fractures discovered in a neonate can be caused by any of the above-mentioned disorders, or from accidental or nonaccidental trauma. One should attempt to determine the cause of the fracture(s) in each case because the medical and social implications and long-term prognoses are so different.

Case Study 11

Ms. J was 28 weeks pregnant, as estimated from her last menstrual period. During a routine prenatal visit, her obstetrician performed an ultrasonographic evaluation because of smaller than normal uterine size. The sonogram indicated a fetus with short limbs. The obstetrician then referred Ms. J to a prenatal diagnostic center. At the center, the perinatologist performed a level-2 ultrasound, an extensive study that measures and looks at most parts of the fetus. At this evaluation, there was shortening and bowing of all the long bones, and an increased prominence of the ventricles of the brain. The perinatologist's diagnosis was a bone dysplasia—specifically, osteogenesis imperfecta (OI) type II.

A radiograph of Ms. J's abdomen indicated very little bone mineralization in the fetus, giving additional credence to the suspected diagnosis. The perinatologist subsequently counseled the parents about the diagnosis and the poor postnatal prognosis. Although he told the parents that OI type II was a lethal neonatal condition, the parents elected to continue the pregnancy.

Because a vaginal delivery of infants with OI type II would significantly increase the risk of fractures and intracranial hemorrhage, the parents chose to have their baby delivered by cesarean section. Immediately after birth, Baby J (Fig. 21-23) developed significant respiratory distress and cyanosis. Because of these problems, the attending neonatologist intubated her and placed her on mechanical ventilation. On physical examination, she had short and bowed limbs (see Fig. 21-23), a very soft skull, dark blue sclerae, midfacial hypoplasia, and although she was alert, little limb movement. Once Baby J was stabilized, the neonatologist consulted a clinical geneticist and a pediatric orthopedist for recommendations on further diagnostic testing and care of the infant. Over the next few days as diagnostic information accrued, the neonatologist met with the family to construct a long-term care plan.

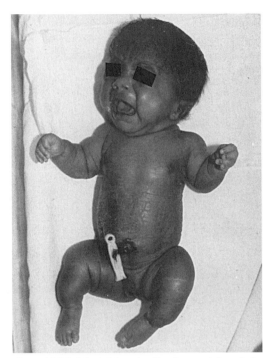

Figure 21-23 Baby J at 1 week with osteogenesis imperfecta type III. Note the short limbs, particularly the upper arms and thighs, and the anterior bowing of the lower legs.

Exercise 16

QUESTION

1. Which course of action will best determine if Baby J had OI type II?
   a. Provide supportive care and wait to see if the baby dies
   b. Order a radiographic skeletal survey
   c. Perform genetic testing
   d. All of the above

ANSWER

1. b.

Even though a number of bone dysplasias can be diagnosed from physical findings alone, the definitive diagnosis normally is established from the radiographic findings, or a combination of physical and radiographic findings. With some bone dysplasias, the physical and radiographic features are not distinctive enough to make a diagnosis in the neonatal period. In these situations, one needs to wait for the skeletal findings to develop (which can take up to 18 months) or go directly to genetic testing if such testing is available.

The radiographs (Figs. 21-24 and 21-25) on Baby J revealed very little calcification of the skull (confined to the base), thin ribs with multiple fractures, mildly flattened vertebral bodies, and thin and distorted long bones with numerous fractures. The broad, ribbon-like bones characteristic of OI type II were not present.

QUESTION

2. Match the description on the right with the types of OI on the left and indicate the type of OI Baby J has.

a. OI type I	1. Fractures but otherwise normal-appearing bones on radiographs, white sclerae after age 1 year
b. OI type II	2. Markedly decreased bone density, ribbon-like long bones, multiple fractures
c. OI type III	3. Fractures but otherwise normal-appearing bones on radiographs, blue sclerae after age 1 year
d. OI type IV	4. Markedly decreased bone density, thin and bowed long bones, multiple fractures

ANSWER

2. a. 3.

   b. 2.

   c. 4. Baby J.

   d. 1.

The radiographic findings in baby J were consistent with a less severe form of OI, OI type III.

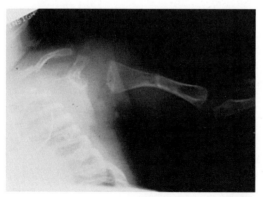

Figure 21-24 Radiograph of the shoulder and upper arm of Baby J, who has osteogenesis imperfecta type III. Note the fractures of the clavicle and humerus, thin ribs, narrow diaphysis and thin cortex of the humerus, and generalized decreased mineralization.

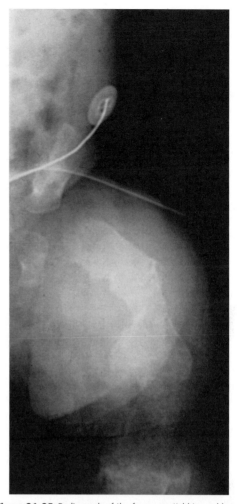

Figure 21-25 Radiograph of the femur, partial hip, and knee of Baby J, who has osteogenesis imperfecta type III. Note the bowing of the femur and the irregular bony contours and markedly decreased mineralization of the bones.

Whereas OI type II is normally lethal in the neonatal period, OI type III frequently is not. The major characteristics of OI type III are a large number of fractures—hundreds during the lifetime of some individuals—and marked distortion, bowing, and shortening of most of the long bones (see Figs. 21-24 and 21-25). In addition, there may be multiple rib fractures and kyphoscoliosis, which may lead to compromised lung volume, respiratory distress, and cardiopulmonary failure. In some infants, the cardiopulmonary failure may lead to death. Because of marked leg bowing, children with this condition are often unable to bear weight or walk, and thus are confined to wheelchairs.

In the case of Baby J, the physicians and parents needed to decide whether to continue to support her with mechanical ventilation.

However, because this condition usually is not fatal in the neonatal period and is not associated with mental deficiency, most physicians (after consultation with the family) would elect to continue full support of such a neonate. Because Baby J's bones were so fragile, she would need to have special care and handling while in the neonatal intensive care unit and probably should be placed on a gel-filled or soft foam-filled mattress. Even the act of rolling her over and changing her diaper could cause fractures. At the time of discharge, she would need to be carried on a pillow, and arrangements for follow-up orthopedic care would need to be made. As Baby J gets older and larger, she may need casting of certain fractures and likely will need various orthopedic surgeries to keep her legs straight. The recent availability of bisphosphonate, which blocks reabsorption of bone by the osteoclasts (thereby increasing bone density), has led to remarkable improvement in the physical condition of most of these children. A number of children with this severe form of OI, who previously could not walk, have became ambulatory after treatment.

Osteogenesis imperfecta is only one category of disorders that results in neonatal fractures. OI is a bone dysplasia caused by a mutation in one of the two genes that code for collagen type 1. However, neonatal fractures can also result from decreased fetal movement. In general, these disorders produce a characteristic and recognizable phenotype called the fetal akinesia sequence (or the fetal akinesia/hypokinesia sequence or the Pena-Shokeir phenotype). The reasons for the decreased fetal movements in fetal akinesia sequence can be classified into neurogenic and myopathic disorders, restrictive dermopathies, teratogen exposures, and intrauterine constraints. There are a number of different syndromes in each of these latter disorders. As a result of the decreased fetal movement, the fetal bones are gracile and lack the strength that is normally seen in bones of a healthy newborn. In turn these fragile bones are more likely to fracture during delivery or with postnatal handling. The final category is that of decreased bone density associated with prematurity, including the rickets of prematurity.

Bone Dysplasias

As discussed earlier, bone dysplasias are primary disorders of bone that affect the growth, density, and shape of bones. Collectively, there are more than 380 recognized disorders with a combined incidence of approximately 1 in 5000. Most are inherited in a mendelian fashion. The most commonly encountered disorders include achondroplasia, osteogenesis imperfecta, and thanatophoric dysplasia; most of the other bone dysplasias are rare with individual incidence being probably less than 1 in 100,000.

Case Study 12

Baby A (Fig. 21-26) was born at 37 weeks' gestation via a cesarean section because of breech presentation. The pregnancy was otherwise uncomplicated. At birth her length was 46 cm (10th percentile), weight 2.6 kg (25th percentile), and OFC 38 cm (>97th percentile). She was mildly unusual in appearance in the newborn period with a large head, short nose, and disproportionately short limbs. A head ultrasound done the first day was normal. Following discharge from the hospital, she did well except that she had poor head control. At 1 week of age, her pediatrician ordered a skeletal survey, which

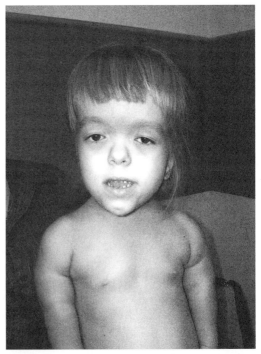

Figure 21-26 Baby A at 6 years old. She has achondroplasia. Note her macrocephaly with a broad forehead, depressed nasal bridge, short nose, and rhizomelic shortening of the upper limbs.

revealed frontal bossing, rhizomelic shortening of all her limbs, and decreased interpedicular height. The consulting radiologist thought that Baby A had spondyloepiphyseal dysplasia congenita. A chromosomal analysis was also done and was normal (46,XX). At 5 and 6 weeks of age she had seizure-like episodes but no EEG was done. At 4 months of age, a clinical geneticist evaluated Baby A and recognized that she had classic achondroplasia.

Exercise 17

QUESTION

1. Which of the following evaluations would be indicated for Baby A at this point?

   a. Do nothing except to follow her on an outpatient basis

   b. Obtain an MRI or CT scan of her brain and cervical spine

   c. Refer her to a neurologist for a neurologic examination

   d. Order a polysomnography

   e. Recommend gene testing to confirm the diagnosis of achondroplasia

ANSWER

1. b and d.

   The three most common significant problems in infants with achondroplasia (ACP) include hydrocephalus, obstructive airway disease, and sudden infant death related to cervical spinal cord necrosis and apnea. To determine if an infant with ACP is at increased risk for sudden infant death, one needs to obtain the following evaluation. First, the primary care physician or a neurologist should do a careful neurologic examination. Next, a polysomnography needs to be done to determine if any apnea or oxygen desaturation is occurring. Finally, an MRI or CT scan of the brain and the cervical spinal cord must be performed. The purpose of these studies is to determine if there is significant foramen magnum or cervical spinal canal stenosis. If so, spinal cord necrosis can ensue, and if this occurs, the infant will most likely die. If any one or all of these tests are abnormal, then a neurosurgeon needs to evaluate the child to determine if a decompression of the spinal cord is needed. The best predictors of spinal cord compression are

lower-limb hyperreflexia or clonus, central hypopnea demonstrated by polysomnography, and foramen magnum measurement below the means for infants with ACP. The neurologic assessment of an infant with ACP may be complicated, as these infants initially often have hypotonia, decreased muscle strength, and poor head control due to their macrocephaly. If pathologic cord compression is present and the problem is properly treated, infants with ACP are unlikely to die from cord necrosis. The risk of death in infants who have not had this evaluation and treatment approaches 7%.

The MRIs done on Baby A demonstrated a pathologically small foramen magnum, cervical stenosis, and ventriculomegaly, but the neurologic examination and the polysomnography were normal. At age 5 months, the neurosurgeon decompressed her with subsequent rapid improvement in motor strength. Even though the ventricles were enlarged, her head size was normal for an infant with ACP and the ventricular size was normal for her brain size. Head sizes in infants and children with ACP normally are larger than for the average child. Subsequently, Baby A's head size has remained within the normal range for individuals with ACP.

Because of the risk of sudden infant death, the diagnosis of ACP needs to be made as soon as possible, preferably in the newborn period. Making the diagnosis early allows for immediate parental counseling, and treatment if needed. The features seen in newborns and neonates with ACP include macrocephaly, frontal bossing, short nose with a depressed nasal bridge, midfacial hypoplasia, upper airway obstruction, mildly shortened arms and legs with the greatest shortening in the upper arms and thighs (rhizomelic shortening), limited elbow extension, and mild brachydactyly. The radiographic findings include a smaller than normal foramen magnum, parallel or decreasing interpedicular distance in the lumbar vertebrae, dysplastic ilia with a narrow sacroiliac groove, flat acetabular roof, ice cream scoop–appearing femoral head, and metaphyseal flaring. Many of the physical and radiographic features may be subtle in the first year, and as such, many newborns with ACP may look completely normal to the parents. This may delay their acceptance of the diagnosis and obtaining appropriate evaluation. ACP is inherited in an autosomal dominant mode with 80% of affected infants having average-sized parents and their condition representing new mutations in the egg or sperm that formed the child. The gene that causes ACP is the fibroblast growth factor receptor 3 gene.

Exercise 17 *Continued*

QUESTION

2. Which of the following statements about bone dysplasias are true?

   a. The majority of bone dysplasias are fatal in the neonatal period.

   b. The usual cause of death in a neonate with a lethal bone dysplasia is spinal cord necrosis.

   c. Some neonates with lethal bone dysplasias can survive long term with ventilator support.

   d. Thanatophoric dysplasia is a deadly bone dysplasia.

ANSWER

2. a. False. About 40 of the 380 or so bone dysplasias are considered fatal in the neonatal period.

   b. False. Respiratory insufficiency is the usual cause of death.

   c. True. Normally, however, these infants become ventilator dependent and do poorly. Some do get off support and survive.

   d. True.

The bone dysplasias are such a heterogeneous group that there is great variation in the features seen and the severity of different disorders. Severe bone dysplasias often cause death immediately after birth or in the neonatal period. Others may have only a few mild findings such as slight shortening of the limbs and asymmetry of the anterior chest. These mild findings are often seen in newborns with spondyloepiphyseal dysplasia congenita. In bone dysplasia with mild features, it may not be possible to make a specific diagnosis in the neonatal period by the clinical and radiographic findings. However, since the severity of most bone dysplasias worsens with age, one often can make the diagnosis later in infancy or in early childhood. In mild and "clinically undiagnosable" cases, the diagnosis can be made by molecular testing in some cases.

The three most common bone dysplasias diagnosed in the newborn and neonatal periods are ACP, osteogenesis imperfecta type 2, and thanatophoric dysplasia, the latter two being fatal in the neonatal period. OI type II is similar to OI type III but more severe and the median survival time is about 2 hours with 90% of patients dying within 4 weeks of birth. In thanatophoric dysplasia, death usually occurs within hours or a few days after birth unless there is intensive medical intervention. In the latter situation infants become ventilator dependent, and if they survive any length of time, they are mentally retarded and have severe growth deficiency. Even with intensive care management, most die during the first year of life. Lethality in bone dysplasias in the neonatal period usually is from respiratory insufficiency caused by a small chest and hypoplastic lungs secondary to the small chest. The small chest is a result of short and often nearly horizontal ribs.

Neuronal Migrational Disorders

Case Study 13

Baby N was a 36-week gestational age female who had multiple joint contractures at birth. She was born to a gravida 6 para 3 (3 abortions) 36-year-old black female. Pregnancy complications included polyhydramnios and preeclampsia. The infant was delivered by cesarean section for fetal decelerations. Baby N was limp and cyanotic at birth and required resuscitation. Birth length, weight, and OFC were 43 cm (15th percentile), 2.31 kg (30th percentile), and 32.5 cm (50th percentile), respectively. Significant findings on physical examination included contractures of all limbs with little movement; limited extension of the elbows, hips, and knees; depressed nasal bridge and micrognathia; camptodactyly of several fingers; mild but generalized reduction in muscle mass; decreased hip abduction; and bilateral clubfoot deformities. She also was hypotonic and had no reflexes. Several laboratory studies were obtained. Thyroxine-stimulating hormone (TSH), lactate, and pyruvate, and blood chromosomes, were normal. Serum creatine kinase was elevated (578 IU/L; normal 50 to 180) and T_4 was slightly elevated (22.06 μg/dL; normal 7.7 to 19.7). Serum cytomegalovirus and toxoplasmosis titers were absent and below 1:16, respectively. A CT scan of the head showed marked gyral malformation, lack of normal sylvian fissure

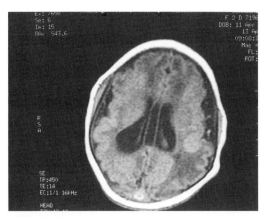

Figure 21-27 CT scan of the brain at 1 week of age of Baby N, who had the perisylvian syndrome. Note marked gyral malformations, lack of normal sylvian fissure development with incomplete opercularization, and prominent subarachnoid spaces and ventricles.

development with incomplete opercularization, and prominent subarachnoid spaces and ventricles (Fig. 21-27). An ophthalmologic examination was normal. Baby N began having seizures at 3 weeks. Because of her ventilatory dependency and poor prognosis, at 1 month of age the parents and attending staff elected to take her off the ventilator and allow her to die.

Exercise 18

QUESTION

1. Which of the following conditions is the most likely diagnosis for Baby N?

   a. Trisomy 13

   b. Arthrogryposis

   c. Miller-Dieker syndrome

   d. Perisylvian syndrome

   e. Fetal akinesia syndrome

ANSWER

1. b and d.

Arthrogryposis, also called congenital contractures, is defined as contractures that are present at birth and involve two or more major joints. The understanding of the underlying pathologic mechanisms producing arthrogryposis and classification of various arthrogrypotic conditions has evolved since the early 1970s, mainly because of the work of Judith G. Hall.[20]

The number of conditions where arthrogryposis is a feature now lists in the hundreds.

Arthrogryposis is produced most commonly by disorders involving the neurologic system, muscles, joints, or connective tissues.[20,21] Neurologic abnormalities are the most common etiologies. The condition develops in the fetus whenever there is prolonged restriction of joint movement. When fetal movement is restricted, the joint becomes "frozen," and at birth the child has contractures. Any condition that causes significant in utero restriction of movement, regardless of the etiology, will likely produce arthrogryposis.

Classic arthrogryposis and amyoplasia-type arthrogryposis are the most common types of arthrogryposis and are related conditions. However, the latter is more severe.[21] Limb involvement in either condition may involve one or any combination of extremities, and typically, the limbs are held in an extended position. Concomitant with the contractures, there is severe hypoplasia of the muscles of the involved limbs. Amyoplasia differs from classic arthrogryposis in that there is absence of muscles in one or more locations. Both of these types of arthrogryposis are thought to be due to congenital loss of anterior horn cells in the spinal cord, secondary to a transitory loss of spinal cord blood supply during fetal development. The segments of spinal cord involved in the ischemic process determine which limbs are affected. These two conditions do not appear to be inherited. Baby N did not have classic or amyoplasia-type of arthrogryposis; her limbs were flexed rather than extended.

The evaluation of a newborn with arthrogryposis normally should include (1) an MRI or CT scan of the head to determine if there are congenital anomalies of the brain; (2) an MRI of the spine; (3) a serum creatine kinase (CK) level to detect muscular dystrophy; (4) nerve conduction studies; (5) an electromyogram; (6) neostigmine challenge test to detect myasthenia gravis; and (7) examination of the baby's mother looking for signs of myotonic dystrophy. If the mother does exhibit signs of myotonic dystrophy, then gene testing should be done on the neonate. If the patient were to die, a complete autopsy should be done. Treatment consists of vigorous physical therapy to gain range of motion of involved joints and to improve the strength of those muscles present. Casting of these patients should be limited, and any cast applied should be removable to allow for frequent physical therapy. Baby N clearly had an abnormal brain, which presumably produced her arthrogryposis.

One of the brain malformations that can cause arthrogryposis is perisylvian syndrome. Although rare, this syndrome is one of three dozen neuronal migrational disorders that have been well characterized. The significant features of the perisylvian syndrome include deficiency of cortex around the sylvian fissures, leading in most cases to pseudobulbar palsy (i.e., limited tongue movement, dysarthria, mastication difficulties, drooling, dysphagia and facial weakness); seizures that are refractory to treatment; poor motor skills; and mild to moderate mental retardation with delayed language acquisition. Limited tongue movement significantly contributes to patients' oral difficulties. In addition to these findings, about 10% of affected individuals have associated arthrogryposis. Baby N had the typical CNS findings as well as arthrogryposis seen in this syndrome and apparently had the disorder. No gene testing is currently available for the perisylvian syndrome.

This case illustrates one type of congenital anomaly of the central nervous system (CNS). There are hundreds of other recognized anomalies of the CNS, with the more common ones being neural tube defects, primarily anencephaly, encephalocele, and meningomyelocele; Dandy-Walker malformation; Arnold-Chiari malformation; agenesis of the corpus callosum and congenital hydrocephaly; holoprosencephaly; porencephaly and its more severe form hydranencephaly. The etiology of each of these defects is heterogeneous, and often genetically or partly genetically determined. The physical and neurologic findings in the neonate with these CNS defects are highly variable but often include microcephaly or macrocephaly, hypotonia or hypertonia, seizures, arthrogryposis, weakness, and paralysis. Younger children with anomalies often exhibit developmental delay, and older children have mental retardation. CT scan or MRI of the brain will detect most of these disorders; however, if a defect is not detected during the neonatal period, one should repeat a brain MRI after the age of 6 months.

The neural migrational disorders (NMDs) are a group of congenital disorders produced when neurons do not migrate to their proper location. This results in a brain that is wired incorrectly and functions abnormally. Some of the better known NMDs are isolated lissencephaly syndrome (ILS); the related disorder, Miller-Dieker syndrome (which is a contiguous gene deletion disorder involving the *LIS1* gene, the gene that causes ILS); X-linked isolated lissencephaly (caused by a mutation in the gene doublecortin [DCX]); Walker-Warburg syndrome, produced by a defect in *O*-mannosyl glycosylation; microlissencephaly, which is associated with severe microcephaly; polymicrogyria disorders, which include the perisylvian syndrome; schizencephaly; and periventricular nodular heterotopia. In all these syndromes there is a lack of normal formation of cerebral gyri and sulci, resulting in a relatively smooth brain surface (lissencephaly), microgyri or pachygyri, or a combination of these abnormalities.

The following should be considered in the evaluation of a neonate with suspected NMD: (1) obtaining an extensive pregnancy and family history; (2) careful dysmorphologic examination including head circumference measurement; (3) ophthalmologic examination; (4) serum creatine kinase, which is elevated in Walker-Warburg syndrome and related disorders; (5) standard chromosomal analysis; and (6) *LIS1* and *DOC* gene testing. Gene testing may also be available for other NMDs.

Teratogens

Exercise 19

QUESTION

1. Which of the following statements about teratogens are true?

    a. Teratogens are environmental agents that adversely affect the embryo or fetus.

    b. Teratogen-related birth defects occur in fewer than 1% of newborns.

    c. The most common human teratogen is ethanol (alcohol).

    d. Consumption of alcohol during a pregnancy can produce fetal alcohol spectrum disorder.

ANSWER

1. a. True.

    b. False.

    c. False.

    d. True.

If one examines the etiology of birth defects, one finds that approximately 10% of all birth defects are produced by recognized environmental exposures during the pregnancy. The most common teratogen is smoking, and about a fifth of all women in the United States smoke during their pregnancies. The most significant teratogen is ethanol. When used in relatively large amounts, ethanol can result in fetal alcohol syndrome (FAS), and in lesser amounts it results in less severe disorders (i.e., partial FAS and alcohol-related neurodevelopmental disorder).[22] Table 21-6 lists a number of other human teratogens.

The following case study illustrates the effects that a teratogen may have on a fetus and the importance of obtaining a detailed pregnancy history.

Case Study 14

Baby U was born at 38 weeks' gestation after a pregnancy complicated by maternal seizures and valproic acid exposure. This was the first pregnancy of the mother, an American Indian, who was 19 years old at the time of the birth. The mother had received anticonvulsant therapy since her early teenage years. When she became pregnant, she was taking valproic acid, 250 mg three times a day, and continued at this dose throughout the pregnancy. A prenatal ultrasound indicated double outlet right ventricle (DORV) defect and absent left radius. The delivery was unremarkable. In addition to these anomalies, Baby U had a small, rudimentary, and low-set right ear (Fig. 21-28); right auricular ear tag (see Fig. 21-28); absent right external auditory canal; prominent nasal bridge (see Fig. 21-28); telecanthus (Fig. 21-29); lateral nasal fullness (see Fig. 21-29); smooth philtrum (see Fig. 21-29); thin upper lip (see Fig. 21-29); hypoplastic right mandible with apparent missing right ramus; hypoplastic left ulna (Fig. 21-30); absence of the left thumb (see Fig. 21-30); syndactyly of the second and third left fingers; and camptodactyly of the second, third, and fourth left fingers. There was an average sized sacral dimple, but the spine and back were otherwise normal. An echocardiogram demonstrated the DORV, a large ventricular septal defect, right ventricle hypertrophy, and an atrial septal defect. The infant's length, weight, and OFC were 46.5 cm (3rd percentile), 2.55 kg (3rd percentile), and 32 cm (3rd percentile), respectively. Problems in the immediate neonatal period included mild respiratory distress, which required mechanical ventilation for 2 days followed by supplemental nasal oxygen, and feeding difficulties, which necessitated nasogastric tube feedings and then a gastric feeding tube. Her cardiac problems were managed with medications; surgery was slated for later in infancy. Laboratory testing that included standard serum chemical tests and

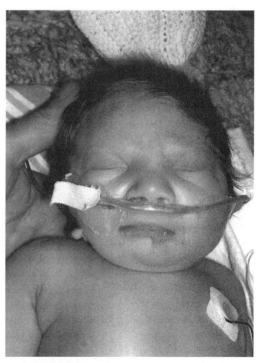

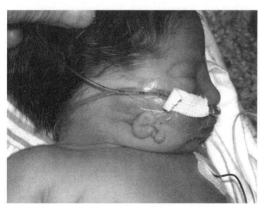

Figure 21-28 Lateral facial view of Baby U with the valproate embryopathy. Observe the small, rudimentary and low-set right ear; right auricular ear tag; and prominent nasal bridge.

Figure 21-29 Facial view of Baby U with the valproate embryopathy. Note the telecanthus, lateral nasal fullness, smooth philtrum, and thin upper lip.

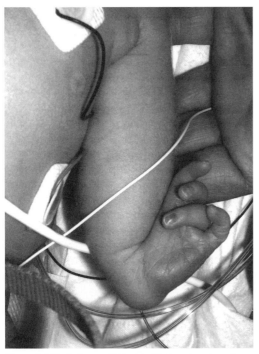

Figure 21-30 Left arm of Baby U with the valproate embry-opathy. Note the shortening of the forearm, absence of the left thumb, and abnormal positioning of the fingers.

7-dehydrocholesterol was normal. A serum fibrinogen was 404 mg/dL with normal being 200 to 400 mg/dL. The family history was remarkable for a maternal grandfather who died from a seizure, and a maternal first cousin who had a congenital heart defect.

Exercise 20

QUESTION

1. What is the most likely cause of Baby U's multiple congenital anomalies?

   a. Fetal alcohol syndrome

   b. Trisomy 13

   c. Oculoauriculovertebral spectrum

   d. Valproate embryopathy

   e. Holt-Oram syndrome

ANSWER

1. d.

It would be unusual for a child with the FAS to have such severe birth defects as were seen in Baby U, although significant defects of the brain and heart can occur in individuals with FAS. Trisomy 13 would be more likely because auricular defects, major congenital heart defects, and radial agenesis have been reported in this condition. However, a subsequent chromosomal analysis on Baby U was normal (46,XX). Oculoauriculovertebral (OAV) spectrum is a condition with marked variation in severity among affected individuals. The common features include colobomata of the eyes, facial asymmetry with one side typically being small, microtia of varying severity, multiple vertebral malformations, and congenital heart defects. Limb defects are not normally a feature of this disorder. Holt-Oram syndrome can have all the limb anomalies seen in Baby U, but the heart defects are not normally as severe, and the ear and facial defects are not typical of Holt-Oram syndrome. Valproate embryopathy, also known as fetal valproate syndrome, is characterized by epicanthal folds, telecanthus, smooth philtrum, thin upper lip, cleft lip, congenital heart defects of varying severity, growth deficiency, mental retardation, and occasionally upper limb defects. Between 1% and 2% of exposed fetuses also will have a lumbar meningomyelocele. Because Baby U does not clearly fit into any other condition and was exposed to valproic acid prenatally, the likely diagnosis is valproate embryopathy.

The case of Baby U illustrates that some teratogens can cause major birth defects. A careful prenatal history including asking about teratogen exposure certainly is warranted for any neonate who has congenital anomalies of unknown etiology.

Inborn Errors of Metabolism

Inborn errors of metabolism are genetically determined biochemical abnormalities of the body. Most disorders are due to a single defective enzyme (protein) that disrupts a metabolic pathway at a specific pathway location. The blockage normally leads to an excessive accumulation of one or more precursor compounds and to a deficiency of the reaction product. The clinical manifestations of a condition depend on the relative deficiency of the enzyme/protein, alternative metabolic pathways that are available, and the actual pathway involved.

On occasion, neonatologists will encounter patients with acute, and sometimes chronic, inborn errors of metabolism. Because of these possibilities, neonatologists and others caring for neonates and infants need to be aware of metabolic conditions and to keep in mind that any patient could have one of these conditions. Failure to diagnoses and properly treat patients with acute metabolic states can ultimately lead to their demise. Untreated chronic metabolic errors, on the other hand, can lead to long-term complications including failure to thrive and mental retardation. The following case illustrates some of these points.

Case Study 15

Baby L was born at term by a spontaneous vaginal delivery to a gravida 2 para 2 mother whose pregnancy was uncomplicated. Birth length and weight were appropriate for gestational age. The OFC was not recorded. The baby was discharged with her mother on the second day of life apparently in good health. On the following day, the neonate ate poorly and was somewhat lethargic. On the fourth day, she began vomiting all feedings and was much more lethargic. At this point her pediatrician evaluated her and recommended an immediate NICU admission. At the time of admission, she was semiconscious, responding only to painful stimulation. She also was moderately dehydrated and was having periodic jerking episodes.

On a quick examination, Baby L appeared to be physically normal (Fig. 21-31) other than for her dehydration. The neonatologist on duty suspected that she had an acute metabolic disorder and wanted to begin treatment immediately.

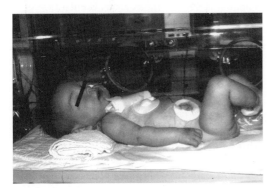

Figure 21-31 Five-day-old female Baby L with methylmalonic acidemia. Other than the micrognathia and posteriorly rotated ears, the neonate was not dysmorphic.

Exercise 21

QUESTIONS

1. Before beginning treatment of Baby L, which of the following samples should be obtained?
   a. Serum electrolytes
   b. Blood glucose
   c. Serum bicarbonate
   d. Serum ammonia
   e. Serum quantitative amino acids
   f. Serum organic and short-chain fatty acids
   g. Serum lactic and pyruvic acids
   h. Urine for genetic screening for metabolic disorders

2. After initial samples have been collected, which of the following life support measures should be started?
   a. Intubation and ventilation
   b. Intravenous fluids with glucose
   c. Hypotensive treatment
   d. Septic workup and treatment with antibiotics
   e. Consult a clinical geneticist/metabolic specialist

ANSWERS

1. All of the above. In suspected cases of acute metabolic disease, it is important to obtain, if possible, blood and urine prior to initiating treatment. Treatment may make it more difficult to determine an exact diagnosis. Urine testing should include spot testing for reducing substances, ketones, specific gravity, pH, ferric chloride, unusual odor, and amino acid and organic acid levels. Additional evaluation will be dictated by the clinical assessment of the patient.

2. a, b, c, and d. A clinical geneticist who has had experience with metabolic disorders should be consulted but doing so would not be an initial step.

Baby L was mildly hypotensive, hypernatremic, hyperkalemic, and acidotic with an arterial pH of 7.1 and a serum bicarbonate of 8 mEq/L. Over the next 24 hours, she was maintained on intravenous fluids with added electrolytes, glucose, and bicarbonate. Her condition stabilized, she stopped seizing, and she became more responsive, although she was now hypotonic.

In addition to numerous other evaluations and consultations, the physicians in charge obtained a metabolic consultation. The consultant agreed that the most likely diagnosis was a metabolic disorder, and recommended several tests to determine what condition she might have. Baby L was found to have hyperammonemia with a serum value of 865 µg/dL (normal range age 0 to 2 weeks = 79 to 130), a serum methylmalonic acid of 38 mmol/L (normal = <0.2 for all ages), decreased level of total and free carnitine, and elevated levels of urine methylmalonic acid, methylcitrate, propionic acid, and 3-hydroxypropionic acid with the highest amounts being methylmalonic acid. Subsequent evaluation showed that Baby L has very low levels of leukocytic methylmalonyl-CoA mutase, confirming her diagnosis of methylmalonic acidemia.

QUESTION

3. From the following list, identify the signs or symptoms of metabolic diseases that can be seen in neonates.

Abnormal odor	Apnea	Coma
Congenital anomalies	Vomiting	Diarrhea
	Hypoglycemia	Hypotension
Hypertonia	Lethargy	Metabolic acidosis
Hypotonia	Poor feeding	
Jaundice	Tachypnea	Seizures
Spasticity		

ANSWER

3. All of these signs and symptoms may be manifestations of inborn errors of metabolism in neonates. When any of these findings are present in a patient, a metabolic derangement must be considered. Diagnosis is important not only to prevent disabilities and death, but also to counsel the family about recurrence risks.

Because the condition of a patient suspected of having a metabolic disorder may be exacerbated by feedings (particularly those containing proteins or amino acids), all oral feedings should be withheld. Rather, support of such a neonate should be by intravenous administration of appropriate electrolytes; serum glucose concentrations should be maintained at the high end of normal, and bicarbonate adminis-

tered if acidosis is present. Once the risk of a metabolic disorder has been eliminated, oral feedings may be introduced. If a metabolic disease is diagnosed, oral feedings may be introduced using a special formula designed for the particular condition, regular formula if there are other means for treating the condition, or formula that does not cause a problem.

Baby L had methylmalonic acidemia (MMA), a paradigm for an inborn error of metabolism. The condition is named for the fact that there are high blood levels of methylmalonic acid in untreated patients who have been ingesting protein in their diet. The elevated methylmalonic acid is due to decreased activity of the adenosylcobalamin-dependent enzyme, methylmalonyl-CoA mutase, which converts l-methylmalonyl CoA to succinyl CoA. l-Methylmalonyl-CoA is in the pathway of the metabolism of the amino acids methionine, isoleucine, valine, and threonine. Methylmalonyl-CoA mutase may be completely absent, which produces the most severe form of MMA. Patients with complete absence of this enzyme rapidly become ill and may die if not treated in the first few days of life. Individuals with partial absence of methylmalonyl-CoA mutase have an intermediate form of the disease. Neonates with the intermediate form normally become sick in the first 2 weeks and with treatment do better than those with complete absence of the enzyme. Since methylmalonyl-CoA mutase is a cobalamin-dependent enzyme, there is a third form of MMA produced by defective intracellular cobalamin metabolism. This form of MMA often has the onset of the illness during infancy precipitated by an acute illness such as a viral infection. This form of MMA often responds to the administration of hydroxyvitamin B_{12}, a form of vitamin B_{12} (cobalamin). In neonates with absence of or partial deficiency of methylmalonyl-CoA mutase, the treatment consists of restricting the intake of methionine, isoleucine, valine, and threonine by limiting protein intact or providing a formula low in these amino acids. Because carnitine is also frequently low in these neonates, supplemental carnitine may be beneficial. Like most enzyme-deficient disorders, MMA is rare, with an incidence of about 1 in 50,000 newborns. It also is inherited as an autosomal recessive disorder.

Methylmalonic acidemia is one of a number of conditions that can be diagnosed by newborn screening techniques. Many states in the United States are now screening for over 30 different conditions, most of which are inborn errors of metabolism. The increased number of disorders that can be detected by newborn screening is made possible by a relatively new technique referred to as tandem mass spectrometry. Not all metabolic conditions that are detected by newborn screening, however, produce an acute metabolic state. Therefore, neonates with these latter conditions normally are not admitted to an NICU and may not be seen by a neonatologist. For example, phenylketonuria (PKU) is associated with a massive buildup of phenylalanine secondary to a block in the conversion of phenylalanine to tyrosine. This blockage occurs because of a deficiency of the enzyme phenylalanine hydroxylase. Although the high levels of phenylalanine seen in phenylketonuria are toxic to brain development and result in mental retardation in the untreated patient, the metabolic derangement does not lead to a metabolic crisis, e.g., acidosis. For more detailed information about this and other metabolic disorders, consult Wappner and Hainline,[23] Scriver and associates,[24] and Nyhan and associates.[25]

Information on Genetic Disorders and Laboratories Doing Specialized Genetic Testing

The pace of discovery of new genetic disorders and genes is incredibly rapid. McKusick's *Online Catalog of Mendelian Inheritance in Man,*[12] a catalogue that lists the recognized genetic conditions and genes in humans, exceeded 16,416 entries as of December 2005. Dozens of new journals, such as *Nature Genetics,* have been established to handle many of the articles reporting new genes and genetic conditions. To make matters even more challenging, for certain genetic disorders hundreds or even thousands of articles have been published. For instance, as of December 2005, there were 952 articles cited in the Ovid Medline database that made reference to the genetics of cystic fibrosis.

Along with the rapid influx of new genetic information has been the development of systems to access this information. Much of this information is now stored in databases that are accessible through the Internet. These various databases address specific informational needs of health care workers, researchers, and lay individuals. So extensive are these reference sources that one can now find specific information on a particular condition, the molecular genetic aspect of the disorder, laboratories doing testing for the condition, and support groups for the family.

Summary

Neonatologists or other neonatal care providers must keep in mind that birth defects and genetic disorders are common and occur in a sizable proportion of their patient population. In today's medical climate, our understanding of and ability to test for genetic disorders changes daily and will continue to do so for the immediate future. It is, therefore, incumbent upon care providers to consult a clinical geneticist or other appropriate clinicians in cases of suspected genetic disorders and birth defects. It is important to establish a diagnosis in order to determine potential complications and the short- and long-term prognosis of the condition. A diagnosis also allows an understanding of the genetics involved, the recurrence risk in subsequent siblings, and the availability of prenatal testing for future pregnancies.

Acknowledgments

The editorial assistance of Pamela Weaver, M.Ed., is greatly appreciated and acknowledged.

References

1. Marden PM, Smith DW, McDonald MJ: Congenital anomalies in the newborn infant, including minor variations. J Pediatr 1964;64:357–371.
2. Kanto WP, Flannery DB: Genetic disorders and major congenital anomalies in a neonatal intensive care unit. Am J Hum Genet 1985;37:A221.
3. Weaver D: Unpublished data, 2005.
4. Hall JG, Powers EK, McIlvaine RT, Ean VH: The frequency and financial burden of genetic disease in a pediatric hospital. Am J Med Genet 1978;1:417–436.
5. Dobyns WB, Filauro A, Tomson BN, et al: Inheritance of most X-linked traits is not dominant or recessive, just X-linked. Am J Med Genet 2004;129A:136–143.
6. Watson JD: The Double Helix: A Personal Account of the Discovery of the Structure of DNA. New York, WW Norton, 1980.
7. Hodes ME: Introduction to molecular genetics. Cancer Invest 1997;15:322–325.

8. McPherson E, Carey J, Kramer A, et al: Dominantly inherited renal adysplasia. Am J Med Genet 1987;26:863–872.

9. Smith DW: Dysmorphology (teratology). J Pediatr 1966;69:1150–1169.

10. Gorlin RJ, Cohen MM Jr, Levin LS: Syndromes of the Head and Neck, 3rd ed. New York, Oxford University Press, 1990.

11. Seashore MR, Wappner RS: Genetics in Primary Care and Clinical Medicine. 1996, Stamford, CT, Appleton & Lange, pp 217–221.

12. McKusick VA: Online Mendelian Inheritance in Man. Accessed at http://www3.ncbi.nlm.nih.gov/Omim/, 2005.

13. Hansmann M, Gembruch U, Bald R: New therapeutic aspects in nonimmune hydrops fetalis based on four hundred and two prenatally diagnosed cases. Fetal Ther 1989;4:29–36.

14. Brown BS: The ultrasonographic features of nonimmune hydrops fetalis: A study of 30 successive patients. J Can Assoc Radiol 1986;37:164–168.

15. Machin GA: Hydrops revisited: Literature review of 1,414 cases published in the 1980s. Am J Med Genet 1989;34:366–390.

16. Philip J: The prenatal diagnosis and management of congenital malformations in the third trimester of pregnancy. In Milunsky A (ed): Genetic Disorders and the Fetus: Diagnosis, Prevention and Treatment, 3rd ed. Baltimore, Johns Hopkins University Press, 1992, pp 693–694.

17. Wheeler PG, Weaver DD, Palmer CG: Familial translocation resulting in Wolf-Hirschhorn syndrome in two related unbalanced individuals: Clinical evaluation of a 39-year-old man with Wolf-Hirschhorn syndrome. Am J Med Genet 1995;55:462–465.

18. Mcdonald-Mcginn DM, Emanual BS, Zackai EH: 22 q11.2 deletion syndrome. Gene Rev 2005. Accessed at http://www.genetests.org.

19. Wheeler PG, Weaver DD, Obeime MO, et al: Urorectal septum malformation sequence: Report of thirteen additional cases and review of the literature. Am J Med Genet 1997;73:456–462.

20. Hall JG: Arthrogryposis. Am Fam Physician 1989;39:113–119.

21. Sells JM, Jaffe KM, Hall JG: Amyoplasia, the most common type of arthrogryposis: The potential for good outcome. Pediatrics 1996;97:225–231.

22. Sampson PD, Streissguth AP, Bookstein FL, et al: Incidence of fetal alcohol syndrome and prevalence of alcohol-related neurodevelopmental disorder. Teratology 1997;56:317–326.

23. Wappner RS, Hainline BE: Inborn errors of metabolism. In McMillan JA, Deangelis CD, Feign RD, Warshaw JB (eds): Oski's Pediatrics: Principles and Practice, 3rd ed. Philadelphia, Lippincott Williams & Wilkins, 1999, pp 1822–1900.

24. Scriver CR, Beaudet AL, Sly WS, et al (eds): The Metabolic and Molecular Basis of Metabolic Diseases. New York, McGraw-Hill, 2001.

25. Nyhan WL, Barshop BA, Ozand PR: Atlas of Metabolic Diseases. London, Hodder Arnold, 2nd ed. London, Hodder Arnold, 2005.

Surgical Emergencies in the Newborn

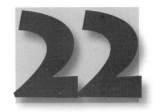

Robert A. Cowles, MD, and Steven Stylianos, MD

Surgical emergencies in newborns are quite varied, and rapid identification of surgically treatable conditions with appropriate surgical consultation can significantly affect the eventual outcome. In this chapter, we will discuss many of the major newborn emergencies that warrant urgent surgical evaluation and treatment. Not all conditions require operative treatment; however, the surgeon remains an important member of the multidisciplinary team. The text is divided in sections based on the common patient presentation. Each section will begin with a descriptive case followed by a discussion of the pertinent issues, options, and expectations. Necrotizing enterocolitis, an important abdominal emergency in the premature newborn, will be discussed in detail in a separate section of this book and therefore will not be covered here.

Emergencies of the Trachea, Esophagus, and Thorax

Case Study 1

A newborn in the nursery is noted to quickly vomit the initial feedings and appears to have excessive drooling. An orogastric tube is placed but cannot be advanced owing to resistance. The infant is nearly full term but no other prenatal history is immediately available. A chest x-ray shows the orogastric tube is coiled in the proximal esophagus (Fig. 22-1).

Exercise 1

QUESTIONS

1. Which of the following are appropriate next step(s) in the care of this newborn?
   a. Re-placement of the orogastric tube until it clearly passes into the stomach
   b. Formal upper gastrointestinal (GI) barium contrast study to assess for patency of esophagus, stomach, and duodenum
   c. Endotracheal intubation
   d. Change in formula and reattempt oral feedings
   e. None of the above

2. Which of the following are important factor(s) that should have been included in his prenatal evaluations?
   a. Presence of polyhydramnios
   b. Size of fetal stomach
   c. Presence of cardiac defects
   d. Presence of renal defects
   e. All of the above

3. Which of the following imaging modalities is appropriate for this baby?
   a. Abdominal x-ray
   b. Renal ultrasound
   c. Echocardiogram
   d. Barium enema
   e. a, b, and c only

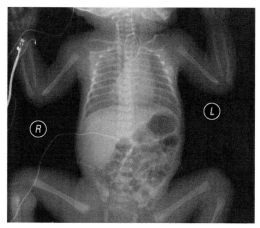

Figure 22-1 Neonate with orogastric tube coiled in the esophagus and a normal distal bowel gas pattern.

The abdominal x-ray shows a normal bowel gas pattern (see Fig. 22-1). Other imaging studies fail to show associated abnormalities. The baby is stable on room air and is prepared for surgical correction.

4. Based on the information you have, what is your diagnosis of the child?

   a. Isolated (pure) esophageal atresia without fistula

   b. Esophageal atresia with distal tracheoesophageal fistula

   c. Esophageal atresia with proximal tracheoesophageal fistula

   d. Pyloric stenosis

   e. Tracheal stenosis

5. Which are the most important factor(s) affecting outcome of a newborn with esophageal atresia and tracheoesophageal fistula?

   a. Presence of imperforate anus

   b. Severe congenital heart disease

   c. Size of the patent ductus arteriosus

   d. Gestational age of 37 weeks

   e. Evidence of a small stomach on prenatal ultrasound

ANSWERS

1. e.

2. e.

3. e.

4. b.

5. b.

Esophageal atresia with tracheoesophageal fistula (EA/TEF) occurs in about 1 in 2500 births and results from abnormal separation of the trachea from the esophagus during development.[1] Newborns with esophageal atresia with (or without) tracheoesophageal fistula most commonly present with excessive drooling and poor tolerance of initial oral feedings. Polyhydramnios with a diminutive fetal stomach can suggest the presence of esophageal atresia but definitive prenatal diagnosis is not routine. Attempts at placement of an orogastric tube that are met with unusual resistance and a chest x-ray showing the tube coiled in the proximal esophagus (see Fig. 22-1) are considered classic findings.[2,3] A dilated, air-filled proximal esophagus can also commonly be appreciated. These findings are sufficient to make a diagnosis of esophageal atresia. Formal upper GI contrast studies or further attempts to pass a nasogastric tube can be hazardous and are discouraged.[3]

A general survey for associated anomalies should be conducted. EA/TEF is part of the VACTERL association and, therefore, a specific search for vertebral, anal, cardiac, renal, and limb anomalies should be undertaken. This evaluation can be completed with a careful physical examination, plain x-rays, ultrasound (spinal and renal), and an echocardiogram. The child's respiratory function should be supported as conservatively as possible. Intubation with positive pressure ventilation should be avoided unless absolutely necessary because much of the tidal volume in this scenario would be lost via the fistula into the stomach. If intubation and mechanical ventilation are felt to be necessary, a surgeon should be contacted in the event that urgent gastrostomy or ligation of the fistula becomes necessary.

EA/TEF can have five different anatomic varieties (Fig. 22-2), with the most common involving esophageal atresia and distal tracheoesophageal fistula. Any configuration that includes a distal fistula should show air in the gastrointestinal tract, often in a normal configuration, while those with pure or isolated esophageal atresia have a gasless abdomen on abdominal x-ray (Fig. 22-3).

Operative repair of EA/TEF most often involves a thoracotomy with esophageal anastomosis and closure of the tracheoesophageal fistula. In pure esophageal atresia without fistula, the first operation is commonly a feeding gastrostomy as there is often a large gap between the two esophageal ends. Newborns with

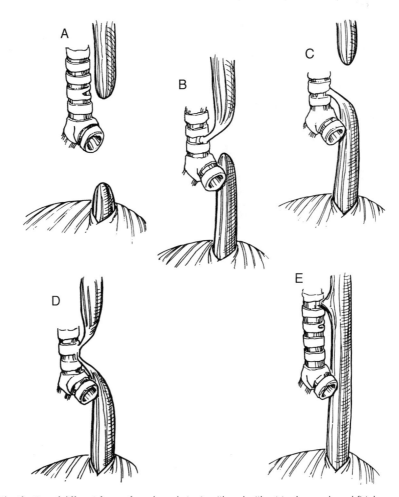

Figure 22-2 Classification of different forms of esophageal atresia with and without tracheoesophageal fistula.

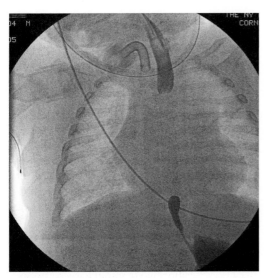

Figure 22-3 Contrast study in a child with isolated esophageal atresia. Note the gap of seven vertebral bodies between the proximal and distal ends of the esophagus.

concurrent EA/TEF, severe congenital heart disease and very low birth weight are particularly challenging cases and have been shown to be poor candidates for full one-stage repair.[4] These frail newborns may benefit from a staged approach beginning with a decompressive gastrostomy, with or without division of the tracheoesophageal fistula, followed by complete repair at a later time.

Case Study 2

You are called to the neonatal intensive care unit (NICU) for a 2-day-old term infant with progressive respiratory distress. Physical examination suggests hyperinflation of the left hemithorax and shift of the apical cardiac impulse to the right. chest x-ray reveals a hyperinflated left upper lobe (Fig. 22-4).

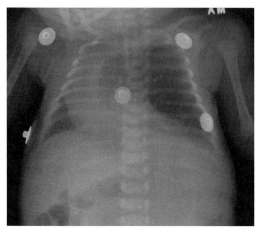

Figure 22-4 Chest x-ray of a newborn showing a hyperinflated left upper lobe with mediastinal shift toward the right.

Exercise 2

QUESTIONS

1. Other expected findings on chest x-ray include which of the following?

   a. Mediastinal shift to the right

   b. Atelectasis of the left lower lobe

   c. Flattening of the left hemidiaphragm

   d. Herniation of the affected lobe across the midline

   e. All of the above

2. What is the most common cause of congenital lobar emphysema?

   a. Aspiration of meconium

   b. Maternal smoking

   c. Deficiency of bronchial cartilage

   d. Vascular ring

   e. Enlargement of the thymus

3. Which of the following treatments can worsen the respiratory insufficiency in infants with congenital lobar emphysema?

   a. Nasal O_2

   b. Stop oral feeds

   c. Selective ventilation of the nonemphysematous lung

   d. Endotracheal intubation and nonselective mechanical ventilation

   e. Bronchodilators

4. *Emergency* thoracotomy and lobectomy are indicated in infants with suspected congenital lobar emphysema (see Fig. 22-4) in which of the following situations?

   a. Even if the infant is asymptomatic

   b. When herniation of affected lobe has caused cardiovascular decompensation

   c. If nasal O_2 is required

   d. When nonbilious emesis occurs

   e. When extrinsic vascular compression of the bronchus is suspected

ANSWERS

1. e.

2. c.

3. d.

4. b.

Infants with congenital lobar emphysema (CLE) have overdistention of one lobe which produces compression and atelectasis of adjacent lobes. If severe, the affected lobe can herniate across the mediastinum and cause mediastinal shift. Fifty percent of infants with CLE present within the first 48 hours of life. The most common cause is deficiency of bronchial cartilage leading to progressive air trapping. Other causes include extrinsic compression of the bronchus by abnormal vascular structures and polyalveolar lobe.[5] The left upper lobe is most commonly affected (see Fig. 22-4), followed by the right middle lobe.[6] Positive pressure ventilation may worsen the air trapping and lead to respiratory decompensation. Selective ventilation of the nonemphysematous lung can be helpful but requires bronchial blockade, which is technically difficult in newborns. Emergency thoracotomy and lobectomy are occasionally needed when unexpected respiratory decompensation occurs (Fig. 22-5).

Lung herniation across the mediastinum due to contralateral pulmonary hypoplasia or agenesis is important to consider. The normal lung that extends across the midline is *not* hyperinflated or emphysematous in cases of pulmonary hypoplasia or agenesis.

The other common congenital lung lesions, such as congenital cystic adenomatoid malformations (CCAMs) and bronchopulmonary sequestrations (BPSs), are sometimes noted in the perinatal period. These do not commonly present as emergencies and can be evaluated by a pediatric surgeon on an elective basis.

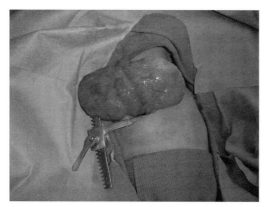

Figure 22-5 Operative photograph taken during resection of an emphysematous lobe. (See also Color Plate.)

Case Study 3

You are called to the NICU for a term baby in severe respiratory distress. The baby has a scaphoid abdomen, and an antenatal ultrasound suggests an abnormal stomach position.

Exercise 3

QUESTIONS

1. What is the best initial diagnostic test?
   a. Chest computed tomography (CT)
   b. Abdominal magnetic resonance imaging (MRI)
   c. Plain radiograph including abdomen and chest
   d. Umbilical vein venogram
   e. Umbilical artery angiogram

2. The pre- and postductal oxygen saturation monitors read 90% and 65%, respectively, while the infant is on the ventilator with an F_{IO_2} of 1.0. The best initial treatment plan would include which of the following?
   a. Emergency thoracotomy in the NICU
   b. Pharmacologic paralysis and high-pressure ventilation
   c. ECMO (extracorporeal membrane oxygenation)
   d. Gentle mechanical ventilation without paralysis to minimize barotrauma
   e. Bilateral chest tubes

ANSWERS

1. c.
2. d.

The most common type of congenital diaphragmatic hernia (CDH) is posterolateral. This occurs in about 1 in every 4000 babies and most (80%) are on the left side. Patients with CDH have respiratory insufficiency due to developmental abnormalities resulting in lung hypoplasia and pulmonary hypertension. Nonoxygenated blood is "shunted" into the systemic circulation via the foramen ovale and the patent ductus arteriosus (PDA). The contralateral lung is compressed and can be damaged by overeager ventilatory pressures. Under the microscope, these lungs look immature as well. Although both lungs are small, the ipsilateral lung demonstrates pulmonary arterial hyperplasia. In selected cases, inhaled nitric oxide can help lower the high pulmonary vascular resistance.

Many diaphragmatic hernias are discovered before birth on routine prenatal ultrasound, which allows for a planned delivery at a neonatal referral center.[7] Prenatal intervention has been studied but is experimental and not commonplace.[8] At birth, a scaphoid abdomen is found and radiographs show intestine in the chest cavity (Fig. 22-6). Cystic lung lesions may occasionally be mistaken for CDH. These conditions can be differentiated by passing a nasogastric tube or by upper GI series.

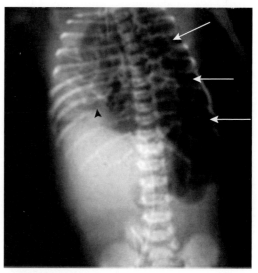

Figure 22-6 Chest x-ray showing loops of intestine in the left chest (*white arrows*) with mediastinal shift toward the right (*arrowhead*).

All newborns with CDH require surgery. The timing of surgery has changed over the past 20 years from an immediate emergency procedure to a planned procedure, days after birth, once evidence of pulmonary hypertension has resolved.[9,10] Monitoring pre- and postductal oxygen saturations is quite useful. ECMO is reserved for those babies who fail all ventilatory and pharmacologic strategies.

Emergencies of the Abdominal Wall

Case Study 4

You are called by a small community hospital where a 34-week gestation, 1900-g boy with an abdominal wall defect was just delivered. The child is vigorous and appears healthy with no other obvious abnormalities. The pediatrician caring for this newborn tells you that there is a large amount of intestine outside the baby's abdomen and that the bowel appears thickened, stiff, and leathery (Fig. 22-7). The actual defect is difficult to visualize under the loops of exposed intestine. The vital signs are stable.

Exercise 4

QUESTIONS

1. This description most classically illustrates what kind of abdominal defect?
   a. Ruptured umbilical hernia
   b. Omphalocele
   c. Gastroschisis

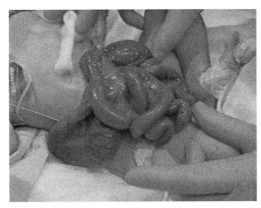

Figure 22-7 Abdominal wall defect with exposed viscera. (See also Color Plate.)

   d. Pentalogy of Cantrell
   e. Epigastric hernia

2. Appropriate instructions for the outside institution prior to transfer include which of the following?
   a. Placement of a nasogastric tube
   b. Placement of an umbilical arterial catheter
   c. Coverage of the exposed intestine with a plastic bowel bag
   d. a and c only
   e. a, b, and c

Upon arrival, the child is stable and you identify the lesion as gastroschisis. The baby is taken to the operating room for attempt at primary closure of the defect.

3. Appropriate preparation of this baby for surgery includes which of the following?
   a. Endotracheal intubation
   b. Establishing secure access for intravenous fluids
   c. Positioning of the bowel to avoid kinking of the mesenteric blood supply
   d. Placing the newborn in a warmed environment
   e. All of the above

4. Which of the following abnormalities are commonly seen in association with gastroschisis?
   a. Hypoplastic left-sided heart syndrome
   b. Jejunal atresia
   c. Malrotation
   d. Biliary atresia
   e. b and c only

5. Which are signs that the baby is developing abdominal compartment syndrome?
   a. Decreased urine output
   b. Increasing P_{CO_2}
   c. Firmness on abdominal examination
   d. Venous congestion of the lower extremities
   e. All of the above

ANSWERS

1. c.
2. d.
3. e.

4. e.

5. e.

The major abdominal wall defects seen in neonates include omphalocele and gastroschisis. Inguinal and umbilical hernias can be considered milder abdominal wall defects but can become a surgical emergency in the NICU. Both types of defects can be seen on prenatal ultrasound, giving the neonatologist and surgeon time to plan the perinatal and postnatal care.[11-13] Gastroschisis can be differentiated from omphalocele based on several aspects.[11] First, the size and location of the defect is different. The defect in gastroschisis is often small and located to the right of the umbilical cord (see Fig. 22-7). Additionally, the herniated abdominal contents are not covered by a membrane in neonates with gastroschisis. In contrast, an omphalocele defect is central and often larger, with a covering membrane (Fig. 22-8).

Immediate postnatal care for children with abdominal wall defects is critical. Evaluation of the defect and its contents is often easy. The defect should be covered to prevent loss of heat and fluid. Placement of a nasogastric tube is required in order to prevent aspiration or gaseous distention of the stomach and bowel. Secure intravenous access and volume resuscitation should be carefully monitored as fluid loss can be significant, especially in gastroschisis. Because the surgical approach to abdominal wall defects involves manipulation of the umbilical cord stump, umbilical vessel catheters are discouraged.

Preoperative care of the newborn with an abdominal wall defect should begin in the deliv-

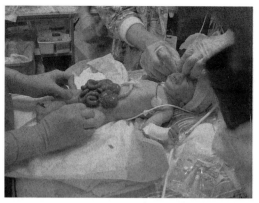

Figure 22-9 Delivery room preparation of a newborn. Intravenous access has been obtained and an orogastric tube is in place. (See also Color Plate.)

ery room (Fig. 22-9). Nasogastric intubation limits gastric and intestinal distention. Intravenous access provides a route for medication and fluid resuscitation. A warm environment minimizes fluid loss and coagulopathy. The herniated abdominal viscera often falls over one side of the child's body. Effort should be made to secure the bowel in a position that avoids kinking of the mesenteric vessels. This will minimize swelling of the viscera.

A screen for concomitant anomalies should be performed, especially when an omphalocele is present. Omphalocele is often associated with congenital heart disease and hypoglycemia, and this information is important to the anesthesiologist and surgeon. Gastroschisis, on the other hand, is associated with intestinal atresia and malrotation.

After successful closure of an abdominal wall defect, the size of the abdominal cavity may not accept the previously herniated viscera without sequelae. When severe, a condition known as abdominal compartment syndrome (ACS) can occur.[13] ACS is due to intra-abdominal hypertension and affects venous return, renal perfusion, and respiratory mechanics. Although no exact intra-abdominal pressure measurement has been correlated with ACS, a decreasing urine output, increasing peak ventilator pressure, increasing P_{CO_2}, and a firm abdomen are clues that ACS may be present. Often, the lower extremities become edematous and develop obvious signs of venous congestion when ACS is present. Reopening the abdomen may be necessary in cases in which ACS is severe.

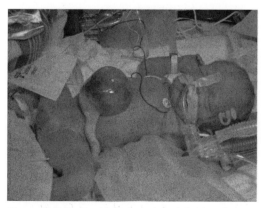

Figure 22-8 Classic centrally located omphalocele with covering membrane. (See also Color Plate.)

Case Study 5

A 30-week gestation, premature newborn has been stable in the NICU and preparations are being made for discharge home. You are alerted by the baby's nurse that he has vomited several times and appears very uncomfortable. When you examine the baby, you notice that the abdomen is nontender but quite distended. There is a reducible umbilical hernia; however, the right groin area appears noticeably larger and firmer than the left. The testes are descended bilaterally.

Exercise 5

QUESTIONS

1. What is the most likely diagnosis?
   a. Hydrocele
   b. Left inguinal hernia
   c. Right inguinal hernia
   d. Intussusception
   e. None of the above

2. What is the most likely cause of the baby's problem?
   a. Straining due to constipation
   b. Failure of closure of the processus vaginalis
   c. Viral infection
   d. All of the above
   e. None of the above

You make the diagnosis at 6 in the evening and attempt to reduce the hernia but without success.

3. At this point, what would you do next?
   a. Request an urgent surgical consultation
   b. Place a nasogastric tube and ask for a surgical consultation first thing in the morning
   c. Reattempt to treat over the next 4 to 6 hours
   d. Administer a suppository
   e. None of the above

4. What is appropriate treatment of an incarcerated inguinal hernia in a newborn?
   a. Always emergent operation
   b. Simple reduction followed by planned operation

   c. Sedation with reduction followed by planned operation
   d. b or c
   e. Reduction, discharge home, followed by elective operation

ANSWERS

1. c.
2. b.
3. a.
4. d.

Vomiting in the newborn can be the result of many conditions. In the case described, the physical findings of a right groin mass are suggestive of an incarcerated right inguinal hernia. Inguinal hernias are common and are the result of a persistently patent processus vaginalis. Crying or straining can often make an inguinal hernia much more obvious but do not cause the hernia.

When a diagnosis of incarcerated inguinal hernia is made, a surgeon should be contacted as soon as possible. Because the incarcerated hernia can contain intestine, bladder, omentum, and the ovary (in girls), it is important to attempt reduction of the hernia as soon as possible. Prolonged incarceration can be detrimental to the incarcerated contents and can make later attempts to reduce the hernia more difficult. Reduction of an incarcerated inguinal hernia is often possible before surgery. Gentle but constant pressure on the incarcerated contents in the direction of the inguinal ring is usually successful. The person reducing the hernia will feel a definite return of the entire contents into the abdominal cavity and resolution of the groin bulge. If simple bedside reduction is not successful, administration of sedation with repeated attempts at reduction is indicated. In cases in which reduction of the hernia is possible either with or without sedation, the hernia should be repaired within 48 hours. Most surgeons would recommend against discharging a newborn with a previously incarcerated inguinal hernia prior to repair because of the high incidence of recurrent incarceration.[14]

Only when a hernia is not reducible, despite sedation and attempts by the pediatric surgeon, is the child taken to the operating room for urgent operative repair. A standard inguinal incision is used. The incarcerated contents are inspected at operation and a decision is made regarding the need for intestinal resection. The operation is often more difficult than a standard inguinal hernia and the internal inguinal ring is sometimes opened. Incarcerated inguinal hernias are associated with higher rates of recurrence and testicular loss.

Gastrointestinal Emergencies

Case Study 6

A 1-week-old newborn is irritable and has several episodes of bilious emesis after the most recent feeding. You are called to ask for new feeding orders. He is tachycardic but otherwise the vital signs are stable. The physical examination reveals a full abdomen but no marked abnormality.

Exercise 6

QUESTIONS

1. What is the appropriate next step in this case?
   a. Consider the possibility of gastroesophageal reflux
   b. Start a proton pump inhibitor
   c. Ultrasound examination of the pylorus
   d. Upper gastrointestinal contrast study
   e. Change oral feedings to a soy-based formula

2. Which of the following is (are) true about intestinal malrotation and volvulus?
   a. They always occur at the same time.
   b. Emergent operation is recommended if either is found to be present.
   c. Neither condition can be asymptomatic.
   d. Both conditions can cause bilious emesis.
   e. Plain abdominal x-rays are very helpful in the diagnosis.

ANSWERS

1. d.
2. d.

Case Study 7

A 2.5-kg newborn has been in the nursery for 2 days for treatment of presumed sepsis. There was no record of prenatal care at your hospital. He initially fed well but had two episodes of green-colored emesis.

Exercise 7

QUESTIONS

1. Bilious emesis can be a sign of which of the following?
   a. Intestinal stenosis
   b. Imperforate anus
   c. Hirschsprung disease
   d. Malrotation with volvulus
   e. All of the above

2. What should be the first initial radiographic study for this baby?
   a. Abdominal ultrasound
   b. Upper GI contrast study
   c. Contrast enema
   d. Chest x-ray
   e. Brain MRI

A nasogastric tube is placed and returns thick, bilious material. The initial radiographic study excludes malrotation but shows significantly dilated loops of bowel.

3. At this point, what is the most appropriate follow-up study?
   a. Abdominal ultrasound
   b. Upper GI contrast study
   c. Contrast enema
   d. Chest x-ray
   e. Brain MRI

4. In this case, what does the presence of an unobstructed small caliber colon on contrast enema suggest?
   a. Small bowel atresia
   b. Imperforate anus
   c. Duodenal atresia
   d. Meconium ileus
   e. a and d

ANSWERS

1. e.
2. b.

3. c.

4. e.

The causes of intestinal obstruction in the newborn are multiple and can be related to either mechanical or functional abnormalities. When bilious emesis is witnessed or when a history of bilious emesis in a newborn is obtained, it is imperative that the physician first exclude malrotation, as this is a potentially life-threatening condition. Although malrotation with or without volvulus is classically associated with bilious emesis, all other forms of mechanical or functional intestinal obstruction distal to the ampulla of Vater can present with bilious emesis as well. A nasogastric tube should be inserted and a list of possible differential diagnoses should be contemplated. The main causes of intestinal obstruction in the newborn include intestinal atresia (duodenal, small intestinal, colonic), malrotation with volvulus, meconium ileus, meconium plug, Hirschsprung disease, and imperforate anus. In general, the diagnosis of most types of anorectal malformations ("imperforate anus") is made after a focused clinical examination of the child's perineum. In the case described, the first radiographic study, after a careful physical examination, should be an upper gastrointestinal (UGI) contrast study to evaluate for anomalies of rotation. On the scout film, the general size of the bowel loops and distribution of enteric gas can hint at the diagnosis. A "double bubble" sign is virtually pathognomonic for duodenal atresia or duodenal stenosis (Fig. 22-10), and a "gasless" abdomen has been described in malrotation with volvulus. The UGI delineates the course of the esophagus, stomach, and duodenum. The fixation of the duodenum in its retroperitoneal location with the ligament of Treitz coursing to the left of the spinal column excludes malrotation (Fig. 22-11). If the ligament of Treitz does not cross the midline, then the child has malrotation (Fig. 22-12). If, in addition, there is a high-grade obstruction of the mid- or distal duodenum, then the malrotation may be complicated by volvulus although malrotation is not necessarily complicated by volvulus every time (Fig. 22-13). The combination of malrotation and volvulus warrants immediate emergency surgical treatment.[15] Ultrasound, CT scan, and MRI should be discouraged as they are not as useful and are much more difficult to obtain than UGI study. On occasion, a UGI study is obtained for an unrelated reason, and a previously unrecognized malrotation is identified. In this scenario,

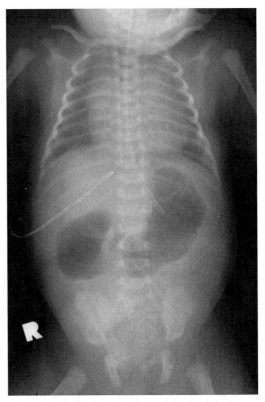

Figure 22-10 "Double bubble" sign of duodenal atresia.

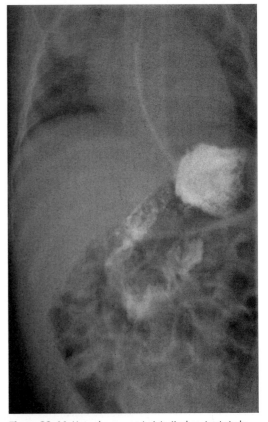

Figure 22-11 Normal upper gastrointestinal contrast study shows the duodenum crossing the midline.

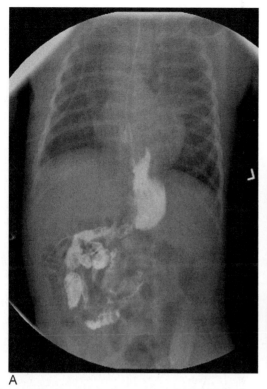
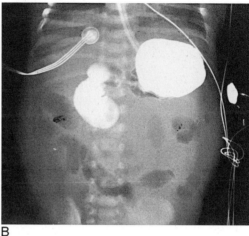

Figure 22-12 A, Abnormal rotation with nonobstructed duodenum. Ligament of Treitz does not cross the midline to the left upper quadrant. The proximal small intestine is seen on the right side of the abdomen. **B,** Abnormal upper gastrointestinal study showing high-grade obstruction of the duodenum in a case of malrotation with midgut volvulus.

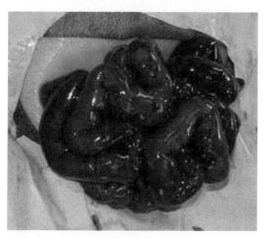

Figure 22-13 Necrotic small bowel due to malrotation with volvulus. (See also Color Plate.)

if the malrotation is not causing symptoms, surgical treatment can be rendered on a nonemergent basis.

If the initial UGI study shows normal rotation or if there is no reason to suspect malrotation at the outset, then a retrograde contrast enema (CE) is the next study of choice. As with the UGI study, the scout film can show dilated small bowel (atresia), calcifications (complicated

meconium ileus), or a dilated colon (Hirschsprung disease). On the CE, the size of the colon is evaluated, as are the presence or absence of transition areas. A microcolon is most commonly associated with small bowel atresia and meconium ileus. In small bowel atresia, the contrast fills the microcolon but does not enter the dilated loops of intestine in a retrograde fashion. In meconium ileus, the CE may demonstrate meconium pellets in the colon, suggesting the diagnosis. In addition, contrast material may enter the dilated proximal bowel, excluding a mechanical atresia with the potential of having a therapeutic effect. In Hirschsprung disease, the CE has been an important diagnostic tool for many years. A transition zone can be identified at the level where aganglionosis begins (Fig. 22-14). If a transition zone is present or if the clinical suspicion is high, a rectal biopsy to secure the diagnosis of Hirschsprung disease is indicated.[16]

Case Study 8

A 2-day-old, 650-g, 25-week gestation newborn has a newly distended abdomen despite the presence of a functioning orogastric tube. The

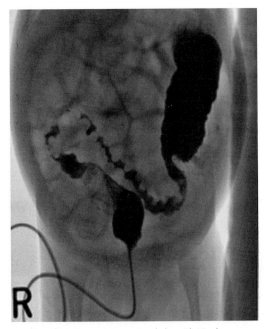

Figure 22-14 Contrast enema in a baby with Hirschsprung disease showing a transition zone in the distal descending colon.

vital signs are stable, oxygen saturation is 95% on nasal CPAP (continuous positive airway pressure), and urine output is adequate. Plain abdominal x-rays, including a cross-table lateral view, reveal a large amount of free intraperitoneal air (Fig. 22-15).

Exercise 8

QUESTIONS

1. What are possible cause(s) of this baby's free intraperitoneal air?

   a. CPAP

   b. Gastric perforation

   c. Spontaneous intestinal perforation

   d. b and c

   e. None of the above

2. What is the next step in the management of this neonate?

   a. Repeat abdominal x-rays in 4 hours

   b. Surgical consultation

   c. Reposition the orogastric tube

   d. Decrease CPAP support

   e. Evacuate the intraperitoneal air with a small percutaneous drain

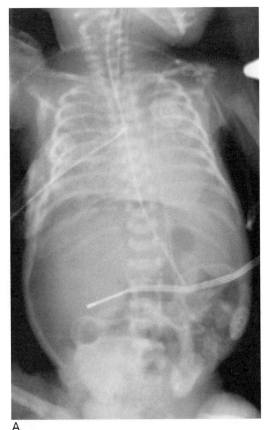

A

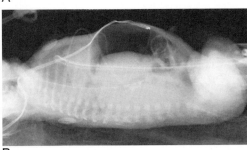

B

Figure 22-15 Abdominal x-rays, flat (**A**) and cross-table lateral (**B**) views, of a 500-g 23-week gestation baby with a large amount of free intraperitoneal air.

ANSWERS

1. d.

2. b.

   Pneumoperitoneum in the severely premature newborn can be due to a variety of conditions. One should assume that the extraluminal air is secondary to a perforated hollow viscus unless there is an obvious reason to believe otherwise. Spontaneous intestinal perforation (SIP), gastric perforation, and necrotizing enterocolitis (NEC) are responsible for a majority of cases.[17] Rarely, intrathoracic air from a pneumothorax can track into the abdomen and cause pneumoperitoneum. Standard endotracheal ventilation and CPAP are not thought to be causes of pneumoperitoneum. NEC is the most common cause of intestinal perforation in premature newborns, but SIP is particularly associated with very low birth weight infants, especially those who receive perinatal steroids and indomethacin.[18–20] A definitive diagnosis of gastric perforation is difficult to make prior to surgery, but massive pneumoperitoneum is often noted on the preoperative abdominal x-rays of neonates with gastric perforation.

When pneumoperitoneum is identified, an urgent surgical consultation should be obtained. In most cases, surgical exploration will be performed, sometimes in the NICU. On selected occasions, when the neonate is unstable or unable to undergo laparotomy, the surgeon will elect to place a small drain in the abdominal cavity. The drain will allow evacuation of air and fluid and will provide a temporary treatment. Placement of the drain can be challenging and should only be performed by a surgeon.

References

1. Moore KL The Developing Human; Clinically Oriented Embryology Philadelphia, WB Saunders, 1988, pp 207–216.
2. O'Neill JA, Grossfeld JL, Fonkalsrud EW, Coran AG (eds): Congenital abnormalities of the esophagus. In Principles of Pediatric Surgery, St. Louis, Mosby, 2004, pp 385–394.
3. Azizkhan RG: Esophageal atresia and distal tracheoesophageal fistula in a neonate. Postgrad Gen Surg 1992;4:1–4.
4. Spitz L, Kiely EM, Morecroft JA, Drake DP: Oesophageal atresia: at-risk groups for the 1990s. J Pediatr Surg 1994;29:723–725.
5. Hishitani T, Ogawa K, Hoshino K, et al: Lobar emphysema due to ductus arteriosus compressing right upper bronchus in an infant with congenital heart disease. Ann Thorac Surg 2003;75:1308–1310.
6. Ozcelik U, Gocmen A, Kiper N, et al: Congenital lobar emphysema: Evaluation and long-term follow-up of thirty cases at a single institution. Pediatr Pulmonol 2003;35:384–391.
7. Adzick NS, Harrison MR, Glick PH, et al: Diaphragmatic hernia in the fetus: Prenatal diagnosis and outcome in 94 cases. J Pediatr Surg 1985;20:357.
8. Harrison MR, Keller RL, Hawgood SB, et al: A randomized trial of fetal endoscopic tracheal occlusion for severe fetal congenital diaphragmatic hernia. N Engl J Med 2003;349:1916–1924.
9. Boloker J, Borteman D, Wung JT, Stolar CJH: Congenital diaphragmatic hernia in 120 infants treated consecutively with permissive hypercapnia, spontaneous respiration and elective repair. J Pediatr Surg 2002;37:357.
10. Clark RH, Hardin WD, Hirschl RB, et al: Current surgical management of congenital diaphragmatic hernia: A report from the Congenital Diaphragmatic Hernia Study Group. J Pediatr Surg 1998;33:1004.
11. O'Neill JA, Grossfeld JL, Fonkalsrud EW, Coran AG (eds): Abdominal wall defects. In Principles of Pediatric Surgery. St. Louis, Mosby, 2004, pp 423–431.
12. Langer JC: Abdominal wall defects. World J Surg 2003;27:117–124.
13. Wilson RD, Johnson MP: Congenital abdominal wall defects: An update. Fetal Diagn Ther 2004;19:385–398.
14. Gahukamble DB, Khamage AS: Early versus delayed repair of reduced incarcerated inguinal hernias in the pediatric population. J Pediatr Surg 1996;31:1218–1220.
15. Rescorla FJ, Shedd FJ, Grosfeld JL, et al: Anomalies of intestinal rotation in childhood: Analysis of 447 cases. Surgery 1990;108:710–715.
16. Swenson O: Hirschsprung's disease: A review. Pediatrics 2002;109:914–918.
17. Grosfeld JL, Molinari F, Chaet M, et al: Gastrointestinal perforation and peritonitis in infants and children: Experience with 179 cases over ten years. Surgery 1996;120:650–655.
18. Gordon PV, Young ML, Marshall DD: Focal small bowel perforation: An adverse effect of early postnatal dexamethasone therapy in extremely low birth weight infants. J Perinatol 2001;21:156–160.
19. Stark AR, Carlo WA, Tyson JE, et al: Adverse effects of early dexamethasone treatment in extremely-low-birth-weight infants. N Engl J Med 2001;344:95–101.
20. Pumberger W, Mayr M, Kohlhauser M, et al: Spontaneous localized intestinal perforation in very-low-birth-weight infants: A distinct clinical entity different from necrotizing enterocolitis. J Am Coll Surg 2002;195:796–803.

Necrotizing Enterocolitis

Ricardo A. Caicedo, MD, Michael D. Weiss, MD,
and Josef Neu, MD

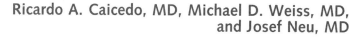

Necrotizing enterocolitis (NEC) is one of the most fearsome diseases in the neonatal intensive care unit (NICU) because it can progress rapidly from mild abdominal distention and feeding intolerance to fulminant septic shock, necrosis of the entire intestine, and death. Mortality rate ranges from 20% to 50% and morbidity includes but is not limited to strictures, adhesions, and short bowel syndrome. The specter of NEC has caused many neonatologists and pediatric surgeons to routinely withhold enteral feedings in neonates for prolonged periods during a highly critical phase of growth and development. The long-term neurodevelopmental and other health consequences of this practice may be significant but not fully realized until these individuals reach maturity. Effective means to prevent both long- and short-term consequences of NEC are yet to be established. The current form of therapy relies on a high index of suspicion, rapid diagnostic evaluation, supportive NICU care, and in some cases surgical treatment. In terms of diagnosis, several conditions, some requiring immediate surgical intervention, may be confused with NEC. This chapter will present the basic background of the pathophysiology of NEC, its clinical presentation, and representative cases that illustrate the differential diagnosis and management of NEC. The chapter will conclude with a brief discussion of potentially promising approaches to the prevention of this disease.

Pathophysiology

A full discussion of the present understanding of NEC pathophysiology is beyond the scope of this chapter, but a brief summary will be presented because it forms the basis of our management. The current thinking regarding the causes of NEC is based primarily on epidemiologic studies from which several important predisposing factors have been dissected. The predominant putative risk factors are prematurity, aggressive enteral feedings, and enteric bacteria.

The primary risk factor for NEC is prematurity; thus, the incidence varies inversely with gestational age. Approximately 90% of cases occur in premature infants, and NEC is rarely seen in older infants and children.[1–3] In fact, NEC became recognized as a distinct clinical entity only after the survival rate of very preterm infants increased over the last three decades. An immature mucosal barrier function and immune response are thought to make premature neonates particularly susceptible to intestinal inflammation and injury.[4,5] The incomplete innervation and poor motility of the premature gastrointestinal (GI) tract leads to stasis and bacterial overgrowth. It also has increased permeability, low levels of protective mucus and secretory immunoglobulin A, and decreased regenerative capabilities, resulting in greater potential for tissue damage.[6]

Necrotizing enterocolitis rarely, if ever, occurs in utero despite the high flux of amniotic fluid through the fetal intestine. The exclusive onset of NEC in the postnatal state may be explained in part by protection of the developing gut by hormones and peptides in amniotic fluid. Moreover, the fetal GI tract is not colonized with bacteria or exposed to a high volume of concentrated nutrients. Although NEC occasionally occurs in infants who have never been fed,[7] over 90% of cases occur in infants receiving enteral feedings, particularly following volume advancement.[8] Timing, volume, and advancement of enteral feedings are key determinants of mucosal injury that trigger the disease process.[9] Although aggressive enteral feedings probably increase the risk of NEC, several studies have shown that "minimal enteral feeding" or priming the GI tract with a very slow intake using food as a trophic agent to stimulate GI mucosal development and motility has not been associated with an increased incidence of NEC or other adverse effects.[10–13] Rather, these studies have demonstrated improved tolerance to subsequent enteral feedings, lower incidence of cholestasis, and higher levels of potentially trophic gut hormones. Human milk feedings appear to be protective against NEC.[14]

Another important factor in the pathogenesis of NEC is the presence of intestinal bacteria that ferment carbohydrate substrates to produce hydrogen gas and can translocate across a compromised epithelial barrier to activate mucosal immune responses. Bacteria commonly isolated from infants with NEC are gram-negative rods, including *Klebsiella* spp., *Escherichia coli*, *Enterobacter* spp., and *Pseudomonas* spp.[15–17] Other microorganisms associated with NEC are *Clostridium difficile*, *Staphylococcus epidermidis*, coronaviruses, and rotaviruses. Whether these microbes are the primary cause of NEC or whether they merely facilitate the disease process is still not understood. Neonatal intensive care measures such as use of broad-spectrum antibiotics and total parenteral nutrition disrupt the normal intestinal colonization with commensal organisms such as lactobacilli and bifidobacteria. This leads to an imbalance in the gut microflora favoring a limited amount of typically virulent organisms and triggering an exaggerated inflammatory response that is ultimately deleterious to the host.[18]

The effects of these major risk factors synergize to produce NEC in susceptible neonates. The immature intestine develops bacterial overgrowth as feedings are advanced, and the mucosal barrier is compromised. Subsequent bacterial translocation and secretion of toxins such as lipopolysaccharide (LPS) activate resident leukocytes in the submucosa. A robust inflammatory cascade ensues, with the release of cytokine/chemokines such as interleukin 8 (IL-8), platelet-activating factor (PAF), tumor necrosis factor (TNF), prostaglandins, leukotrienes, and oxygen radicals.[19] These mediators propagate the mucosal injury by producing vasoconstriction, ischemia/reperfusion injury, apoptosis, and further disruption of interepithelial tight junctions.[20] Bacteria that enter the submucosa continue to ferment dietary carbohydrates, producing intraluminal gas (pneumatosis intestinalis), a leading sign of NEC. The final pathway is coagulation necrosis of the bowel wall, which can progress to perforation, peritonitis, sepsis, and death. Thus, NEC more likely represents a *secondary* hypoxic-ischemic injury in response to uncontrolled inflammation, and is not the product of primary asphyxia or hypoxia-ischemia, as is sometimes postulated.[21]

Clinical Presentation

The age of onset of NEC is highly variable, but it rarely occurs in the first 3 days of life. Many cases of NEC occur in premature infants who have had only mild illness and who are convalescing as "feeders and growers" in an intermediate intensive care setting.[3,22–24] Our experience (Fig. 23–1) is that infants at the lowest gestational age (24 to 28 weeks) tend to develop NEC after the second week of life, whereas those at an intermediate age (29 to 32 weeks) develop it between 1 and 3 weeks, and the most mature infants develop it in the first week of life (see Fig. 23–1). NEC in term infants may be related more to perinatal ischemia in comparison to the preterm, but the term infant is also usually fed enterally and colonized with bacteria more rapidly.[25]

The clinical signs of NEC can vary markedly, with the earliest signs often being nonspecific. An instrument, originally developed by Bell and associates,[24] that has been helpful in the diagnosis and management of NEC stages the severity of disease based on clinical, radiographic, and laboratory criteria (Table 23-1).

Stage I includes a broad spectrum of signs that should lead the clinician to be suspicious of NEC but are not specific for the disease and

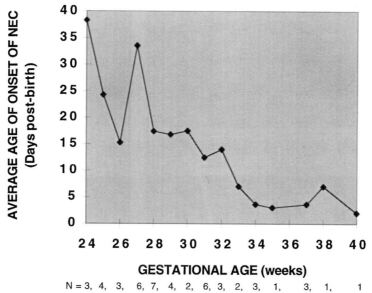

Figure 23-1 The experience at Shands Teaching Hospital at the University of Florida from 1994 to 1997 concerning age of onset of necrotizing enterocolitis (NEC). The x-axis represents gestational age in weeks, and the y-axis the average day of onset of NEC after birth. The number of cases for each gestational age is shown in the N row. The onset of NEC is later with decreasing gestational age.

may represent a myriad of problems, including simple feeding intolerance, sepsis, ileus, intestinal trauma due to feeding tubes, or metabolic problems such as hypoglycemia (Fig. 23–2). Signs of stage II and III NEC (i.e., pneumatosis intestinalis, ascites, grossly bloody stools, pneumoperitoneum, altered hematologic indices, and metabolic acidosis) are more definitive but still may represent diagnoses other than NEC (Figs. 23–3 and 23–4). The context in which these signs occur is critical when making a diagnosis and deciding on treatment.

Case Study 1

Baby D is a 1250-g male infant born following a 29-week gestation to a mother with a cervical culture positive for group B streptococcus. The baby was born via emergent cesarean section because of preterm labor and transverse lie. Apgar scores were 7 at 1 minute and 8 at 5 minutes. He was admitted to the NICU for respiratory distress and prematurity. Ampicillin and gentamicin were administered intravenously for 48 hours and discontinued after cultures were reported as negative. His respiratory symptoms resolved after several hours, and enteral feedings were begun on day 2 of life using a 24 kcal/oz "premature" formula. Feedings were initiated at a volume of 10 mL/kg/day (divided into feedings every 3 hours) and advanced by that amount daily as tolerated.

On day 6, while in the intermediate care nursery, the bedside nurse noted an episode of bradycardia and a 25-mL gastric residual that contained bile. You are called to the bedside. Upon arrival you note that the neonate's vital signs are significant for tachycardia, a capillary refill time of about 4 seconds, and a blood pressure of 28/17 mm Hg. The pertinent findings on your physical examination included a grayish-appearing infant with cool extremities. His abdomen is tender and distended; bowel sounds are absent. During the examination, the neonate is noted to have labored respirations with occasional apnea.

Exercise 1

QUESTIONS

1. Based on the foregoing history and physical examination, which of the following actions should receive the highest priority?

   a. Consult pediatric surgery

   b. Order a complete blood count (CBC) with differential count, blood cultures, and an arterial blood gas

   c. Obtain a radiograph of the abdomen

TABLE 23-1

MODIFIED BELL'S STAGING CRITERIA FOR NEONATAL NECROTIZING ENTEROCOLITIS (NEC)

Stage	Systemic Signs	Intestinal Signs	Radiologic Signs	Treatment
IA—suspected NEC	Temperature instability, apnea, bradycardia, lethargy	Elevated pregavage residuals, mild abdominal distention, emesis, guaiac-positive stool	Normal or intestinal dilation, mild ileus	Nothing by mouth, antibiotics for 3 days pending cultures
IB—suspected NEC	Same as IA	Bright red blood from rectum	Same as IA	Same as IA
IIA—definite NEC, mildly ill	Same as IA	Same as IB, *plus* diminished or absent bowel sounds with or without abdominal tenderness	Intestinal dilation, ileus, pneumatosis intestinalis	Nothing by mouth, antibiotics for 7–10 days if examination is normal in 24–48 hr
IIB—definite NEC; moderately ill	Same as IA, *plus* mild metabolic acidosis and mild thrombocytopenia	Same as IIA, *plus* definite abdominal tenderness with or without abdominal cellulitis or right lower quadrant mass, absent bowel sounds	Same as IIA, with or without portal vein gas, with or without ascites	Nothing by mouth, antibiotics for 14 days, NaHCO$_3$ for acidosis
IIIA—advanced NEC; severely ill, bowel intact	Same as IIB, *plus* hypotension, bradycardia, severe apneas, combined respiratory and metabolic acidosis, disseminated intravascular coagulation (DIC), neutropenia, anuria	Same as IIB, *plus* signs of generalized peritonitis, marked tenderness, distention of abdomen, abdominal wall erythema	Same as IIB, with definite ascites	Same as IIB, *plus* 200 mL/kg/day fluids, fresh frozen plasma, inotropic agents; intubation; ventilation therapy; paracentesis; surgical intervention if patient fails to improve with medical management within 24–48 hr
IIIB—advanced NEC; severely ill, bowel perforation	Same as IIIA	Same as IIIA	Same as IIB, *plus* pneumoperitoneum	Same as IIIA, *plus* surgical intervention

Modified from Bell MJ, Ternberg JL, Feigin RD, et al: Neonatal necrotizing enterocolitis: Therapeutic decisions based upon clinical staging. Ann Surg 1978;187:1–7.

    d. Intubate the neonate, administer 20 mL/kg of normal saline (over 30 minutes), and place a nasogastric tube to low intermittent suction

2. Other than NEC, what diagnoses would you consider in this infant?

ANSWERS

1. d. Although all the other choices should be performed, stabilization should receive the highest priority. This infant is in shock and is exhibiting signs of respiratory failure. Signs indicative of shock in this patient include his gray appearance, tachycardia, hypotension, and prolonged capillary refill time. Respiratory failure is suggested by the labored respirations, poor air exchange, and apnea. Regardless of the cause of these findings, this infant needs to be resuscitated immediately with volume (20 mL/kg of 0.9 N saline) to support blood pressure and

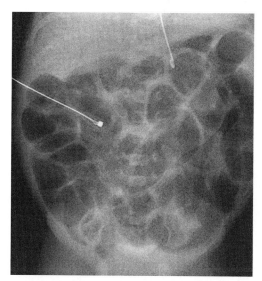

Figure 23-2 Stage I necrotizing enterocolitis exhibits dilated loops of bowel throughout the abdomen. This paralytic ileus may be focal, may involve only one quadrant of the abdomen, or may display dilated gas-filled loops of bowel throughout the entire abdomen.

intubation for the respiratory failure. If the perfusion does not improve, he will likely require inotropic agents such as dopamine to support his cardiovascular status.

In NEC, large amounts of extracellular fluids commonly leak out of the damaged bowel, depleting the intravascular space of volume. Additionally, tissue necrosis and systemic hypoperfusion can lead to a capillary leak syndrome throughout the body.[26] These pathophysiologic processes contribute to the urgent need for volume resuscitation in neonates with NEC. A nasogastric tube should be placed immediately to low intermittent suction. This benefits the infant in two ways. First, it decompresses the bowel, decreasing wall tension and improving perfusion of the bowel wall. Second, decompression of the bowel decreases intra-abdominal pressure and allows the infant to ventilate more efficiently with greater tidal volumes.

All the other choices listed are important, but should be performed only after initial stabilization has occurred. A CBC with differential count provides useful information regarding the possibility of infection, and, if the hemoglobin is low, volume expansion may be undertaken with packed red blood cells rather than crystalloid. Thrombocytopenia is also frequently observed in NEC. Portable radiographs of the abdomen are

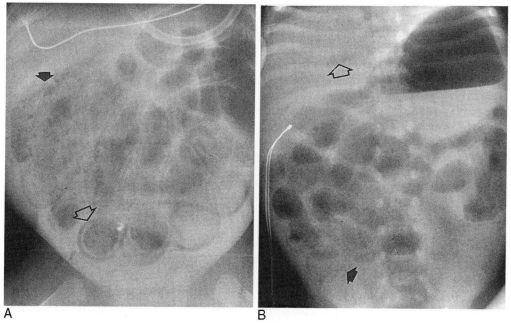

A   B

Figure 23-3 A, Stage IIA necrotizing enterocolitis (NEC) illustrates diffusely dilated bowel, as well as submucosal air in multiple loops of ischemic gut. A few loops have scattered small cysts (*solid arrowhead*) of air in the wall, but most show confluent streaks of air (*open arrowhead*) dissecting along the submucosal plane. Both patterns are examples of pneumatosis intestinalis. **B,** Stage IIB/IIIA NEC presents with diffuse dilatation of bowel with air. Intramural air (*solid arrowhead*) is present in the right lower quadrant. Air is also present within the portal vein (*open arrowhead*) and its branches in the liver. The air-filled loops of adjacent bowel are separated from a combination of mural thickening and ascites.

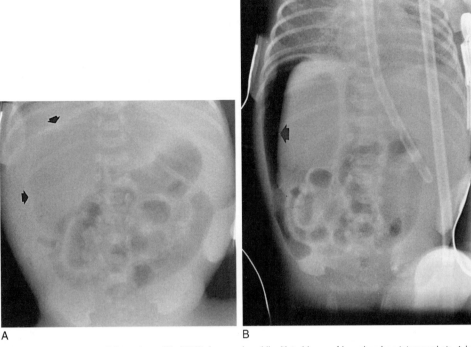

A   **B**

Figure 23-4 A, Stage IIIB necrotizing enterocolitis (NEC) shows only mildly dilated loops of bowel and no intramural air. A large bubble of free intraperitoneal air (*arrowheads*) is superimposed over the liver. The patient is in the supine position, and the free air rises to the epigastric region. **B,** With the patient in the left lateral decubitus position, free intraperitoneal air is seen rising over the lateral liver margin (*arrowhead*). The presence of free air indicates that an intestinal perforation has occurred and surgical exploration is indicated.

essential for the diagnosis of NEC, and two views should be obtained. Pneumatosis intestinalis is usually evident on an antero-posterior radiograph of the abdomen. However, a left lateral decubitus view is most helpful in diagnosing free air in the peritoneal cavity. A surgical consultation should also be obtained as soon as possible. By involving the pediatric surgeon early in the course of NEC, he or she becomes knowledgeable about the patient's history and is better able to care for the neonate if surgery is required.

Although this infant's primary disease process is in the intestine, multiple organ systems are commonly affected. Sonntag and associates[27] reviewed the medical records of 150 very low birth weight (VLBW) neonates with stage II NEC or higher over a 14-year period in order to evaluate the incidence of multisystem organ failure and capillary leak syndrome in these neonates. Only 16% of these neonates demonstrated isolated gastrointestinal symptoms. Most had at least three organ systems affected. The lungs, microvasculature,

cardiovascular, coagulation, and renal systems were most likely to be affected. Therefore, in infants with stage IIA or higher NEC, multisystem involvement should be expected.

2. The differential diagnosis for this neonate includes an ileus secondary to sepsis and NEC.[28] Because this infant has a distended abdomen and a bilious aspirate, intestinal obstruction needs to be ruled out. Common causes of intestinal obstruction in newborns are listed in Table 23-2.

After stabilizing the neonate, you review the results of the abdominal radiograph which reveal pneumatosis intestinalis.

QUESTIONS

3. What conditions other than NEC might cause pneumatosis intestinalis?

4. After blood cultures are obtained and you have made the radiographic and clinical diagnosis of NEC, which antibiotics would you choose and why?

TABLE 23-2

CAUSES OF NEONATAL INTESTINAL OBSTRUCTION

I. Mechanical
  A. Congenital
    1. Intrinsic
      a. Atresia
      b. Stenosis
      c. Meconium ileus
      d. Anorectal malformation
      e. Enteric duplication
    2. Extrinsic
      a. Volvulus
      b. Peritoneal band
      c. Annular pancreas
      d. Cyst and tumor
      e. Incarcerated hernia
  B. Acquired
    1. Necrotizing enterocolitis
    2. Intussusception
    3. Peritoneal adhesion
II. Functional
  A. Hirschsprung disease
  B. Meconium plug syndrome
  C. Ileus
  D. Peritonitis
  E. Intestinal pseudo-obstruction syndrome

Adapted from Byrne WJ: Disorders of the intestines and pancreas. In Taeusch HW, Ballard RA, Avery ME (eds): Diseases of the Newborn, 6th ed. Philadelphia, WB Saunders, 1991, pp 346–347.

ANSWERS

3. See Table 23-3 for a differential diagnosis of pneumatosis intestinalis.

4. NEC may be associated with a wide variety of organisms (see earlier discussion under "Pathophysiology"). Bacteremia occurs in 30% to 50% of infants with NEC. Therefore, broad-spectrum antibiotics should be started

TABLE 23-3

DIFFERENTIAL DIAGNOSIS OF NEONATAL PNEUMATOSIS INTESTINALIS

Necrotizing enterocolitis*
Midgut volvulus
Acute or chronic diarrhea
Gastrointestinal surgery
Hirschsprung disease
Short bowel syndrome
Neutropenia
Idiopathic
Mesenteric thrombosis
Imperforate anus
Congenital malignancy
Congenital heart disease (postcatheterization)

*Common cause.
Adapted from Crouse DT: Necrotizing enterocolitis. In Pomerance JJ, Richardson CJ (eds): Neonatology for the Clinician. Norwalk, CT, Appleton & Lange, 1993, pp 368–370.

as soon as blood cultures are obtained. The authors usually begin with ampicillin and gentamicin and replace the ampicillin with vancomycin if *S. epidermidis* is suspected. If the baby continues to worsen while receiving these antibiotics or there are clear signs of peritonitis, clindamycin or metronidazole is usually begun to improve coverage of anaerobic organisms.

Baby D is taken to the operating room because "free air" is seen on the radiograph of his abdomen. A diagnosis of NEC with small bowel necrosis is made, and approximately a third of his small bowel is resected.

QUESTION

5. What is the major cause of significant long-term morbidity in babies who have had intestinal resection for NEC?

ANSWER

5. There is no definitive answer. Co-morbidities, systemic inflammation, and poor nutrition are all likely to be contributing factors. NEC requiring bowel resection may result in short bowel syndrome, with a diminished capacity to absorb nutrients and support growth. In general, for a neonate to survive on enteral nutrition, 8 to 15 cm of bowel must be left if the ileocecal valve remains intact. If the valve is removed, 25 to 40 cm must remain intact for successful enteral supplementation.[29]

Case Study 2

Baby T is a 1500-g 30-week gestation infant, born via spontaneous vaginal delivery. The mother's prenatal course was complicated by preterm labor and treated with magnesium sulfate. In addition, she was given two doses of betamethasone to accelerate the baby's lung maturity. Apgar scores were 8 at 1 minute and 9 at 5 minutes.

The neonate is noted to have mild retractions in the delivery room and is admitted to the NICU with a diagnosis of mild respiratory distress syndrome. He initially requires an increase in the inspired oxygen concentration to 60% and use of nasal continuous positive airway pressure (CPAP), but over the next 9 days he is weaned to room air. Ampicillin and gentamicin are administered for 2 days, and both are stopped when cultures reveal no growth.

On day 2 of life, feedings are started at an initial volume of 20 mL/kg/day and gradually advanced to full enteral feeds over the next 7 days. On day 12 of life, baby T has a bile-stained gastric aspirate totaling 20 mL. Physical examination at that time reveals an increase in his abdominal girth from 22 to 26 cm, a firm and distended abdomen, and a stool that tested positive for blood. Laboratory studies reveal a white blood cell (WBC) count of 3000/mm^3 with 5% mature neutrophils and 23% band forms. The absolute neutrophil count is 8260, the immature to total (I:T) neutrophil ratio is 0.4, and the absolute band count is 2714. The hemoglobin concentration is 11.2 g/dL, and the platelet count is 46×10^9/L. An arterial blood gas determination reveals pH 7.17, Paco$_2$ 47 mm Hg, Pao$_2$ 147 mm Hg, and base excess 8. Serum electrolyte values are normal. An anteroposterior abdominal radiograph reveals right intestinal intramural and portal venous air, consistent with NEC. The baby is started on vancomycin and gentamicin, a nasogastric tube is placed to low intermittent suction, and a surgery consultation is sought.

Over the next several hours, the baby's condition worsens and he requires intubation, mechanical ventilation, and packed red blood cells to correct hypovolemia and a mild anemia. Following these interventions, the baby's condition stabilizes, and is managed medically without surgical intervention. A blood culture obtained at the time of the bilious residual grows Enterobacter cloacae.

After a week of total parenteral nutrition, baby T becomes completely asymptomatic. Enteral feedings are begun at that time and advanced slowly. The baby tolerates the feedings well, until a full feeding volume is reached. He then develops feeding intolerance manifested by increased gastric residuals and abdominal distention. He is otherwise asymptomatic.

Exercise 2

QUESTIONS

1. Which features in the case history should increase your suspicion of NEC?

2. Which indicators from the physical examination, laboratory values, and x-rays are suggestive of NEC?

3. What complication of NEC could the feeding intolerance represent? What steps could you take to confirm your suspicion?

4. What is the significance of the portal venous gas seen on the lateral decubitus x-ray?

ANSWERS

1. Several details from the history should increase the suspicion of NEC, including the gestational age of the infant (30 weeks), the onset of symptoms on day 12 of life, the recent advancement of enteral feedings, and the bilious gastric aspirate.

   Most babies with NEC are born prematurely. In a large, 25-year retrospective study involving 266 cases of NEC, Snyder and associates[30] found that the mean birth weight of affected infants was 1529 g and the mean gestational age was 31.1 weeks. This suggests that gut immaturity almost certainly plays a role in the development of NEC. Interestingly, the Apgar scores of neonates who developed NEC in Snyder's study were 5 and 7 at 1 and 5 minutes of life, respectively, suggesting that adverse perinatal events are not important etiologic factors in the preterm population. Risk factors associated with NEC in full-term neonates include asphyxia, intrauterine growth restriction, chronic malabsorption, polycythemia, exchange transfusion, myelomeningocele, and congenital heart disease.

   The second important indicator in the history is the age of presentation (12 days). In Snyder's study, the average age of onset of NEC was 14.9 days. As noted previously, there is an inverse correlation between the time of presentation of NEC and gestational age.

   The third finding from the history that should alert the clinician to the possibility of NEC is that the neonate recently had his feedings advanced.[31] There is a strong (albeit unproved) association between the rate of feeding advancement and risk for NEC.[7] Therefore, it is recommended that feedings not be advanced more than approximately 20 mL/kg/day. NEC has also been observed in infants receiving formula or medications with a high osmolality and in infants receiving nasojejunal feedings.

The last significant item in the history is the finding of a bilious gastric aspirate of 27 mL. The presence of bile in a gastric aspirate of a neonate of that magnitude should always raise concern. Although it is important to make sure that the tip of the nasogastric tube is not through the pylorus (and therefore sampling secretions from the duodenum), bile should always be considered an abnormal finding. Furthermore, the volume of the gastric residual in this infant was clearly in excess of normal. Both findings are indicative of a gastrointestinal process, and NEC should be included in the differential diagnosis.

2. Findings on physical examination suggestive of NEC include an increase in abdominal girth of 4 cm; a firm, distended abdomen; and a stool specimen that tests positive for blood. The last two signs have been observed in 70% and 54% of patients with NEC, respectively; however, they are far from specific.

   The laboratory data are significant for neutropenia and thrombocytopenia. It is noteworthy that there was no evidence of a metabolic acidosis, and the serum electrolyte values and platelet count were normal. Infants with NEC commonly exhibit a metabolic acidosis (occasionally in association with a respiratory acidosis), neutropenia, thrombocytopenia, and hyponatremia (secondary to third-space losses).

   The x-ray findings of intestinal intramural and portal venous air are highly suggestive of NEC. The entire constellation of findings is consistent with stage IIB NEC (see Table 23-1).

3. The feeding intolerance is suggestive of stricture formation. Less common signs of stricture formation include the persistence of blood in the stool and recurrent episodes of bacteremia. The presence of stricture can be confirmed by a contrast study of the bowel. However, it is controversial whether contrast studies should be obtained in all babies with NEC who have been medically managed. It is essential that all these patients be evaluated if they develop gastrointestinal symptoms in the future. The primary pediatrician and parents should be informed of the possibility of future symptoms from strictures, because some babies can become symptomatic months after discharge from the hospital.

4. This finding indicates a severe form of NEC that frequently requires surgery for resection of dead bowel.[32] However, portal venous gas by itself is not an indication for surgical intervention.

Case Study 3

Baby K is the 1150-g infant born at 29 weeks' gestation to a 29-year-old mother whose pregnancy was complicated by preterm labor. A cesarean section was performed because of breech presentation. Apgar scores were 5 at 1 minute and 7 at 5 minutes.

Baby K initially requires intubation due to worsening respiratory symptoms and receives two doses of surfactant. She is weaned rapidly to nasal CPAP (6 cm H_2O pressure) and 30% oxygen by day 2 of life. She is started on breast milk at a feeding volume of 10 mL/kg/day on day 2 of life. On day 3 of life, the baby is noted to have a small bilious gastric residual with a slight increase in abdominal girth of 1 cm. The neonate is also noted to have hyperglycemia.

Exercise 3

QUESTIONS

1. What is the major abnormality and differential diagnosis of the finding in the radiograph shown in Figure 23-5?

2. Based on radiographic findings, what steps should be taken in management?

ANSWERS

1. The left lateral decubitus radiograph demonstrates free intraperitoneal air. The differential diagnosis of free intraperitoneal air is extensive. The five most common causes are gastric perforation (either spontaneous or secondary to a nasogastric tube), NEC, meconium peritonitis, intestinal atresias, and barotrauma with extension of intrathoracic air into the abdomen. See Table 23-4 for complete differential diagnosis.

2. As with all neonatal emergencies, management begins with the ABCs of intensive

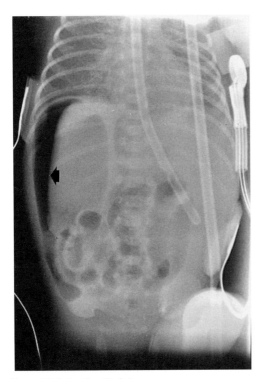

Figure 23-5 See Case Study 3.

TABLE 23-4

TABLE 23-4

DIFFERENTIAL DIAGNOSIS OF NEONATAL PNEUMOPERITONEUM

Gastrointestinal perforation secondary to obstruction
Meconium ileus*
Spontaneous ileal perforation*
Atresia*
Stenosis
Midgut volvulus (malrotation)
Hirschsprung disease
Gastroschisis
Duplication
Incarcerated hernia
Imperforate anus
Small left colon syndrome
Intussusception
Meconium plug
Necrotizing enterocolitis*
Spontaneous gastric perforation*
Catheter-associated intestinal infarction
Peptic ulceration (duodenum)
Meckel's diverticulum
Appendicitis
Drugs (indomethacin, dexamethasone)
Gastric lactobezoar
Traumatic
   Barotrauma with extension of intrathoracic air into
     the abdomen*
   Nasogastric tube*
   Suction catheter
   Thermometer
   Enema
   Ventriculoperitoneal shunt
   Gastric perforation with tracheoesophageal fistula
     requiring ventilation

*Common causes.
Adapted from Kleigman RM: Necrotizing enterocolitis: Differential diagnosis and management. In Polin RA, Yoder MC, Burg FD (eds): Workbook in Practical Neonatology, 2nd ed. Philadelphia, WB Saunders, 1993, p 457.

care (airway, breathing, and circulation). In the absence of respiratory distress, attention should first be directed to assessment of circulation (i.e., perfusion) and correction of any abnormalities. In view of the baby's history, it must be assumed that the free air represents a gastrointestinal perforation and that additional intravenous crystalloid will be required because of third-space losses. Therefore, it is important to establish intravenous access and provide fluids as needed to maintain adequate peripheral perfusion, blood pressure, and urine output. Gastric decompression and broad-spectrum antimicrobial therapy are also indicated, for the reasons stated in Case Study 1.

Surgical intervention is mandatory in a newborn with pneumoperitoneum secondary to a gastrointestinal perforation. In an extremely premature neonate with marked cardiorespiratory compromise, intervention may consist of simple peritoneal drainage under local anesthesia at the baby's bedside.[32,33] A discussion of the surgical options for NEC with perforation are beyond the scope of this chapter but range from simple drainage to resection of nonviable bowel and primary repair to resection of nonviable bowel and proximal diversion.[34–37]

Spontaneous perforation of the bowel, not associated with NEC,[38] occurs most commonly in the distal ileum. The frequency of ileal perforation appears to be increasing and has been associated with prenatal administration of indomethacin.[39] The clinical characteristics of this disease process are very similar to NEC (Table 23-5). It is interesting to note that a majority of patients have never been fed before they develop spontaneous ileal perforations. The physical

CLINICAL CHARACTERISTICS, TREATMENT
MODALITIES, AND FEEDING HISTORY IN
NEONATES WITH INTESTINAL PERFORATION

Characteristics	NEC (*n* = 21)	Localized Perforation (*n* = 21)
Patent ductus arteriosus	12	15
Hyaline membrane disease	14	15
Intravenous indomethacin	10	15
Mean dose of indomethacin, mg/kg/patient	0.26	0.34*
UAC	14	15
UAC in place within 48 hr of perforation	4	12†
Fed before perforation	18	8‡
Umbilical venous catheter	9	7
Nasogastric tube	19	20
Intravenous aminophylline	9	9
Mean days of mechanical ventilation	10.8	7.1
Range of days of mechanical ventilation	0–3	10–18
Mean days of nasal cannula oxygen	1.8	0.05
Range of days of nasal cannula oxygen	0–11	0–1
Exchange transfusion	0	1
Confirmed sepsis before perforation	2	0

*$P < 0.05$.
†$P < 0.02$.
‡$P < 0.005$.
NEC, necrotizing enterocolitis; UAC, umbilical artery catheter.
Adapted from Bucheit JQ, Stewart DL: Clinical comparison of localized intestinal perforation and necrotizing enterocolitis in neonates. Pediatrics 1994;93:32–36.

PHYSICAL EXAMINATION, LABORATORY,
AND RADIOLOGIC FINDINGS PRECEDING THE
DIAGNOSIS OF INTESTINAL PERFORATION

Findings	NEC (*n* = 21)	Localized Perforation (*n* = 21)
Clinical		
Abdominal distention	20	21
Abdominal discoloration	7	9
Apnea	4	2
Bradycardia	4	2
Hypotension	6	7
Temperature instability	1	1
Laboratory		
Metabolic acidosis (pH < 7.25 with base deficit > 7)	9	2*
Central hematocrit (>65%)	0	0
Thrombocytopenia (<100,000/µL)	9	6
Leukopenia (<5000/µL)	8	1†
Hematest-positive stools	6	4
Positive screen for cocaine metabolites	0	1
Radiologic		
Pneumoperitoneum	21	19
Pneumatosis intestinalis	14	0‡
Portal venous air	6	0‡

*$P < 0.02$.
†$P < 0.01$.
‡$P < 0.001$.
NEC, necrotizing enterocolitis.
Adapted from Bucheit JQ, Stewart DL: Clinical comparison of localized intestinal perforation and necrotizing enterocolitis in neonates. Pediatrics 1994;93:32–36.

findings of spontaneous intestinal perforations (Table 23-6) are also very similar to NEC, with the marked exception of a lack of pneumatosis intestinalis on the abdominal radiograph.[40] Unlike NEC, in which infants commonly have positive blood cultures for enteric organisms, neonates with spontaneous intestinal perforations are more likely to demonstrate positive cultures for *S. epidermidis* and *Candida*.[39,41] The prognosis for neonates with spontaneous intestinal perforations is excellent when diagnosis and treatment are early.

Baby K is taken to the operating room where she is found to have an ileal perforation. An enterostomy is performed and is reanastamosed 1 month later.

Case Study 4

Baby Z is a 600-g male infant born at 25 weeks' gestation to a 25-year-old mother who had preterm premature rupture of membranes for 10 days. Apgar scores are 1 at 1 minute, 1 at 5 minutes, and 5 at 10 minutes. He receives mechanical ventilation, surfactant, broad-spectrum antibiotics, and indomethacin for prophylaxis against intraventricular hemorrhage. Over the next several days, his condition improves, and on day 5 of life he is begun on enteral feedings (<10 mL/kg). He tolerates the feeds well until day 9, when the bedside nurse notes abdominal distention and a bilious gastric residual. You arrive at the neonate's bedside and find that the neonate is on modest *ventilator settings (F$_{IO_2}$ 0.3, rate 20, peak inspiratory pressure 16 cm H$_2$O, and positive end-expiratory pressure 5 cm H$_2$O). Physical examination reveals a heart rate of 170 beats per minute, a blood pressure of 48/32 mm Hg, and marked abdominal distention. Laboratory studies are remarkable for an elevated WBC count of 22,800 (69% mature neutrophils, 1% band forms), a platelet count of 265,000, and a hematocrit of 30.2%.*

Exercise 4

QUESTIONS

1. What are the notable findings on the abdominal radiograph shown in Figure 23-6? Based on this study and the physical examination, what is the differential diagnosis for this patient?
2. How should you proceed in managing this neonate's care over the next several hours?

ANSWERS

1. There are dilated loops of bowel, and there is no intramural air or "free" air. The differential diagnoses are the same as those listed for the neonate presented in case study 1.
2. After evaluating and stabilizing the neonate's airway, breathing, and circulation,

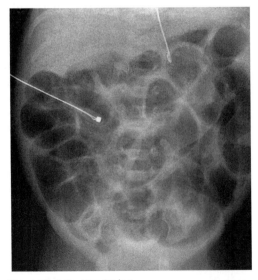

Figure 23-6 See Case Study 4.

the key is to monitor the infant for progression of the disease, shock, and intestinal perforation. This is best accomplished by serial physical examinations, abdominal radiographs, and laboratory studies. A carefully performed physical examination should be done at least every 2 hours. As part of the assessment, there should be close monitoring of vital signs, urine output, and perfusion, in addition to a careful examination of the abdomen for evidence of worsening peritonitis. Serial left lateral decubitus films should be performed every 6 to 8 hours to determine whether a perforation has occurred. Last, serial laboratory studies should be performed for signs of worsening thrombocytopenia, a decreased WBC count, or worsening metabolic acidosis.

Baby Z does not have any evidence of pneumatosis intestinalis on the initial abdominal x-ray. Furthermore, two follow-up films are read as normal. However, he eventually develops the radiographic findings of "free" air, as shown in Figure 23-4B. The lack of pneumatosis intestinalis on the initial x-ray and the follow-up films increases the likelihood of a disease process other than NEC. At the time of operation, the baby is found to have a malrotation with midgut volvulus and perforation of the dilated proximal bowel loop. Malrotation with midgut volvulus is a less common cause of intestinal perforation, but is a surgical emergency. In addition to signs of obstruction, these infants can occasionally present with pneumatosis intestinalis and bloody stools secondary to vascular compromise of the bowel. This case demonstrates how the clinician needs to be vigilant in considering other pathologic states that can present like NEC.

Prevention of Necrotizing Enterocolitis

Currently, the most widely used and probably efficacious practices to prevent NEC include careful infection control measures, judicious fluid administration, the use of human milk, and a high index of suspicion with early intervention. Additionally, several preventive strategies show promise but their efficacy is unproved or is based on limited data.[9]

Retrospective studies[9] have shown that the rate of advancement in feeding volume is proportional to incidence of NEC, but delayed or reduced volume advancement has not proved efficacious in preventing NEC in prospective trials.[42] A more recent trial[43] concluded that prolonged (≥ 10 days) minimal enteral feedings reduced the incidence of NEC in very low birth weight neonates, supporting the idea that trophic feeds are protective against NEC.

The osmolarity, carbohydrate composition, and pH of the enteral intake have also been implicated in the pathogenesis of NEC.[44,45] Formulas with high osmolarity have been shown to increase the incidence of NEC in human infants.[44] Some oral medications, such as vitamin preparations, use hyperosmolar vehicles that potentially could cause osmotic injury to the bowel. Many premature infants do not respond as quickly to a meal with brisk production of gastric acid and peptic protease.[5,46] A prospective masked study showed a lower incidence of NEC in a group of infants fed an acid-supplemented formula (to pH 3 to 4) compared to standard formula.[47] As with several of these interventions, these findings should be replicated before considering adopting them as routine practice.

The safety of preventive strategies must also be evaluated. Administration of enteral aminoglycosides produced a significant decrease in the incidence of NEC in early studies.[48–50] However, the long-term use of these antibiotics was associated with the emergence of resistant strains of *Staphylococcus*, *Klebsiella*, and *E. coli*.[48] This finding has discouraged the routine use of long-term oral antibiotic therapy for the prophylaxis for NEC. Further studies of oral aminoglycosides should probably not be undertaken unless the problems of microbial resistance can be overcome. Oral administration of immuoglobulins A and G together was efficacious in one prospective trial; however, other trials have not been confirmatory and safety data are lacking.[51]

Future approaches to NEC prevention are directed at the components of the developing intestine, an "ecosystem" consisting of host cells, nutrents, and microflora (Figs. 23-7 and 23-8). Supplementation of enteral feedings with individual nutrients such as glutamine has been demonstrated to be protective against various forms of enterocolitis in animals. One study of glutamine supplementation in low-birth-weight infants demonstrated a decreased incidence of hospital-acquired sepsis, putatively as a result of decreased translocation through mucosal surfaces.[52] However, there were not enough patients to analyze differences in the incidence of NEC and a subsequent multicenter trial of glutamine supplementation did not demonstrate efficacy. Another study showed decreased NEC in patients receiving supplemental arginine, but this study has not been repeated.[53] Testing of IL-11[54] and recombinant platelet activating factor acetylhydrolase[55] have demonstrated protection against ischemic bowel damage in rodents. However, it remains questionable whether animal models of NEC in which intestinal ischemia predominates actually represent the same pathophysiologic progression of NEC as seen in low-birth-weight human infants.

Another agent which shows theoretical promise is recombinant lactoferrin, a highly effective inhibitor of bacterial growth that appears to exert a trophic effect on the small intestinal crypt cells.[56] Intestinal trefoil factor, a protein produced throughout the small intestine and colon and secreted onto the luminal surface where it forms the viscoelastic mucus layer by interaction with mucin glycoproteins, is involved in the protection of the intestinal barrier in mice.[57] However, there are no studies of the effects of intestinal trefoil factor on mucosal barrier function in human infants.

Probiotics, or microbes/microbial products that exert a beneficial and nonpathogenic effect on the host, may protect against NEC by preventing gut colonization with pathogenic organisms, by maintaining homeostasis of the intestine, and by modulating inflammatory responses. Colonization of the GI tract with *Lactobacillus* spp. has been attempted in humans with negative results,[58] although more recent preliminary data using an infant rat model of NEC suggest that enteric instillation of probiotic bifidobacteria may prevent intestinal injury via modulation of the inflammatory cascade.[59] In animal models, the incidence of NEC was decreased by supplementation with bifidobacteria.[60] Randomized prospective trials of probiotic administration in humans have very recently been published, and these show a modest absolute risk reduction for NEC.[51] No adverse events have been reported, but caution is advised because of the risk of infection with probiotic organisms such as lactobacilli and bifidobacteria in the

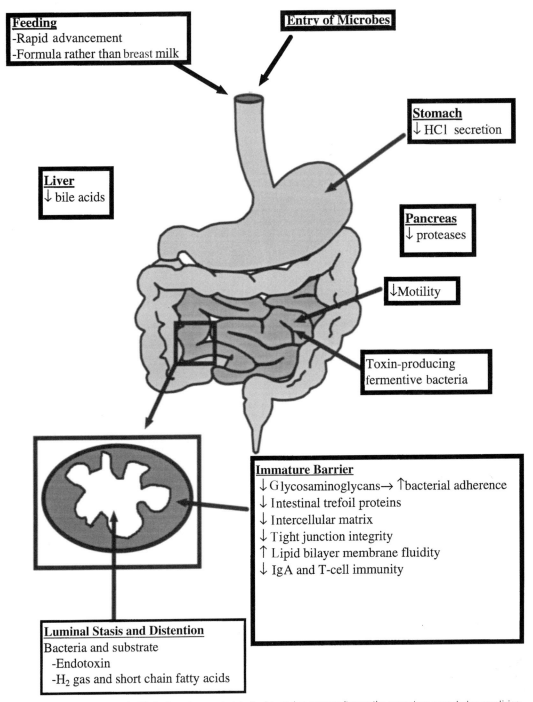

Feeding
-Rapid advancement
-Formula rather than breast milk

Entry of Microbes

Stomach
↓ HCl secretion

Liver
↓ bile acids

Pancreas
↓ proteases

↓Motility

Toxin-producing fermentive bacteria

Immature Barrier
↓ Glycosaminoglycans→ ↑bacterial adherence
↓ Intestinal trefoil proteins
↓ Intercellular matrix
↓ Tight junction integrity
↑ Lipid bilayer membrane fluidity
↓ IgA and T-cell immunity

Luminal Stasis and Distention
Bacteria and substrate
-Endotoxin
-H$_2$ gas and short chain fatty acids

Figure 23-7 Factors associated with the immature gastrointestinal tract that may predispose the premature neonate to necrotizing enterocolitis.

immunocompromised host, a description that may befit the preterm neonate. Human milk, in addition to containing antioxidants, lactoferrin, and secretory IgA, contains lactobacilli as well as oligosaccharides that promote GI colonization with probiotic organisms.

As it stands today, NEC remains a difficult disease to prevent. The most beneficial strategies include avoidance of preterm birth, stringent infection control, use of human milk and trophic feedings, and vigilance in watching for presenting symptoms and signs. Further progress

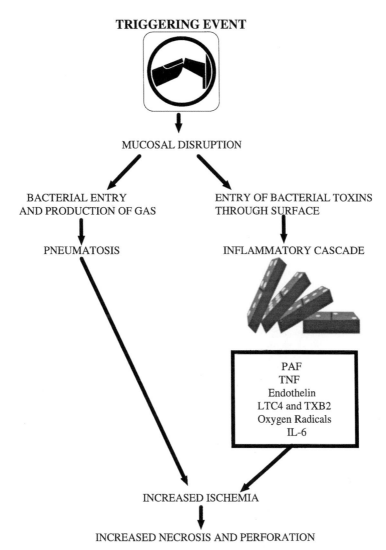

Figure 23-8 A proposed series of events that may result in necrotizing enterocolitis. IL-6, interleukin 6; LTC4, a leukotriene; PAF, platelet-activating factor; TNF, tumor necrosis factor; TXB2, thromboxane B2.

relies on a better understanding of the developing intestinal "ecosystem" and its role in modulating the risk and development of NEC.

References

1. Bell MJ, Rudinsky M, Brotherton T, et al: Gastrointestinal microecology in the critically ill neonate. J Pediatr Surg 1984;19(6):745–751.
2. Israel EJ: Neonatal necrotizing enterocolitis, a disease of the immature intestinal mucosal barrier. Acta Paediatr Suppl 1994;396:27–32.
3. Kliegman RM, Fanaroff AA: Necrotizing enterocolitis. N Engl J Med 1984;310(17):1093–1103.
4. Kliegman RM: Models of the pathogenesis of necrotizing enterocolitis. J Pediatr 1990;117(1 Pt 2): S2–S5.
5. Neu J: Functional development of the fetal gastrointestinal tract. Semin Perinatol 1989;13(3):224–235.
6. Neu J: Necrotizing enterocolitis: the search for a unifying pathogenic theory leading to prevention. Pediatr Clin North Am 1996;43(2):409–432.
7. Anderson DM, Kliegman RM: The relationship of neonatal alimentation practices to the occurrence of endemic necrotizing enterocolitis. Am J Perinatol 1991;8(1):62–67.
8. Stoll BJ: Epidemiology of necrotizing enterocolitis. Clin Perinatol 1994;21(2):205–218.
9. Lee JS, Polin RA: Treatment and prevention of necrotizing enterocolitis. Semin Neonatol 2003;8(6):449–459.
10. LaGamma EF, Ostertag SG, Birenbaum H: Failure of delayed oral feedings to prevent necrotizing enterocolitis. Results of study in very-low-birth-weight neonates. Am J Dis Child 1985;139(4):385–389.
11. Lucas A, Bloom SR, Aynsley-Green A: Gut hormones and 'minimal enteral feeding.'. Acta Paediatr Scand 1986;75(5):723.

12. Meetze WH, Valentine C, McGuigan JE, et al: Gastrointestinal priming prior to full enteral nutrition in very low birth weight infants. J Pediatr Gastroenterol Nutr 1992;15(2):163–170.

13. Slagle TA, Gross SJ: Effect of early low-volume enteral substrate on subsequent feeding tolerance in very low birth weight infants. J Pediatr 1988; 113(3):526–531.

14. Lucas A, Cole TJ: Breast milk and neonatal necrotising enterocolitis. Lancet 1990;336(8730):1519–1523.

15. Chan KL, Saing H, Yung RW, et al: A study of pre-antibiotic bacteriology in 125 patients with necrotizing enterocolitis. Acta Paediatr Suppl 1994; 396:45–48.

16. Kosloske AM: Pathogenesis and prevention of necrotizing enterocolitis: A hypothesis based on personal observation and a review of the literature. Pediatrics 1984;74(6):1086–1092.

17. Kosloske AM: A unifying hypothesis for pathogenesis and prevention of necrotizing enterocolitis. J Pediatr 1990;117(1 Pt 2):S68–S74.

18. Claud EC, Walker WA: Hypothesis: inappropriate colonization of the premature intestine can cause neonatal necrotizing enterocolitis. Faseb J 2001; 15(8):1398–1403.

19. Hsueh W, Caplan MS, Tan X, et al: Necrotizing enterocolitis of the newborn: Pathogenetic concepts in perspective. Pediatr Dev Pathol 1998;1(1):2–16.

20. Kinugasa T, Sakaguchi T, Gu X, Reinecker HC: Claudins regulate the intestinal barrier in response to immune mediators. Gastroenterology 2000; 118(6):1001–1011.

21. Neu J: The 'myth' of asphyxia and hypoxia-ischemia as primary causes of necrotizing enterocolitis. Biol Neonate 2005;87(2):97–98.

22. Covert RF, Neu J, Elliott MJ, et al: Factors associated with age of onset of necrotizing enterocolitis. Am J Perinatol 1989;6(4):455–460.

23. Stoll BJ, Kanto WP Jr, Glass RI, et al: Epidemiology of necrotizing enterocolitis: A case control study. J Pediatr 1980;96(3 Pt 1):447–451.

24. Bell MJ, Ternberg JL, Feigin RD, et al: Neonatal necrotizing enterocolitis. Therapeutic decisions based upon clinical staging. Ann Surg 1978; 187(1):1–7.

25. Maayan-Metzger A, Itzchak A, Mazkereth R, Kuint J: Necrotizing enterocolitis in full-term infants: Case-control study and review of the literature. J Perinatol 2004;24(8):494–499.

26. Crouse D: Necrotizing Enterocolitis. Norwalk, CT, Appleton & Lange, 1993.

27. Sonntag J, Wagner MH, Waldschmidt J, et al: Multisystem organ failure and capillary leak syndrome in severe necrotizing enterocolitis of very low birth weight infants. J Pediatr Surg 1998;33(3):481–484.

28. Byrne W: Disorders of the Intestines and Pancreas, 6th ed. Philadelphia, WB Saunders, 1991.

29. Dorney SF, Ament ME, Berquist WE, et al: Improved survival in very short small bowel of infancy with use of long-term parenteral nutrition. J Pediatr 1985;107(4):521–525.

30. Snyder CL, Gittes GK, Murphy JP, et al: Survival after necrotizing enterocolitis in infants weighing less than 1,000 g: 25 years' experience at a single institution. J Pediatr Surg 1997;32(3):434–437.

31. Caplan MS, MacKendrick W: Necrotizing enterocolitis: A review of pathogenetic mechanisms and implications for prevention. Pediatr Pathol 1993; 13(3):357–369.

32. Albanese C, Rowe M Necrotizing Enterocolitis, 5th ed. St Louis, Mosby, 1998.

33. Ein SH, Shandling B, Wesson D, Filler RM: A 13-year experience with peritoneal drainage under local anesthesia for necrotizing enterocolitis perforation. J Pediatr Surg 1990;25(10):1034–1036; discussion 1036–1037.

34. Robertson JF, Azmy AF, Young DG: Surgery for necrotizing enterocolitis. Br J Surg 1987;74(5): 387–389.

35. Pokorny WJ, Garcia-Prats JA, Barry YN: Necrotizing enterocolitis: incidence, operative care, and outcome. J Pediatr Surg 1986;21(12):1149–1154.

36. O'Neill JA Jr, Holcomb GW Jr: Surgical experience with neonatal necrotizing enterocolitis (NNE). Ann Surg 1979;189(5):612–619.

37. Kosloske AM: Indications for operation in necrotizing enterocolitis revisited. J Pediatr Surg 1994;29 (5):663–666.

38. Reed DN Jr, Polley TZ Jr, Rees MA: Jejunal atresia secondary to intrauterine intussusception, presenting as acute perforation. Can J Surg 1987;30 (3):203–204.

39. Uceda JE, Laos CA, Kolni HW, Klein AM: Intestinal perforations in infants with a very low birth weight: A disease of increasing survival? J Pediatr Surg 1995;30(9):1314–1316.

40. Buchheit JQ, Stewart DL: Clinical comparison of localized intestinal perforation and necrotizing enterocolitis in neonates. Pediatrics 1994;93(1): 32–36.

41. Mintz AC, Applebaum H: Focal gastrointestinal perforations not associated with necrotizing enterocolitis in very low birth weight neonates. J Pediatr Surg 1993;28(6):857–860.

42. Kennedy KA, Tyson JE, Chamnanvanikij S Early versus delayed initiation of progressive enteral feedings for parenterally fed low birth weight or preterm infants. Cochrane Database Syst Rev(2):2000(2) CD001970.

43. Berseth CL, Bisquera JA, Paje VU: Prolonging small feeding volumes early in life decreases the incidence of necrotizing enterocolitis in very low birth weight infants. Pediatrics 2003;111(3):529–534.

44. Book LS, Herbst JJ, Atherton SO, Jung AL: Necrotizing enterocolitis in low-birth-weight infants fed an elemental formula. J Pediatr 1975;87(4):602–605.

45. deLemos R: The Role of Hyperosmolar Formulas in Necrotizing Enterocolitis—Animal Studies. Columbus, Ross Laboratories, 1975.

46. Grand RJ, Watkins JB, Torti FM: Development of the human gastrointestinal tract. A review. Gastroenterology 1976;70(5 Pt1):790–810.

47. Carrion V, Egan EA: Prevention of neonatal necrotizing enterocolitis. J Pediatr Gastroenterol Nutr 1990;11(3):317–323.

48. Egan EA, Nelson RM, Mantilla G, Eitzman DV: Additional experience with routine use of oral kanamycin prophylaxis for necrotizing enterocolitis in infants under 1,500 grams. J Pediatr 1977;90 (2):331–332.

49. Grylack LJ, Scanlon JW: Oral gentamicin therapy in the prevention of neonatal necrotizing enterocolitis. A controlled double-blind trial. Am J Dis Child 1978;132(12):1192–1194.

50. Egan EA, Mantilla G, Nelson RM, Eitzman DV: A prospective controlled trial of oral kanamycin in the prevention of neonatal necrotizing enterocolitis. J Pediatr 1976;89(3):467–470.

51. Bell EF: Preventing necrotizing enterocolitis: What works and how safe? Pediatrics 2005;115(1): 173–174.

52. Neu J, Roig JC, Meetze WH, et al: Enteral glutamine supplementation for very low birth weight
infants decreases morbidity. J Pediatr 1997;131
(5):691–699.

53. Amin HJ, Zamora SA, McMillan DD, et al: Arginine
supplementation prevents necrotizing enterocolitis
in the premature infant. J Pediatr 2002;140(4):
425–431.

54. Du X, Liu Q, Yang Z, et al: Protective effects of interleu-
kin-11 in a murine model of ischemic bowel necrosis.
Am J Physiol 1997;272(3 Pt 1):G545–G552.

55. Caplan MS, Lickerman M, Adler L, et al: The role of
recombinant platelet-activating factor acetylhydrolase in a neonatal rat model of necrotizing enterocolitis. Pediatr Res 1997;42(6):779–783.

56. Levay PF, Viljoen M: Lactoferrin: A general review.
Haematologica 1995;80(3):252–267.

57. Mashimo H, Wu DC, Podolsky DK, Fishman MC:
Impaired defense of intestinal mucosa in mice lacking
intestinal trefoil factor. Science 1996;274(5285):
262–265.

58. Reuman PD, Duckworth DH, Smith KL, et al: Lack
of effect of Lactobacillus on gastrointestinal bacterial colonization in premature infants. Pediatr Infect
Dis 1986;5(6):663–668.

59. Caplan MS, Amer M, Kaup S: Bifidobacteria suple-
mentation prevents NEC in newborn rats by modulation of the inflammatory cascade. Pediatr Res
1998;43:99A.

60. Caplan MS, Miller-Catchpole R, Kaup S, et al: Bifi-
dobacterial supplementation reduces the incidence
of necrotizing enterocolitis in a neonatal rat model.
Gastroenterology 1999;117(3):577–583.

Early Discharge of the Premature Infant

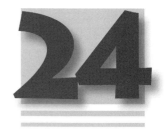

Eric C. Eichenwald, MD

Few hospitalized patients have as long, and variable, hospital stays as premature infants. In contrast to many situations in medicine, the majority of premature infants remain hospitalized not because of acute illness but because of immaturity. Immaturity in respiratory control, feeding, and thermoregulatory behavior will prolong hospital stays. Most neonatologists agree that premature babies should remain hospitalized until physiologic maturity in these functions is demonstrated. These "skills" develop in a somewhat predictable pattern in most premature infants. However, recognition of when a premature infant is mature enough to go home may differ among caregivers, and additional hospital policies surrounding discharge may also affect total length of stay. As pressures increase to limit the costs of medical care, programs to promote the earlier discharge of premature infants have been developed and tested. Earlier discharge for selected premature infants may be advantageous in that it reduces exposure to a potentially adverse intensive care unit environment, promotes more parent involvement, and reduces costs. Within single institutions, it has been possible to successfully alter practice to allow earlier discharge, but broader applicability of these programs remains uncertain.

In this chapter, current data about when premature babies are usually discharged and the clinical and practice factors that influence the duration of hospitalization in premature infants will be discussed. Several clinical vignettes will be used to focus the discussion of discharge timing.

Case Study 1

You are asked to do a prenatal consult on a woman in preterm labor at 26 weeks' gestation. Fetal testing, including an ultrasound, has been normal, and the estimated fetal weight is appropriate for gestational age. After reviewing some of the short- and long-term issues of extremely preterm birth, the mother and father ask when they can expect their baby to go home if everything goes smoothly in the newborn intensive care unit (NICU).

Exercise 1

QUESTION

1. Which of the following statements about discharge timing are true?
   a. It is unpredictable.
   b. The baby will go home at about 35 weeks' postmenstrual age.
   c. The baby will likely remain hospitalized until around the original due date.
   d. Discharge timing will likely be influenced by any complications of prematurity that develop.

ANSWER

1. c and d.

Discharge Timing of Premature Infants

One of the most common questions parents have about their premature infant's hospitalization is when their baby can come home. Although discharge timing is affected by many factors, data are available to help set expectations. Discharge policies have evolved over the last 30 years to allow earlier, safe discharge of premature infants.[1-3] In the 1960s and 1970s, most premature infants who were otherwise medically stable were kept in the hospital until they reached a predetermined weight, usually about 2300 to 2500 g. Randomized trials later demonstrated the safety of discharging premature infants at lower weights as long as they were medically stable and acting mature,[4-7] were able to maintain a normal temperature in an open crib, took all feedings by mouth, and were free of clinically significant apnea events. Most NICUs rely on achievement of maturity as the deciding factor in discharge timing, although some continue to require a minimum weight for discharge.

Length of hospital stay can be expressed in two ways—the number of days from birth to discharge or the postmenstrual age (PMA) at discharge. As expected, infants with lower birth weights and gestational ages have longer and more variable hospital stays as measured by the number of days in the hospital.[8-10] Expressing discharge timing as the postmenstrual age allows better comparisons between hospitals and different gestational age groups (Fig. 24-1). Extremely premature infants tend to be discharged at a later postmenstrual age compared with gestationally older infants.[11] Although not systematically studied, data suggest that infants born at less than 28 weeks' gestation are discharged closer to term gestation (38 to 42 weeks PMA), and those above 28 weeks can be expected to be discharged closer to 35 to 36 weeks PMA.[11,12] The variability in the PMA at discharge is highest in infants delivered at the lowest gestational ages, and narrows as gestational age at birth increases.[8] In one study of a medically homogeneous population of infants delivered at 30 to 34 weeks, infants were discharged home at a nearly identical PMA of slightly less than 36 weeks.[12] This expected discharge time is consistent with data reported from large databases collected from multiple NICUs.[3]

Case Study 2

You are asked to present data to your hospital administration on hospital length of stay for premature infants at two hospitals in which your pediatric staff attends. You are surprised to find that at one of your hospitals, infants delivered at 24 to 28 weeks' gestation go home at a postmenstrual age almost 2 weeks later than at your other hospital, and those delivered at 30 to 34 weeks go home almost a week later.

Exercise 2

QUESTION

1. What is the possible cause of these differences?

   a. A higher rate of nosocomial sepsis at one of your hospitals

   b. Practice differences among your pediatric staff surrounding discharge

   c. Different monitoring practices to detect apnea of prematurity

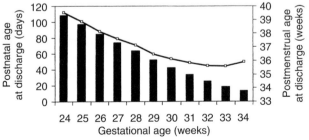

Figure 24-1 Length of hospital stay shown as chronological age and postmenstrual age. Infants delivered at earlier gestational ages are discharged at a later postmenstrual age compared with gestationally older infants. (Data based on 90,000 infant discharges from Pediatrix nurseries; from written communication, R. Clark, 2002.)

d. Different feeding practices

e. Differences in illness severity and complications of prematurity at the two institutions

f. All of the above

ANSWER

1. f.

Variation in Discharge Timing

Several studies have shown that NICUs differ significantly in length of hospital stay for similar groups of patients (Fig. 24-2).[12–14] Both the Vermont Oxford Network and the NICHD Neonatal Network have reported wide variations between member NICUs in the average length of stay for surviving infants delivered with a birth weight between 501 and 1500 g.[3] Reasons for these differences are multifactorial and include both clinical and procedural issues. Although it has not been systematically studied, it is likely that individual NICUs continue to delay discharge until an infant has reached a specified weight or postmenstrual age despite evidence that earlier discharge is safe. In addition, common complications of prematurity, including necrotizing enterocolitis, nosocomial infections, and chronic

lung disease, all increase the average length of hospital stay for affected infants by as long as 2 to 3 weeks.[15] Thus, units with higher rates of certain complications would be expected to have, on average, longer lengths of hospital stays for a given population of infants.

There is also inherent biologic variability concerning when premature infants reach mature behavior (Fig. 24-3). For example, apnea of prematurity resolves at a later postmenstrual age in infants delivered prior to 28 weeks' gestation compared with those delivered later (Fig. 24-4).[11,16] In one study, 20% of infants delivered between 24 and 26 weeks continued to have recurrent apneic and bradycardic events recorded beyond 40 weeks PMA.[11] Because the resolution of apnea is usually a precondition for discharge, this delayed onset of mature cardiorespiratory behavior explains, in part, the longer and greater variability in hospital stays in this extremely preterm population. In addition, most neonatologists agree that some time should pass between the last documented apneic spell and discharge. This discretionary delay in discharge has been termed the "apnea countdown" or the "margin of safety."[11,12,16] A 1996 survey of neonatologists revealed that 74% of practitioners discharged premature infants using a criterion of 5 to 7 days free of apnea, but answers ranged from as little as 1 to more than 10 days.[16] Thus, individual practitioner differences in the required

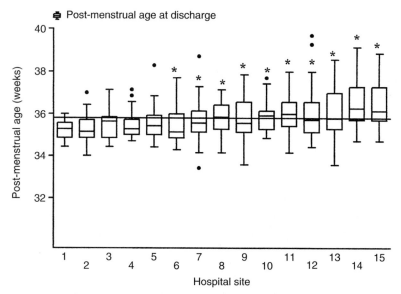

Figure 24-2 Variation in timing of hospital discharge of healthy infants delivered between 30 and 34 completed weeks between 10 NICUs. Box and whiskers plot of the postmenstrual age at discharge by hospital site. (From Eichenwald EC, Blackwell M, Lloyd JS, et al: Inter-neonatal intensive care unit variation in discharge timing: Influence of apnea and feeding management. Pediatrics 2001;108:928–933.)

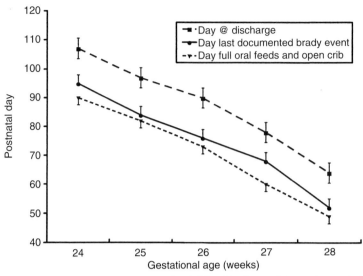

Figure 24-3 Postnatal day that 24- to 28-week infants reached both full oral feedings and temperature control in an open crib, last documented bradycardic event, and postnatal day at discharge home. Gestationally younger infants reach developmental maturity at older ages. (From Eichenwald EC, Aina A, Stark AR: Apnea frequently persists beyond term gestation in infants delivered at 24 to 28 weeks. Pediatrics 1997;100:354–359.)

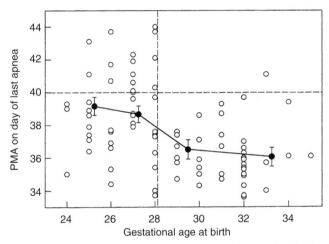

Figure 24-4 Relationship between the gestational age at birth and the postmenstrual age (PMA) on the day of last apnea. (From Darnall RA, Kattwinkel J, Nattie C, Robinson M: Margin of safety for discharge after apnea in preterm infants. Pediatrics 1997;100:795–801.)

apnea-free period prior to discharge also likely affect average discharge timing among institutions. In addition, in-hospital monitoring and documentation practices for apnea of prematurity may affect its diagnosis, and in turn may influence length of stay. Several studies have shown that continuous event monitoring with pneumograms reveal many more apneic, bradycardic, and oxygen desaturation events compared with nursing documentation alone.[17] Longer use of pulse oximeters in convalescent premature infants was associated with a later postmenstrual age at last recorded apnea event, and later discharge.[12] Eichenwald and associates recently reported that in a homogeneous population of 33- to 34-week infants in 10 different NICUs, the proportion of infants diagnosed with apnea of prematurity ranged from 24% to 76%.[14] In this study, there were no other clinical or demographic factors that explained the variability in diagnosis of apnea between NICUs. Centers with a higher incidence of apnea also had longer length of stays, presumably because of policies requiring an apnea-free period prior to discharge.

These results suggest that policies or procedures surrounding the type of monitoring used to detect apnea and its documentation also may be important in influencing interinstitutional differences in discharge timing.

Persistent apnea events in preterm infants may delay the time of home discharge. As a strategy to address this issue, home cardiorespiratory monitors are frequently recommended for premature infants with resolving apnea. However, home monitoring is used inconsistently, and there is minimal data supporting its routine use. Moreover, it does not prevent fatal cardiorespiratory events at home.[19,20] In one study, white infants were significantly more likely to be discharged home on a monitor than black infants; infants sent home with a monitor were also significantly more likely to be rehospitalized compared with those at home without monitoring.[21] In addition, despite the hypothetical effect home monitoring might have on length of hospital stays for infants with apnea of prematurity, data suggest that more aggressive use of home monitoring in convalescent preterm infants does not affect discharge timing in this population.[18]

Feeding practices also have an impact on hospital length of stay in premature infants. Although little is known about developmental aspects of feeding behavior, mature cardiorespiratory and feeding behaviors often develop in parallel.[12] Transition to full oral feedings in premature infants is influenced by a number of factors, some of which may be controlled by the clinician. It is not clear whether specific feeding practices can shorten the transition time from gavage to full oral feedings. Use of early oral motor stimulation or earlier offering of oral feedings may lead to more rapid attainment of full oral feedings in premature infants.[22,23] In one small study, infants delivered at less than 30 weeks' gestation were randomized to receive oral feedings 48 hours after reaching full volume tube feedings regardless of weight or postmenstrual age.[23] This earlier feeding practice was compared with a group of infants orally fed at the attending physician's discretion. Infants in the early oral feeding group were transitioned to full oral volumes 12 days sooner, and were discharged home 10 days earlier compared with the standard fed infants. These results suggest that hospital policies which restrict oral feedings to a certain postmenstrual age or weight may serve to delay development of this skill, and prolong hospital stays for premature infants.

However, earlier termination of gavage feedings may be associated with slower growth velocity and a higher incidence of postnatal growth restriction, offsetting the potential benefits of earlier discharge.[24]

Other factors also affect variability in discharge timing among NICUs. One study showed that infants were more likely to be discharged on a weekday than on a weekend, indicating significant physician discretion in the timing of discharge.[25] Preparation of families for discharge, arrangements for appropriate follow-up for infants once they are home, and complex social situations, which often go hand in hand with premature birth, may also contribute to length of stay, especially for more medically fragile infants.

Case Study 3

After reviewing the data on hospital discharge in the two hospitals, you determine that the main reason why premature babies have a longer length of stay at one of the hospitals is that they are tube fed an average of 2 weeks longer. The hospital administration suggests that you set up a program for home gavage feeding to shorten length of hospital stay. You are perplexed as to what you would need to do to successfully develop such a program.

Earlier Discharge of the Premature Infant

Over the last 30 years, several studies have been published, reporting sets of policies aimed at "early" or "accelerated" discharge of the premature infant.[4–7,26–28] These early discharge programs generally have combined more intensive parent teaching with stronger community-based supports, and are limited to premature infants who have demonstrated physiologic maturity, regardless of weight or postmenstrual age. Most studies have demonstrated the effectiveness of these programs within single institutions, with significant reductions in length of stay and hospital costs without adverse postdischarge outcomes. In one randomized trial of an early discharge program, significant reductions in length of hospital stay were observed only in infants with birth weights between 1500 and

2000 g.[6] Other studies of early discharge programs for premature infants have accomplished shorter hospital stays for even the smallest, most immature infants.[4,5]

These studies are important because they have consistently demonstrated that infants can be sent home safely at lower weights and younger ages than previously were thought advisable. However, the significant limitations to these programs make their applicability restrictive. Each of the successful early discharge programs, including randomized trials, involved selected infants and families with stable home environments, with extensive parent preparation prior to discharge, as well as postdischarge skilled nursing care, often directed by neonatologists. None of the programs have reported extensive experience with shifting low acuity medical care to the home, including home gavage feeding, or incubator care; thus, their routine use in the home cannot be recommended. However, these studies do provide guidance for neonatologists in developing a discharge process. Common themes in the earlier discharge programs published to date include a multidisciplinary approach to discharge planning, involving nursing, medicine, and social work, and early intensive parent involvement in the care of their infant. It is likely that this team approach, including the parents, will result in shorter length of hospital stays for premature infants for individual units. In-hospital caregivers have much less influence over availability of home care services, and thus, decisions about what can be accomplished in the home will continue to be driven by local factors.

Practical Guidelines for Discharge of the Premature Infant

Case Study 4

You are getting ready to discharge a former 25-week infant who is now 39 weeks postmenstrual age on a Friday afternoon. The infant has been taking full nipple feedings for 4 days, and has been apnea-free for a week off medication. The infant suffers from chronic lung disease (being treated with diuretics and oxygen therapy) and retinopathy of prematurity (stage 2, zone 2) that has been slowly improving,

as assessed with recommended weekly ophthalmologic examinations. You have arranged for home oxygen and a twice-weekly visiting nurse, and the parents have been trained in administering the medications.

Exercise 3

QUESTION

1. You have been unable to schedule the follow-up ophthalmologic examination. Should you:
   a. Wait to discharge the baby on Monday
   b. Ask the parents to schedule the ophthalmology examination themselves, with a follow-up phone call to be sure it is scheduled
   c. Keep the baby in the hospital until the baby does not require such frequent eye examinations
   d. Continue to try to schedule the examination and call the parents when it has been arranged
   e. Schedule a 6-month ophthalmology follow-up visit because the retinopathy has been improving

ANSWER

1. a or c.

The wide variability among NICUs in discharge timing of premature infants indicates a significant degree of physician discretion in the discharge process. Discharge timing of premature infants is a complex process affected by both medical and nonmedical factors, which explains some of the variation in discharge timing between NICUs. However, a significant amount of the variation is influenced by discretionary clinical practices that may accelerate or delay discharge. This suggests that a coherent process for determining when a baby is ready to be discharged could result in shorter length of hospital stay, and cost savings.[29,30] Based on clinical experience and randomized and nonrandomized trials of NICU discharge timing, generalized guidelines and criteria for appropriate and safe discharge of the premature infant have emerged and have been published by the American Academy of Pediatrics (AAP) and other organizations.[1,3] Common elements in assessing an infant's readiness for discharge include the following:

1. A sustained pattern of weight gain rather than a specific achieved weight.

2. Physiologic maturity defined as (1) the ability to suckle feed using breast or bottle without cardiorespiratory compromise, (2) maintenance of normal body temperature in an open environment, and (3) stable cardiorespiratory function of sufficient duration.

3. Appropriate immunizations administered and metabolic screening performed.

4. Hematologic status assessed and appropriate therapy instituted.

5. Nutritional risks assessed and therapy and dietary modification instituted.

6. Sensorineural assessments and hearing and ophthalmologic examinations.

7. Review of hospital course completed, unresolved medical problems identified, and plans for treatment instituted. Education and assessment of family readiness to care for infant, especially if discharged with medical needs.

8. Mechanism for medical follow-up of the infant arranged, and communication with the receiving medical provider.

9. Assurance of automobile safety/car seat.

These guidelines provide the minimal degree of guidance to caregivers, and purposely leave much to the discretion of the discharging physician, depending on the medical and social needs of the infant and family. Early family involvement in their infant's care, anticipation of discharge needs, and frequent communication with community-based medical caregivers are the cornerstones of discharge planning. To avoid unwarranted variation and delay in discharge, each unit should establish local guidelines based on medically sound, evidence-based discharge criteria. The goal for NICU discharges should not necessarily be an "early" discharge, but rather a hospital stay that is as short as possible with a safe discharge to home.

References

1. American Academy of Pediatrics, Committee on Fetus and Newborn: Hospital discharge of the high-risk neonate—Proposed guidelines. Pediatrics 1998;102:411–417.

2. Merritt TA, Raddish M: A review of guidelines for the discharge of premature infants: Opportunities for improving cost effectiveness. J Perinatol 1998; 18:527–537.

3. Merritt TA, Pillers D, Prows SL: Early NICU discharge of very low birth weight infants: A critical review and analysis. Semin Neonatol 2003;8: 95–115.

4. Brooten D, Savitri K, Brown L, et al: A randomized clinical trial of early hospital discharge and home follow-up of very-low-birth-weight infants. N Engl J Med 1986;315:934–939.

5. Casiro OG, McKenzie ME, McFadyen L, et al: Earlier discharge with community-based intervention for low birth weight infants: A randomized trial. Pediatrics 1993;92:128–134.

6. Kotagal UR, Perlstein PH, Gamblian V, et al: Description and evaluation of a program for the early discharge of infants from a neonatal intensive care unit. J Pediatr 1995;127:285–290.

7. Gibson E, Medoff-Cooper B, Nuamah IF, et al: Accelerated discharge of low birth weight infants from neonatal intensive care: A randomized, controlled trial. J Perinatol 1998;18:517–523.

8. Rawlings JS, Scott JS: Postconceptional age of surviving preterm low-birth-weight infants at hospital discharge. Arch Pediatr Adolesc Med 1996;150: 260–262.

9. Bannwart D, Rebello CM, Sadeck L, et al: Prediction of length of hospital stay in neonatal units for very low birth weight infants. J Perinatol 1999;19: 92–96.

10. Zernikow B, Holtmannspotter K, Michel E, et al: Predicting length-of-stay in preterm neonates. Eur J Pediatr 1999;158:59–62.

11. Eichenwald EC, Aina A, Stark AR: Apnea frequently persists beyond term gestation in infants delivered at 24 to 28 weeks. Pediatrics 1997;100: 354–359.

12. Eichenwald EC, Blackwell M, Lloyd JS, et al: Interneonatal intensive care unit variation in discharge timing: Influence of apnea and feeding management. Pediatrics 2001;108:928–933.

13. Adams JM, Moreno J, Reynolds K, et al: Resource utilization among neonatologists in a University Children's Hospital. Pediatrics 1997;99:E2.

14. Eichenwald EC, Escobar GJ, Zupancic JAF, et al: Inter-NICU variability in diagnosis of apnea of prematurity predicts variability in length of stay (abstract). Pediatr Acad Soc 2005;57:1599.

15. Bisquera JA, Cooper TR, Berseth CL: Impact of necrotizing enterocolitis on length of stay and hospital charges in very low birth weight infants. Pediatrics 2002;109:423–428.

16. Darnall RA, Kattwinkel J, Nattie C, Robinson M: Margin of safety for discharge after apnea in preterm infants. Pediatrics 1997;100:795–801.

17. Razi NM, Humphreys J, Pandit PB, Stahl GE: Predischarge monitoring of preterm infants. Pediatr Pulmon 1999;27:113–116.

18. Sychowski SP, Dodd E, Thomas P, et al: Home apnea monitor use in preterm infants discharged from newborn intensive care units. J Pediatr 2001;139:245–248.

19. Subhani M, Katz S, DeCristofaro J: Prediction of postdischarge complications by predischarge event recordings in infants with apnea of prematurity. J Perinatol 2000;2:92–95.

20. Cote A, Hum C, Brouillette R, Themens M: Frequency and timing of recurrent events in infants

using home cardiorespiratory monitors. J Pediatr 1998;312:783–789.

21. Malloy MH, Graubard B: Access to home apnea monitoring and its impact on rehospitalization among very low birth weight infants. Arch Pediatr Adolesc Med 1995;149:326–332.

22. Fucile S, Gisel E, Lau C: Oral stimulation accelerates the transition from tube to oral feeding in preterm infants. J Pediatr 2002;141:230–236.

23. Simpson C, Schanler R, Lau C: Early introduction of oral feeding in preterm infants. Pediatrics 2002; 110:517–522.

24. Blackwell MT, Eichenwald EC, McAlmon K, et al: Interneonatal intensive care unit variation in growth rates and feeding practices in healthy moderately premature infants. J Perinatol 2005;25: 478–485.

25. Touch SM, Greenspan JS, Kornhauser MS, et al: The timing of neonatal discharge: An example of unwarranted variation? Pediatrics 2001;107:73–77.

26. Cruz H, Guzman N, Rosales M, et al: Early hospital discharge of preterm very low birth weight infants. J Perinatol 1997;17:29–32.

27. Gunn TR Thompson JMD, Jackson H, et al: Does early hospital discharge with home support of families with preterm infants affect breastfeeding success? A randomized trial. Acta Paediatr 2000; 89:1358–1363.

28. Ortenstrand A, Waldenstrom U, Winbladh B: Early discharge of preterm infants needing limited special care, followed by domiciliary nursing care. Acta Paediatr 1999;88:1024–1030.

29. Perlmutter DF, Suico C, Krauss A, Auld PAM: A program to reduce discharge delays in a neonatal intensive care unit. Am J Managed Care 1998; 4:548–552.

30. Richardson DK, Zupancic JAF, Escobar GJ, et al: A critical review of cost reduction in neonatal intensive care. II. Strategies for reduction. J Perinatol 2001;21:121–127.

Index

Note: Page numbers followed by f indicate figures and those followed by t indicate tables.